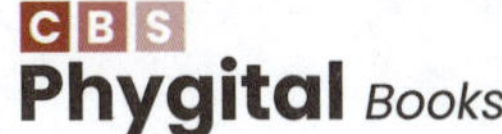

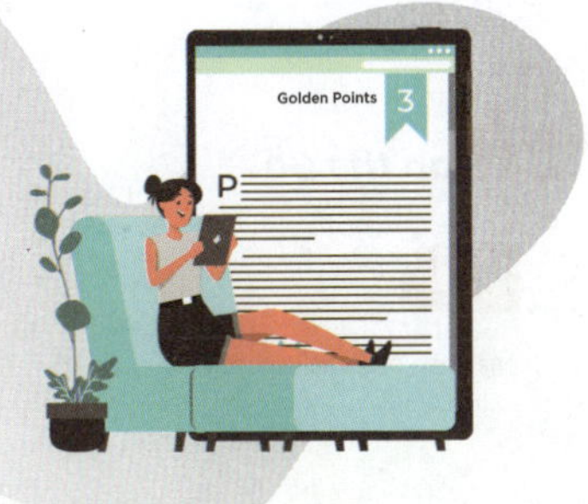

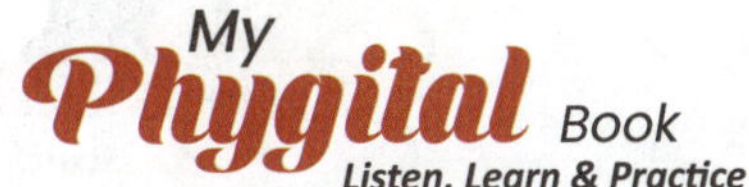

Reading is not enough, Now ***Listen, Learn & Practice*** Every Chapter

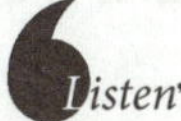

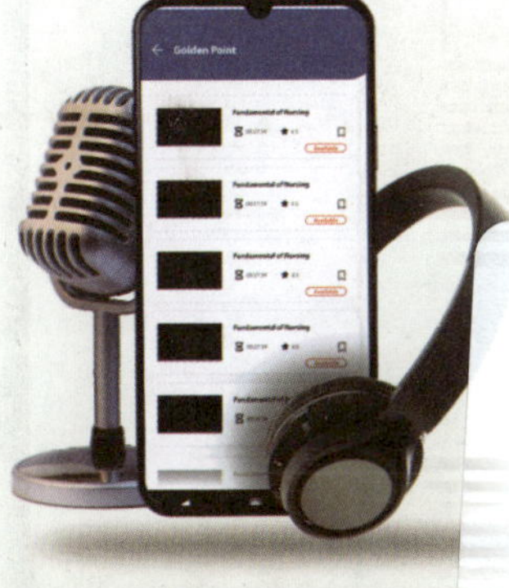

i. Golden Points

Get **500+** Chapter-wise One-Liners in **PODCAST form** (audio) for quick revision of chapters

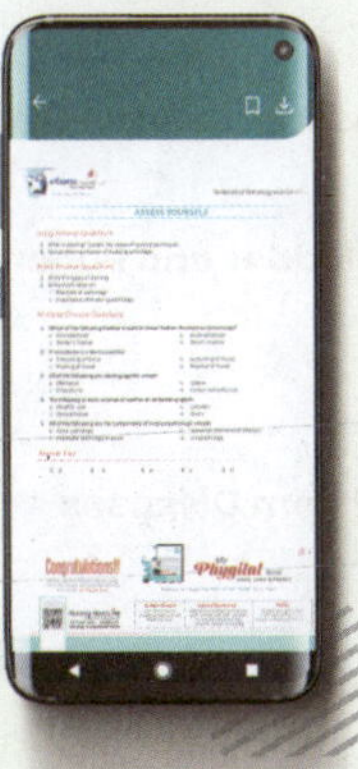

ii. Solved Exercises

Subjective and Objective exercises of the book have been given with their solutions (in PDF) to evaluate and assess the complete chapter knowledge

- **20+** Long Answer Questions
- **20+** Short Answer Questions
- **50+** Multiple Choice Questions

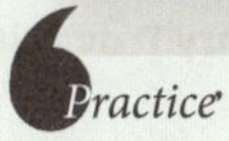

iii. MCQs

100+ Chapter-wise Multiple Choice Questions in Practice and Review mode to provide in-depth concept clarity

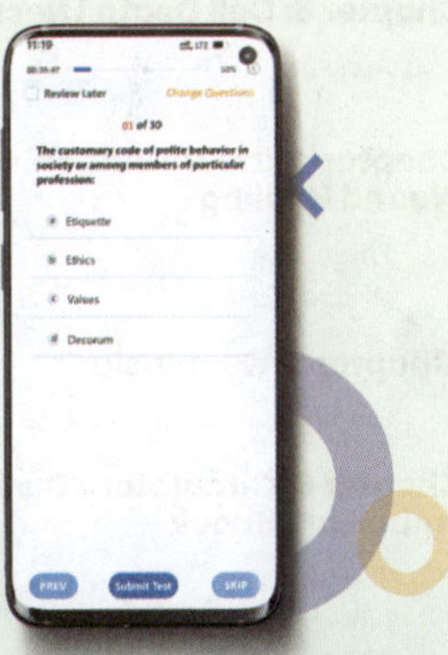

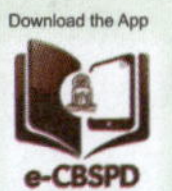

CBS Phygital Books >
Textbook of Pathology and Genetics
PHYGITAL

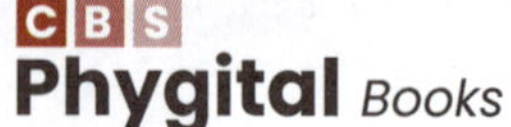

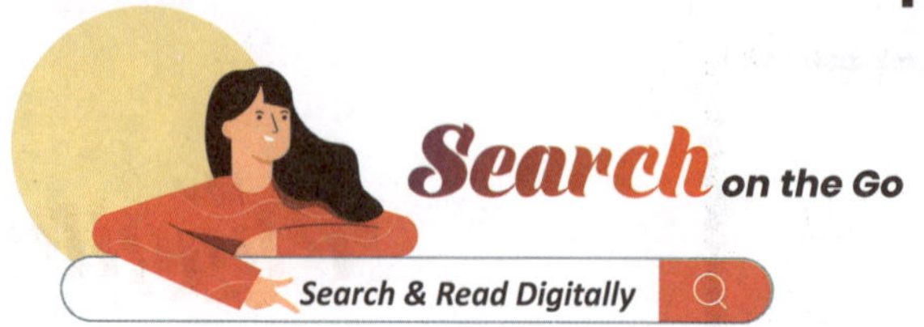

Mapping of the most important topics from the Book at one place with one click search
Get 50+ Important topics of the book at one click

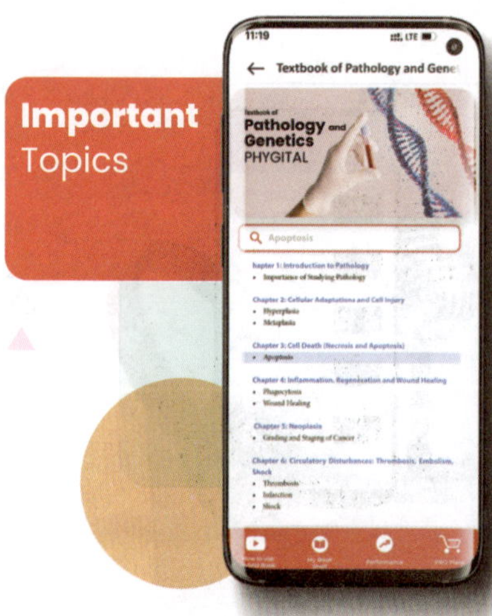

Chapter 1: Introduction to Pathology

- Importance of Studying Pathology

Chapter 2: Cellular Adaptations and Cell Injury

- Hyperplasia
- Metaplasia

Chapter 3: Cell Death (Necrosis and Apoptosis)

- Apoptosis

Chapter 4: Inflammation, Regeneration and Wound Healing

- Phagocytosis
- Wound Healing

Chapter 5: Neoplasia

- Grading and Staging of Cancer

Chapter 6: Circulatory Disturbances: Thrombosis, Embolism, Shock

- Thrombosis
- Infarction
- Shock

Chapter 7: Disturbances of Body Fluids and Electrolytes

- Disturbances in Body Fluid
- Acid-Base Imbalances

Chapter 8: Respiratory System Diseases

- Chronic Obstructive Pulmonary Disease
- Pleural Effusion
- Lung Tumors

Chapter 9 Cardiovascular System Diseases

- Atherosclerosisis
- Ischemic Heart Disease

Chapter 10: Gastrointestinal System Diseases

- Gastric Cancer

Chapter 11: Liver, Gallbladder and Pancreas Diseases

- Jaundice
- Liver Function Tests

Chapter 12: Skeletal System Diseases

- Bone Healing
- Osteoporosis

Chapter 13: Endocrine System Diseases

- Thyroid Neoplasm
- Diabetes Mellitus

Chapter 14: Kidneys and Urinary Tract Diseases

- Glomerulonephritis

Chapter 15: Male Genital System Diseases

- Cryptorchidism

Chapter 16: Female Genital System Diseases

- Carcinoma Cervix
- Uterine Fibroid or Leiomyoma

and many more...

Scan the QR Code to Download the App

Download the App

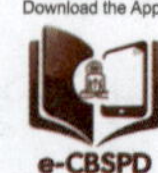

CBS Phygital Books >
Textbook of Pathology and Genetics
PHYGITAL

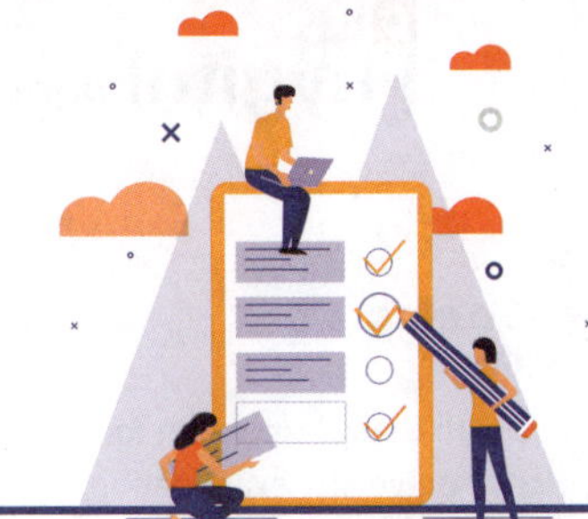

My Exam Center
Read & Learn

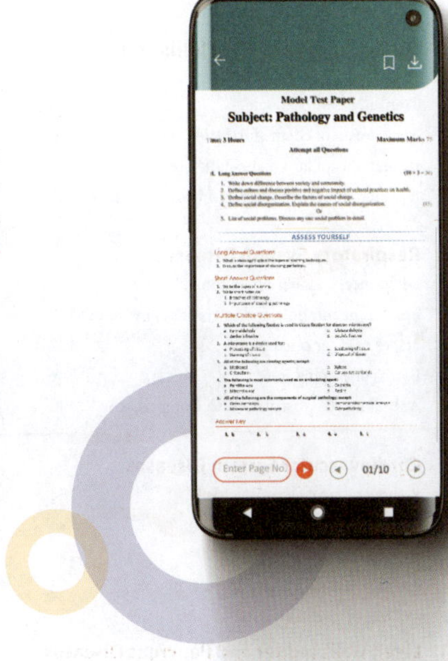

Solved Papers

Get Qs Bank covering the complete subject in the form of subjective exercises and extra exercises with their solutions

- 20+ Long Essay Questions
- 20+ Short Essay Questions

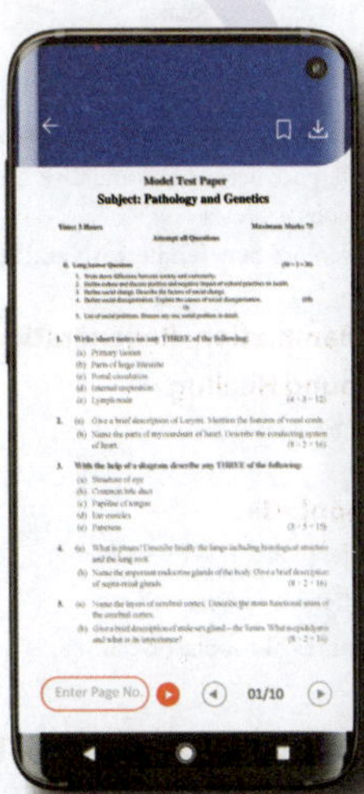

Unsolved Papers

Explore the pool of 20+ unsolved previous year exam papers of top Universities, like Delhi University, RUHS, KUHS, CCS University, MGR University and many more (Semester-wise in PDF Format)

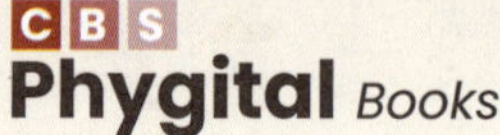

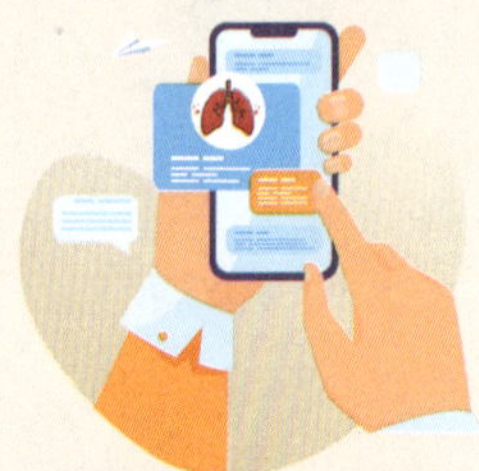

High Yield Topics

Revise on the Go

Get **50+** Topic-wise Selective Images & Tables with their description for LMR and Quick reference, based on the topics of University examination

List of High Yield Topics

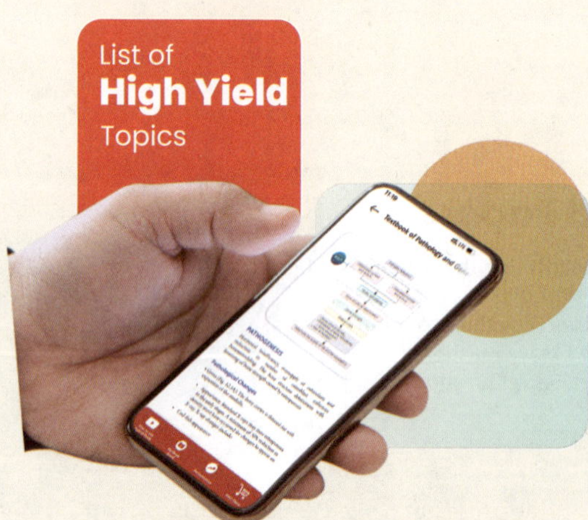

and many more...

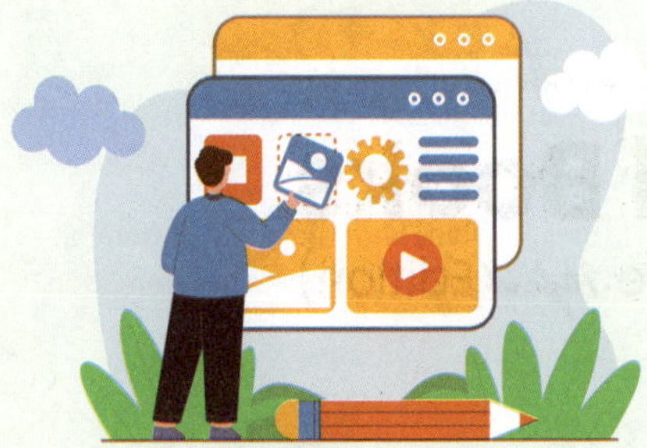

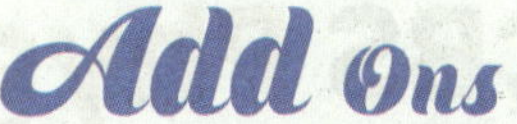

Add Ons

Dil Mange More Content

Don't settle for less, go beyond with Conceptual Videos, Recent Updates, E-books & much more...

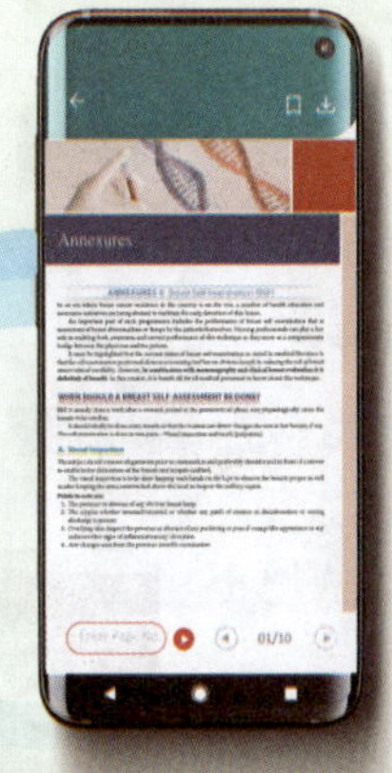

i. Recent Update

Regular updates related to **Recent advancement** and **Book Errata**

ii. E-book

Get PDFs of important chapters/sections **(Annexures/ Appendices)** of book

(This feature is for Institutions and pro-users)

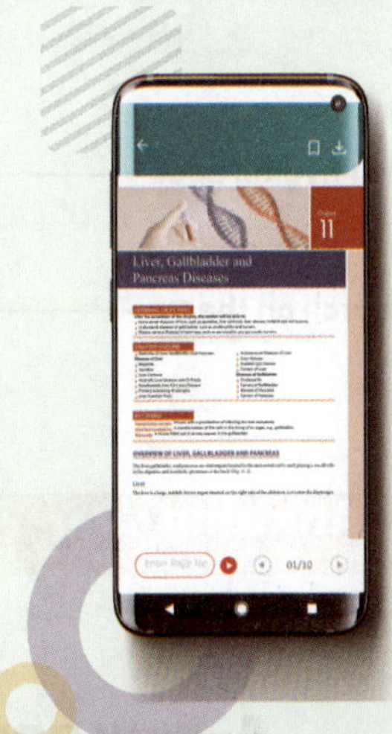

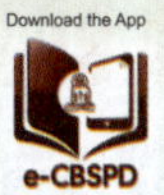

CBS Phygital Books >
Textbook of Pathology and Genetics PHYGITAL

Textbook of

Pathology and Genetics

for BSc Nursing Students

As per the Revised INC Syllabus (2021-22)

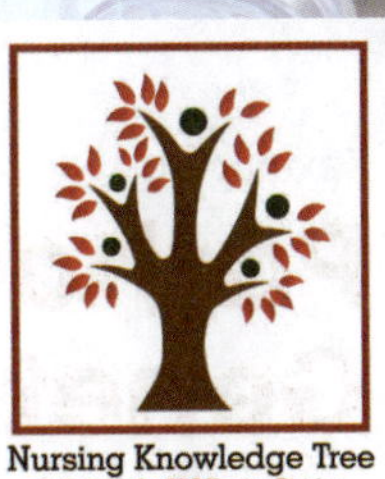

Textbook of

Pathology and Genetics

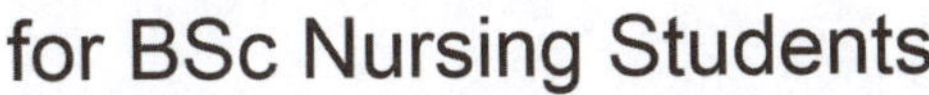

for BSc Nursing Students

As per the Revised INC Syllabus (2021-22)

Vandana Puri
MBBS, MD (Pathology), DNB (Pathology), MNAMS,
DM (Resident) Hematopathology (AIIMS, New Delhi)
Professor
Department of Pathology
Lady Hardinge Medical College, New Delhi

Kavita Gaur
MBBS, MD (Pathology), DNB (Pathology), MNAMS
Assistant Professor
Department of Pathology
Lady Hardinge Medical College, New Delhi

CBS Publishers & Distributors Pvt Ltd

• New Delhi • Bengaluru • Chennai • Kochi • Kolkata • Lucknow • Mumbai
• Hyderabad • Jharkhand • Nagpur • Patna • Pune • Uttarakhand

Textbook of

Pathology and Genetics

for BSc Nursing Students

As per the Revised INC Syllabus (2021-22)

ISBN: 978-93-90619-87-0

Reprint: 2026, 2025

First Edition: 2024

Published by **Satish Kumar Jain** and produced by **Varun Jain** for

CBS Publishers and Distributors Pvt Ltd

4819/XI Prahlad Street, 24 Ansari Road, Daryaganj, New Delhi 110 002, India.

Ph: +91-11-23289259, 23266861, 23266867 Website: www.cbspd.com

Fax: 011-23243014

e-mail: delhi@cbspd.com; cbspubs@airtelmail.in.

Corporate Office: 204 FIE, Industrial Area, Patparganj, Delhi 110 092

Ph: +91-11-4934 4934 Fax: 4934 4935

e-mail: feedback@cbspd.com

Branches

- **Bengaluru:** Seema House 2975, 17th Cross, K.R. Road, Banashankari 2nd Stage, Bengaluru-560 070, Karnataka
  Ph: +91-80-26771678/79 Fax: +91-80-26771680 e-mail: bangalore@cbspd.com
- **Chennai:** 7, Subbaraya Street, Shenoy Nagar, Chennai-600 030, Tamil Nadu
  Ph: +91-44-26680620, 26681266 Fax: +91-44-42032115 e-mail: chennai@cbspd.com
- **Kochi:** 68/1534, 35, 36-Power House Road, Opp. KSEB, Cochin-682018, Kochi, Kerala
  Ph: +91-484-4059061-65 Fax: +91-484-4059065 e-mail: kochi@cbspd.com
- **Kolkata:** Hind Ceramics Compound, 1st Floor, 147, Nilganj Road, Belghoria, Kolkata-700056, West Bengal
  Ph: +91-033-2563-3055/56 e-mail: kolkata@cbspd.com
- **Lucknow:** Basement, Khushnuma Complex, 7-Meerabai Marg (Behind Jawahar Bhawan), Lucknow-226001, Uttar Pradesh
  Ph: +0522-4000032 e-mail: tiwari.lucknow@cbspd.com
- **Mumbai:** PWD Shed, Gala No. 25/26, Ramchandra Bhatt Marg, Next to J.J. Hospital Gate No. 2, Opp. Union Bank of India, Noor Baug, Mumbai-400009, Maharashtra
  Ph: +91-22-66661880/89 Fax: +91-22-24902342 e-mail: mumbai@cbspd.com

Representatives

- **Hyderabad** +91-9885175004
- **Nagpur** +91-9421945513
- **Pune** +91-9623451994
- **Jharkhand** +91-9811541605
- **Patna** +91-9334159340
- **Uttarakhand** +91-9716462459

Printed at : Goyal Offset Works Pvt. Ltd. Haryana

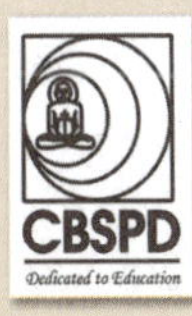

CBS Nursing Knowledge Tree

Extends its Tribute to

Florence Nightingale

For glorifying the role of women as nurses,
For holding the title of "The Lady with the Lamp,"
For working tirelessly for humanity–
Florence Nightingale will always be
remembered for her
selfless and memorable services to the
human race.

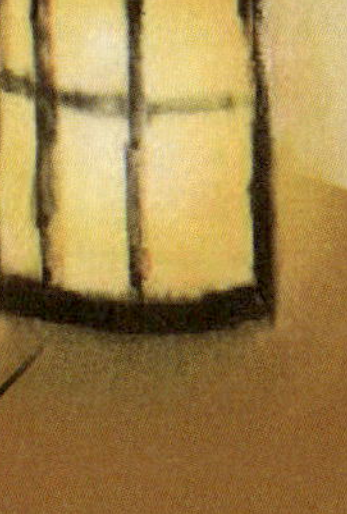

Florence Nightingale
(May 1820 – August 1910)

Dedication

Dedicated to My Soulmate Dr Shakti Tiwari,
My Kids Arsh and Amaira,
My parents for their Unconditional Support, and
My Teachers and Students for their Inspiration.

—Vandana Puri

Dedicated to Sriji and Thakurji, the ceaseless oceans of Divinity and mercy that keep me going with their infinitesimal blessings, my spiritual preceptors who have held my hand at every step of my journey, my parents who have supported me through thick and thin and my students who serve as my continuous source of inspiration.

—Kavita Gaur

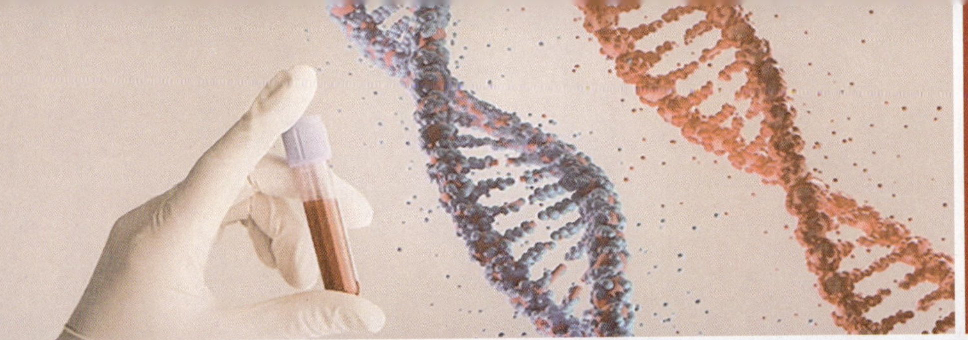

About the Authors

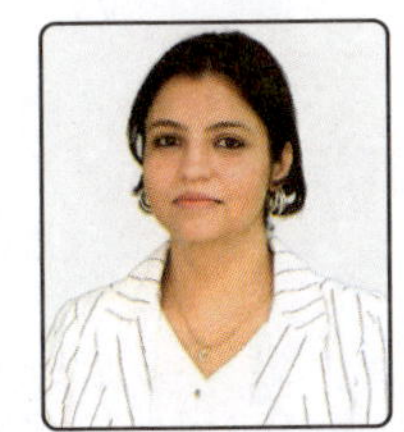

Vandana Puri, MBBS, MD (Pathology), DNB (Pathology), MNAMS, DM (Resident) Hematopathology (AIIMS, New Delhi), is presently working as a Professor of Pathology at Lady Hardinge Medical College, New Delhi. She did her MBBS from CMC, Coimbatore, and MD and senior residency from Lady Hardinge Medical College, New Delhi. She completed her senior research associateship and DM in Hematology from AIIMS, New Delhi. She has also worked as an Assistant Professor at UCMS, New Delhi.

The author holds a distinguished academic record and is the recipient of numerous awards for her work, especially in national and international quizzes organized at various academic platforms. She has authored over 50 national and international publications and has contributed to book chapters in specialized areas of Pathology. She believes in developing building blocks of Pathology to learn medicine in the best way. Her unique style of teaching is highly popular among students across the country. She has 60,000 followers on Instagram channel @drvandanapathology.

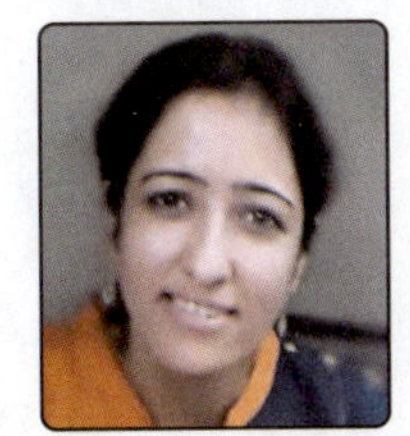

Kavita Gaur, MBBS, MD (Pathology), DNB (Pathology), MNAMS, is presently working as an Assistant Professor (Pathology) at Lady Hardinge Medical College, New Delhi. She did her MBBS and MD from Jawaharlal Nehru Medical College, and Aligarh Muslim University (AMU), following which she pursued her senior residency from the prestigious Govind Ballabh Pant Institute of Postgraduate Medical Education and Research (GIPMER), MAMC, New Delhi.

The author is an avid researcher and has keen interest in research activities. She did her senior research associateship in Hepatopathology from GIPMER. She has also worked at Batra Hospital and Medical Research Center, New Delhi. She has a distinguished academic record and is the recipient of numerous awards at various academic platforms for her work. She has authored over 70 national and international publications and has contributed to book chapters in specialized areas of pathology.

The author is keenly interested in anatomic pathology, autopsy pathology, medical education, museology and innovative workspace design. She is NAMS task force member for education and is known for passionately mentoring students on how to manage their academic life and well-being simultaneously. Her unique style of teaching the basics and nuances of pathology is admired by students across all disciplines. She is a firm believer in work-life balance and in her free time, she shows interests in spirituality, meditation, literature, writing poetry and traveling.

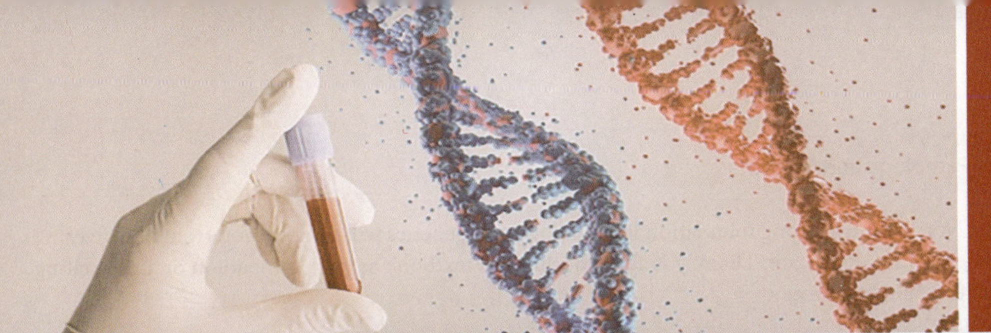

Preface

Welcome to the dynamic and ever-evolving field of Pathology and Genetics in nursing practice! As caregivers on the frontlines of healthcare, nurses play a crucial role in understanding and applying the principles of pathology and genetics to provide comprehensive and patient-centered care.

This textbook is crafted with the aim of equipping nursing students and professionals with a solid foundation in pathology and genetics, empowering them to navigate the intricacies of disease processes and genetic variations. The integration of these two disciplines is essential in today's healthcare landscape, where advancements in genetics are rapidly influencing our understanding of diseases and their management.

Pathology, the study of the nature and causes of diseases, is fundamental to identifying, treating, and preventing illnesses. As the role of genetics in healthcare continues to expand, nurses need to be adept at integrating genetic information into their practice. This includes understanding the genetic basis of diseases, assessing risk factors, and participating in genetic counseling.

Key Features of this Textbook Include:

Learning resources: Engaging learning resources with **detailed yet concise presentation,** which include illustrations, tables, and self-assessment tools, designed to enhance understanding and facilitate active learning.

Recent updates, facts and research: Integration of the latest research findings and technological advancements in pathology and genetics, ensuring that readers are **up-to-date** with the rapidly evolving landscape of healthcare.

Relevant techniques: Studded with **all major tests** that nursing student will come across, like routine hemogram, semen analysis, urine analysis, etc. The nuances of preanalytic, analytical and postanalytic testing are covered to make nurses well aware of the technological demands of tests.

Clinical relevance: Emphasis has been laid on the practical application of pathology and genetics in real-world nursing scenarios. Case studies and examples will help bridge the gap between theory and clinical practice.

Comprehensive coverage: A thorough exploration of fundamental concepts in pathology and genetics, providing a comprehensive understanding of the principles that underpin nursing practice.

Interdisciplinary approach: Recognition of the interdisciplinary nature of healthcare, with insights into how pathology and genetics intersect with other healthcare disciplines.

Whether you are a nursing student embarking on your educational journey or a seasoned professional seeking to expand your knowledge base, this textbook is tailored to meet your needs. We hope that this resource will inspire curiosity, critical thinking, and a lifelong commitment to learning in the realm of pathology and genetics. Nurses with a strong foundation in pathology and genetics will be at the forefront of delivering high-quality, evidence-based care. Thank you for choosing this textbook as your companion on this exciting and essential educational journey.

Happy Learning!

Vandana Puri
Kavita Gaur

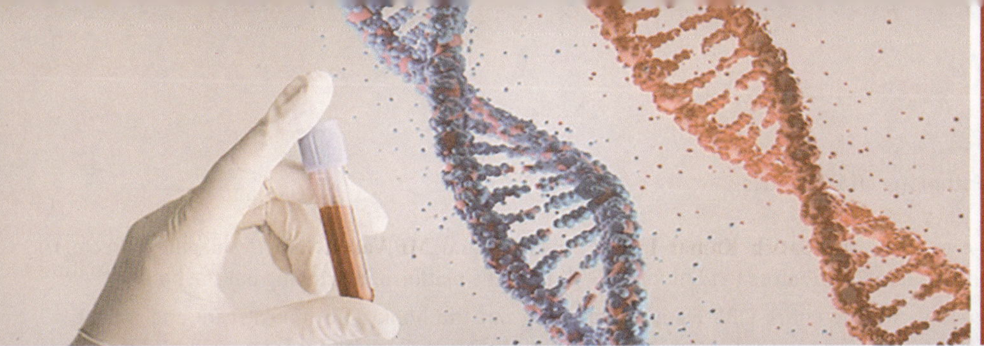

Acknowledgments

Firstly, we would like to express our eternal gratitude for the blessings of The Almighty God. We thank our parents for their blessings, everlasting love, and support. We wish to sincerely thank our teachers and faculty for being the source of our inspiration and knowledge, and for helping us to achieve a lot in our personal and professional life:

1. Professor Manjula Jain, Director Professor, Department of Pathology, LHMC, New Delhi
2. Professor Sunita Sharma, Director Professor, Department of Pathology, LHMC, New Delhi
3. Professor Kiran Agarwal, Director Professor and Head, Department of Pathology, LHMC, New Delhi
4. Professor Shilpi Agarwal, Director Professor, Department of Pathology, LHMC, New Delhi
5. Professor Anita Nangia, Director Professor, Department of Pathology, LHMC, New Delhi
6. Professor Shailaja Shukla, Professor, Department of Pathology, LHMC, New Delhi
7. Dr Smita Singh, Professor, Department of Pathology, LHMC, New Delhi
8. Dr Jasmita Dass, Associate Professor, AIIMS, New Delhi

We thank our friends, students and well-wishers, for their invaluable contributions and support in writing this book.

Dr Himil Parekh, SR, Hematology, AIIMS, New Delhi
Dr Mousami Kar, consultant Hematology, BLK, New Delhi

—Vandana Puri

I would also like to acknowledge my mentors—Late Dr Mehar Aziz and Late Dr Md. Naim, Dr Rana K Sherwani Director Professors, Department of Pathology, AMU, Dr Ranjana Gondal, Ex HOD GIPMER, Dr Shashi Narayan, Senior Consultant Hematopathologist, Dr Pramila Bajaj, Ex Senior Histopathologist, Batra Hospital, Dr Puja Sakhuja, Director Professor and Head, GIPMER, New Delhi, Dr Ravindra Kumar Saran, Director Professor, GIPMER, Dr Vineeta Batra, Director Professor, GIPMER, New Delhi, Dr Kaushik Majumdar, Consultant Histopathologist, Al Sabah Hospital, Kuwait, and Dr Vikas Kashyap, Consultant Histopathologist, Apollo Hospital, New Delhi.

—Kavita Gaur

We would like to express our gratitude and appreciation for the support of our wonderful colleagues and juniors who add joy and inspiration to our workfront.

We would like to thank **Mr Satish Kumar Jain** (Chairman) and **Mr Varun Jain** (Managing Director), M/s CBS Publishers and Distributors Pvt Ltd for providing us the platform in bringing out the book.

We sincerely thank the entire CBS team for bringing out the book with utmost care and attractive presentation. We would like to thank Ms Nitasha Arora (Assistant General Manager – Publishing) and Dr Anju Dhir (Sr. Product Manager cum Commissioning Editor) for their publishing support. We would also like to extend our thanks to Ms Surbhi Gupta (Sr. Editor cum Team Lead), Mr Ashutosh Pathak (Assistant Production Manager cum TL) and all the production team members for devoting laborious hours in editing, designing and typesetting the book

All the suggestions and critical evaluation by readers and academicians are highly appreciated.

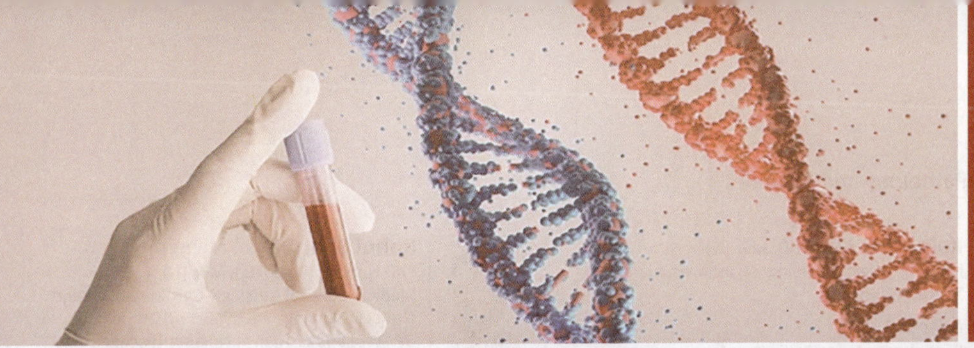

Contributors and Reviewers

Special Contribution

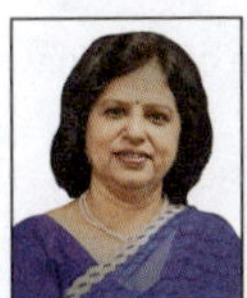

Anju Dhir
PhD, MSc (Micro), BSc (Med)
Ex-Lecturer (Microbiol)
Shivalik Institute of Nursing
Shimla, Himachal Pradesh
Sr. Product Manager cum Commissioning Editor
CBS Publishers & Distributors Pvt Ltd.

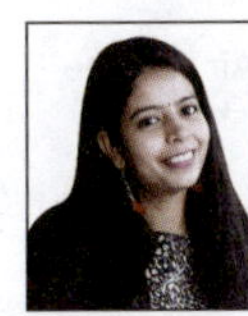

Saumya Srivastava
MSc (Oncology Nursing), RM, RN
Nursing Tutor
Vivekananda College of Nursing
Lucknow, Uttar Pradesh

Contributors

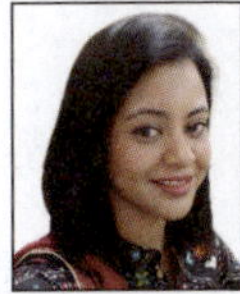

Mousami Kar MD (Pathology), DM (Hematopathology), AIIMS, New Delhi
Consultant
Hematopathology, BLK Hospital
New Delhi

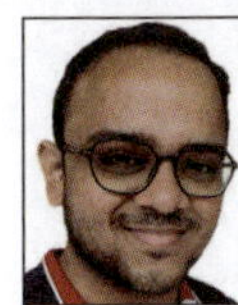

Himil Parikh MBBS (Government Medical College, Surat), MD (GCS Medical College, Ahmedabad)
DM Hematopathology (Trainee)
AIIMS, New Delhi

Reviewers

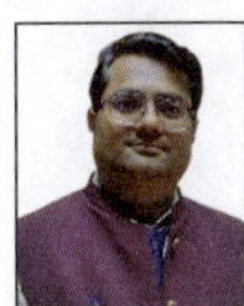

Hemant Tyagi PhD, MSc (N), RM, RN
Medical-Surgical Nursing
Principal
Imperial College of Nursing
Jaipur, Rajasthan

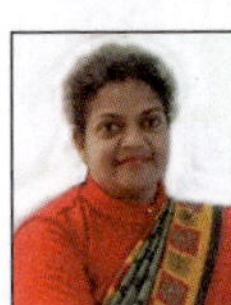

Janet J PhD, MSc (N)
Medical-Surgical Nursing
Principal
Yatharth Nursing College and Paramedical Institute
Chandauli, Uttar Pradesh

The names of the contributors and reviewers are arranged in alphabetical order.

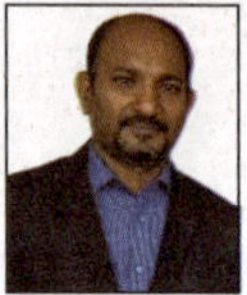

Kalpesh K Jain PhD, MSc (N)
Medical-Surgical Nursing – Cardiovascular and Thoracic Nursing

Principal
Sevashram Nursing College
Bharuch, Gujarat

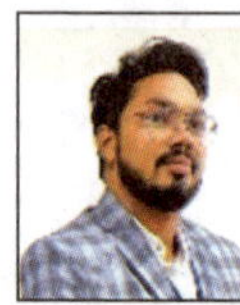

Rahul Sharma
PhD Nursing (Pursuing), MSc (N)
Medical-Surgical Nursing – Cardiovascular and Thoracic Nursing
UP State Spokesman at Nursing Teacher's Association of India
Co-chair Person of the South East Asia Regional Hub within the Challenger's Committee, Nursing Now Challenge, London, UK

Professor and Principal
Ruma Institute of Medical Sciences
Pratapgarh, Uttar Pradesh

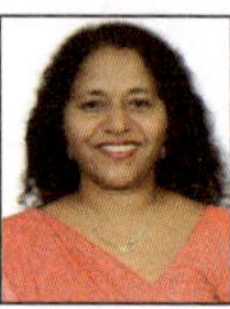

Priyadarsini John
PhD Nursing (Pursuing), MSc (N)
Medical-Surgical Nursing

Principal
Indian Red Cross Society's Bel-Air College of Nursing, Panchgani, Maharashtra

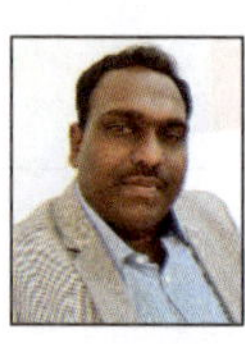

Vijayreddy Vandali
PhD Scholar, MSc (N), MPA, PGDHA, PGCDE
Medical-Surgical Nursing

Professor and Principal
Shree Gopaldev Jadhav College of Nursing
Kalaburagi, Karnataka

The names of the contributors and reviewers are arranged in alphabetical order.

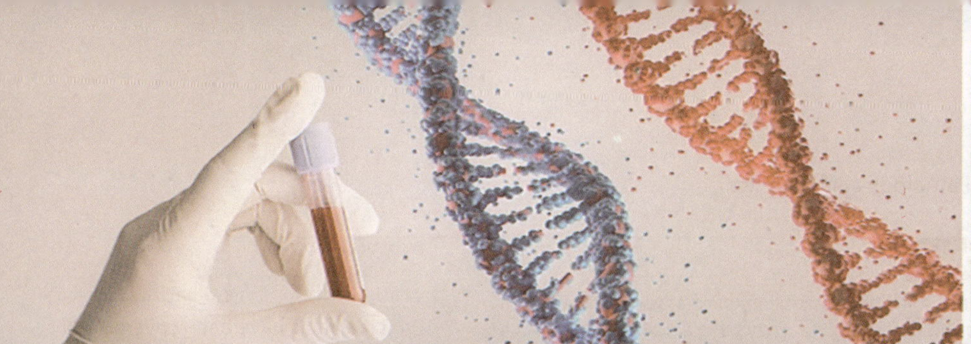

Special Features of the Book

LEARNING OBJECTIVES

After the completion of the chapter, the readers will be able to:

- Develop a clear idea about the field of pathology.
- Understand the importance of studying pathology.
- Know the important branches within pathology.
- Awareness of important terms used by pathologists,used throughout this book.
- Understand various staining techniques and their utility.

Learning Objectives given in the beginning of each chapter enable the student to know what he/she will learn after reading it.

CHAPTER OUTLINE

- Introduction
- Aspects of Disease
- Important Terminology in the Study of Pathology
- Historical Background
- Importance of Studying Pathology
- Branches of Pathology
- Histopathological Examination

Every chapter begins with a **Chapter Outline** to provide a glimpse of the topics discussed.

KEY TERMS

Cytopathology: Cytopathology refers to specialized diagnostic procedures for studying individual cells removed from tissues.

Disease: A derangement in the structure/function of an organ or system adversely affecting a part of or the entire body.

Histopathology: Histopathology is the diagnosis and study of diseases of the tissues, and involves examining tissues and/or cells under a microscope.

Microtome: A microtome is a specialized precision cutting tool that cuts sections from a block of implanted tissue repeatedly and accurately.

Important terms of the respective chapters have been summarized under **Key Terms**.

MUST KNOW

Oxidizing agents: It includes potassium permanganate, potassium dichromate, osmium tetra-oxide. They have a definite action such as osmium tetra-oxide is used for electron microscopy.

Principal facts have been covered under **Must Know** boxes.

CASE SCENARIO 1

A 60-year-old elderly female slips in the bathroom and cannot move her right leg. X-ray revealed a fracture at the neck of femur. A surgery was performed and the patient was advised 2 months of bed rest. After 2 months, the right leg appeared wasted with loss of muscle mass. The cellular adaptation fitting this case scenario is?

Each and every topic starts with **Clinical Case Scenario** with explanation from theoretical and clinical integration point of view.

NURSING CONSIDERATIONS

In elderly patients who are bedridden, disuse atrophy may be seen. Nursing practitioners must:

- Assist the patient in their activities of daily living till recovery, with patience and compassion.
- Help in increasing mobility through light exercises.
- Keep a check on adequate nutrition, especially protein intake to prevent further reduction in muscle mass.
- Keep the skin moisturized to prevent bedsores.

Nursing Consideration boxes are covered for implementation of better clinical practices.

CLINICAL CORRELATION

- Protein calorie malnutrition leads to muscle wasting.
- Pressure due to tumor growth compresses adjacent tissue and can lead to compromised blood supply and atrophy of surrounding tissues.
- Lack of estrogen stimulation postmenopause can lead to vaginal atrophy.

Theoretical and clinical integrated aspects have been covered under **Clinical Correlation** boxes throughout the book.

EXTRA EDGE

Oncotic necrosis is a process of cell swelling and thereby distinct from cell death by apoptosis, which is a process of cellular shrinkage and fragmentation. If an acutely swollen cell fails to correct the electrolyte imbalance and loss of volume control, then potentially reversible cell injury can become the initial stage of oncotic necrosis.

Content of utmost importance are covered under **Extra Edge** boxes for better understanding of the concept.

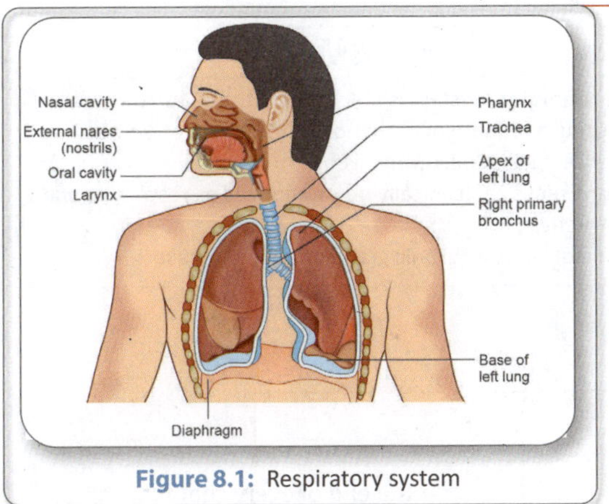

Figure 8.1: Respiratory system

Numerous Clinical **Figures** are used to make the learning easy to understand.

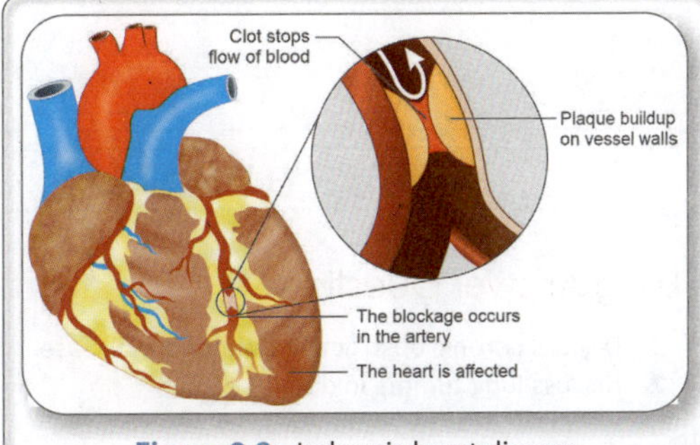

Figure 9.8: Ischemic heart disease

Various **Tables and Flowcharts** are used to help students grasp the concepts quickly.

Table 8.2: Stages of lobar pneumonia

Stage	Characteristics
Congestion (1–2 days)	• **Grossly:** Lung is heavy, boggy and red. • **Microscopically: Vascular engorgement**, intra-alveolar fluid with **neutrophils** and bacteria
Red hepatization (2–4 days)	• **Grossly: Red**, firm and **airless**, with a **liver-like consistency**, hence, the term **hepatization** • **Microscopically:** Confluent **exudation** with neutrophils, **RBCs**, **fibrin** filling alveoli

Flowchart 25.1: Algorithm for managing recurrent spontaneous abortions

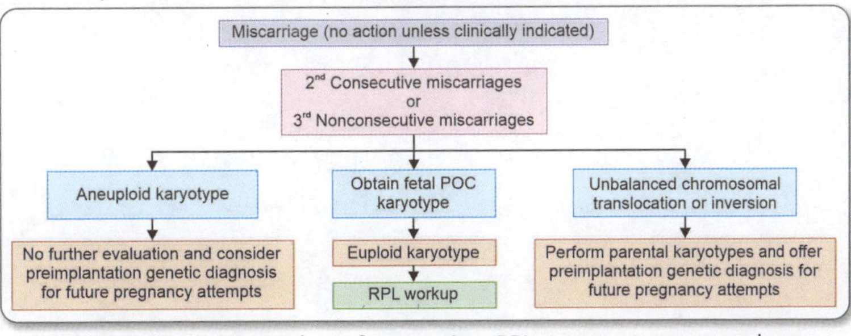

Abbreviation: POC, product of conception; RPL, recurrent pregnancy loss

Each and every chapter ends with **Summary** containing one-liners for quick revision of the chapter.

SUMMARY

- The respiratory system is entrusted with the function of ensuring adequate oxygenation of the blood as well as defence against microorganisms.
- Lung disease can clinically be categorized as restrictive and obstructive.
- Tuberculosis is a chronic granulomatous disease.

ASSESS YOURSELF

Long Answer Questions

1. Discuss chronic obstructive pulmonary disease.
2. Discuss lung tumors in detail.

Short Answer Questions

1. Write about adenocarcinoma of lungs.
2. What is lobar pneumonia?

Multiple Choice Questions

1. **Asthma, a respiratory disease, is caused due to:**
   a. Infection of trachea
   b. Infection of lungs
   c. Bleeding into pleural cavity
   d. Spasm in bronchial muscles
2. **Smokers have shorter breath due to:**
   a. Arteriosclerosis
   b. Emphysema
   c. Hypertension
   d. Cough

At the end of every chapter, **Assess Yourself** section has been included to help the students assess their understanding of the discussed topics.

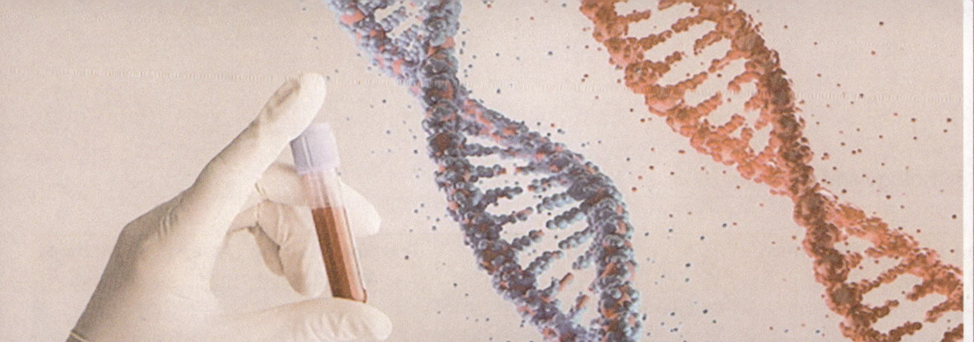

Syllabus

PATHOLOGY – I

Placement: BSc Nursing (IIIrd Semester) **Theory:** 1 Credit (20 hours)

Unit	Time (Hrs)	Learning Outcomes	Content	Teaching/Learning Activities	Assessment Methods
I	8 (T)	• Define the common terms used in pathology. • Identify the deviations from normal to abnormal structure and functions of body system.	**Introduction** • Importance of the study of pathology • Definition of terms in pathology • **Cell injury:** Etiology, pathogenesis of reversible and irreversible cell injury, necrosis, gangrene • **Cellular adaptations:** Atrophy, hypertrophy, hyperplasia, metaplasia, dysplasia, apoptosis • **Inflammation:** ▪ Acute inflammation (Vascular and cellular events, systemic effects of acute inflammation) ▪ Chronic inflammation (granulomatous inflammation, systemic effects of chronic inflammation) • Wound healing • **Neoplasia:** Nomenclature, normal and cancer cell, benign and malignant tumors, carcinoma *in situ*, Tumor metastasis: General mechanism, routes of spread and examples of each route	• Lecture • Discussion • Explain using slides • Explain with clinical scenarios	• Short answer • Objective type

Contd...

Unit	Time (Hrs)	Learning Outcomes	Content	Teaching/Learning Activities	Assessment Methods
			• **Circulatory disturbances:** Thrombosis, embolism, shock • **Disturbance of body fluids and electrolytes:** Edema, transudates and exudates		
II	5 (T)	Explain pathological changes in disease conditions of various systems	**Special Pathology** Pathological changes in disease conditions of selected systems: **1. Respiratory system** ▪ Pulmonary infections: Pneumonia, lung abscess, pulmonary tuberculosis ▪ Chronic obstructive pulmonary disease: Chronic bronchitis, emphysema, bronchial asthma, bronchiectasis ▪ Tumors of lungs **2. Cardiovascular system** ▪ Atherosclerosis ▪ Ischemia and infarction ▪ Rheumatic heart disease ▪ Infective endocarditis **3. Gastrointestinal tract** ▪ Peptic ulcer disease (gastric and duodenal ulcer) ▪ Gastritis—*H. pylori* infection ▪ Oral mucosa: Oral leukoplakia, squamous cell carcinoma ▪ Esophageal cancer ▪ Gastric cancer ▪ Intestinal: Typhoid ulcer, inflammatory bowel disease (Crohn's disease and ulcerative colitis), colorectal cancer **4. Liver, gallbladder and pancreas** ▪ **Liver:** Hepatitis, amoebic liver abscess, cirrhosis of liver ▪ **Gallbladder:** Cholecystitis ▪ **Pancreas:** Pancreatitis ▪ Tumors of liver, gallbladder and pancreas **5. Skeletal system** ▪ **Bone:** Bone healing, osteoporosis, osteomyelitis, tumors ▪ **Joints:** Arthritis—rheumatoid arthritis and osteoarthritis	• Lecture • Discussion • Explain using slides, X-rays and scans • Visit to pathology lab, endoscopy unit and OT	• Short answer • Objective type

Contd...

Unit	Time (Hrs)	Learning Outcomes	Content	Teaching/Learning Activities	Assessment Methods
			6. Endocrine system ▪ Diabetes mellitus ▪ Goiter ▪ Carcinoma thyroid		
III	7 (T)	Describe various laboratory tests in assessment and monitoring of disease conditions	**Hematological tests for the diagnosis of blood disorders** • **Blood tests:** Hemoglobin, white cell and platelet counts, PCV, ESR • **Coagulation tests:** Bleeding time (BT), prothrombin time (PT), activated partial prothrombin time (APTT) • Blood chemistry • **Blood bank:** ▪ Blood grouping and cross matching ▪ Blood components ▪ Plasmapheresis ▪ Transfusion reactions **Note:** Few lab hours can be planned for observation and visits (Less than 1 credit, lab hours are not specified separately)	• Lecture • Discussion • Visit to clinical lab, biochemistry lab and blood bank	• Short answer • Objective type

PATHOLOGY – II

Placement: BSc Nursing (IVth Semester) **Theory:** 1 Credit (2 hours)

Unit	Time (Hrs)	Learning Outcomes	Content	Teaching/Learning Activities	Assessment Methods
I	5 (T)	Explain pathological changes in disease conditions of various systems	**Special pathology:** Pathological changes in disease conditions of selected systems: **1. Kidneys and urinary tract** ▪ Glomerulonephritis ▪ Pyelonephritis ▪ Renal calculi ▪ Cystitis ▪ Renal cell carcinoma ▪ Renal failure (acute and chronic) **2. Male genital systems** ▪ Cryptorchidism ▪ Testicular atrophy ▪ Prostatic hyperplasia ▪ Carcinoma penis and prostate	• Lecture • Discussion • Explain using slides, X-rays and scans • Visit to pathology lab, endoscopy unit and OT	• Short answer • Objective type

Contd...

Unit	Time (Hrs)	Learning Outcomes	Content	Teaching/Learning Activities	Assessment Methods
			3. Female genital system ▪ Carcinoma cervix ▪ Carcinoma of endometrium ▪ Uterine fibroids ▪ Vesicular mole and choriocarcinoma ▪ Ovarian cyst and tumors **4. Breast** ▪ Fibrocystic changes ▪ Fibroadenoma ▪ Carcinoma of the breast		
			5. Central nervous system ▪ Meningitis ▪ Encephalitis ▪ Stroke ▪ Tumors of CNS		
II	5 (T)	Describe the laboratory tests for examination of body cavity fluids, urine and feces	**Clinical Pathology** • **Examination of body cavity fluids:** ▪ Methods of collection and examination of CSF and other body cavity fluids (sputum, wound discharge) specimen for various clinical pathology, biochemistry and microbiology tests • **Analysis of semen:** ▪ Sperm count, motility and morphology and their importance in infertility • **Urine:** ▪ Physical characteristics, analysis, culture and sensitivity • **Feces:** ▪ Characteristics ▪ Stool examination: Occult blood, ova, parasite and cyst, reducing substance, etc. ▪ Methods and collection of urine and feces for various tests	• Lecture • Discussion • Visit to clinical lab and biochemistry lab	• Short answer • Objective type

GENETICS

T – Theory

Unit	Time (Hrs)	Learning Outcomes	Content	Teaching/Learning Activities	Assessment Methods
I	2 (T)	Explain nature, principles and perspectives of heredity	**Introduction:** • Practical application of genetics in nursing • Impact of genetic condition on families • Review of cellular division: Mitosis and meiosis • Characteristics and structure of genes • Chromosomes: Sex determination • Chromosomal aberrations • Patterns of inheritance • Mendelian theory of inheritance • Multiple allots and blood groups • Sex-linked inheritance • Mechanism of inheritance • Errors in transmission (mutation)	• Lecture • Discussion • Explain using slides	• Short answer • Objective type
II	2 (T)	Explain maternal, prenatal and genetic influences on development of defects and diseases	**Maternal, prenatal and genetic influences on development of defects and diseases** • Conditions affecting the mother: Genetic and infections • Consanguinity atopy • Prenatal nutrition and food allergies • Maternal age • Maternal drug therapy • Prenatal testing and diagnosis • Effect of radiation, drugs and chemicals • Infertility • Spontaneous abortion • Neural tube defects and the role of folic acid in lowering the risks • Down syndrome (Trisomy 21)	• Lecture • Discussion • Explain using slides	• Short answer • Objective type
III	2 (T)	Explain the screening methods for genetic defects and diseases in neonates and children	**Genetic testing in the neonates and children** • Screening for ▪ Congenital abnormalities ▪ Developmental delay ▪ Dysmorphism	• Lecture • Discussion • Explain using slides	• Short answer • Objective type

Contd...

Unit	Time (Hrs)	Learning Outcomes	Content	Teaching/Learning Activities	Assessment Methods
IV	2 (T)	Identify genetic disorders in adolescents and adults	**Genetic conditions of adolescents and adults** • Cancer genetics: Familial cancer • Inborn errors of metabolism • Blood group alleles and hematological disorder • Genetic hemochromatosis • Huntington's disease • Mental illness	• Lecture • Discussion • Explain using slides	• Short answer • Objective type
V	2 (T)	Describe the role of nurse in genetic services and counseling	**Services related to genetics** • Genetic testing • Gene therapy • Genetic counseling • Legal and ethical issues • Role of nurse	• Lecture • Discussion	• Short answer • Objective type

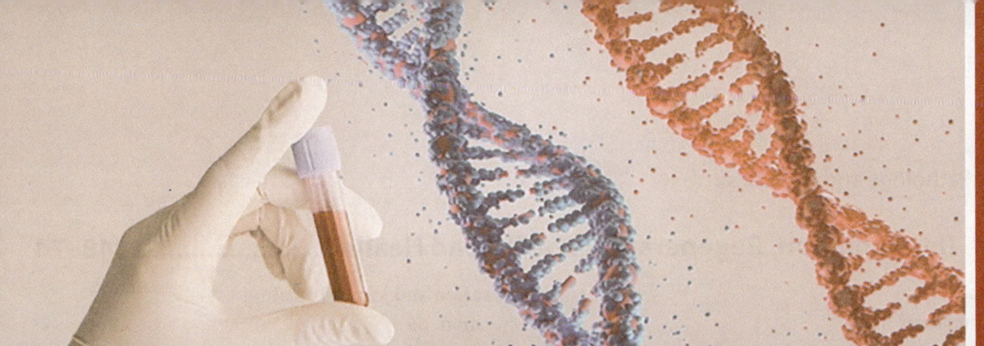

Contents

SECTION II SYSTEMIC PATHOLOGY

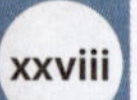

Chapter 23 Examination of Feces 432–440

SECTION IV GENETICS

Chapter 24 Basics of Genetics 443–469

Chapter 25 Maternal and Genetic Influences on Development of Defects and Diseases 470–503

Chapter 26 Prenatal Testing 504–515

Chapter 27 Genetic Testing in the Neonates and Children 516–534

Chapter 28 Genetic Conditions of Adolescent and Adults 535–564

SECTION I

General Pathology

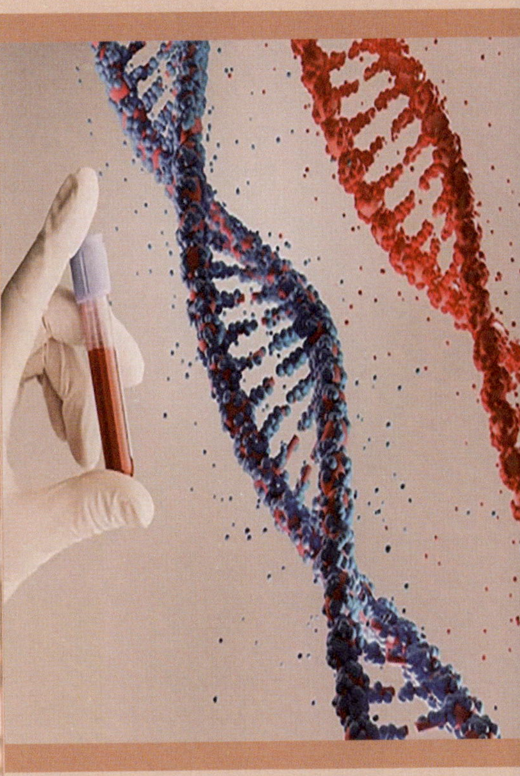

SECTION OUTLINE

Chapter 1

Introduction to Pathology

LEARNING OBJECTIVES

After the completion of the chapter, the readers will be able to:

- Develop a clear idea about the field of pathology.
- Understand the importance of studying pathology.
- Know the important branches within pathology.
- Awareness of important terms used by pathologists,used throughout this book.
- Understand various staining techniques and their utility.

CHAPTER OUTLINE

- Introduction
- Aspects of Disease
- Important Terminology in the Study of Pathology
- Historical Background
- Importance of Studying Pathology
- Branches of Pathology
- Histopathological Examination

KEY TERMS

Cytopathology: Cytopathology refers to specialized diagnostic procedures for studying individual cells removed from tissues.

Disease: A derangement in the structure/function of an organ or system adversely affecting a part of or the entire body.

Histopathology: Histopathology is the diagnosis and study of diseases of the tissues, and involves examining tissues and/or cells under a microscope.

Microtome: A microtome is a specialized precision cutting tool that cuts sections from a block of implanted tissue repeatedly and accurately.

Pathology: Pathology (from the Greek word *pathología*, meaning the study of suffering) refers to the speciality of medical science concerned with the cause, development, structural/functional changes, and natural history associated with diseases.

Sectioning: Sectioning refers to cleanly and consistently cutting paraffin embedded or frozen tissue into a thin slice.

INTRODUCTION

Pathology is the branch of medicine which deals with the study of disease. This includes identification (diagnosis) of the patient's disease, recognizing the most likely causes, understanding the underlying cellular and molecular mechanisms leading to disease development and predicting treatment (therapeutic) response.

ASPECTS OF DISEASE

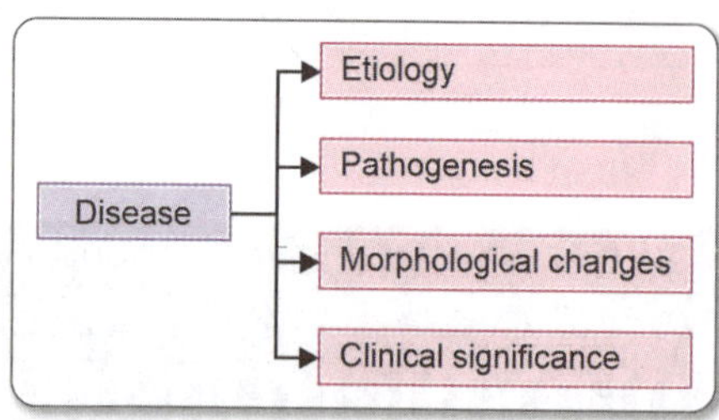

Figure 1.1: Four major aspects of pathology

The four aspects of a disease which comprise pathology are as follows (Fig. 1.1):

1. **Etiology:** It is referred to as 'cause' of a disease.
2. **Pathogenesis:** It is a process/mechanism leading to disease.
3. **Morphological changes:** The structural alterations in cells or tissues that are often characteristic of the disease process.
4. **Clinical significance:** It is referred to as functional consequence of morphological changes.

Advancements in pathology, especially over the last decade have been tremendous with the advent of molecular diagnostics and the incorporation of genetic testing. The pathology laboratory serves as the ultimate link between clinical medicine and experimental science, thus making it one of the most exciting and innovative areas to work in for a healthcare professional. Some of the most critical questions essential for successful management of patient disease are answered in the pathology laboratories.

Before proceeding, it is important to know about the key terminology that has been used throughout the text, commonly used in all healthcare settings, especially in the context of pathology and diagnostics.

IMPORTANT TERMINOLOGY IN THE STUDY OF PATHOLOGY

- **Disease:** A derangement in the structure/function of an organ or system adversely affecting a part of or the entire body.
- **Symptoms:** The physical or mental disturbance experienced by the patient himself/herself, indicating the presence of disease, e.g., fatigue, vomiting and shortness of breath.
- **Signs:** Evidence of disease detected by the physician, e.g., an enlarged liver.
- **Diagnosis:** To know/identify the disease.
- **Lesion:** Changes in cells/tissues/organs occurring due to disease that is the actual pathology, e.g., a skin boil.
- **Etiology:** The why of disease or the cause of disease.
- **Pathogenesis:** The how of the disease or the mechanism of how a disease develops.
- **Etiopathogenesis:** To understand the cause and mechanisms behind disease.
- **Morphology:** The visual study of the structural features of a disease. This can be macroscopic or microscopic.
- **Gross examination/macroscopic features:** The structural changes seen in an organ/lesion in a diseased state, visualized *by the naked eye*. For example, the presence of an enlarged kidney.
- **Microscopic examination:** The structural changes seen in cells/tissues/organs in a diseased state, visualized *under the microscope, e.g., fatty change of the liver*.
- **Light microscope:** The most commonly used type of microscope which uses visible light to magnify structures otherwise invisible to the naked eye.
- **Electron microscope:** A type of microscope using a beam of accelerated electrons rather than visible light to visualize structures after enhanced magnification. This is used to examine structures not seen with the light microscope such as mitochondria, endoplasmic reticulum.
- **Ultrastructural features:** Features of subcellular organelles seen using an electron microscope.
- **Prognosis:** To predict the outcome of disease on the basis of the clinical/diagnostic features.
- **Therapy/Treatment:** Steps taken to cure/bring relief to a diseased condition.

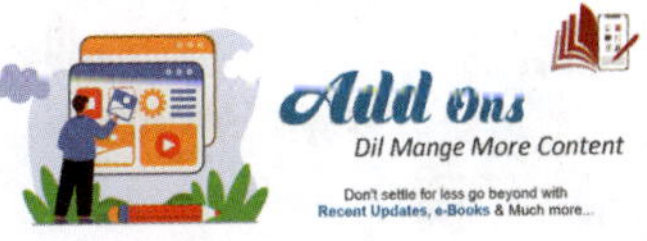

HISTORICAL BACKGROUND

- **Hippocrates** (460–370 BC) is considered the Father of Modern Medicine. He proposed the modern theory of disease.
- **Giovanni Morgagni** (1682–1771) described the finding of over 600 autopsies. He correlated his pathological findings with the clinical features exhibited by the patients prior to their demise.
- **Antonie van Leeuwenhoek,** 'the Father of Microbiology', used handcrafted microscopes to observe and report on what he described as animalcules.
- **Robert Hooke** (1636–1703) later used the microscope to document the existence of 'little boxes' or cells.
- **Thomas Willis** (1621–1675) pioneered the best qualitative analysis of urine at this time. He was the first to notice the characteristic sweet taste of diabetic urine.
- **Richard Lower** (1631–1691) was the first to perform direct transfusion of blood from one animal to another.
- Moving on to the nineteenth century, many scientists were making great strides in bacteriology, microbiology and histology. Improvements in the microscope allowed further exploration of the cellular and microbial worlds.

IMPORTANCE OF STUDYING PATHOLOGY

- **Diagnosis of disease:** The word "diagnosis" has been derived from the Greek root word (dia+ gignosko), which means *to know apart or to thoroughly know.* The most important role of the pathologist is to diagnose or identify a disease. This is done by testing samples taken from patients (blood/sputum/tissue/pus/fluids, etc). Sometimes, the clinician suspects a particular disease on the basis of the patient's symptoms and signs, which requires confirmation, whereas in other cases, pathologists give a diagnosis which was not suspected at all.
- **Understanding the cause of disease:** Disease can be caused due to any of or a combination of multiple factors, like infectious agents, genetic mutations, deficiency or excess of hormones/nutrients, reduced blood supply, etc. In some instances, removal of an injurious agent or addition of a specific nutrient can completely cure disease. For example, supplementation of vitamin C can cure scurvy. Identifying the cause is thus important, as appropriate therapy can be given ensuring optimum management.
- **Understanding the mechanisms of disease:** This is essential for developing pharmacotherapeutic and other dietary/lifestyle interventions which can aid in better treatment.
- **Predicting the course of disease:** With various advances in the field of molecular genetics, we have entered the era where we can also predict the course of disease or *prognosis* in different patients.
- **Identifying the molecular profile of a disease:** This is of increasing relevance, especially in the field of cancer therapy. Scientists observed that patients with a similar tumor diagnosis, e.g., breast carcinoma were performing differently with treatment. Different molecular types of various tumors have now been described enabling targeted therapy aiding in better outcomes.

  Understanding the fundamentals of both pathology as well as genetics is critical for managing patients well as well as predicting treatment outcomes and is an essential foundation to become a successful nursing practitioners.

BRANCHES OF PATHOLOGY

- **General pathology:** General pathology deals with understanding the general mechanism of injury in cells and tissues, as well as the body's response to these injurious stimuli.
- **Systemic pathology:** The study of pathological changes in disease specifically involving a particular organ/body system, e.g., myocardial infarction (heart attack).

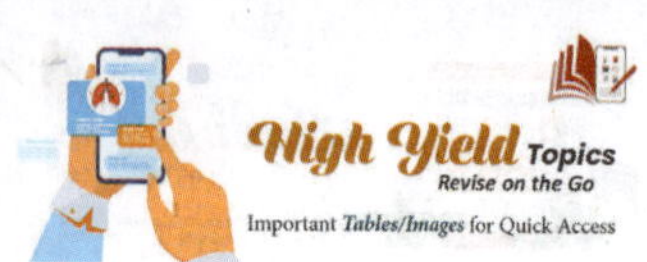

- **Histopathology:** The study of pathological changes occurring in tissues, seen by examining both gross and microscopic features.
- **Surgical pathology:** The study of pathological changes occurring in tissues—either small pieces (biopsies) or entire organs/parts (resection specimens) during the course of surgery to remove a disease.
- **Cytopathology/cytology:** The study of pathological changes at a cellular level. It involves examination of fine needle aspirates (FNAC)/fluids into which cells are shed off (effusion cytology).
- **Hematology:** The study of pathological changes occurring in the blood and/or bone marrow as part of a disease process.
- **Autopsy:** The study of pathological changes in a tissue/organ which is removed after the death of a person for evaluation with the aim of understanding the cause of death.
- **Forensic pathology:** This involves the application of pathological techniques to aid in the investigation of crime. This includes autopsy work, DNA studies for confirming parentage, identity and toxicological study of samples where poisoning is suspected.
- **Immunopathology:** The study of pathological changes, specifically in diseases caused by abnormalities in the functioning of the immune system.
- **Clinical pathology:** The branch of pathology dealing with the study of body fluids including blood, semen, urine, cerebrospinal fluid with a specific clinical context.
- **Chemical pathology:** Chemical pathology deals with the biochemical basis of disease and the use of biochemical assays for screening, diagnosis, prognosis, and management.
- **Genetic pathology:** It includes cytogenetics, molecular genetics and biochemical genetics. Cytogenetics involves the microscopic analysis of numerical and structural chromosomal anomalies such as increase or decrease in the number of chromosomes. Molecular genetics deals with analysis of structure and function of genes at the molecular level. Biochemical genetics deals with evaluation of molecular aspect of genetic evolution, mutation, gene action and regulation.
- **Molecular pathology:** The study of detecting and diagnosing pathological changes at the level of DNA/RNA/proteins.

HISTOPATHOLOGICAL EXAMINATION

Steps of Histopathological Examination

Specimen Receiving

A histology requisition form with complete patient information, clinical findings, a provisional clinical diagnosis, and previous investigations must accompany every tissue specimen brought into the surgical pathology lab. The individual accessing the specimen must match the information on the requisition form and specimen container. A unique number should be given to each specimen in order to identify it.

Gross Examination

The specimen should be subjected to a thorough examination in a clean area with good ventilation, adequate lighting, and convenient tissue disposal facilities. Gross examination entails carefully inspecting the item, describing it on the requisition form, and packing it entirely or partially into a small plastic cassette that is then placed in an appropriate fixative.

Fixation

Fixation of tissue can be done by physical or chemical means. Physical methods include heating, microwaving and cryopreservation. Chemical fixation is achieved by immersing the specimen in fixative. Fixation is done to provide stability to the tissues for easy handling.

MUST KNOW

Oxidizing agents: It includes potassium permanganate, potassium dichromate, osmium tetra-oxide. They have a definite action such as osmium tetra-oxide is used for electron microscopy.

Tissue Embedding

It is a process of infiltrating or surrounding the tissue with a medium, which is similar in density to that of the tissue. Paraffin wax is the most commonly used followed by celloidin, nitrocellulose and various type of resins. It can be done manually or by automation. Paraffin-embedded tissue can be sectioned at a thickness varying from 4 μm to 10 μm.

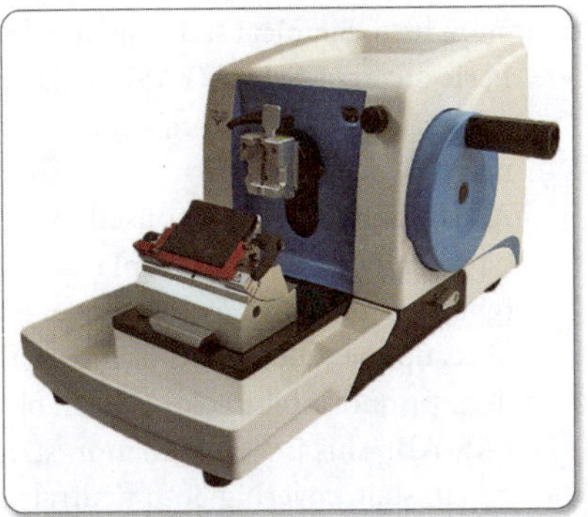

Figure 1.2: Microtome for tissue cutting

Sectioning

Once the tissue has been embedded, it must be sliced into sections with appropriate thickness. Microtomes are the mechanical devices used for cutting uniform section of tissue of desired thickness (Fig. 1.2).

Staining

The staining process uses a variety of dyes to check their ability to stain cellular components. Hematoxylin and eosin (H&E) stain is used routinely. The sections should be "deparaffinized" by treating them with xylene to alcohol and then with water. Routine staining is referred to as Hematoxylin and eosin (H&E) stain, special stains are employed in specific situations according to the diagnostic needs.

Visualizing tissue and cell architecture requires the use of histological staining. There aren't many natural colors in living or fixed cells, and there aren't many variations in the refractive indices of their individual sections. Pathologists and scientists can view tissue morphology (structure) or search for the existence or prevalence of specific cell types, structures, or even microorganisms under a microscope by staining tissue sections.

Both standard and unique staining are used in histology. The H&E stain is the primary example of routine staining. Special staining is the term used to describe additional staining techniques to the standard H&E stain that provide the precise information needed by researchers or pathologists.

Routine Staining

Tissue-based diagnosis is built on routine H&E staining. The nucleus and a few other components are stained blue, and the cytoplasm, and eosinophilic structures are then counterstained with an aqueous or alcoholic solution of eosin for a preliminary microscopic examination of the tissues. If used correctly, this method can offer extraordinary insights about tissue composition and cell structure. For tissue-based diagnosis, particularly in the identification and categorization of cancer, this information is crucial. The primary technique in histology is H&E staining, which is also known as the "gold standard" for brightfield microscopy.

Special Stains

In addition to routine histopathological evaluation which is performed with hematoxylin and eosin staining (commonly referred to as H&E staining), a number of ancillary or "special" stains are used by pathologists to arrive at a correct diagnosis.

Special stains may further be:

Histochemical: In which special combinations of specific reagents are applied on tissue slides to delineate morphology.

Immunohistochemical: In which specific antibodies are used to detect antigenic proteins on cells within a tissue. This is done by using the principle of specificity of antigen-antibody binding, if an antigen is present the binding will occur, which is visualized by a chromogenic reagent commonly 3,3′-Diaminobenzidine (DAB).

Common histochemical stains include:

- **Periodic acid-Schiff (PAS):** This is used to detect the presence of glycogen, fungal structures, neutral mucin (seen in the stomach and duodenum), basement membranes. PAS positivity is highlighted by a magenta color.
- **Alcian blue:** This stain is used to highlight acidic mucins (both sulfated and sialated). Alcian blue stain is typically done at different pH. Staining at pH 0.5 picks up the sulfated acid mucins of the large intestine (goblet cells). This capability gives it the ability to diagnose Barrett's metaplastic change. Staining at pH 2.5 picks up the sialomucins of the small and large intestine. Alcian blue positivity is reflected by a beautiful deep turquoise blue color. Alcian blue also picks up stromal origin mucins comprising of hyaluronic acid.
- **PAS-AB:** This is a combination stain with a dual color of magenta and turquoise blue serving as a pan-mucin stain covering both neutral and acidic mucins.
- **Mucicarmine:** Used to highlight epithelial mucin and gives a rose color to mucin. It is sometimes used for the diagnosis of mucoepidermoid carcinoma of the salivary gland.
- **Masson's trichrome**: As the name suggests, the word trichrome means three colors. This stain is a connective tissue stain used to highlight fibrosis. It is also used to highlight muscle from surrounding connective tissue, muscle taking up a red stain and the collagen either blue or green depending on the counterstain used. It is commonly used on liver biopsies to document the presence or absence of cirrhosis.
- **Reticulin stain:** This is a silver impregnation technique commonly used to highlight fibrosis. It helps highlight reticulin, which are actually type III collagen fibers and form the framework of organs such as the liver and spleen. Reticulin stain is commonly used to confirm cirrhosis and demonstrate collapse as seen in liver failure. Another frequent application is to highlight fibrosis in the bone marrow (myelofibrosis).
- **Van-Gieson (VG stain):** It is a stain used to highlight collagen using picric acid and acid fuschin. Collagen is highlighted as red in this technique.
- **Perl's stain (Prussian blue):** Stains iron in the ferric form bound to protein (hemosiderin). This is based on the reaction of ferric iron with potassium ferrocyanide generating an insoluble potassium ferri-ferrocyanide complex which stains deep blue.
- **Sudan black, Oil red O:** Both stains are used to highlight fat, however, tissue used must be fresh. Frozen sections are usually used for this purpose. This is because lipids dissolve in the organic solvents used in tissue processors.
- **Masson's fontana:** It used to highlight melanin, which is seen as black in color.
- **Congo red:** It used to stain amyloid.
- **Toluidine blue:** It used as a rapid staining alternative as this is quick to perform. Used to highlight mast cells.
- **Grocott-Methenamine stain:** It is used to demonstrates fungi, nocardia and actinomyces.
- **Gram's stain:** Gram-positive bacteria typically stain blue to purple, while Gram-negative bacteria stain pink or red.
- **Ziehl-Neelsen staining:** Acid-fast bacteria, such as *Mycobacterium tuberculosis*, that do not stain with Gram's staining are stained using the Ziehl-Neelsen method. Methylene blue serves as a counterstain while carbol fuchsin serves as a stain (Fig. 1.3).
- **Lepra stain (Wade Fite stain):** It used to highlight *Mycobacterium lepra*.

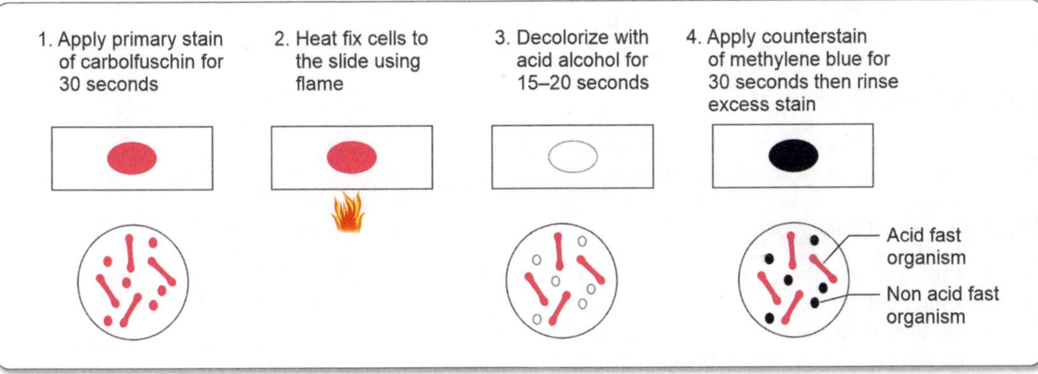

Figure 1.3: Procedure of Ziehl-Neelsen staining

Mounting

This is the final step which involves placing the prepared specimen onto a microscope slide, often with the addition of mounting medium and a coverslip for further microscopical study.

MUST KNOW

Xylene (DPX) or Canada Balsam, Permount, Glycerol, Gelatin, Fluoromount, Vectashield, Mounting Medium with DABCO, Clear Mounting Media, Entellan, Hoyer's Solution are some commonly used mounting media.

SUMMARY

- Pathology is the *branch of medicine which deals with the study of disease.*
- Histology is the study of pathological changes occurring in tissues, seen by examining both gross and microscopic features.
- Systemic pathology is study of pathological changes in disease specifically involving a particular organ/body system, e.g., myocardial infarction ("heart attack").
- Histopathology is study of pathological changes occurring in tissues, seen by examining both gross and microscopic features.
- Surgical pathology is study of pathological changes occurring in tissues—either small pieces or entire organs/parts during the course of surgery to remove a disease.
- Cytopathology/cytology is the study of pathological changes at a cellular level.
- Hematology is the study of pathological changes occurring in the blood and/or bone marrow as part of a disease process.
- Autopsy is the study of pathological changes in a tissue/organ which is removed after the death of a person for evaluation with the aim of understanding the cause of death.
- Forensic pathology involves the application of pathological techniques to aid in the investigation of crime.
- Immunopathology is the study of pathological changes, specifically in diseases caused by abnormalities in the functioning of the immune system.
- Clinical pathology is branch of pathology dealing with the study of body fluids including blood, semen, urine, cerebrospinal fluid with a specific clinical context.
- Genetics is the branch of medicine dealing with the study of hereditary disease.
- Molecular pathology is study of detecting and diagnosing pathological changes at the level of DNA/RNA/proteins
- Bacteria can be classified as Gram-positive or Gram-negative based on the two different forms of Gram's staining.
- Fixation is done to provide stability to the tissues for easy handling.
- Carbohydrate molecules are stained using the Periodic Acid-Schiff (PAS) method.

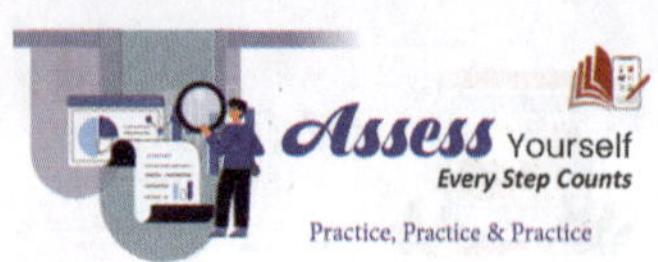

ASSESS YOURSELF

Long Answer Questions

1. What is staining? Explain the types of staining techniques.
2. Discuss the importance of studying pathology.

Short Answer Questions

1. Write the types of staining.
2. Write short notes on:
   i. Branches of pathology
   ii. Importance of studying pathology

Multiple Choice Questions

1. **Which of the following fixative is used in tissue fixation for electron microscopy?**
   a. Formaldehyde b. Glutaraldehyde
   c. Zenker's fixative d. Bouin's fixative
2. **A microtome is a device used for:**
   a. Processing of tissue b. Sectioning of tissue
   c. Staining of tissue d. Disposal of tissue
3. **All of the following are clearing agents; except:**
   a. Methanol b. Xylene
   c. Chloroform d. Carbon tetrachloride
4. **The following is most commonly used as an embedding agent:**
   a. Paraffiin wax b. Colloidin
   c. Nitrocellulose d. Resins
5. **All of the following are the components of surgical pathology; except:**
   a. Gross pathology b. Immunohistochemical analysis
   c. Molecular pathology analysis d. Cytopathology

Answer Key

1. b **2.** b **3.** a **4.** a **5.** d

Chapter 2

Cellular Adaptations and Cell Injury

LEARNING OBJECTIVES

After the completion of the chapter, the readers will be able to:

- Know the definitions of cellular adaptations and cell injury.
- Discuss the types of cellular adaptations, their mechanisms and the case settings in which they occur.
- Understand the types of cell injury.
- Describe the distinguishing features of the types of cell injury.
- Learn about various intracellular accumulations.

CHAPTER OUTLINE

KEY TERMS

Apoptosis: A controlled series of events resulting in cell death during the physiological process. It results in the planned removal of the targeted cells.

Cellular adaptations: It refers to the changes made by cells in response to various stimuli or changes in their local environment.

Dysplasia: It is a precancerous state, it refers to an increased amount of immature cell types, often abnormal.

Homeostasis: A biological creature can maintain its internal stability while adjusting to changing environmental conditions through a process known as homeostasis.

Intracellular accumulations: These are abnormal levels of different substances accumulating in cells, which may be harmless or cause varying degrees of cell injury.

Mallory bodies: Mallory bodies (MB) are cytoplasmic hyaline inclusions of hepatocytes.

Necrosis: Necrosis is the term for irreversible cell damage and eventual cell death caused by pathogenic processes.

Neurofibrillary tangles: These are abnormal accumulations of a protein called tau which is collected inside neurons. Neurofibrillary tangles are a fundamental neuropathological hallmark of Alzheimer disease.

Russell bodies: These are eosinophilic, homogeneous immunoglobulin (Ig)-containing inclusion bodies that are typically detected in abnormal plasma cells.

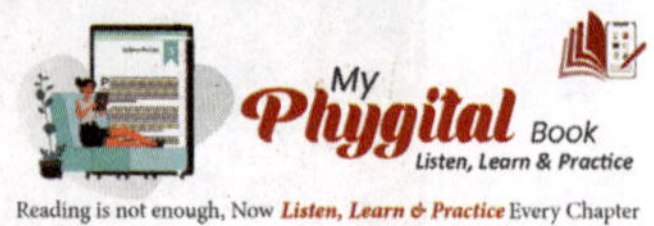

INTRODUCTION

Cellular adaptations are the changes that occur as a result of numerous stimuli or changes in the immediate environment. This could involve changing the quantity of cells or their morphological characteristics. It can be either pathological—occurring in disease states—or physiological, occurring in healthy tissues or organs.

CELLULAR ADAPTATION AND RESPONSE

Depending on the cell-replicative properties that make up the tissue, tissues adapt in various ways. For instance, labile tissue, such as the skin, can replicate quickly and can also regenerate after injury, in contrast to permanent tissue, like brain and heart tissue, which cannot. Cell death occurs physiologically in the form of apoptosis or pathologically in the form of necrosis if cells cannot adapt to the unfavorable environmental changes. Figure 2.1 exhibits spectrum of cellular response to stress.

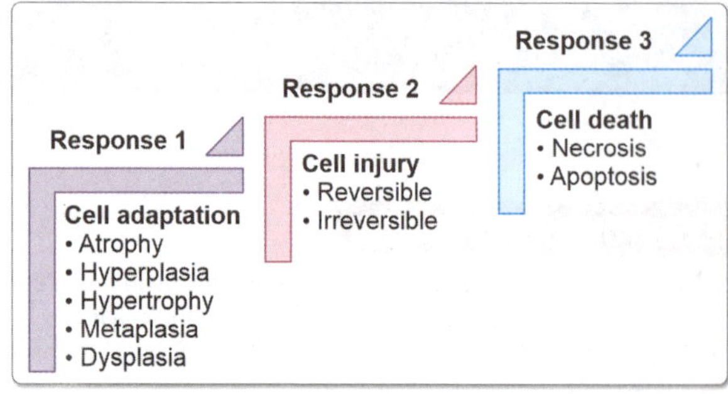

Figure 2.1: Spectrum of cellular response to stress

The phenomenon of cellular response to stress/injurious stimuli, for continued survival in altered conditions, is referred to as cellular adaptation.

Cellular adaptation can be caused by physiological (such as increase in muscle mass after exercise or an increase in the number of epithelial breast cells during pregnancy) or pathological factors such as acid reflux to the esophagus (e.g., Barrett's esophagus) factors due to persistent stomach acid exposure to stimuli.

Cells can typically survive harsh surroundings better as a result of these alterations. Cell damage can result from ongoing stress (such as critical hypertrophy of left ventricle resulting in myofibril damage and heart failure).

The types of cellular adaptation are (Fig. 2.2):

- Atrophy
- Hyperplasia
- Hypertrophy
- Metaplasia
- Dysplasia

The important point to note is that except moderate and severe dysplasia these changes are *reversible.*

Figure 2.2: Types of cellular adaptation

ATROPHY

CASE SCENARIO 1

A 60-year-old elderly female slips in the bathroom and cannot move her right leg. X-ray revealed a fracture at the neck of femur. A surgery was performed and the patient was advised 2 months of bed rest. After 2 months, the right leg appeared wasted with loss of muscle mass. The cellular adaptation fitting this case scenario is?

The word atrophy is derived from the Latin word atrophia which means 'not fed or unnourished'. On a cellular level, this implies a reduction in size and/or reduction in the number of cells in a tissue, resulting in reduced metabolic activity. While the adaptation of atrophy is *acquired,* it must be differentiated from congenital conditions seen at birth.

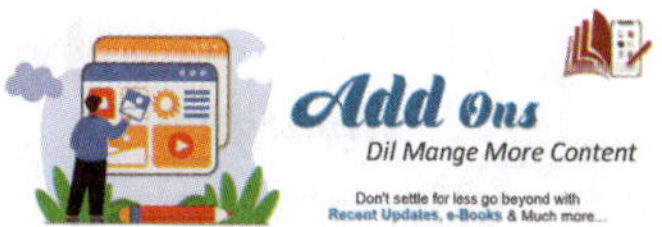

Hypoplasia must be distinguished from atrophy, which is the reduction of an organ due to its insufficient development.

Agenesis or aplasia can be referred to as organ's inability to grow.

Increased protein degradation is an underlying mechanism behind atrophy. This can occur through:
- Digestion of cellular components by lysosomal enzymes present within the same cell, known as autophagy.
- Ubiquitin mediated pathways of degradation.
- External protease mediated digestion of cellular components.

Types

Physiological

- It is commonly seen under normal conditions, in the normal development of embryological structures.
  - Atrophy of notochord or thyroglossal duct during fetal development.
  - Postmenopausal atrophy of the uterus.
  - Regression of the thymus in adolescence.
  - Involutional of embryonal structures, e.g., notochord, branchial cleft, etc., during the process of development.

Pathological

Atrophy in disease states can be local, i.e., confined to a particular site or area (localized) or generalized. Generalized atrophy occurs due to:
- Deficiency of nutrients.
- Reduced workload/use, such as the atrophy of skeletal muscles caused by post-fracture denervation and a reduction in skeletal muscle volume.
- Decreased stimulation of the endocrine and neuroendocrine systems.
- Ischemia, or a decrease in blood flow.

Atrophy confined to a particular site can be because of:
- **Disuse:** E.g., wasting of muscles seen in bedridden patients.
- **Denervation:** Any injury to the nerves leads to wasting of the muscle supplied by that nerve.
- **Pressure effect:** A large growing tumor can cause atrophy of the surrounding structures.
- **Reduced blood supply leading to ischaemia:** Renal hypoperfusion leads to renal tubular atrophy.

Pathological Features (Figs 2.3A to C)

- **Gross examination:** Reduction in weight, size of organ, the organ appears shrunken.
- **Microscopic examination:** Reduction in cell size.

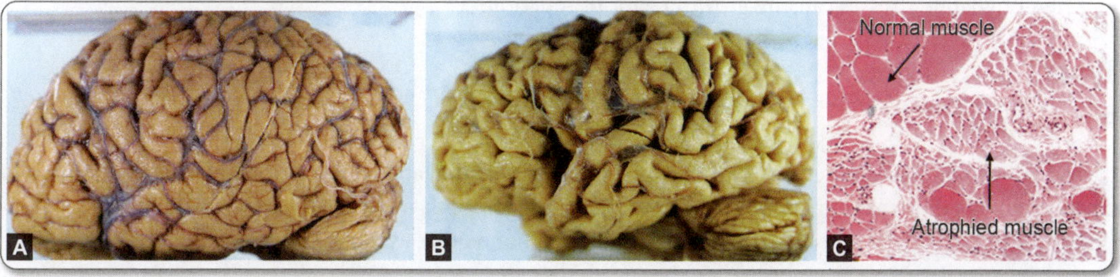

Figures 2.3A to C: **A.** Gross normal brain; **B.** Atrophic brain; **C.** Microscopic image showing muscle atrophy

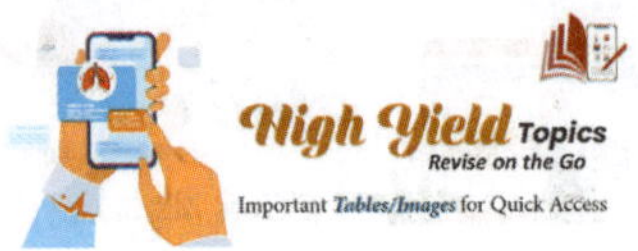

Mechanism

In atrophy, balance between protein synthesis and breakdown is altered. Protein synthesis is either inhibited or protein breakdown by various proteolytic mechanisms is boosted.

NURSING CONSIDERATIONS

In elderly patients who are bedridden, disuse atrophy may be seen. Nursing practitioners must:
- Assist the patient in their activities of daily living till recovery, with patience and compassion.
- Help in increasing mobility through light exercises.
- Keep a check on adequate nutrition, especially protein intake to prevent further reduction in muscle mass.
- Keep the skin moisturized to prevent bedsores.

CLINICAL CORRELATION

- Protein calorie malnutrition leads to muscle wasting.
- Pressure due to tumor growth compresses adjacent tissue and can lead to compromised blood supply and atrophy of surrounding tissues.
- Lack of estrogen stimulation postmenopause can lead to vaginal atrophy.

HYPERTROPHY

CASE SCENARIO 2

A 20-year-old thin otherwise healthy male, weighing 50 kg, starts exercising in the gym and also increases his protein intake with the intention of increasing his body weight. After 6 months of following this routine, his weight increases to 59 kg and his muscle mass also increased. Which cellular adaptation is responsible behind this change?

The word hypertrophy is derived from the Latin words—"hyper" and "trophos" which means excessive nourishment. On a cellular level, this implies an increase in size of an organ due to an increase in cell size owing to increased synthesis of structural components.

Nondividing cells can only undergo hypertrophy, whereas dividing cell can undergo both hypertrophy and hyperplasia.

How does Hypertrophy Occur?

- Cellular stretching.
- Due to the action of hormones or growth factors.
- Proteins active in the embryo causing growth stimulation are subsequently re-activated after some time in an adult.
- Hemodynamic stresses causing growth factor production.

Types

Physiological

It occurs due to increased functional demand, hormonal stimulation and effect of growth factors. For example, ductal elements of breast during pregnancy and lactation, smooth muscle of the uterus during pregnancy (Figs 2.4A to D), skeletal muscle of body builders engaged in regular exercise undergo hypertrophy.

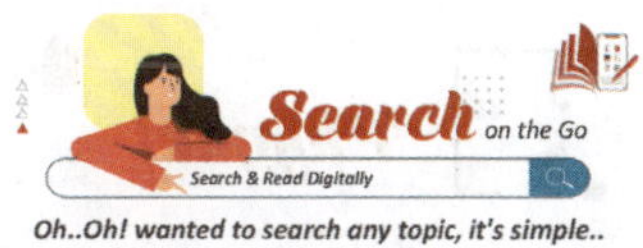

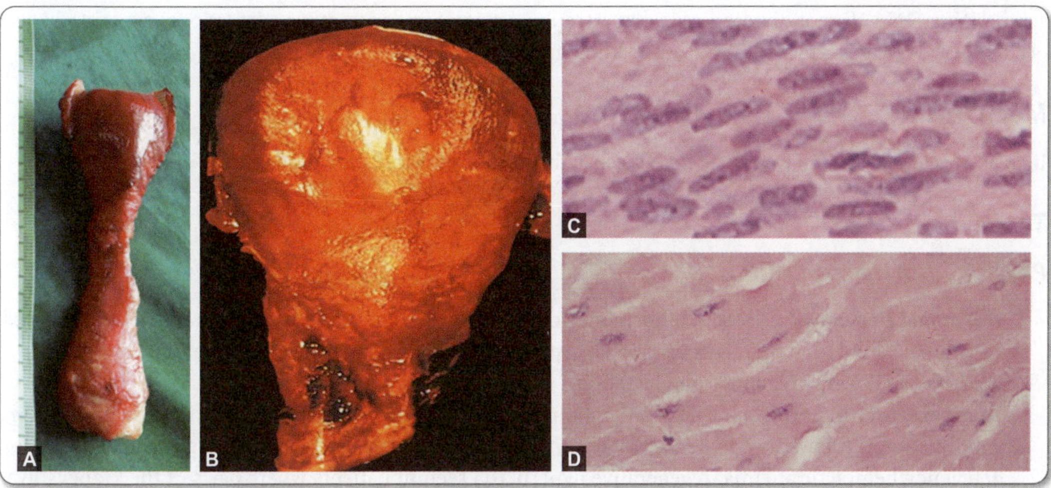

Figures 2.4A to D: **A.** Normal uterus; **B.** Hypertrophied uterus; **C.** Microscopic image of smooth muscle (uterus); **D.** Microscopic image of Hypertrophied muscle (uterus)

Pathological

It occurs due to increased workload of the body:

- **In the presence of any obstructive pathology, the natural response is to expand to maintain function, e.g.:**
  - Urinary bladder muscle hypertrophy with outflow obstruction due to an enlarged prostate.
  - Arterial medial layer hypertrophy in case of hypertension.
  - Intestinal wall hypertrophy seen proximal to a malignant lesion.
- **Hemodynamic/pressure effect:**
  - Left ventricular hypertrophy seen in systemic hypertension and aortic valvular disease.
  - Right ventricular hypertrophy seen in chronic lung disease, mitral stenosis and tricuspid valve lesions.

Pathological Features

- **Gross examination:** Increase in weight, size of organ.
- **Microscopic examination:** Increase in cell size.

HYPERPLASIA

CASE SCENARIO 3

A 65-year-old male presents to the surgical OPD with complaints of increased frequency of urination, urinating more frequently at night and pain during micturition. Digital rectal examination revealed an enlarged prostate. Prostate specific antigen was mildly elevated. The cellular adaptation fitting this case scenario is?

Hyperplasia is an increase in the number of cells in a tissue resulting in an increase in the size of an organ. Hyperplasia is often accompanied by hypertrophy. It only takes place, when the cells are capable of synthesizing DNA. In nondividing cells, hypertrophy occurs. Similar to other adaptations, hyperplasia also occurs in two settings—physiological and pathological.

Mechanism

Increased cellular proliferation due to stem cell activation or growth factor production.

Types

Physiological Hyperplasia

- **Hormonal hyperplasia:** In this, a hormone acts as a growth factor and triggers transcription of genes. Hormonal stimulation increases functional capacity of tissues when needed. For example, hyperplasia of breast tissue during pregnancy and lactation.
- **Compensatory hyperplasia:** The proliferation of cells while they preserve their differentiated structure and function is known as compensatory hyperplasia. For example, erythroid hyperplasia in case of iron deficiency/hemolytic anemia, regenerative hyperplasia seen in patients where parts of the kidneys/liver are removed.

Pathological Hyperplasia

Excessive hormonal stimulation and excessive generation of growth factors lead to pathological hyperplasia. For example, benign prostatic hyperplasia in response to androgen mediated growth factor secretion, endometrial hyperplasia in response to excess estrogen states (Figs 2.5A to C).

Pathological Features

- **Gross examination:** Increase in weight, size of organ.
- **Microscopic examination:** Increase in cell number.

METAPLASIA

The reversible process of cellular switching in which one adult cell type is replaced with another, due to stem cell reprogramming in response to injurious stimuli. Chronic stress causes stem cells to be reprogrammed into a different type of epithelium (like squamous metaplasia), which can withstand the stressful environment better. Cells may completely regress or result in malignant transformation and ongoing insult. Therefore, such change in differentiation makes the cell more resistant to the insult.

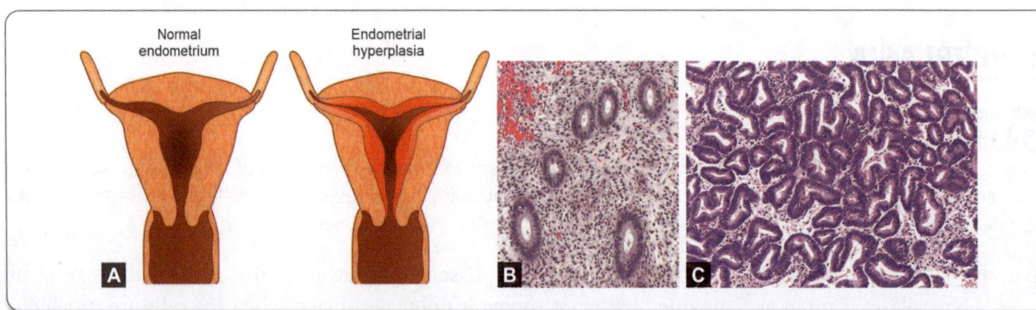

Figures 2.5A to C: **A.** Endometrial hyperplasia in response to excessive estrogen states; **B.** Microscopic appearance of normal endometrium; **C.** Microscopic appearance of endometrial hyperplasia

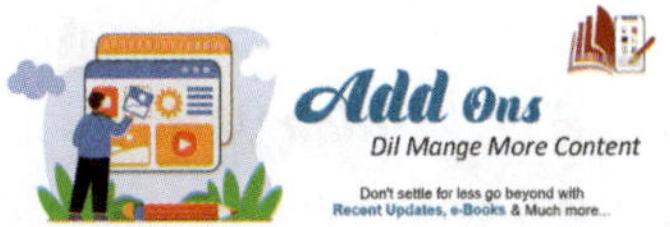

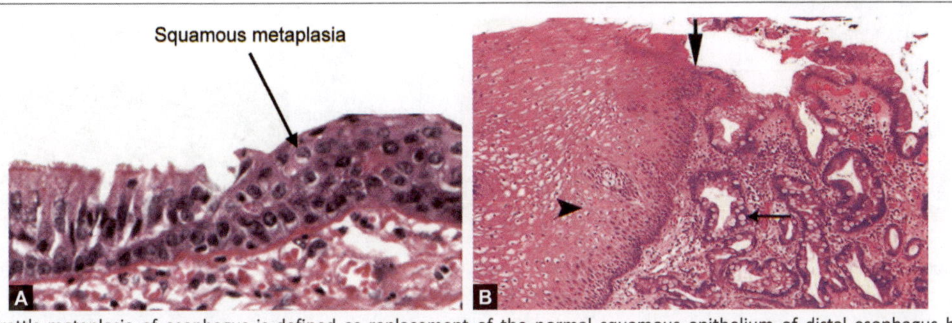

Barrett's metaplasia of esophagus is defined as replacement of the normal squamous epithelium of distal esophagus by metaplastic glandular epithelium containing intestinal-type goblet cells. Note the squamous epithelium on the left (arrow head) is continuous with the metaplastic epithelium containing goblet cells (long thin arrow) on the right. The transition is shown by downward arrow on the top.

Figures 2.6A and B: A. Squamous metaplasia, respiratory system; **B.** Barrett's metaplasia

Types of Metaplasia

Physiological Metaplasia

Cervical ectopy: This condition is commonly seen among the women who are in the reproductive age. The columnar epithelium, which lines the endocervix, is present on the ectocervix in this situation, exposing the columnar cells to the vaginal milieu.

Pathological Metaplasia

- Intestinal metaplasia also known as Barrett's metaplasia, which occurs due to chronic exposure to gastric acid, that can progress into adenocarcinoma (Figs 2.6A and B).
- Metaplasia of corneal squamous cells due to deficiency of vitamin A.
- Squamous metaplasia of the bronchi due to smoking, which causes replacement of ciliated pseudostratified columnar epithelium with stratified squamous epithelium.

Epithelial Metaplasia

Squamous Metaplasia

Any cell type becomes a squamous cell from other cell types (e.g., pseudostratified columnar epithelium) (respiratory type epithelium) (Figs 2.7A and B):

- In chronic smokers squamous switch occurs for cellular protection and adaptability.
- In chronic sinusitis—respiratory tract lining epithelial cells can show squamous metaplasia.
- In vitamin A deficiency:
  - **From transitional lining epithelium:** Epithelium lining the urinary bladder and pelvis can show squamous metaplasia in the presence of stones and chronic inflammation.
  - **From columnar epithelium:** Endocervical lining epithelium in chronic cervicitis, prostatic duct epithelium with aging.

Columnar Metaplasia

Intestinal metaplasia is the term for a change in cell type in which the nonkeratinized squamous epithelium that typically covers the esophagus changes into nonciliated columnar epithelial cells. E.g., intestinal

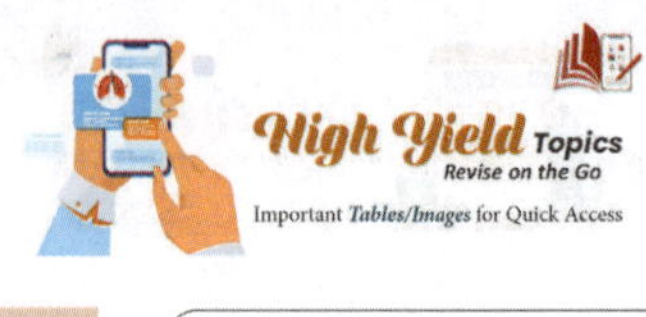

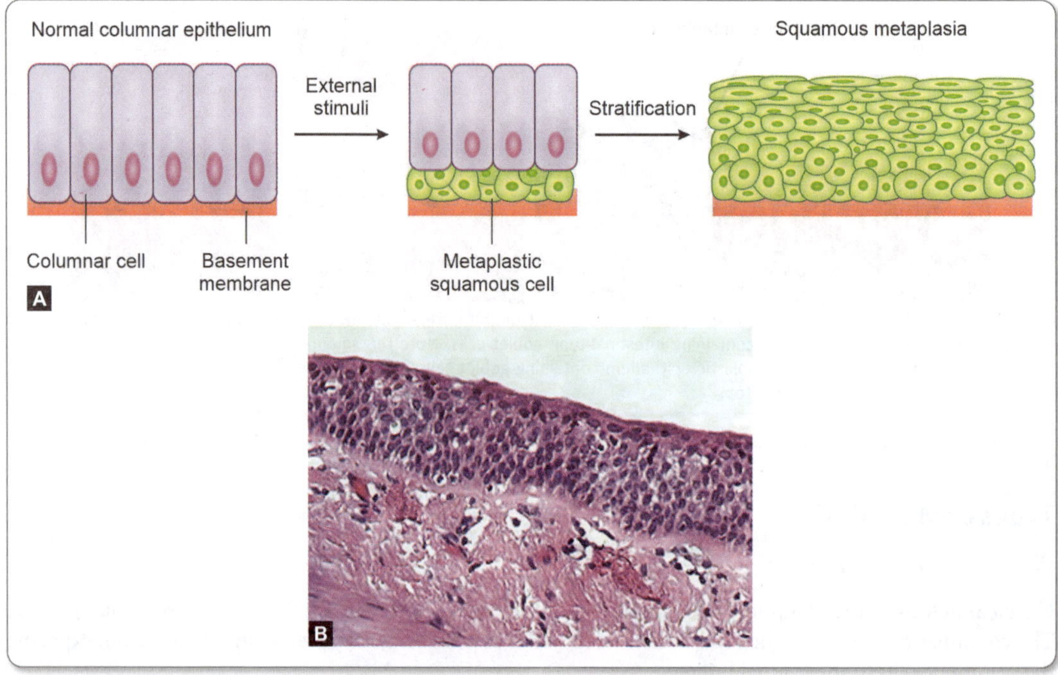

Figures 2.7A and B: Squamous metaplasia. **A.** Diagrammatic representation; **B.** Microscopic apperance

metaplasia in chronic gastritis, Barrett's esophagus-replacement of squamous epithelium by columnar epithelium with goblet cells (Figs 2.8A and B).

Figures 2.8A and B: Columnar metaplasia: **A.** Diagrammatic representation; **B.** Note specialized intestinal metaplasia with characteristic goblet cells

Mesenchymal Metaplasia

Osseous Metaplasia

Formation of bone from other cell types, e.g., previous cases of tuberculosis, medial calcification of arteries and postsurgery/post-trauma scars, endometrial osseous metaplasia, is a rare pathological condition in which a mature bone is formed in the endometrium (Fig. 2.9).

Cartilaginous Metaplasia

This can be seen in healing fractures.

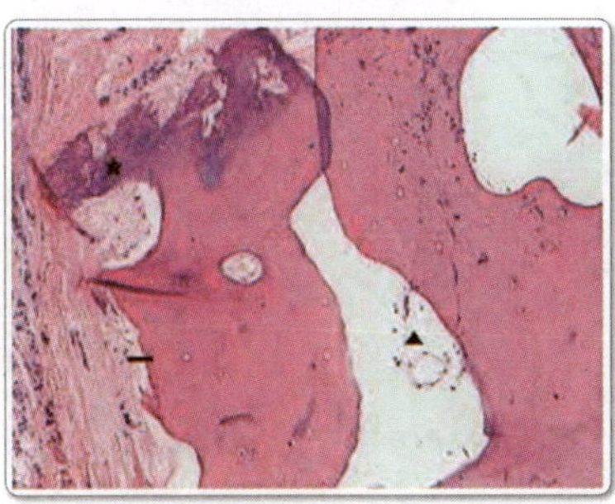

Figure 2.9: Osseous metaplasia (microscopic appearance)

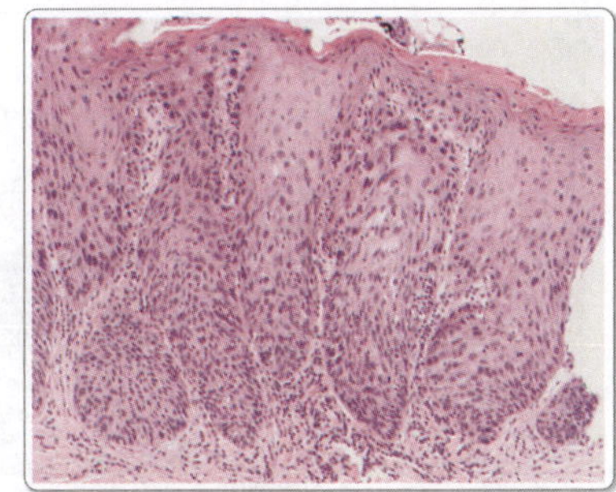

Figure 2.10: Dysplasia; note atypia, loss of polarity, increased nuclear size, hyperchromasia and pleomorphism

DYSPLASIA

Dysplasia refers to disordered cellular growth. It is characterized by: Loss in the uniformity of cellular size, shape, orientation and nuclear features, which is generally considered a premalignant state. The key features to diagnose dysplasia include (Fig. 2.10):

- **Cellular pleomorphism:** Cells are of variable sizes, shapes and orientation.
- **Nuclear hyperchromasia:** The nucleus takes up an increased basophilic hue.
- **Increased mitotic activity:** Reflecting increased cellular proliferation.
- **Loss of normal maturation pattern within the lining epithelium:** As one proceeds to the surface of a lining epithelium cells flatten, this is lost in the case of dysplasia.
- **Loss of nuclear polarity or orientation:** In the case of severe dysplasia.
- But the hallmark of dysplasia differentiating it from frank malignancy is NO invasion into the underlying tissue, that is the basement membrane remains intact.
- Severe dysplasia often becomes irreversible and develops into carcinoma in situ.
- Common organs where dysplasia is described includes the cervix (CIN-1, 2, 3), esophagus, biliary tract and prostate.

Major Types of Dysplasia (Fig. 2.11)

- **Mild:** When ⅓ or less of the epithelial lining is involved
- **Moderate:** When ⅓–⅔ of the thickness of the epithelial lining is involved
- **Marked:** When >⅔ of the thickness of the epithelial lining is involved, however the dysplastic features are still not full thickness
- **Carcinoma in situ:** When the entire thickness of the lining epithelium shows dysplastic features but there is no breach in the basement membrane.

EXTRA EDGE

Type IV collagen and laminin are basement membrane markers which can be demonstrated immunohistochemically, loss of these markers points to...INVASION

NURSING CONSIDERATIONS

Nursing professionals have an important role to play in both the preventive and curative phases of cancer:

- **Preventive phase:** Counseling on lifestyle modifications, taking HPV vaccine for the prevention of cervical cancer, encouraging women to participate in screening programs.
- **Curative phase:** To provide compassionate first point information when the patient receives a diagnosis of dysplastic change and preliminary counseling before surgery/other therapy.

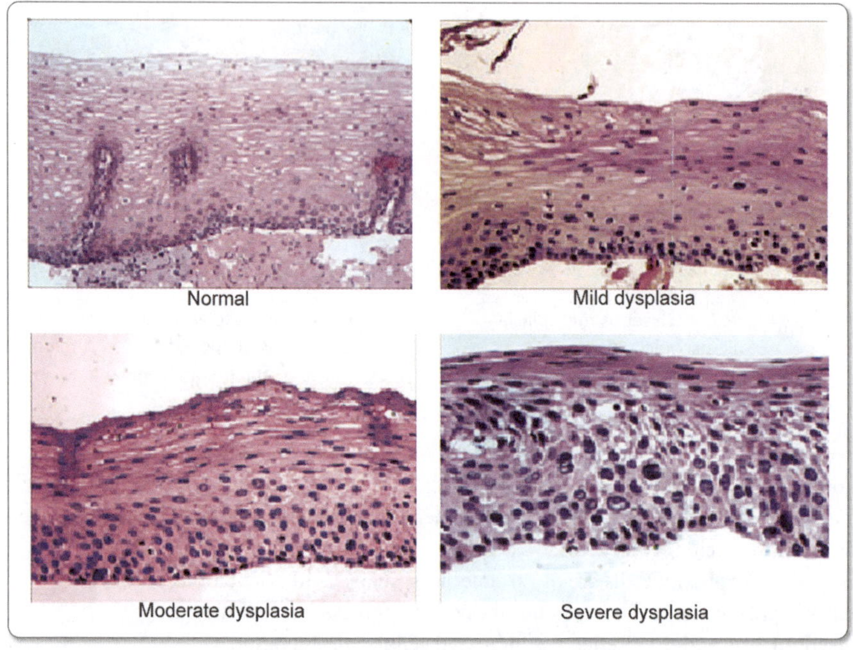

Figure 2.11: Histologic appearance of normal squamous epithelium and mild, moderate, and severe esophageal squamous dysplasia

Mechanism

Reprogramming of local tissue stem cells: Affected cells are directed by external stimuli toward a specific differentiation pathway. The affected organ or tissue is colonized by differentiated cell populations from adjacent.

Table 2.1 presents the difference between metaplasia and dysplasia and Table 2.2 presents difference between hyperplasia and dysplasia.

Table 2.1: Difference between metaplasia and dysplasia

Feature	Metaplasia	Dysplasia
Definition	Replacement of one differentiated adult cell type with another	Cellular disorder with loss in the uniformity of cellular size, shape, orientation and nuclear features
Type of response	Adaptive	Oncogenetic
Mechanism	Stem cell reprogramming	Genetic and epigenetic alterations
Trigger	Usually environmental	Environmental/hormonal/genetic/viral
Type of cell	Epithelial/mesenchymal	Usually epithelial
Reversibility	Reversible	Usually irreversible
Progression	Low grade dysplasia	Invasive cancer
Examples	Barrett metaplasia, esophagus	Cervical intraepithelial neoplasia (CIN)

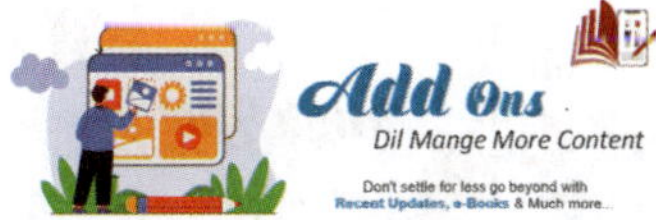

Table 2.2: Difference between hyperplasia and dysplasia

Feature	Hyperplasia	Dysplasia
Definition	Increase in the number of cells in a tissue resulting in an increase in the size of an organ	Cellular disorder with loss in the uniformity of cellular size, shape, orientation and nuclear features
Physiological/pathological	Both in physiological and pathological states	In pathological states
Cellular polarity	Usually maintained	Lost
Type of response	Adaptive	Oncogenetic
Progression	Reversible	Moderate and severe grades are irreversible
Examples	Benign prostatic hyperplasia	Dysplastic esophageal lining epithelium

CELL INJURY

Cell injury refers to changes seen in cells as a result of derangement in structure or function of a tissue/organ, due to disruption of normal steady state or homeostasis.

When a cell can no longer adapt to stress, cell injury occurs. It can be reversible, meaning that once the stress is removed, the cell can return to its original state. It can also be irreversible, meaning that the cell dies when the stress is excessive or continues for too long.

The principal targets for cell injury are: Cell membrane, mitochondrion, protein synthesis machinery and DNA.

FACTORS CAUSING CELL INJURY

- **Infectious organisms:** Bacteria, viruses, fungi, parasites.
- Hypoxia/reduction in oxygen supply.
- Drugs/chemicals/toxins.
- Physical agents, like heat/cold/radiation/trauma.
- Immune dysfunction—allergies/autoimmune disease.
- Nutritional deficiencies and excess resulting in malnutrition and obesity respectively.
- Chemical causing electrolyte derangements (e.g., glucose).

Most disease is a result of the combination of one or many of the above-mentioned factors, that is disease commonly has a multifactorial etiology.

Biochemical Basis of Cell Injury

Depletion of ATP

Depletion of ATP leads to dysregulation of energy-dependent mechanisms such as membrane transport. Other functions which may be altered which include (Fig. 2.12):

- Reduced protein synthesis, as the ribosomes detach from the rough endoplasmic reticulum.
- Proteins formed are defective and misfolded.
- Accumulation of sodium in the cell leads to influx of water into the cell, it occurs due to failure of sodium dependent pump.
- The calcium pump fails, increasing intracellular calcium favouring cell death by necrosis.
- Anaerobic glycolysis is activated leading to accumulation of lactic acid reducing the cell pH leading to reduced activity of many cellular enzymes.

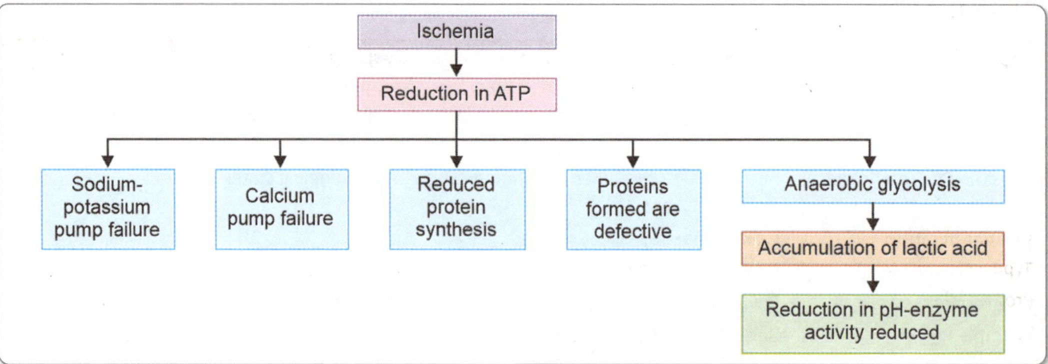

Figure 2.12: Effects of reduction in ATP

Membrane Damage

Damage to cell membranes results in increased cell membrane permeability causing leak of lysosomal enzymes leading to cell death by necrosis.

Free Radical Mediated Injury

Generation of free radicals damages the cellular lipids in the cell membrane (lipid peroxidation) and also causes DNA damage.

Mitochondrial Damage

This leads to leakage of cytochrome c causing cell death *via* apoptosis.

Loss of Calcium Homeostasis

Normal cytosolic calcium levels are very low and majority of which is sequestered in endoplasmic reticulum and mitochondrion. Injury causes increased release of calcium leading to activation of enzymes resulting in cell injury.

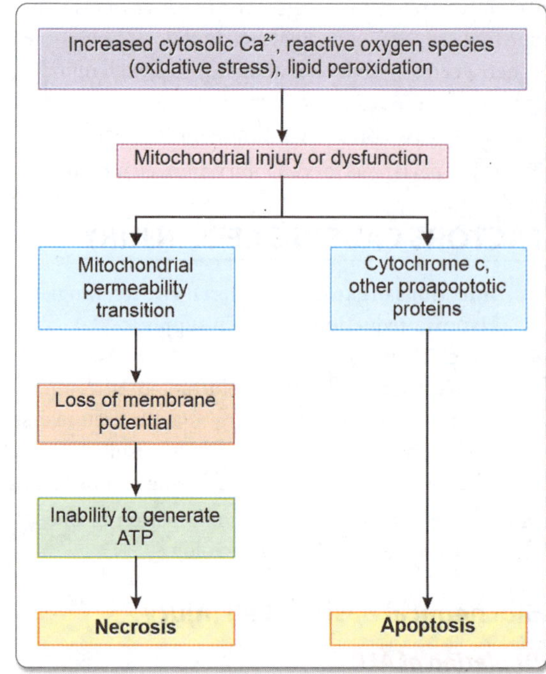

Figure 2.13: Cell injury by mitochondrial damage

Cell Injury by Mitochondrial Damage

Mitochondria is a major site of synthesis of ATP. Increased mitochondrial permeability leads to formation of transition pores which causes loss of membrane potential and oxidative phosphorylation.

ATP depletion leads to: Cell swelling, reduced cytosolic enzyme activity, reduced protein synthesis (Fig. 2.13).

Cell Injury by Abnormal Calcium Homeostasis

Intracellular calcium is normally low as it is sequestered in mitochondria and ER. Release of calcium from intracellular stores, increased calcium influx through plasma membrane. It leads to activation of enzymes such as: Phospholipases, proteases, endonucleases, ATPase which lead to cell injury (Fig. 2.14).

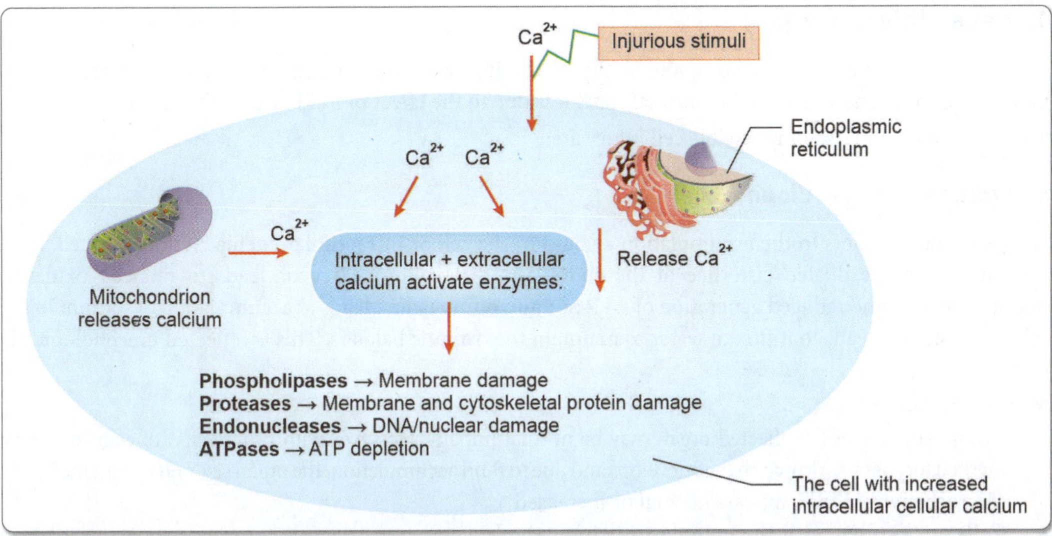

Figure 2.14: Abnormal calcium homeostasis leads to cell injury

Cell Injury by DNA and Membrane Damage

Membranes are normally made up of lipids, with phospholipids being the most abundant form. Membrane damage can be caused by: Oxygen-free radicals, calcium dependent phospholipases, calcium-dependent proteases. Increased permeability of plasma membrane causes influx of fluids and ions and leads to loss of osmotic balance. Injury to lysosomal membrane causes release of lysosomal enzymes which disrupts cytoplasmic organelles.

Cell Injury by Oxidative Stress

Free radicals have a single unpaired electron in their outer orbit. Reactive oxygen species attacks unsaturated fatty acid of the membrane and causes DNA damage and fragmentation. Also, it causes protein degradation by increasing protein cross-linking and causing oxidative modification.

EXTRA EDGE

- Hypoxia is the most common cause of cell injury.
- Ischemia is the most common cause of hypoxia.

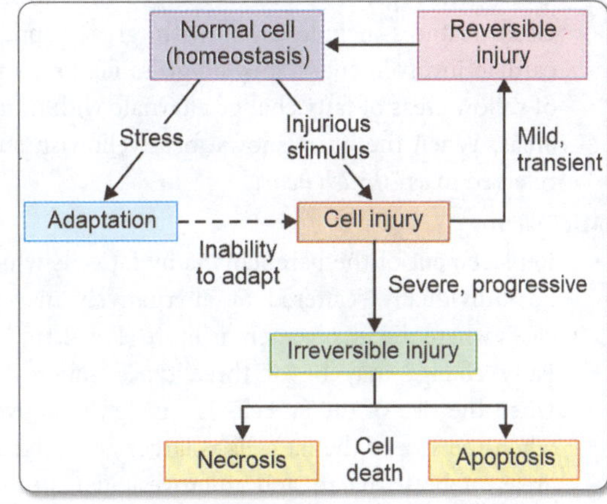

Figure 2.15: Reversible and irreversible responses to injurious stimuli

TYPES OF CELL INJURY

There are two types of cell injury (Fig. 2.15).

1. Reversible Cell Injury

Reversible cell damage is defined as the ability of the injured cell to regain homeostasis and return to a morphologically (and functionally) normal state. It is due to the effect of mild or transient injury.

The two main hallmarks of reversible cell injury are:

I. Hydropic Change (Cloudy Swelling)

Hydropic change refers to the accumulation of fluid in the cell or intracellular edema. Within the cell, fluid accumulates in the dilated cisternae of the endoplasmic reticulum. Hypoxia leads to reduced oxidative phosphorylation and reduced generation of ATP. Sodium pump failure leads to accumulation of sodium in the cell which in turn leads to influx of water to maintain the osmotic balance. This is reflected morphologically as hydropic change.

Morphological features

- **Gross:** The size of the affected organ may be normal initially. However with progression of cellular injury, marked turgor or hydropic change develops and due to fluid accumulation, the organ size and weight increases.
- **Microscopy:** Cell size appears normal or increased
- **Cells are swollen with the cytoplasm being pale:** In later stages the cell cytoplasm show vacuolation which is visible on light microscopy.
- **Ultrastructural changes include:** Blebbing of the cell membrane and dilatation of the endoplasmic reticulum.

II. Fatty Change

Fatty change refers to the accumulation of fat (triglycerides) within the cytoplasm and is also called *steatosis*. Steatosis can be demonstrated using special stains such as oil red O and Sudan black. Fatty change is commonly seen in cells of the liver. It can additionally be seen in other metabolically active organs such as the heart, kidney and skeletal muscle.

Morphological features

- **Gross:** The organ involved is enlarged and shows an increased weight.
- Gross features include a yellowish, greasy appearance with a solid and firm consistency. In cases of cardiac involvement, a specific gross feature is the *tabby cat/tigered heart appearance* in which bands of yellow areas of fatty change alternate with uninvolved areas. When the heart shows focal yellowish streaks is referred to as *"thrush heart"*.

Microscopy

- Replacement of the parenchyma by fat cells which may be individually scattered or alternatively may fuse in cases where the involvement is more (Fig. 2.16).
- Fatty change may be of three types—microvesicular, when the size of the fat cells is smaller, macrovesicular when the size of the fat cells is larger and mixed, when areas of both macro and microvesicular steatosis are noted.

  Individual cells show a vacuolated appearance with nucleus pushed to the periphery, giving a "signet ring" appearance. The vacuolated appearance is due to tissue processing.

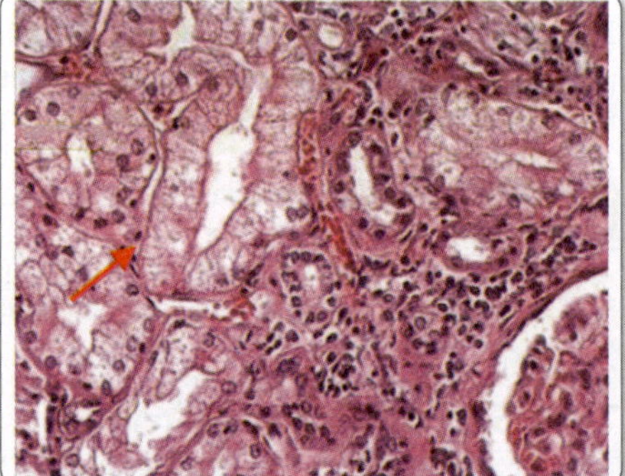

Figure 2.16: Light microscope findings showing hydropic change/cellular swelling in proximal convoluted tubule (PCT) of kidney (reversible cell injury)

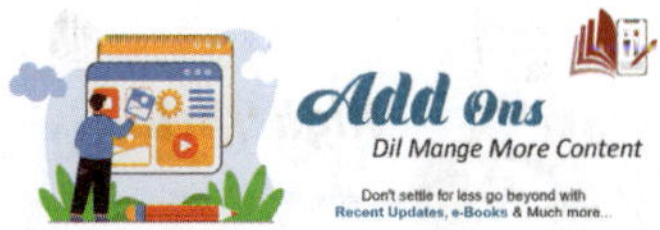

EXTRA EDGE

Features of reversible cell injury (Fig. 2.17):

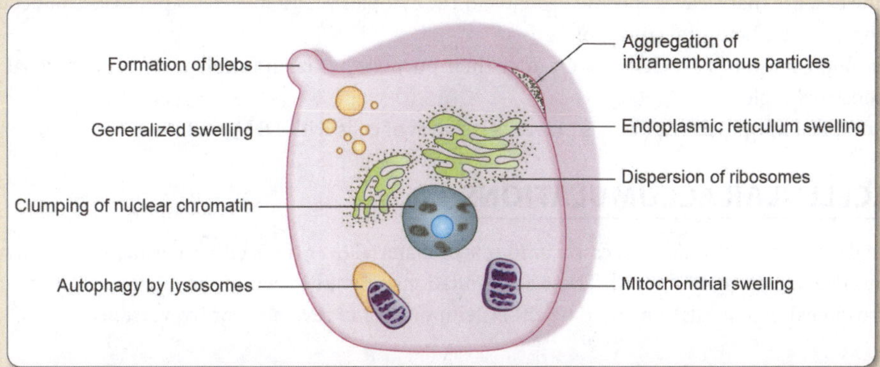

Figure 2.17: Morphological features of reversible cell injury

- Water influx causing cellular swelling is the earliest sign of cell damage.
- Vacuolar degeneration or hydropic change causing tiny, transparent vacuoles within the cytoplasm.
- Alterations to the plasma membrane characterized by formation of blebbing, blunting and loss of microvilli.
- Amorphous densities and swelling of the mitochondria.
- ↑ cytosolic myelin figure formation (phospholipids from damaged membranes).
- Nucleus alterations (disaggregation of granular and fibrillar components).
- Fatty change caused by lipid vacuole buildup (in organs involved in lipid metabolism).

2. Irreversible Cell Injury

Irreversible cell injury is one of the more severe and pervasive cell injuries that results in necrosis or apoptosis. It occurs when the cell has reached the point of no return. The swelling of the mitochondria and lysosomes, lysosomal membrane damage that causes enzyme leakage, cell membrane damage, and increased acidity in the cellular environment are all signs of permanent cell injury. Necrosis and apoptosis are the two biological responses caused by irreversible cell injury.

MUST KNOW

Electron microscopic features of irreversible injury are large amorphous densities in mitochondria.

Features

- Inability to recover from mitochondrial malfunction (lack of oxidative phosphorylation and ATP synthesis).
- Significant membrane function damage.

Necrosis

Necrosis is a type of cell death characterized by cytoplasmic swelling, damage to cell membrane, and organelle breakdown. The components of the cytosol are leaked into the extracellular space as a result of necrosis and show loss of nuclei (Fig. 2.18).

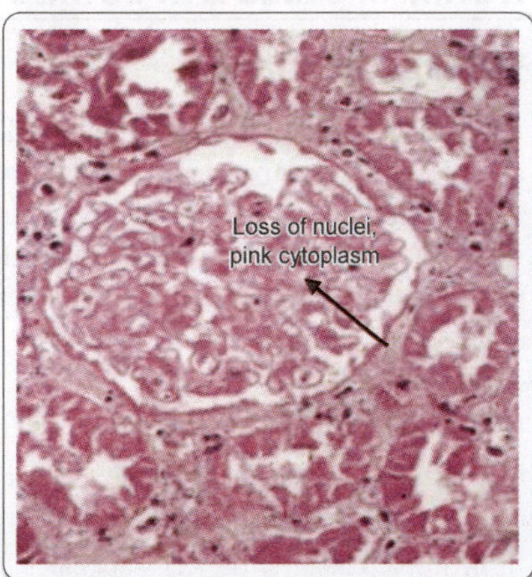

Figure 2.18: Coagulative necrosis kidney

Apoptosis

Apoptosis is programmed cell death of harmful cells. The process depends on the energy and is mediated by the enzyme caspase that cleaves specific proteins in the cytoplasm and nucleus. Apoptosis can occur in both physiological and pathological conditions.

- **Physiological apoptosis:** Cells die off after their purpose has been fulfilled, e.g., endometrial shedding in menstrual cycle.
- **Pathological apoptosis:** Apoptosis prevents survival of cells with DNA mutation.

INTRACELLULAR ACCUMULATIONS

The normal cell may accumulate excessive amounts of material over time, either permanently or temporarily, which could be damaging to the cell. These accumulations might be seen in the nucleus or in the cytoplasm (phagolysosomes). Accumulation could be either temporary and reversible or irreversible.

Types of Accumulated Substances

- **Normal cellular components:** Normal cellular components which are accumulated in excess such as water, lipids, protein and carbohydrate.
- **Abnormal substances:** It can be endogeneous such as product of abnormal synthesis or metabolism or exogeneous such as mineral or result of pathogenic infection.
- Pigments.

Accumulation of various substances occurs by following mechanism:

- Accumulation of normal substances, either as a result of an increase in their production or as a result of the failure of metabolism to remove them, as in the case of fatty changes in the liver.
- A normal or abnormal endogenous material builds up as a result of inherited or acquired metabolic disorders, such as storage diseases or an insufficient level of alpha-1 antitrypsin (mutations cause faulty folding and transport of this protein).
- Cells acquire an aberrant exogenous material without the defects, similar to silica or carbon buildup.

NORMAL CELLULAR COMPONENTS

Water Accumulation

Excessive accumulation of water in the cells leads to cloudy swelling or hydropic/vacuolar degeneration. It results due to the defect in the cell's ability to regulate sodium. When sodium enters the cell, water follows to maintain the iso-osmotic pressure, which causes parenchymal cellular swelling. The liver, kidney, and heart are examples of paranchymus organs which undergo this form of cellular degeneration.

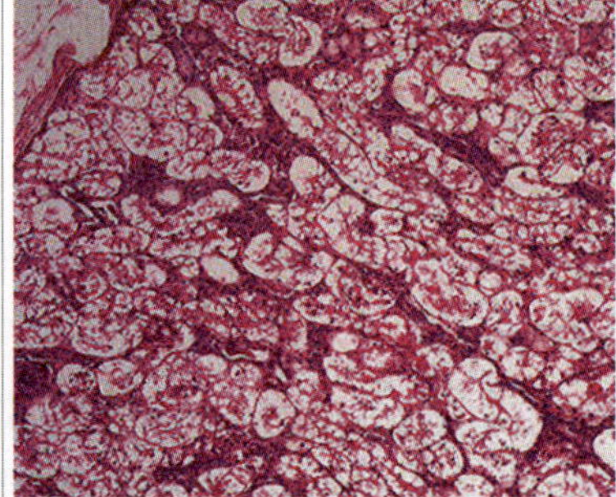

Figure 2.19: Hydropic swelling of renal tubular epithelial cells

Gross examination: The organ appears enlarged, soft and pale.

Microscopic appearance: There is an accumulation of proteinaceous small granules due to abnormal protein metabolism.

In hydropic changes, the cells appear ballooned, pale, watery and vacuolated, due to the cellular swelling nucleus is pushed toward the periphery and eventually the cell bursts and nucleus undergoes lysis (Fig. 2.19).

It occurs where water transfer is most active, such as the renal tubular epithelium following intravenous administration of hypertonic glucose or in case of hyperkalemia.

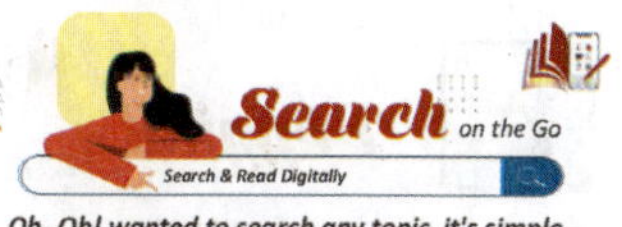

Fat Accumulation

Abnormal triglyceride accumulations within the hepatocytes (the main site because the liver plays a central role in fat metabolism) are referred to as fatty alterations (steatosis) (Fig. 2.20) and can also affect the heart, skeletal muscles, and kidney.

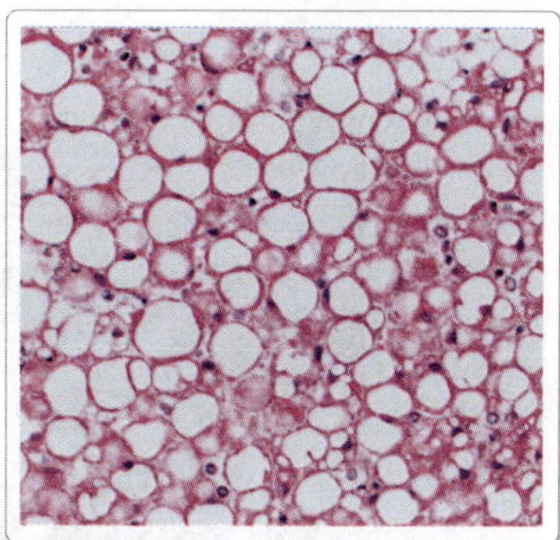
Figure 2.20: Image showing macrovascular steatosis

Etiology

- Starvation and alcoholism—promote fatty acid mobilization from peripheral stores.
- Protein deficiency which causes decreased apoprotein production.
- Diabetes mellitus, tetracycline toxins, liver toxins including CCL4 and estrogen, steroid, and hypoxia are all linked to obesity.
- Mild fatty changes may not have any impact on cellular function.
- Severe fatty changes may lead to liver cirrhosis and hepatocellular carcinoma.

Mechanisms

- *Excessive entry of free fatty acids in the cell*, seen in obesity, increased fat in the diet and starvation where peripheral fat is broken down to provide for energy.
- **Reduced conversion of fat to lipoprotein:** This conversion step is mediated by apoprotein. In conditions such as protein energy malnutrition and carbon tetrachloride poisoning, apoprotein production is hampered in the body, hence triglycerides are not converted to lipoprotein and accumulate in the liver.
- **Reduced fatty acid metabolism (oxidation):** Toxins, alcohol and any cause of hypoxia alters mitochondrial function affecting oxidative processes. This, in turn, hampers the oxidation of fatty acids to ketone bodies.

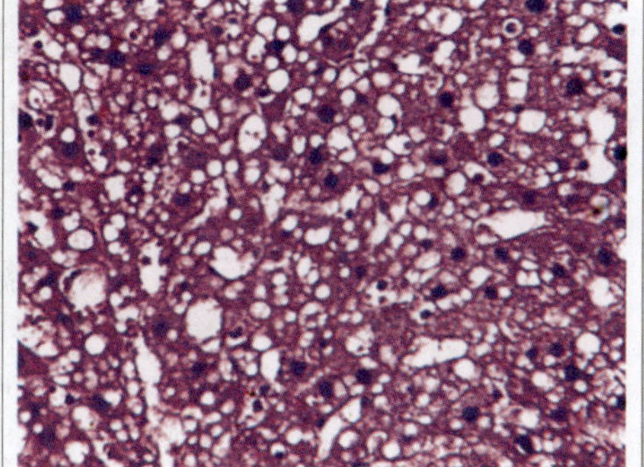
Figure 2.21: Liver cells showing fat accumulation

Morphological changes show fat accumulation in the form of clear vacuoles within the parenchymal cells. Progressive fatty changes cause the liver to become enlarged and yellowish and in extreme instances, liver appears greasy, yellowish and soft (Fig. 2.21).

Protein Accumulation

Intracellular accumulations of proteins typically manifest as spherical, eosinophilic droplets, vacuoles, or clumps in the cytoplasm, though protein accumulation is less frequent than lipid accumulation.

Examples of protein accumulation:

- In the rough endoplasmic reticulum (RER) of some plasma cells, there is a notable buildup of newly synthesized immunoglobulins that can result in rounded, eosinophilic **Russell bodies** (Figs 2.22A and B).
- Intracellular proteins (**Mallory bodies:** Keratin intermediate filaments) (Fig. 2.23) accumulate in alcoholic liver disorders and are visible in the liver cells as eosinophilic inclusions.
- **Neurofibrillary tangle**, which is an accumulation of proteins found in Alzheimer's disease of the brain (Fig. 2.24).

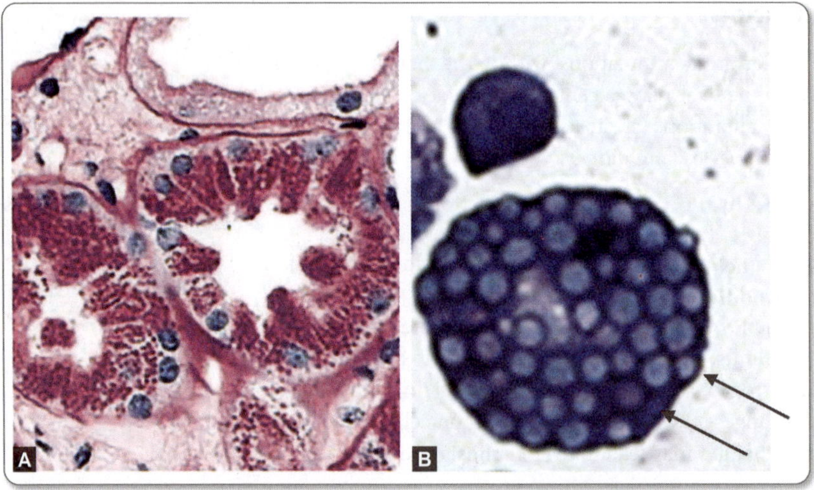

Figures 2.22A and B: **A.** Image showing reabsorption droplets in PCT; **B.** Russell bodies

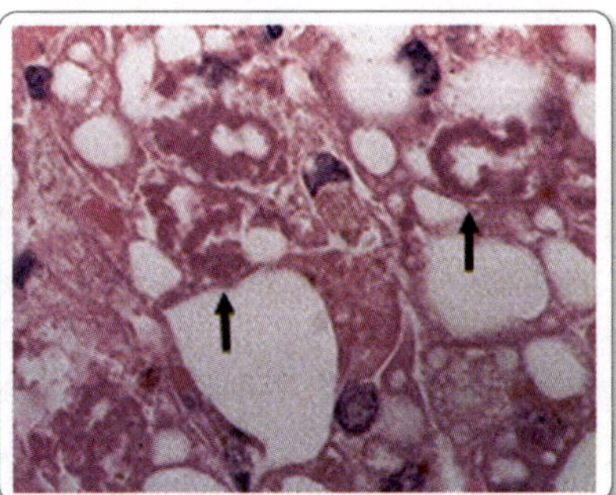

Figure 2.23: Mallory bodies as seen in alcoholic hepatitis which are appearing pink in H&E stain

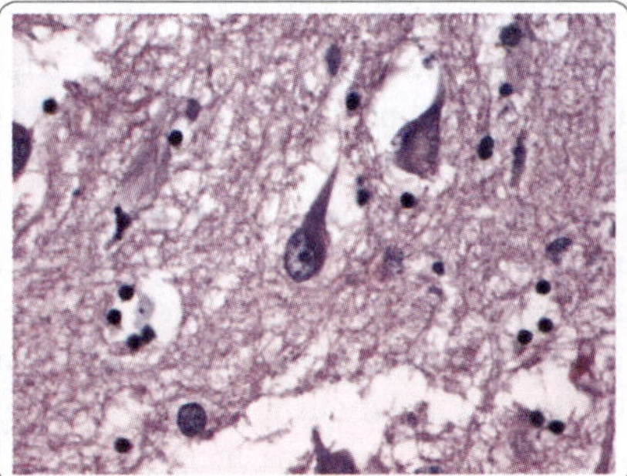

Figure 2.24: Neurofibrillary tangles as seen in Alzheimer's disease

Glycogen Accumulation

Glycogen overproduction can be seen in the following ways:

- Glycogen will build up in the heart muscles, pancreatic beta cells, and renal tubular epithelium in poorly controlled diabetes mellitus.
- Glycogen storage diseases occur due to an enzymatic defects that cause an accumulation of glycogen in the different cells of the body.

ACCUMULATION OF ABNORMAL SUBSTANCES

Hyaline Change

It is defined as accumulation of glassy, homogenous, eosinophilic substances resulting from variety of pathologic conditions. It can be of two types:

1. **Intracellular:** Hyaline deposition is usually seen in epithelial cells. Examples include: Hyaline droplets, hyaline degeneration, Mallory's hyaline.
   - **Hyaline droplets:** It occurs because of excess reabsorption of plasma proteins, these can be observed in proximal convoluted tubules.
   - **Hyaline degeneration:** These are deposits in voluntary muscle, as seen in degeneration of rectus abdominis.
   - **Mallory's hyaline:** These are accumulations of intermediate filament seen in hepatocytes in alcoholic hepatitis.
   - **Hyaline inclusions:** These are cytoplasmic and nuclear inclusions seen in various viral infections.
   - **Russell bodies:** Russell bodies, also known as Mott cells, are eosinophilic immunoglobulin containing inclusion bodies that are typically detected in abnormal plasma cells.
2. **Extracellular:** Extracellular hyaline is seen in connective tissues. For example, hyaline degeneration in leiomyomas, hyaline arteriosclerosis and hyalinization of glomerulus in chronic kidney disease.

Pathologic Calcification

It is an abnormal tissue deposition of calcium salts, together with trace levels of iron, magnesium, and other mineral salts. The two types of pathologic calcifications are:

1. **Dystrophic calcification:** It is commonly seen in dying tissues. For example, areas of necrosis, atheromas, aging or damaged heart valves, tuberculous lymph nodes. Typical serum calcium levels are normal in dystrophic calcification.
   - **Gross appearance:** White granules, which are often felt as gritty deposits.
   - **Microscopic appearance:** On H&E staining, calcium deposits appear as basophilic, granular and clumped appearance (Fig. 2.25).
2. **Metastatic calcification:** It is a type of soft tissue calcification caused by an increased serum calcium levels. It is characterized by deposition of calcium in viable tissue. For example, blood vessels, kidneys and lungs (Fig. 2.26). It is usually seen in cases of hypercalcemia.

Etiology of Pathologic Calcification

- **Hypercalcemia:** Excess calcium intake, due to milk-alkali syndrome, renal stones caused by milk and antacid self-therapy.

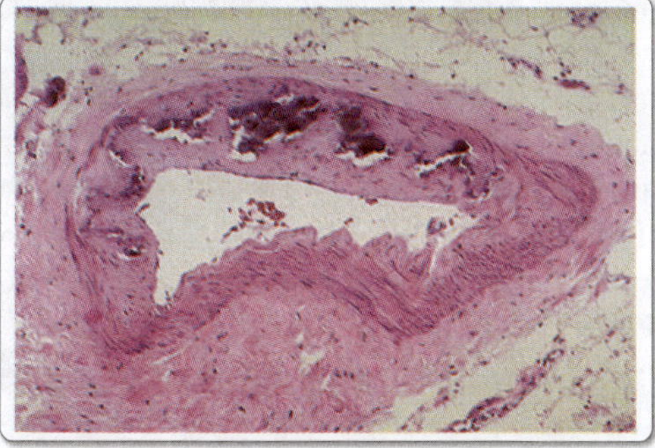

Figure 2.25: Dystrophic calcification of an artery from a patient with arteriosclerosis

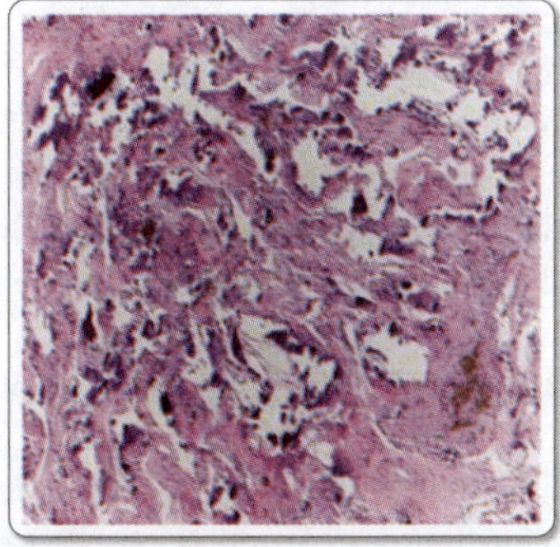

Figure 2.26: Showing interstitial metastatic calcifications along the alveolar septa, perivascular space and within bronchioles

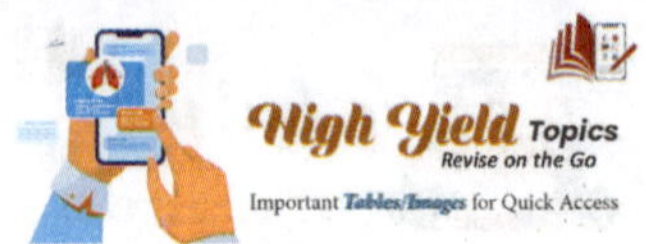

- **Hyperparathyroidism:** It occurs due to primary hyperthyroidism or caused by other tumors.
- **Destruction of bone tissue:** It occurs due to primary tumors of bone marrow (e.g., multiple myeloma).
- **Vitamin-D related disorders:** Such as vitamin-D intoxication, sarcoidosis.
- **Renal failure:** Which may cause retention of phosphate, leading to secondary hyperparathyroidism.

Table 2.3 presents a list of differences between metastatic and dystrophic calcification:

Table 2.3: Difference between metastatic and dystrophic calcification

Features	Metastatic calcification	Dystrophic calcification
Description	Diffuse (intracellular and extracellular) calcification of normally noncalcified tissue	Localized (intracellular and extracellular) calcification of normally noncalcified tissue
Tissues involved	Kidney, lung, gastric mucosa, and blood vessels' interstitial tissues are otherwise normal tissues. Acid is rapidly lost by affected tissues. Increased pH levels encourage calcium deposition.	Tissues that are ageing or dying, or inflammatory or ageing tissues
Etiology	Secondary to hypercalcemia, caused by, for instance • Primary hyperthyroidism • Hypervitaminosis-D • Bone mineralization due to immobility • Increased bone resorption (due to bone metastasis, multiple myeloma, immobilization, paget disease)	Secondary to local injury or necrosis due to: • Cardiovascular condition • Fat necrosis • Infarct • Chronic granulomatous disease • Tuberculosis
Histology	Finely-speckled calcium through soft tissues	• Psammoma bodies (extracellular) • Deeply basophilic on H&E stain

PIGMENTS

Pigments are colored substances, which are either exogenous or endogenous.

Endogenous Pigment

- **Lipofuscin:** These are composed of lipids and phospholipids complexed with proteins. It is not injurious to the cell or its function. It is typically seen in the liver and the heart of the ageing patients or patients who are severely malnourished, cancer cachexia. Lipofuscin in heart is called brown atrophy (Fig. 2.27).
- **Melanin:** It is non-hemoglobin derived brown-blackish pigment formed when the enzyme tyrosinase catalyses the oxidation of tyrosine to dihydroxyphenylalanine in melanocytes in various organs. Excess melanin is evident can be seen in malignant melanoma.
- **Hemosiderin:** These pigments typically appear intracellularly and are visible as yellow to brown granules. They contain ferric hydroxide, which is iron coupled to a protein framework and is revealed by a variety of chemicals. Since red blood cells, which contain 60% of the body's total iron content, are where oxygen is carried

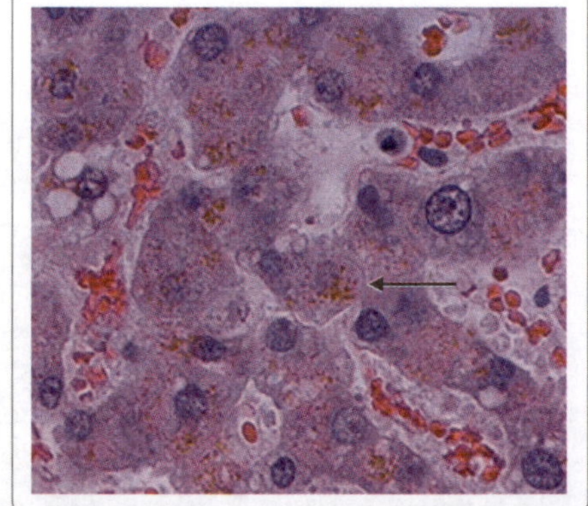

Figure 2.27: Lipofuscin is characterized by pale golden brown finely granular pigment seen in hepatocytes

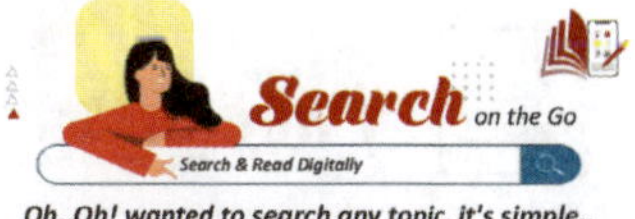

by haemoglobin, iron is a crucial component of the human body. Myoglobin and several enzymes, including cytochrome oxidase and the peroxidases, also exhibit it (Fig. 2.28).

- **Porphyrin:** These are the chemicals often existing in trace concentrations in tissues. They are thought to be the heme component of hemoglobin's precursors. The biosynthesis of heme and porphyrins is disrupted by the rare pathological illnesses known as porphyrias.

    Porphyrin pigment can be detected as localized deposits in liver sections of people with erythropoietic protoporphyria. The pigment is a rich, dark brown pigment that, when freshly frozen, fluoresces brilliantly red before quickly fading when exposed to ultraviolet light. The pigment appears bright red in color with a dark Maltese cross in the middle when observed in paraffin slices and under polarized light.

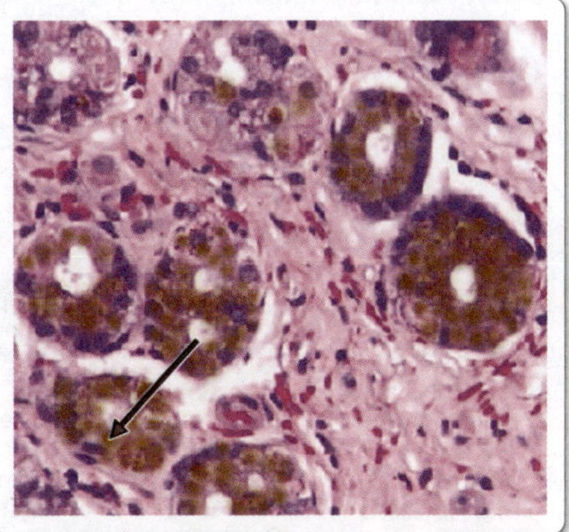

Figure 2.28: Patchy hemosiderin deposition in gastric glandular cells

- **Bile pigments:** Bile pigments are the byproducts of haemoglobin breakdown. These are excreted in bile. The bile pigments are biliverdin and bilirubin in its oxidized form. The color of bilirubin and biliverdin are orangish yellow and green, respectively.

Exogenous Pigment

It refers to storage of chemicals that do not naturally occur in the body, such as tattoo ink, coal dust, or smoke.

- **Carbon:** it is stored in the lysosomes of macrophages *via* phagocytosis
- **Copper deposits:** Wilson's disease is characterized by accumulation of copper in the liver. Typically, copper is not visible on tissue slides that have been hematoxylin and eosin (H&E) stained. For the purpose of positively identifying copper in liver biopsy tissue, stains like rhodanine or rubeanic acid can be utilized.

For more concise details about pigments please refer to Flowchart 2.1.

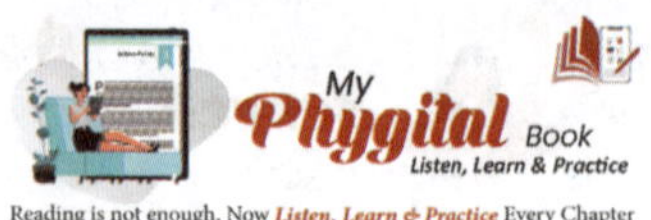

Flowchart 2.1: Classification of pigments

Pigments

- **Exogenous**
  - **Carbon**
    - **Most common** exogenous pigment
    - Phagocytosed by **lung macrophages**
  - **Tattooing**
    - Localized, exogenous pigmentation of the skin
    - Phagocytosed by **dermal macrophages**
- **Endogenous**
  - **Lipofuscin (Wear and tear pigment)**
    - Insoluble pigment
    - Also called lipchrome or wear and tear pigment
    - Derived by **lipid peroxidation** of **polyunsaturated lipids of subcellular membranes**
    - **Tell-tale sign** of free radical injury to the cell and lipid peroxidation
    - **Yellow brown, Perinuclear** pigment
    - Responsible for **brown atrophy of liver and heart**
    - Seen in **aging, protein energy malnutrition and cancer cachexia**
    - **Stain-long ZN stain**
  - **Melanin**
    - Non-heme derived pigment
    - Normally present in hair, skin, iris, stria vascularis of inner ear, zona reticularis of adrenal gland and substantia nigra of brain
    - Only naturally occurring endogenous black pigment derived from **tyrosine**
    - **Special stain: Masson Fontana**
    - IHC stain-S100, **HMB45** (Specific)
    - Albinism-Little or no melanin synthesis
    - Tumor of melanocytes-melanoma
  - **Hemosiderin**
    - Heme derived pigment
    - **Golden yellow to Brown,** granular or crystalline pigment
    - Seen at sites of – Local hemorrhage or bruise
    - Systemic overload of iron hemosiderin is called hemosiderosis
    - Hemosiderin-aggregates of ferritin micelles
    - **Special stain: Perls Prussian blue stain –** Converts soluble ferrocyanide to ferric ferrocyanide
    - Perls stain detects **Ferric iron** deposits in tissue

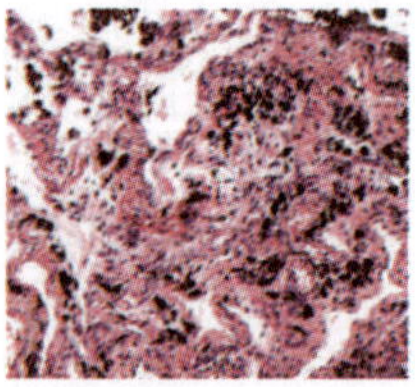

Black carbon pigment inside the cytoplasm of the macrophages in the alveolar wall

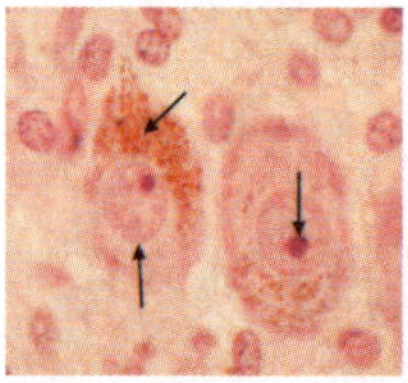

Mic: Perinuclear pigment

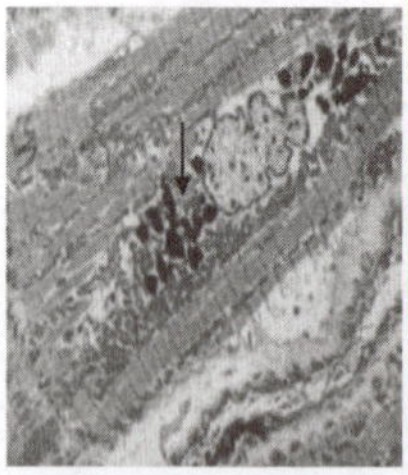

(Electron microscopy showing perinuclear pigment)

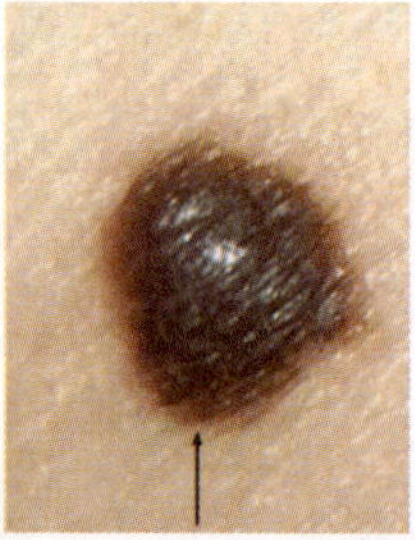

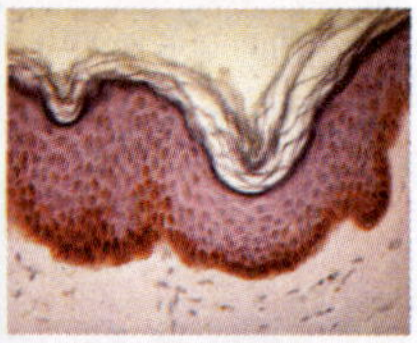

Melanin in **basal** layer of **epidermis**

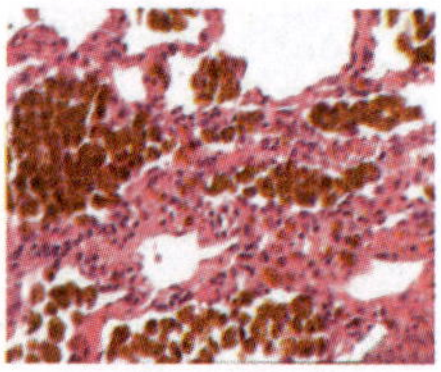

Hemosiderin Laden Macrophages in Lung Alveoli

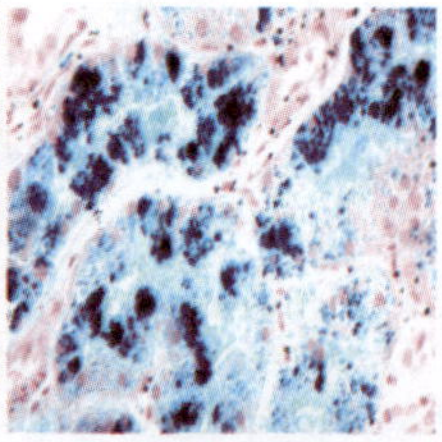

Perls stain showing hemosiderin pigment

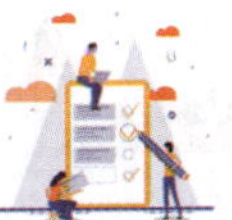

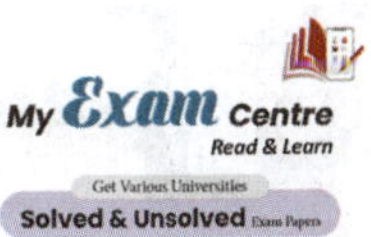

SUMMARY

- This phenomenon of cellular response to stress/injurious stimuli, for continued survival in altered conditions, is referred to as cellular adaptation.
- Atrophy implies a reduction in size and/or reduction in the number of cells in a tissue.
- Hypertrophy implies an increase in size of an organ due to an increase in cell size.
- Hyperplasia is an increase in the number of cells in a tissue resulting in an increase in the size of an organ.
- Metaplasia is the reversible process of cellular switching in which one adult cell type is replaced with another, due to stem cell reprogramming in response to injurious stimuli.
- Dysplasia is a premalignant state characterized by the loss in the uniformity of cellular size, shape, orientation and nuclear features.
- Carcinoma in-situ is characterized by the dysplastic feature involving the entire thickness of the lining epithelium but there is no breach in the basement membrane.
- Cell injury refers to changes seen in cells as a result of derangement in structure or function of a tissue/organ, due to disruption of normal steady state or homeostasis.
- Reversible cell injury is the type of cell injury where damage is potentially reversible and the steady state or cellular homeostasis can be re-achieved, if the injurious stimulus is withdrawn.
- Hydropic change refers to the accumulation of fluid in the cell or intracellular edema.
- The accumulation of fat (triglycerides) within the cytoplasm and is also called *steatosis*.
- Irreversible cell injury is one of the more severe and pervasive cell injuries that results in necrosis or apoptosis.
- Necrosis is a type of cell death characterized by cytoplasmic swelling, damage to cell membrane, and organelle breakdown.
- Apoptosis is the programmed cell death of the harmful cells.
- Reactive oxygen species attacks unsaturated fatty acid of the membrane and causes DNA damage and fragmentation
- Excessive accumulation of water in the cells leads to cloudy swelling or hydropic/vacuolar degeneration.
- Neurofibrillary tangle is an accumulation of proteins found in Alzheimer's disease brain tissue.
- Russell bodies are eosinophilic, homogeneous immunoglobulin (Ig)-containing inclusions usually found in cells undergoing excessive synthesis of Ig.
- Mallory bodies (MB) are cytoplasmic hyaline inclusions of hepatocytes.
- Hyaline changes can be defined as accumulation of glassy, homogenous, eosinophilic substances resulting from variety of pathologic conditions.
- Dystrophic calcification is commonly seen in dying tissues.
- Metastatic calcification is a type of soft tissue calcification caused by an increased serum calcium levels.
- Pigments are colored substances, which are either exogenous or endogenous.

ASSESS YOURSELF

Long Answer Questions

1. Discuss cellular adaptations and its types with appropriate examples.
2. Explain cell injury and its types along with mechanism of cell injury.

Short Answer Questions

1. Define hypertrophy.
2. Write the types of metaplasia.
3. Write about morphological features of fatty changes.
4. Differentiate between dysplasia and metaplasia.
5. Differentiate between necrosis and apoptosis.

6. Write short notes on:
   i. Intracellular accumulations
   ii. Pathologic calcifications
   iii. Vacuolar degeneration

Multiple Choice Questions

1. **Hyperplasia generally means:**
   a. An organ will increase in size due to excessive formation of extracellular fluids
   b. Increase in the number of cells
   c. Blebbing at the periphery
   d. Shrinkage in cell size
2. **What would be an example of hypertrophy?**
   a. Breast development at puberty
   b. Enlargement of uterus during pregnancy
   c. Enlargement of uterus during menstruation
   d. Papillomavirus induced skin wart
3. **In hypoxic cell injury, cell swelling occurs because of increased intracellular....**
   a. Lipid
   b. Water
   c. Protein
   d. Lipofuscin
4. **All of the following are true about dysplasia; except:**
   a. It is characterized by disorderly arrangement of cells
   b. Its constituent cells show cellular pleomorphism
   c. It always progresses to invasive carcinoma
   d. It can be seen in both epithelial and mesenchymal cells
5. **All of the following are true about metaplasia; except:**
   a. It is a reversible change
   b. It results from reprogramming of stem cells
   c. It makes the cells more resistant to the ongoing insult
   d. It always progresses to dysplasia

Answer Key

1. b **2.** b **3.** b **4.** c **5.** d

Chapter 3

Cell Death (Necrosis and Apoptosis)

LEARNING OBJECTIVES

After the completion of the chapter, the readers will be able to:

- Know the important forms of cell death (necrosis, apoptosis).
- Understand the different types of necrosis and the morphological features seen in these types.
- Understand the process of apoptosis, the pathogenetic mechanisms/pathways involved.
- Distinguish between necrosis and apoptosis.

CHAPTER OUTLINE

- Introduction
- Necrosis
- Gangrene
- Apoptosis

KEY TERMS

Apoptosis: Apoptosis is the process of programmed cell death, which is used to eliminate unwanted cells.

Gangrene: Gangrene is characterized by ischemia and necrotic tissue, frequently involving a finger or other extremity.

Homeostasis: Homeostasis is defined as a self-regulating process by which a living organism can maintain internal stability while adjusting to changing external conditions.

Karyolysis: Karyolysis is disintegration and dissolution of the nucleus of a necrotic cell.

Karyorrhexis: Karyorrhexis is the destructive fragmentation of a dying cell's nucleus, resulting in an irregular distribution of chromatin throughout the cytoplasm.

Necrosis: It is an uncontrolled cell death that leads to tissue damage by causing the intracellular contents to leak into the surrounding tissue, enlargement of the cell organelles, plasma membrane rupture, and eventual cell lysis.

Pyknosis: Pyknosis is the process by which a cell contracts or condenses as a result of an increase in nuclear compactness or density.

INTRODUCTION

A multicellular organism's life cycle must include cell death. Basic life processes include cell death, survival, proliferation, and differentiation. During embryonic development, cell death is crucial for maintaining the body's equilibrium and getting rid of damaged cells. Initial classification of cell death includes: Type I cell death (apoptosis), type II cell death (autophagy), and type III cell death (necrosis).

The term, 'necrosis' refers to cell enlargement (oncosis) and eventual membrane rupture, which is how cells die. Necrotic cell death often affects clusters or zones of cells, and the discharge of cell contents into the ECM causes an inflammatory response. Contrarily, apoptosis normally affects single cells and is controlled by cellular signaling cascades. Apoptosis is a process that causes the cell and its organelles to condense and shrink, eventually resulting in cell disintegration.

NECROSIS

Definition

It is an uncontrolled cell death that leads to tissue damage by causing the intracellular contents to leak into the surrounding tissue, enlargement of the cell organelles, plasma membrane rupture, and eventual cell lysis.

Necrosis, differs from the apoptosis in the way that it results from external signals, is almost always accompanied by inflammatory responses because of the release of nuclear proteins, ATP, DNA, and heat shock proteins which cause the release of proinflammatory cytokine interleukin-1 β (IL 1).

Causes

- **Hypoxia:** This can occur due to shock, ischemia, or respiratory failure.
- **Physical agents:** These include external wounds such as trauma, temperature extremes, radiation exposure, or electric shock.
- **Chemical agents:** These include poisons, occupational exposure, drug toxicity, or illicit substances.
- **Biological agents:** These are fungi, viruses, or bacteria.
- **Immunologic reactions:** These are autoimmune responses.

Mechanism

- Necrotic cells typically demonstrate by swelling of organelles such the endoplasmic reticulum and mitochondria, rupturing of the plasma membrane, and cell lysis (Fig. 3.1).
- Cells become more eosinophilic, glassy, and vacuolated as a result of these modifications.
- This is worsened by organelle membrane breakdown and loss of cell membrane integrity.
- A lack of oxygen delivery to cells causes necrosis linked to hypoxia or chemical damage, which lowers ATP synthesis.

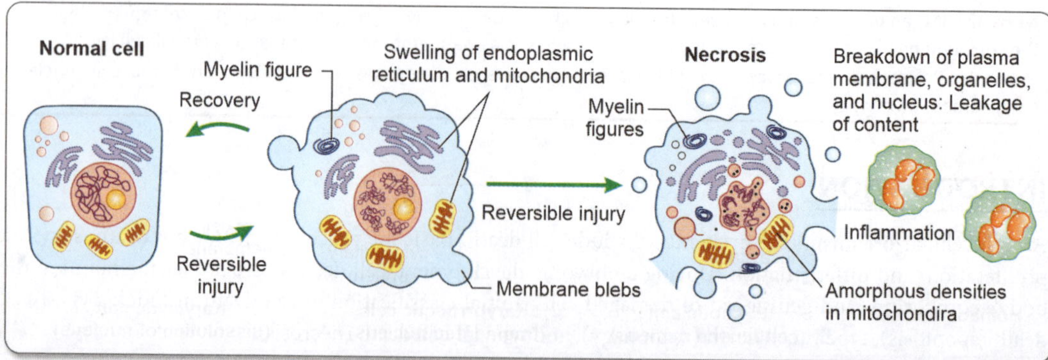

Figure 3.1: Mechanism of necrosis

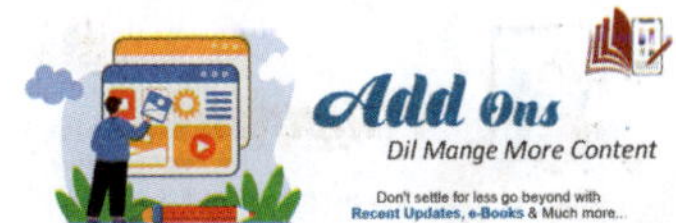

- This shortage of ATP causes the energy-dependent sodium pump in the plasma membrane to malfunction, resulting in an inflow of calcium and water, which causes cells to expand and ribosomes to detach from the endoplasmic reticulum.
- Various cytosolic enzymes, such as phospholipases and proteases, can be activated by cytosolic calcium, including those that break down proteins and membranes (including lysosomal membranes).

Features of Necrosis

- Swelling of the cell.
- Swelling of the nucleus.
- Nuclear dissolution which is called Karyolysis (Fig. 3.2).
- Nuclear fragmentation also known as Karyorrhexis (Fig. 3.2).
- Nuclear shrinkage and increased basophilia–pyknosis (Fig. 3.2).
- Pale eosinophilic cytoplasm.
- Cytoplasmic vacuoles may be present in areas of necrosis.
- Adjacent cellular debris and inflammatory cells may be present if there is leakage of the cell membrane.

EXTRA EDGE

Necroptosis is a combination of necrosis and apoptosis. Necroptosis causes the membrane to rupture, allowing intracellular chemicals to escape and killing the target cells. The immune system uses necroptosis as a defence against pathogen-mediated infections.

Types

Coagulative Necrosis

- It is the most common type of necrosis, caused by ischemic injury causing hypoxic death of the cells.
- In this form of necrosis, cell death is present but cellular outline/architecture is maintained giving rise to a *"tombstone" appearance.*

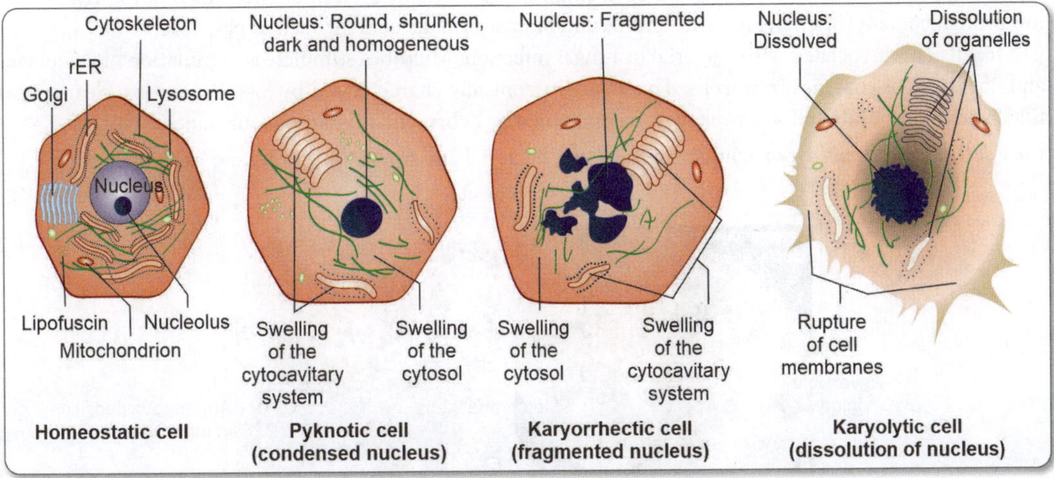

Figure 3.2: Necrotic cells: Pyknosis, karyorrhexis and karyolysis
Abbreviation: rER, rough endoplasmic reticulum

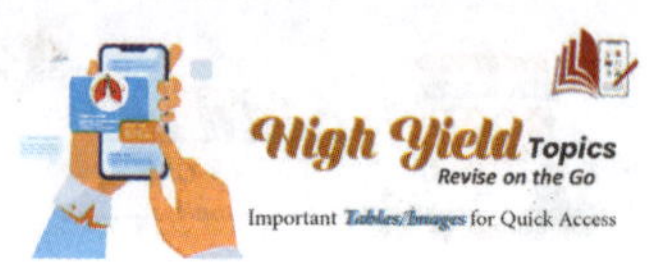

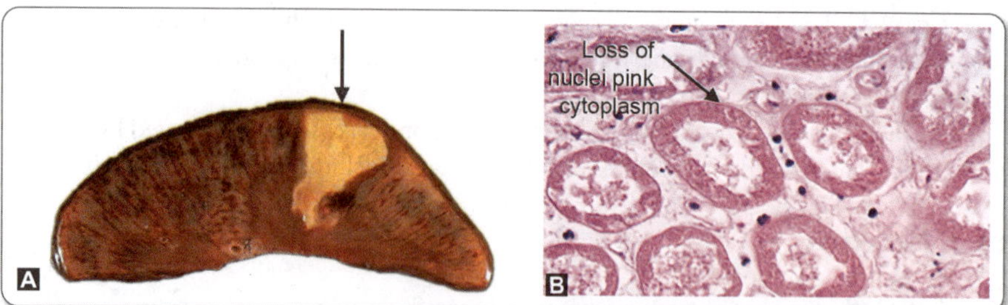

Figures 3.3A and B: Coagulative necrosis: **A.** Gross appearance; **B.** Microscopic appearance

- Here, cell injury leads to destruction of all proteins including enzymes.
- As enzymes lyse the cell membranes, in their absence, cellular outline is preserved.

Case setting: Frequently seen in **ischemic/hypoxic injury in all organs except the brain,** e.g., myocardial infarction seen in patients of ischemic heart disease (heart attack) and infarction in kidney (Figs 3.3A and B).

Gross examination: The organ size usually is normal with the necrotic areas appearing pale and firm.

Microscopic examination: Individual cell outline is identifiable.

Cellular content however is lost.

Cytoplasm is deeply eosinophilic due to protein denaturation.

Cell nuclei may show any of the following or one or more of the following:

- **Pyknosis:** Small, condensed nuclei.
- **Karyorrhexis:** Fragmented nuclei.
- **Karyolysis:** Dissolution of the nuclei.

Liquefactive/Colliquative Necrosis

This type of necrosis is due to the release of lysosomal/bacterial hydrolytic enzymes and is characterized by a complete loss of structural details, involved tissue being completely destroyed to rapidly soften and form a liquified mass (encephalo-malacia-brain softening). It is commonly seen in organs which have high fat and low protein content (brain), (Figs 3.4A and B) and high enzymatic content such as pancreas.

It is usually associated with bacterial or fungal infection. Microbes stimulate accumulation of leucocytes and liberation of enzymes from cells. This is microscopically characterized by loss of neurons, clear spaces filled with neutrophils and macrophages, accompanied by debris and lipidaceous substance.

Case setting: Ischemic/hypoxic injury in the brain, bacterial and fungal infections and gangrene.

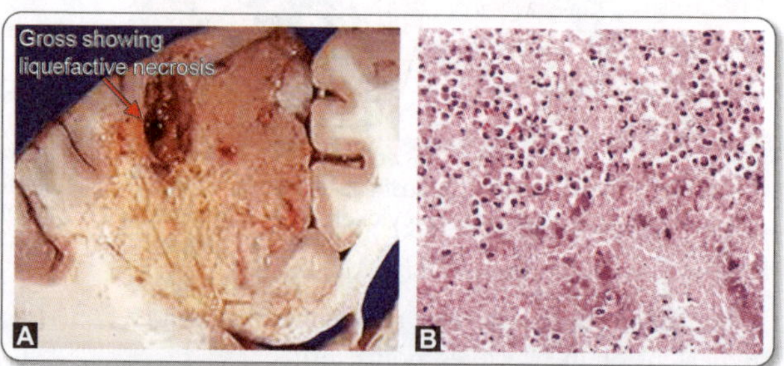

Figures 3.4A and B: Liquefactive necrosis of brain: **A.** Gross appearance; **B.** Microscopic appearance

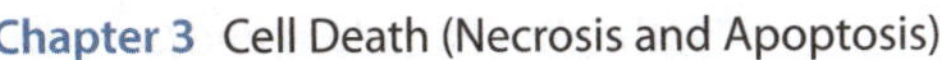

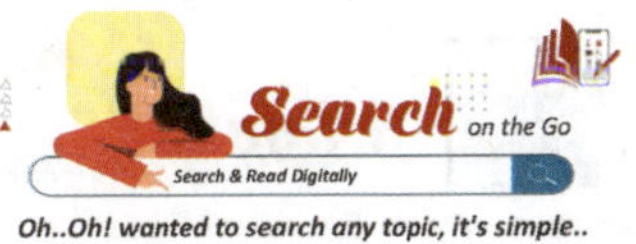

In Table 3.1 the difference between coagulative and caseous necrosis is given.

Table 3.1: Difference between coagulative and caseous necrosis

Characteristic features	Coagulative necrosis	Caseous necrosis
Pathogenesis	It is typically caused by ischemia or infarction.	It is typically caused due to delayed hypersenstivity reaction to mycobacterium tubercular antigens
Cause	Hypoxia	Tuberculosis infection of lungs, lymph nodes
Morphology	Pale and firm tissue segment that contrasts with the surrounding well-vascularized tissue and is dry on the cut surface.	Affected tissue is cheesy white in texture

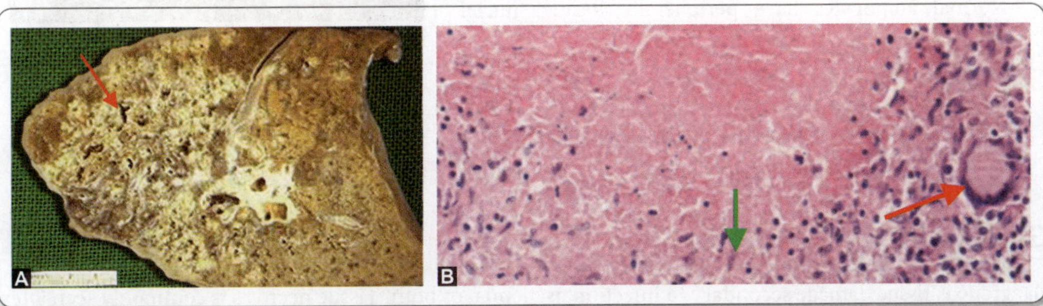

Figures 3.5A and B: Caseous necrosis of lungs: **A.** Gross appearance; **B.** Microscopic appearance

Caseous Necrosis

This is a unique type of necrosis associated with tubercular infection. It is a form of coagulative necrosis but cellular outlines are lost.

Gross examination: Distinct gross appearance of tissue—"cheese" like/white.

Microscopic examination: This form of necrosis is characterized by an amorphous, dirty granular quality. In cases of tuberculosis, caseous necrosis may be the only feature or may be seen in association with other microscopic features of tuberculosis such as epithelioid cell granulomas or Langhan's giant cells (Figs 3.5A and B).

Fibrinoid Necrosis

This form of necrosis is seen in the case of vascular damage and is associated with exudation of plasma proteins including eosinophilic fibrin. The vessel wall may be infiltrated by inflammatory cells (Fig. 3.6).

Gross examination: No specific gross features are seen.

Microscopic examination: Bright pink, amorphous material deposited in the vessel wall, can be visualized on H&E and also by special stains such as *Masson's trichrome, PTAH, Martius scarlet blue*

Case setting: Malignant hypertension in arterioles, polyarteritis nodosa, vasculitis, lupus nephritis.

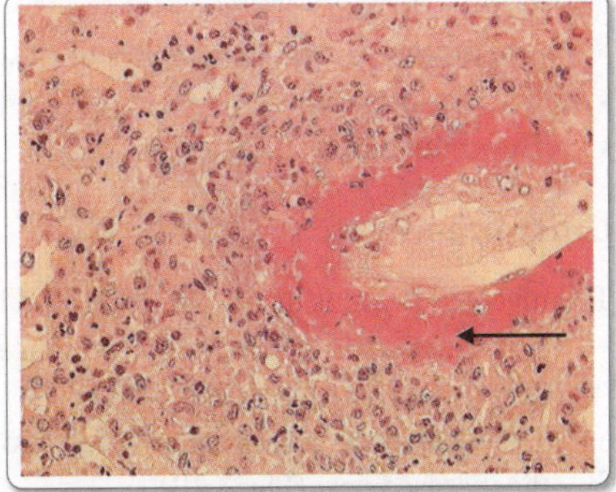

Figure 3.6: Microscopy-wall of artery showing fibrinoid necrosis (arrow)

Fat Necrosis

When fatty organs are inflammed, lipases are released. These convert the fat of the adipocytes into fatty acids, which in turn, combine with calcium leading to saponification (soap formation). This appears as chalky white deposits, e.g., traumatic fat necrosis of the breast, pancreatic fat necrosis secondary to pancreatitis.

Gross examination: Chalky white areas which are soft to firm in consistency (Fig. 3.7).

Microscopic examination:

- Cellular outlines of adipocytes are lost.
- Normal adipocytes have peripherally located nuclei which are lost in this type of necrosis.
- Cytoplasm appears smudgy due to necrotic fat, inflammation may also be seen.
- Calcific deposits which are basophilic may be seen.

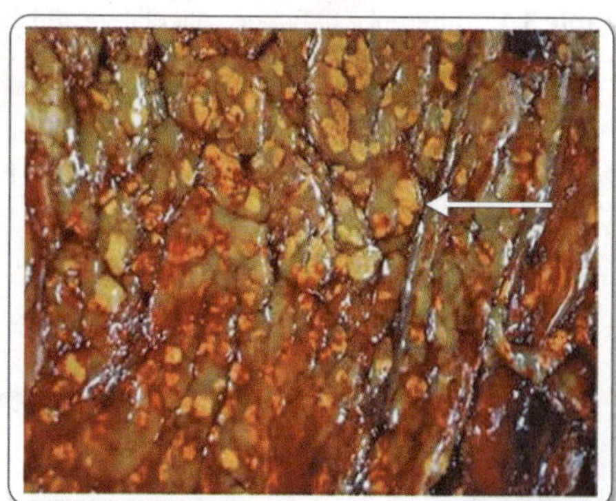

Figure 3.7: Chalky white appearance in fat necrosis

Case setting: Traumatic fat necrosis of the breast, fat necrosis of the pancreas.

GANGRENE

Gangrene is tissue damage secondary to infection, ischemia, or both. Tissue necrosis is commonly seen after loss or reduction of blood supply (ischaemia) due to any cause. Gangrene is characterized by ischemia and necrotic tissue, frequently encircling a finger or other extremity. It can be recognized by the blackened or discolored tissue. The three main types of gangrene are:

1. Dry Gangrene

This is a type of gangrene frequently occurring in distal extremities due to a gradual blockage of vessels. Dry gangrene is dehydrated, ischemic tissue induced by increasing ischemia distal to arterial blockage.

Causes

- Raynaud's disease.
- Berger's disease.
- Atherosclerosis and progressive occlusion of the peripheral arterial blood supply to distal tissue.
- Vascular occlusions.
- Thromboembolic diseases.

Gross Appearance

The involved organ is dried, shrunken and black in color.

- A characteristic feature is the presence of a clear-cut line of demarcation between the gangrenous and non-gangrenous area (Fig. 3.8A).
- The involved area may show a "Mummified" appearance with subsequent shedding (autoamputation) of the diseased part (Fig. 3.8B).

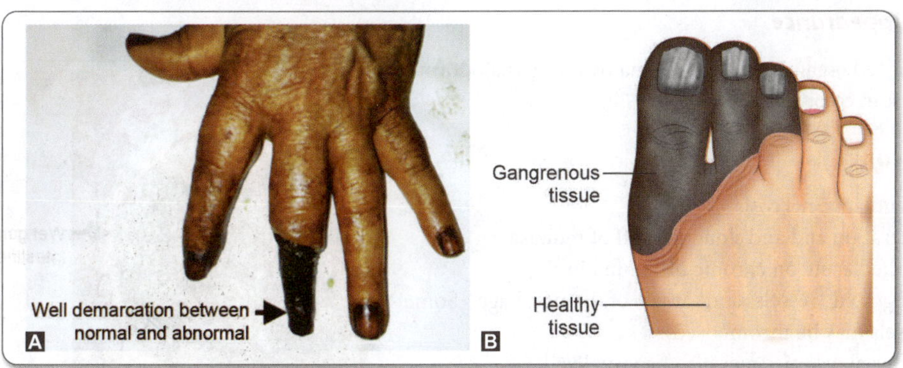

Figures 3.8A and B: Dry gangrene: **A.** Clinical presentation; **B.** Illustration

Microscopic Features

- Ischemic/coagulative necrosis.
- Mild/minimal inflammation around the line of demarcation only.

EXTRA EDGE

The symptoms of acute limb ischemia are classically identified by the 6 Ps mnemonic:

1. **P**aresthesia
2. **P**ain
3. **P**allor
4. **P**ulselessness
5. **P**oikilothermia (disorder temperature regulation)
6. **P**aralysis

2. Wet Gangrene

This usually occurs in organs that are normally well-vascularized, such as the lungs, intestine and any pressure points. In comparison to dry gangrene, tissue damage occurs more rapidly and is often accompanied by bacterial superinfection. There is no clear cut demarcation between the affected and unaffected part. As bacterial infection results in toxin production, a possible consequence is systemic inflammation or septicemia making this condition potentially life-threatening, if not managed in time. Wet gangrene has accompanying edema and erythema but no crepitus, and it may also be dry and worsened by a secondary infection.

Causes

- **Bed sores:** In bed-ridden (immobilized) patients.
- Intestinal intussusception and volvulus.
- Strangulated hernia.
- **Diabetics:** Naturally predisposed to infections and vascular blockage due to atherosclerosis.

Gross Appearance

The involved organ is swollen, edematous, soft, malodorous and black in color (Fig. 3.9).

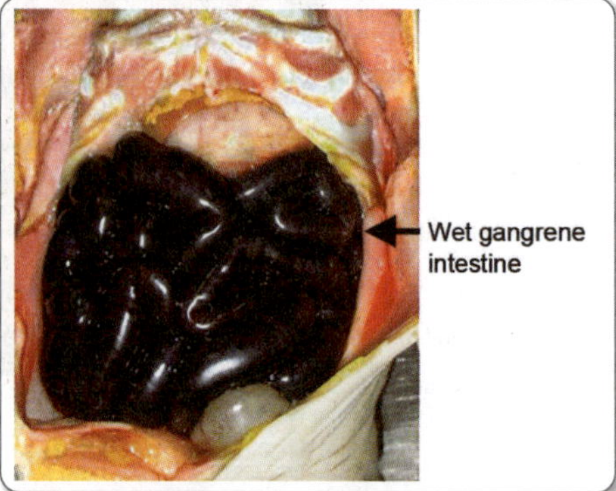

Figure 3.9: Wet gangrene

Microscopy

- Coagulative necrosis.
- Ulceration and and sloughing off of mucosa.
- Marked acute on chronic inflammation.
- Congested vessels and areas of hemorrhage. Some vessels may be thrombosed.
- Bacterial colonies may also be visualized.

3. Gas Gangrene

This represents a special type of wet gangrene, specifically caused by *Clostridium perfringens*, a gram-positive anaerobic bacteria.

In addition to all the gross features seen in cases of wet gangrene, here tissue is crepitant, i.e., having a crackling sound on touch, due to accumulation of gas bubbles (Fig. 3.10).

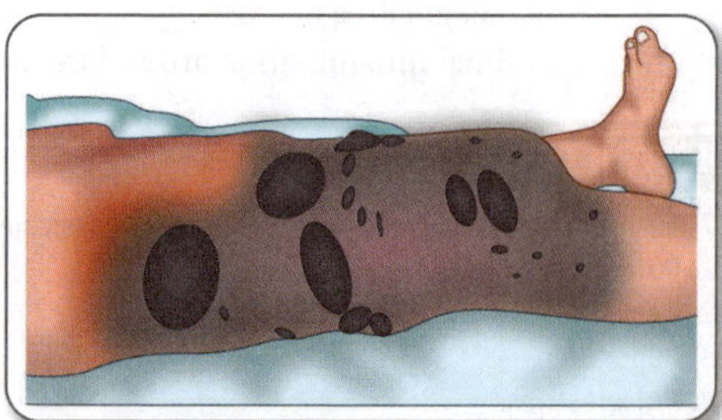

Figure 3.10: Gas gangrene

Symptoms of gas gangrene includes: Pain, edema, the development of hemorrhagic bullae, and color changes ranging from pale coloration to a bronze-purplish red colored tissue. The patient frequently has a trauma or recent surgical intervention history.

Case setting: Victims of road traffic accidents, any traumatic injury, military explosions, bullet injuries. Patients undergoing surgeries on the intestine also are predisposed to this type of gangrene.

Table 3.2 presents difference between dry gangrene and wet gangrene.

Table 3.2: Difference between dry gangrene and wet gangrene

Features	Dry gangrene	Wet gangrene
Type of vessel occluded	Arterial involvement more frequent	Arterial and venous
Line of demarcation	Present at the junction between healthy and gangrenous part	Not clearly defined
Rate of tissue damage	Slow	Rapid
Bacterial superinfection	Absent	Present
Mummification	Present	Absent
Degree of inflammation	Minimal	Marked
Gross appearance	Dry, shrunken and black	Moist, swollen, edematous
Septicemia	Infrequent	More common
Examples	Atherosclerosis, Raynaud's disease, Berger disease	Bedsores, diabetic ulcers, intestinal volvulus

NURSING CONSIDERATIONS

- Be watchful of the developmental of bed sores so that timely management can be started.
- Observe any discoloration of any extremity carefully.
- Always be extra vigilant for diabetics and immunocompromised patients who are prone to developing gangrene and infection.
- In the case of gas gangrene, strict aseptic precautions are to be maintained while performing wound care.
- Nursing practitioners should be especially thorough with procedures of autoclaving linen and waste segregation and disposal in such cases.

APOPTOSIS

Definition

Apoptosis or cell suicide is a tightly controlled, genetically programmed form of cell death which can eliminate unwanted host cells through activation of coordinated series of events such as necrosis. It is energy dependent, involving a sequence of steps mediated and activated by enzymes called caspases. It characteristically does not induce accompanying inflammation.

Apoptotic form of cell death can be seen in two settings:

1. *Physiological*

- Involution of fetal structures in development.
- Involution of the thymus at puberty.
- Reduction in breast size on cessation of lactation.
- Cell death with completion of cell lifespan as a natural process.

2. *Pathological*

- Councilman bodies of liver disease.
- Chemotherapy induced damage to cells.
- After inflammation has subsided.
- Neurodegenerative disease - neurons.

EXTRA EDGE

Oncotic necrosis is a process of cell swelling and thereby distinct from cell death by apoptosis, which is a process of cellular shrinkage and fragmentation. If an acutely swollen cell fails to correct the electrolyte imbalance and loss of volume control, then potentially reversible cell injury can become the initial stage of oncotic necrosis.

Microscopic Features (Fig. 3.11)

- Cell size is small (shrunken appearance).
- Cytoplasm is condensed, eosinophilic.
- Highly condensed nuclear chromatin (pyknosis).
- No accompanying inflammation.
- Blebs or protrusion of the cytoplasm may be seen.
- Membrane bound cellular bodies (apoptotic bodies) with condensed nuclear chromatin appearing as solitary cells or as groups of few cells amidst viable cells.

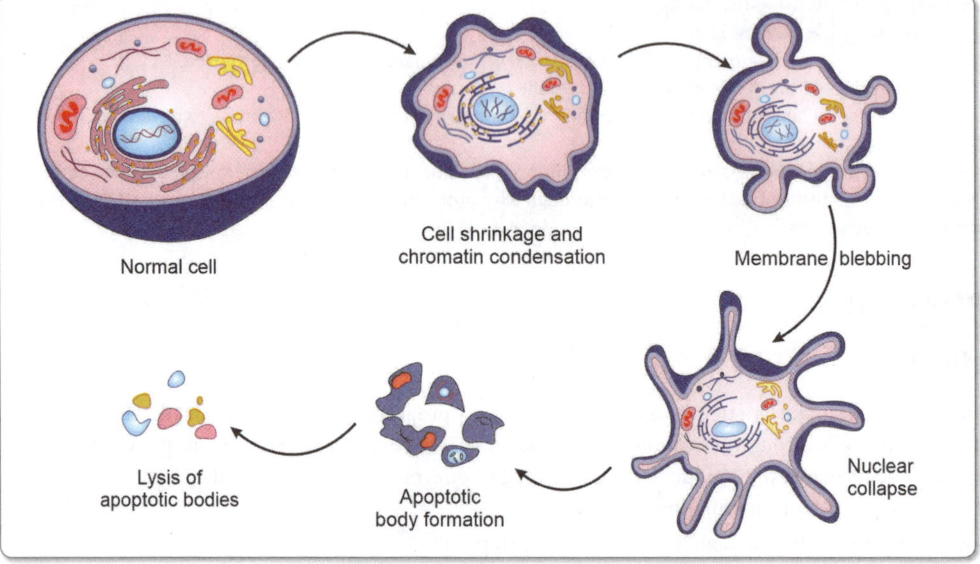

Figure 3.11: Cell apoptosis

Pathogenesis

Apoptosis is characteristically caused by a multistep sequence of events (cascade) which includes initiation, execution (similar to the ignition of a car and then its subsequent setting into motion) and ultimately phagocytosis.

- **Initiation** is achieved through two pathways—extrinsic and intrinsic (Fig. 3.12).
- **Extrinsic pathway:** This pathway is mediated through receptors on the surface of the cell (as these receptors are not within the cell, hence the terminology—extrinsic).
  - This pathway is also called the *death receptor pathway* and involves **caspase-8.**
  - The extrinsic pathway involves binding of the death receptor molecules with their ligands.

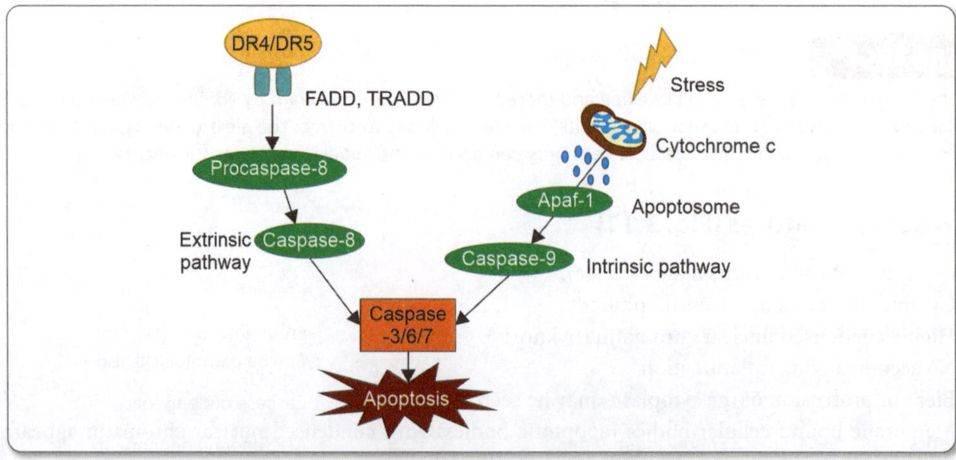

Figure 3.12: Intrinsic and extrinsic pathway of apoptosis

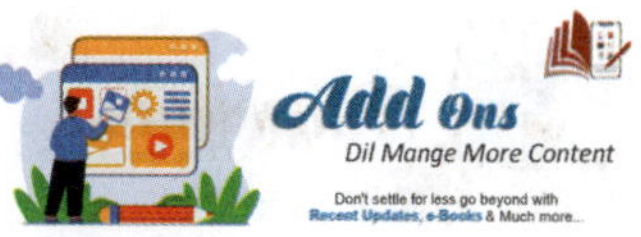

- **The specific cell receptors associated with apoptosis in the extrinsic pathway include:** Tumor necrosis factor receptor type 1(TNFR1) and CD 95 (also called Fas). Their respective binding ligands are TNF receptor ligand and Fas ligand (FasL). The death receptors span or cross-over the cell membrane. In the intracellular portion, there is space for binding another class of proteins called the adaptor proteins, such as TNF receptor-associated death domain (TRADD) and Fas-associated death domain (FADD). When the death receptor ligands bind with the corresponding death receptor molecule, a specific binding site on the adaptor protein becomes available and the complex of ligand, receptor and adaptor protein together called death inducing signalling complex (DISC) activates procaspase 8 which is converted to caspase-8 leading to cell death.
- **Intrinsic/mitochondrial pathway:** This pathway occurs within the cell itself, hence the name intrinsic. Any injurious stimuli or a reduction of growth factors triggers this pathway, characterized by an increase in mitochondrial permeability. With injury, there is loss of the molecules Bcl-2, Bcl-XL, Mcl-1 from the mitochondrial membrane which are anti-apoptotic. At the same time pro-apoptotic proteins bax, bim, bak are activated. Cytochrome c leaks out of the mitochondria due to the increased permeability. This binds to apoptosis activating factor 1, forming the complex called apoptosome, in turn activating **caspase-9 ultimately activating caspase-3 and 6 leading to the execution phase of apoptosis.**

Anti-apoptotic Proteins	Pro-apoptotic Proteins	Proteins-Mitochondrial Intermembrane space
Bcl-2, Bcl-XL, Mcl-1	Bax, Bak, Bad, Bid, Bim, Bcl-XS	Cytochrome c, apoptosis inducing factor

- **Execution phase:** The intrinsic and extrinsic pathways ultimately cause activation of **caspases-3 and 6.** This in turn leads to activation of protease enzymes and endonucleases These cleave the cell proteins and nucleus leading to cell disintegration.
- **Phagocytosis:** With cell death, all debris generated release molecules that attract macrophages which ultimately remove the debris through the process of phagocytosis.

Table 3.3 lists various kinds of differences between necrosis and apoptosis.

Table 3.3: Difference between necrosis and apoptosis

Features	Necrosis	Apoptosis
Cell size	Increased	Shrunken/reduced
Inflammation	Present	Absent
Nuclei	Pyknosis, karyolysis, karyorrhexis	Pyknosis, nuclear fragmentation
Type of cell death	Uncontrolled	Controlled/programmed
Cells involved	Individual cells/small clusters	Larger groups of cells are frequently involved
Cell membrane	Disrupted	Maintained
Cytoplasmic blebs	Infrequent	Present
Physiological/pathological	Pathological	Frequently physiological Can be pathological also
Mediator	Caspase independent	Caspase dependent
Energetics	Energy independent	ATP (energy) dependent

Refer to Figures 3.13A and B for diagrammatic comparison between nerosis and apoptosis.

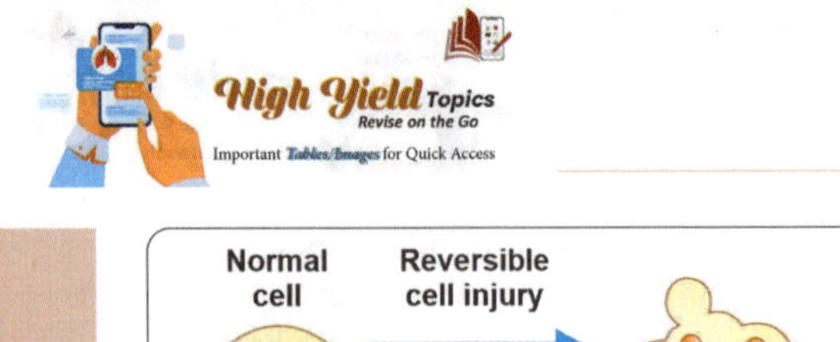

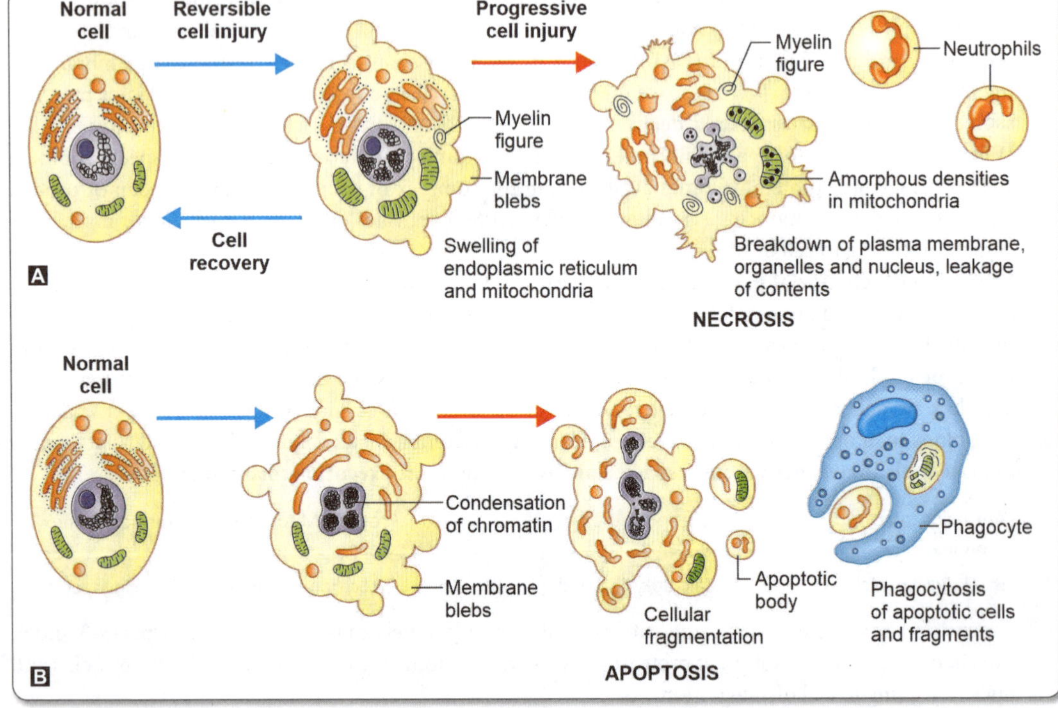

Figures 3.13A and B: Diagrammatic comparative between apoptosis and necrosis: **A.** Inflammation is caused by the release of cellular contents into the extracellular matrix through ruptured plasma membranes; **B.** Cellular fragments that have undergone apoptosis are released as plasma membrane-bound apoptotic entities that phagocytes can recognize but that do not result in inflammation

SUMMARY

- Basic life processes include cell death, survival, proliferation, and differentiation.
- Necrosis refers to cell enlargement (oncosis) and eventual membrane rupture, which is how cells die.
- Necrotic cells morphologically shows swelling of organelles such the endoplasmic reticulum and mitochondria, rupturing of the plasma membrane, and cell lysis.
- Apoptosis is a process that causes the cell and its organelles to condense and shrink, eventually resulting in cell disintegration.
- In coagulative necrosis, cell death is present but cellular outline/architecture is maintained giving rise to a "tombstone" appearance.
- Liquefactive necrosis is due to the release of lysosomal/bacterial hydrolytic enzymes and is characterized by a complete loss of structural details.
- Caseous necrosis is associated with tubercular infection.
- Fibrinoid necrosis is seen in the case of vascular damage and is associated with exudation of plasma proteins including eosinophilic fibrin.
- Gangrene is characterized by ischemia and necrotic tissue, frequently encircling a finger or other extremity.
- Dry gangrene is dehydrated, ischemic tissue induced by increasing ischemia distal to arterial blockage.
- Apoptosis or cell suicide is a genetically programmed form of cell death which eliminate unwanted host cells through activation of coordinated series of events such as necrosis.
- Apoptosis is characteristically caused by a multistep sequence of events which include initiation, execution and ultimately phagocytosis.

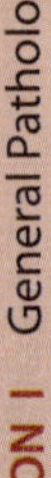

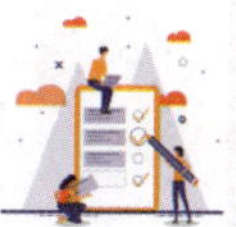

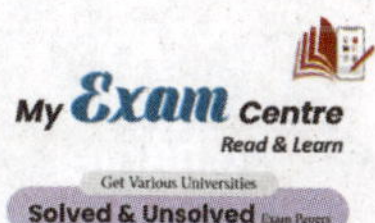

ASSESS YOURSELF

Long Answer Questions

1. Explain the types of necrosis with example.
2. Explain the the pathogenesis of apoptosis.

Short Answer Questions

1. Define apoptosis and nacrosis.
2. What is wet gangrene?
3. Write short notes on:
   i. Caseous necrosis
   ii. Morphological features of apoptotic cells
   iii. Cell death

Multiple Choice Questions

1. **This is an extracellular messenger of apoptosis:**
   a. Tumor necrosis factor
   b. Serine
   c. Translation inhibitor
   d. Ribozyme
2. **This is concerned with the intrinsic pathway of apoptosis:**
   a. Cytochrome d
   b. Cytochrome c
   c. Cytochrome b
   d. Cytochrome a
3. **This is an antiapoptotic protein:**
   a. Bim
   b. Bcl-Xs
   c. Bfl 1
   d. NOXA
4. **This is an active cell death process:**
   a. Necrosis
   b. Lysis
   c. Apoptosis
   d. Senescence
5. **This cell organelle participates actively in animal apoptosis:**
   a. Nucleus
   b. Vacuoles
   c. Mitochondria
   d. Chloroplast

Answer Key

1. a **2.** b **3.** c **4.** c **5.** c

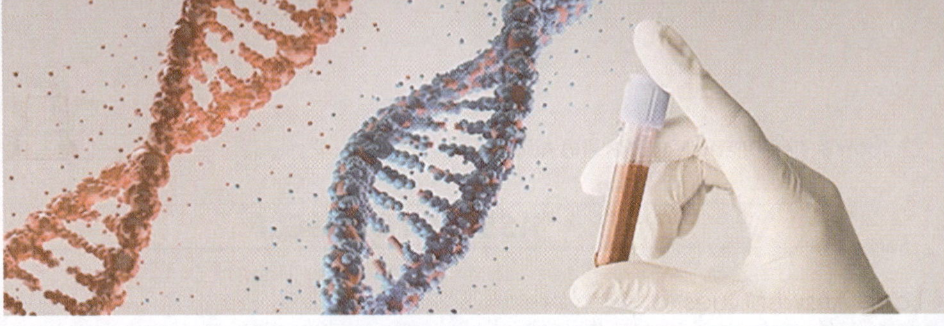

Chapter 4

Inflammation, Regeneration and Wound Healing

LEARNING OBJECTIVES

After the completion of the chapter, the readers will be able to:

- Understand the process of inflammation.
- Learn about the types of inflammation.
- Understand the sequence of events in acute inflammation.
- Know the salient features of the chemical mediators of inflammation.
- Learn the outcomes of acute inflammation.
- Learn about the features of chronic inflammation.
- Know the diagnostic features of granulomatous inflammation.
- Distinguish between acute and chronic inflammation.
- Understand the terms—healing, repair and regeneration.
- Know the types of wound healing.
- Differentiate between the two major types of wound healing.
- Know the steps involved in the types of wound healing.
- Know the age of a wound.
- Understand the factors influencing wound healing.
- Learn about the complications of wound healing.

CHAPTER OUTLINE

KEY TERMS

Chemotaxis: It is the movement of leukocytes to a specific area of the body along a chemical gradient mediated by specific molecules known as chemokines.

Contracture: A contracture is a shortening of the skin, tendons, muscles, and other soft tissues around the joints that results in extreme stiffness and limits normal movement.

Dehiscence: Dehiscence is a partial or total separation of previously approximated wound edges, due to a failure of proper wound healing.

Epithelialization: It is the process of returning the site of injury to its original state.

Contd...

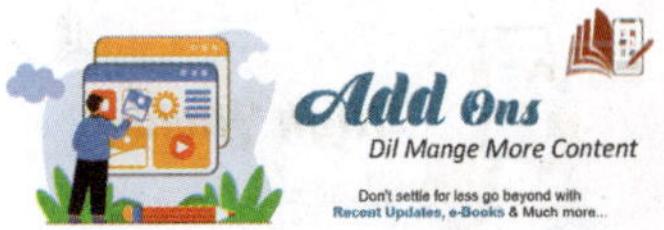

Granulation tissue: Granulation tissue is a type of new connective tissue which is granular, deeply red, and extremely fragile.

Inflammation: The intricate biological reaction of body tissues to damaging stimuli, such as infections, damaged cells, or irritants, includes inflammation.

Keloid: Keloids appear as hard, rubbery lumps in areas where there has previously been skin damage.

Marjolin ulcer: Marjolin ulcer is a type of skin cancer that develops on previously damaged skin, persistent scars, and open wounds.

Repair: It is the process of generating a scar or less functional tissue with a different form and/or composition of the original tissue.

INFLAMMATION

The local reaction of living mammalian tissues to damage caused by any agent is known as inflammation. It is the body's defensive response to eliminate injurious agent or prevent it from spreading, after which the necrosed tissues and cells are removed.

The following potential agents could be responsible for producing inflammation:

- Infectious agents, such as fungus, viruses, bacteria, and their toxins;
- Immunological agents, such as antibody responses to antigen and cell-mediated immunity.
- Physical agents, such as radiation, heat, cold, and mechanical damage.
- Chemical agents, such as poisons, both inorganic and organic.
- Inert substances, like foreign objects.

MUST KNOW

Inflammation versus Infection

In contrast to infection, which is the outcome of pathogenic bacteria entering the body and causing toxins to have an adverse effect, inflammation is the body's defensive reaction to a variety of etiologic agents, whether infectious or not.

SIGNS OF INFLAMMATION

Four cardinal signs of inflammation as named by a Roman writer Celsus includes:

1. Rubor (redness)
2. Tumor (swelling)
3. Calor (heat)
4. Dolor (pain)

Virchow subsequently added the fifth sign functio laesa (loss of function) to these.

TYPES OF INFLAMMATION

Inflammation can be classified as acute and chronic, depending upon the duration of response and defense mechanism of host.

ACUTE INFLAMMATION

The immediate and rapid response of the body to an injurious agent/injury, accompanied by the formation of a protein-rich cellular exudate. Acute inflammation is usually characterized by early resolution and repair. Acute inflammation is characterized by three primary features:

1. Buildup of fluid and plasma at the site of injury.
2. Platelet activity within the vessel.
3. Polymorphonuclear neutrophils acting as inflammatory cells.

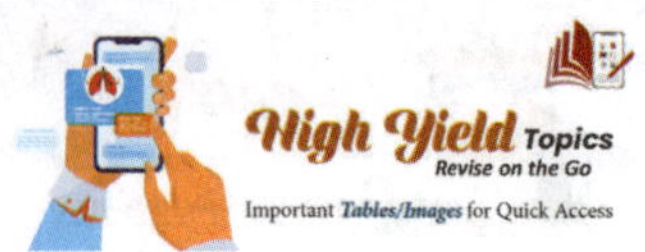

It is an active process comprising a number of steps or *events* which are classified as vascular and cellular.

This highlights the importance of the two key players in acute inflammation (Fig. 4.1):

1. The blood vessel **(vascular)**
2. Various cells both within the vessel and outside in the extracellular matrix **(cellular)**

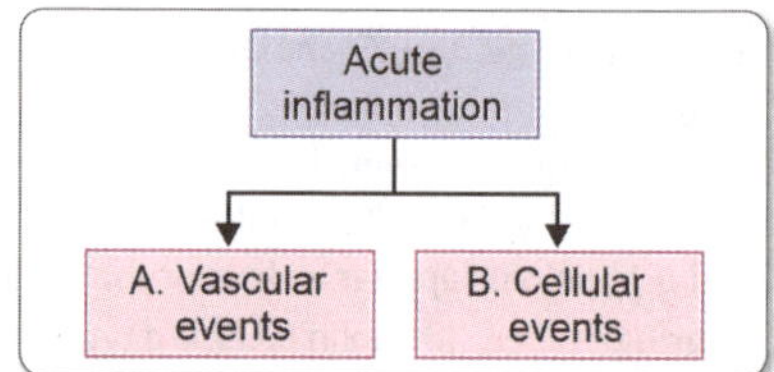

Figure 4.1: Events of acute inflammation

Vascular Events (Fig. 4.2)

The aim of this phase of acute inflammation is to initiate the movement of cells and plasma proteins within the vessels to the injury site. This is accomplished by increasing blood flow and vessel wall permeability.

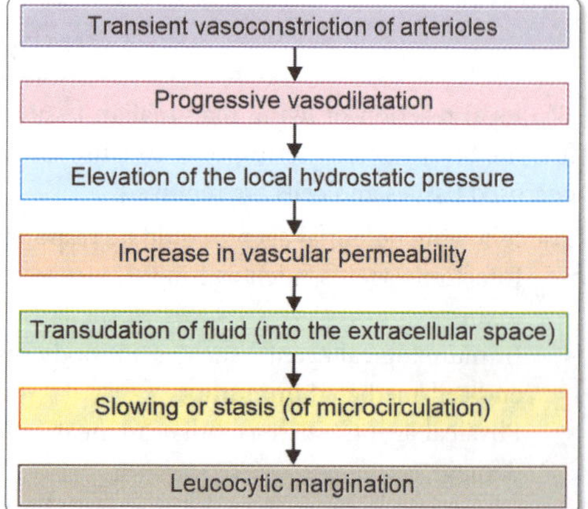

Figure 4.2: Vascular events

Hemodynamic Changes

- **Injury and immediate transient vasoconstriction of arterioles:** Whatever the nature of the injury, the initial vascular response results in temporary arteriole vasoconstriction. When there is a little injury, blood flow can be re-established within three to five seconds, but with more severe injury, vasoconstriction may last for about 5 minutes.
- **Progressive vasodilation:** Subsequently, there is a progressive dilation of the blood vessels, mostly affecting the arterioles, but also affecting the venules and capillaries to a lesser degree. Within 30 minutes of the damage, this change becomes obvious. Warmth and redness at the site of acute inflammation are caused by vasodilatation, which increases the volume of blood in the microvascular bed of the affected area.
- **Increased microvasculature permeability:** Involves structural changes in the vessels primarily at the level of the endothelium enabling plasma proteins and leukocytes to leave the circulation.
- **Transudation of fluid:** Progressive vasodilatation may therefore cause fluid to transude into the extracellular space by raising the local hydrostatic pressure. This is responsible for the swelling at local site of acute inflammation.
- **Slowing or stasis:** Slowing down or stasis of the microcirculation, raises the concentration of red blood cells and, consequently, the viscosity of the blood.
- **Leucocytic margination**, or the peripheral orientation of leucocytes (mostly neutrophils) along the vascular endothelium, follows stasis or slowdown. Leucocytes adhere to the vascular endothelium for a brief period of time before migrating and moving through the spaces created by the endothelial cells into the extravascular space.

EXTRA EDGE

The Lewis experiment provides the clearest illustration of the characteristics of hemodynamic alterations in inflammation. The triple response, also referred to as the red line response, includes the following:

- The ***red line***, which develops a few seconds after stroking, is caused by localized venule and capillary vasodilatation.
- ***Flare*** is the bright reddish appearance that surrounds the red line and is caused by the nearby arterioles' vasodilatation.
- ***Wheal*** is the enlargement, or edema, of the skin around it caused by fluid seeping into the extravascular space.

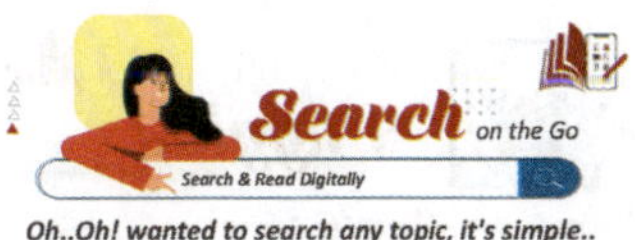

Altered Microvasculature Permeability

The formation of edema fluid in the interstitial compartment within and around the inflammatory tissue is caused by blood plasma leaking through the peripheral vascular bed's endothelium wall.

The impermeable endothelium layer of the microvasculature becomes leaky during acute inflammation. The most frequent cause of increased leakiness that just affects venules and has no effect on capillaries or arterioles is contraction of endothelial cells. Vascular leakiness results from the endothelial cells' contraction-induced transient gaps between them. Histamine, bradykinin, and other chemical mediators are released to mediate it.

The enhanced permeability may develop 2–12 hours after the damage and continue for hours or days (***delayed prolonged leakage***), or it may start immediately after the injury and last for several hours or days (***rapid sustained leakage***).

Severe bacterial infections are examples of immediate sustained leaking, while moderate thermal and radiation injuries may result in delayed prolonged leakage.

MUST KNOW

Vascular events also include changes to the lymphatics during the course of inflammation. This includes inflammation of the lymphatic vessel (lymphangitis) as well as reactive lymph node enlargement.

Table 4.1 exhibits the mechanism of increased vascular permeability:

Table 4.1: Mechanism of increased vascular permeability

Name of mechanism	How it acts
Endothelial cell retraction	Mediated by actin cytoskeleton
Trans-endothelial cell migration (Transcytosis):	By formation of vesiculo-vacuolar organelle, possibly mediated by caveolin
Direct endothelial injury—**When injury is severe**	Direct damage to endothelial cells
Leukocyte mediated endothelial injury	Activated leukocytes cause endothelial injury and detachment
Loosening of endothelial cell—cell adherens junction	Vascular endothelial-cadherin internalization

Cellular Events

The two mechanisms that consists of the cellular phase of inflammation are—leucocyte exudation and phagocytosis.

Recruitment of Leukocytes (Calling the Army)

The primary characteristic of the inflammatory reaction is the leucocytes' escape from the microvasculature lumen into the interstitial tissue. Polymorphonuclear neutrophils (PMNs) are the body's initial line of defence in acute inflammation, with monocytes and macrophages appearing later on.

A multistep process involving attachment of circulating leukocytes to endothelial cells and their migration through the endothelium (*extravasation)* (Fig. 4.3).

- **In the lumen:**
  - Margination
  - Rolling
  - Adhesion to endothelium—Transient and firm
- **Trans-luminal:** Transmigration across the endothelium (also called *diapedesis*)

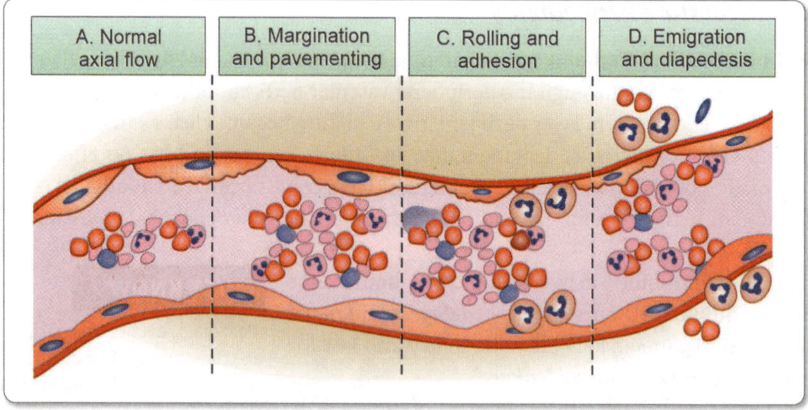

Figure 4.3: Sequence of changes in the exudation of leukocytes

- **Extraluminal:**
  - Migration in interstitial tissues
  - Chemotaxis

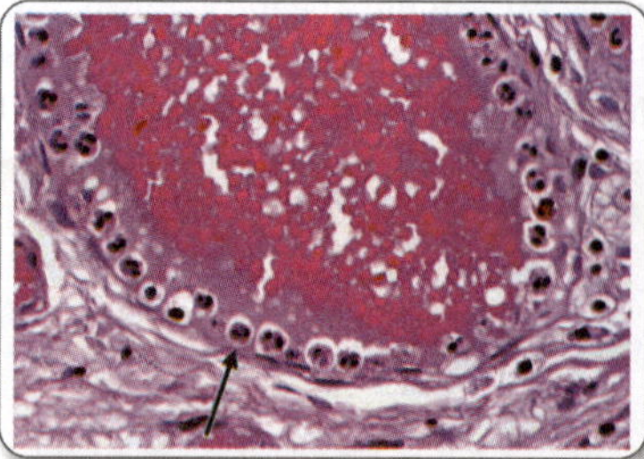

Figure 4.4: Margination of WBCs (Arrow showing)

Margination

Central axial flow of WBCs surrounded peripherally by red blood cells (Fig. 4.4). After slowing of blood flow (stasis), the normal flow distribution is changed. RBC viscosity increases and they move centrally as they cluster with each other. WBCs start flowing near the endothelium (pavementation).

Rolling

The neutrophils that are marginated at the periphery slowly move along the endothelial surface, a process referred to as "rolling". The interaction between the endothelial cells is initially transient which means the neutrophils intermittently attach to the activated endothelial surface and then detach. The activated endothelial cells recognize the neutrophils by sensing a carbohydrate molecule on the rolling neutrophil, this molecule is sialyl-lewis-X. Once this recognition is achieved, selectins are produced that help the neutrophils stick or adhere to the endothelium.

Adhesion

The interactions between the neutrophils and the endothelial cells are transient in the beginning and gradually become stable so that the neutrophils firmly park or "pavement" on the endothelial surface. This phase is called adhesion and is mediated by the selectins as well as other molecules—the integrins and immunoglobulin derived adhesion molecules (Table 4.2).

EXTRA EDGE

Leukocyte adhesion defects (LAD) is of two types:

1. LAD type 1 is due to a deficiency of β_2-integrin
2. LAD type 2 is due to mutations in fucosyl transferase required for synthesis of sialylated oligosaccharide.

These normally bind selectins.

Clinical findings:

- Delayed separation of umbilical cord.
- Increased circulating neutrophils (leukocytosis due to loss of the marginating pool).
- Recurrent bacterial infection that lacks pus formation.
- Poor wound healing.

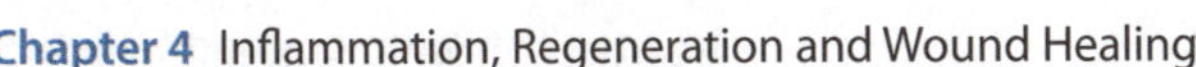
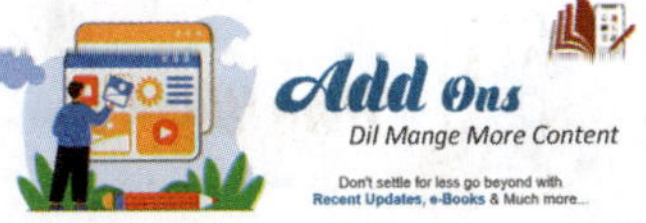

Table 4.2: Summary of molecules involved in rolling and adhesion

Name of selectin	Expressed by	Action
L-selectin	Leukocytes	Directs lymphocytes toward the endothelial cells
E-selectin	Endothelial cells	Rolling, adhesion
P-selectin	Preformed in platelets and endothelial cells	Rolling
Integrins	Expressed on surface of endothelial cells, pericytes	Adhesion (facilitates strong adhesions between leukocytes and endothelial surface)
Intercellular adhesion molecule (ICAM-1)	Endothelial cells, some lymphocytes	Strengthens adhesion Binds β_2 integrin
Vascular cell adhesion molecule (VCAM-1)	Endothelial cells	Strengthens adhesion Binds β_1 integrin

Transluminal Migration of Neutrophils

Once the neutrophils adhere to the endothelial surface they migrate across the endothelium through gaps between the endothelial cells. The neutrophils achieve this by amoeboid movement with the help of cytoplasmic processes called pseudopods. This process is also called *diapedesis*. This is mediated by CD 31 or platelet endothelial cell adhesion molecule **(PECAM-1)**.

Emigration

Once the neutrophils move through endothelial gaps outside the vessel into the interstitial space, they produce matrix metalloproteinases and collagenases which dissolve the extracellular matrix, allowing the neutrophils to freely move through the extravascular areas required.

Chemotaxis

Leukocytes are required for recruitment to the area of cell injury. This is to both destroy the offending agent and control further cellular damage. The process by which leukocytes move to a specific area of the body along a chemical gradient mediated by specific molecules is called *chemotaxis*. The molecules that facilitate this movement are called chemoattractants or chemokines.

The most frequently involved chemaoattractants are:

- Exogenous bacterial products
- Complement products—C5a, C3a
- Leukotrienes-LTB_4
- Interleukin-8

Leucocyte Activation

In order to perform specialized functions, neutrophils require additional activation.

Phagocytosis

The process by which cells absorb solid particulate matter is known as phagocytosis (cell-eating). The term "phagocyte" refers to the cells that carry out this task. Once the neutrophils reach the site of injury, their main role is to destroy a microbial pathogen, if present and remove all debris in the area as well as limit the cellular damage.

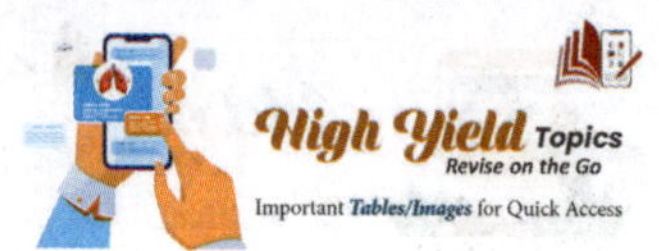

Phagocytic cells are primarily divided into two types:

1. Early-stage acute inflammatory reaction polymorphonuclear neutrophils (PMNs), also known as microphages.
2. Fixed tissue mononuclear phagocytes and circulating monocytes, also referred to as macrophages.

When neutrophils and macrophages enter tissue spaces, they release a variety of proteolytic enzymes, including acid hydrolases, lysozyme, protease, collagenase, elastase, lipase, and proteinase. These enzymes break down the extracellular matrix and collagen. The following three phases are involved in the phagocytosis process:

1. Recognition and Engulfment

The expression of mannose receptor and scavenger receptor, two surface receptors on macrophages that detect bacteria, triggers phagocytosis. The bacteria or organism is made ready (or tastier!) for scavenging by a process called *opsonization* in which the bacteria is coated by proteins called opsonins, e.g., **IgG and C3b opsonin** and molecules called **lectins** which have the property of binding to bacterial polysaccharides, enabling them to bind to the microbial cell wall.

2. Engulfment

The leukocyte forms pseudopods around the targeted particle that is to be ingested. This, in turn, forms a vesicle called the phagosome. The membrane of the phagosome fuses with the membrane of the lysosome to form the phagolysosome.

The opsonized particle that has attached itself to the phagocyte's surface is prepared for ingestion. This is achieved by the actin filaments under the cell membrane activating and forming cytoplasmic pseudopods around the particle, encasing it in a phagocytic vacuole.

3. Killing and Degradation

Hydrolytic enzymes break down the microbes after they are killed by antibacterial agents. Nevertheless, certain bacteria, such as tubercle bacilli, are not killed or broken down by this method. Within the neutrophils and macrophages, killing of the ingested molecule is facilitated by reactive oxygen species. The mechanism of killing may be oxygen dependent or oxygen independent. The *oxygen dependent* H_2O_2*–MPO-Halide system* is the most potent bactericidal mechanism and works by halogenation and peroxidation.

Oxygen independent mechanisms of killing bacteria include through the action of substances stored in neutrophil granules including enzymes and proteins such as defensins, lactoferrin, lysozymes.

Chemical Mediators of Inflammation

Chemical mediators of inflammation are substances produced during inflammation inducing and regulating specific events in the inflammatory response (Fig. 4.5).

Chemical mediators may be **cell derived** or **plasma derived.**

Their action is usually **short-lived**, triggered by agents causing the inflammation such as microbial products, drugs/environmental stimuli. Chemical mediators serve to recruit inflammatory cells and direct their movement to the site of injury.

An exaggerated production of chemical mediators could be harmful for the body and hence the mediators undergo spontaneous decay or are inactivated *via* enzymatic action.

A brief overview of the various mediators is as follows:

Cell-derived

- These type of mediators can be synthesized as needed (prostaglandin) or preformed, sequestered and released (e.g., histamine and serotonin).

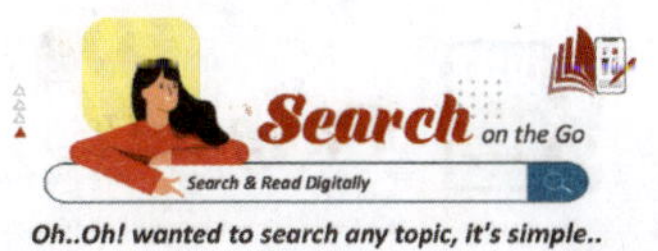

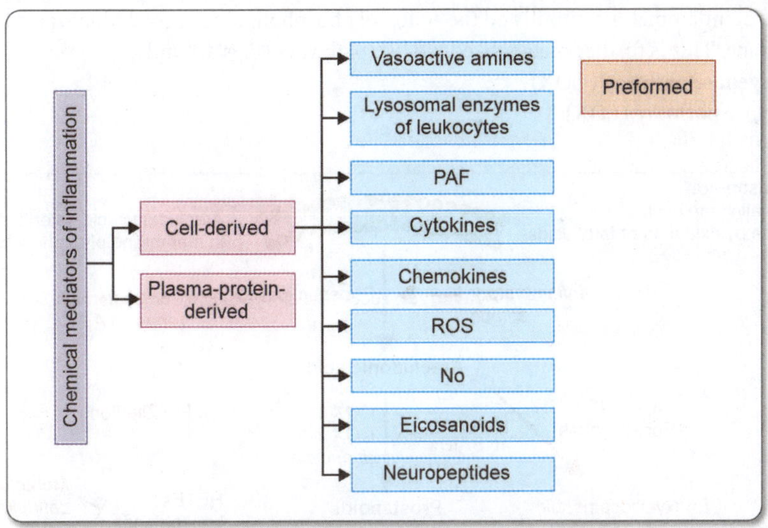

Figure 4.5: Chemical mediators of inflammation

- The various cells that act as sources for these molecules include epithelial/mesenchymal cells along with key hematopoietic cells such as platelets, cells of the monocyte-macrophage system and mast cells. The various cell-derived mediators are enlisted in Figure 4.5. Salient features of the important chemical mediators of inflammation are as follows:

Histamine

It is produced as a preformed mediator and is stored in the granules of mast cells, eosinophils, basophils and platelets.

Histamine is released by:

- IgE antibody binding to Fc receptors on mast cells.
- Activated complement products—C3a, C5a.
- By the action of white blood cells (leukocytes).
- Physical injury/heat/exercise.

Actions:

- Vasodilatation-increasing the blood flow
- Endothelial cell activation and creation of gap between them.
- Increased vascular permeability.

Serotonin

Similar to histamine it is preformed and has similar actions..However, the source of serotonin is primarily platelets and platelet aggregation promotes their release. Histamine and serotonin are together called the **vasoactive amines**.

Arachidonic Acid-Derived Mediators (Eicosanoids)

These are mediators derived from 20 carbon atom fatty acid-arachidonic acid, e.g., prostaglandins, leukotrienes and lipoxins. Normally, arachidonic acid is present in the cell membrane in an esterified form, i.e., it is not free.

In the presence of inflammatory stimuli and the action of phospholipase A_2, arachidonic acid is liberated from the cell membrane. This is further metabolized *via* two pathways (Figs 4.6 and 4.7):

1. **Cyclo-oxygenase pathway (COX)**
2. **Lipoxygenase pathway (LOX)**

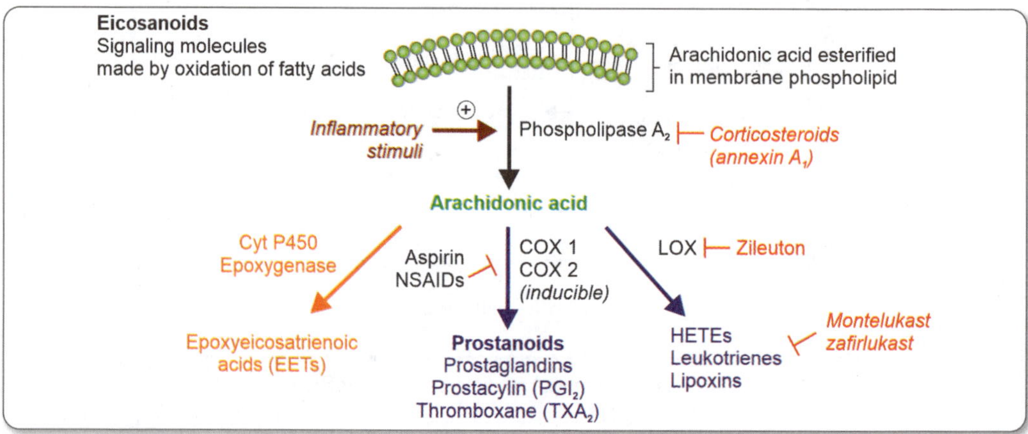

Figure 4.6: Cyclo-oxygenase pathway

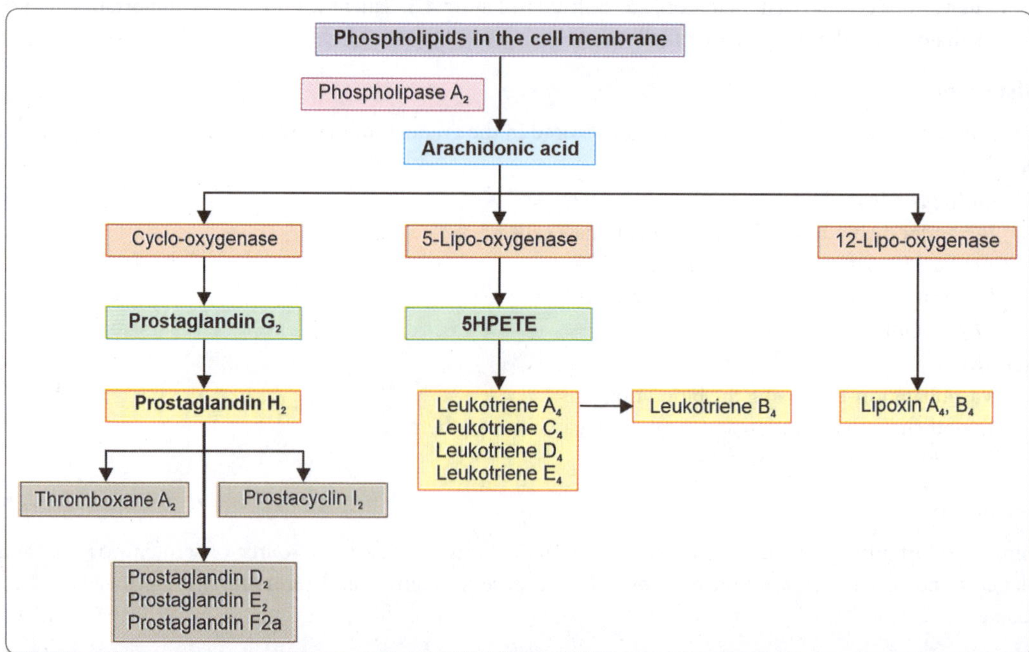

Figure 4.7: Lipoxygenase pathway

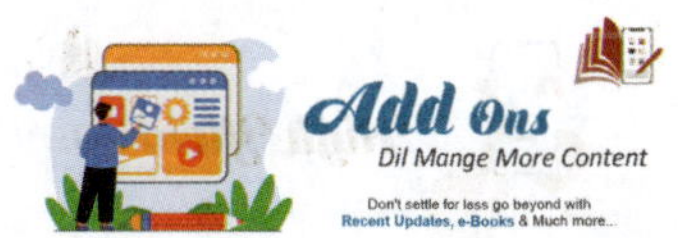

By the action of the cyclooxygenase pathway, prostaglandins are formed. By the action of lipoxygenase pathway, leukotrienes and lipoxins are liberated. The entire pathway of synthesis of these mediators is illustrated in Figures 4.6 and 4.7.

Cytokines and Chemokines

The term "chemokines" refers to a group of substances that are released by activated macrophages and platelets, including interleukin-8 and platelet factor-4. These substances are powerful chemoattractants for inflammatory cells. Polypeptide compounds known as cytokines are produced by both activated monocytes and activated lymphocytes. Activated macrophages produce TNF-α and IL-1, whereas activated T-cells create TNF-β and IFN-γ.

Cytokines are soluble protein molecules liberated by:

- Activated lymphocytes.
- Activated monocytes/macrophages.
- Endothelial cells.
- Epithelial/mesenchymal ie connective tissue cells.

The important cytokines involved as chemical mediators of inflammation include IL-1, IL-2, TNF-α and IFN-γ.

Interleukins and TNF–α

They represent acute phase reactants and have the following effects which can be memorized by correlating with the phases of inflammation:

- Recruit neutrophils.
- Endothelial cell activation, increasing adhesion to the endothelial cells.
- Releasing growth factors.
- Releasing other cytokines.
- Laying down of fibroblasts and collagen.

Interferon-γ

It causes activation of macrophages and neutrophils and is important in the development of granulomatous inflammation.

Chemokines: These mediators help in recruiting various cells of inflammation. They direct or help these cells to move to the site of injury. Important chemokines include:

- **MCP-1:** Monocyte chemoattractant protein.
- **IL-8:** Chemoattractant for neutrophils.
- **C5a:** Neutrophils.

Nitrous oxide: This chemical mediator is released by the endothelial cells. It can also be produced by macrophages as well as neurons. They act as a potent mediator of inflammation.

Actions:

- Vasodilation.
- It inhibits the recruitment of inflammatory cells.
- It inhibits platelet aggregation.
- It inhibits mast cell induced inflammation.
- It kills bacteria.

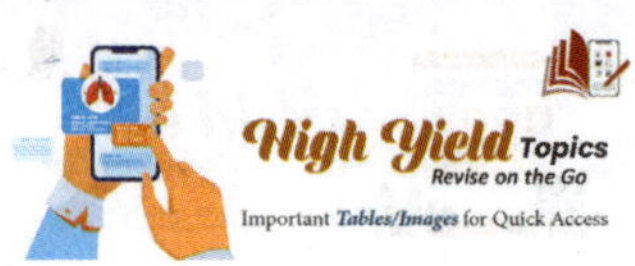

Plasma-derived

These mediators exist in an inactive latent state and are also converted to active forms. They include proteins of the complement system, clotting system and kinin system. Each of these systems has its own plasma-based accelerators and inhibitors, along with corresponding positive and negative feedback processes.

Kinin System

Bradykinin is produced when this system is activated by factor Xlla. It is named after the slow contraction of smooth muscle that it causes. Initially, prekallikrein activator, a piece of factor Xlla, converts plasma prekallikrein into kallikrein. Bradykinin is then created by the action of kallikrein on high molecular weight kininogen. Early on in the inflammatory process, bradykinin acts and has the following effects:

- Smooth muscle contraction;
- Vasodilation;
- Increased vascular permeability; and
- Pain

Clotting System

Factor Xlla initiates the clotting system's cascade, which produces fibrinogen. Thrombin then acts on fibrinogen to produce fibrin and fibrinopeptides.

The actions of fibrinopeptides in inflammation are:

- Increased vascular permeability.
- Chemotaxis for leucocyte.
- Anticoagulant activity.

The Fibrinolytic System

Plasminogen activator, which is derived from endothelial cells, leucocytes, and kallikrein of the kinin system, activates fibrinolytic system. In order to create plasmin, plasminogen which is a part of plasma proteins is activated by plasminogen activator. Fibrinopeptides or fibrin split products are created when fibrin is further broken down by plasmin.

Action of plasmin in inflammation are as follows:

- Prekallikrein activator, which is formed by activating factor XII and stimulating the kinin system to produce bradykinin.
- Fibrin degradation, which results in fibrin split products that are chemotactic to leucocytes and increase vascular permeability.
- Complement C3 splitting off to form C3a, a permeability factor.

The Complement System

There are two ways that the complement system can be activated:

1. Via the classical channel, which involves antigen-antibody complexes.
2. Via an alternative pathway, which involves non-immunologic substances such IgA, cobra venom, and bacterial toxins.

Actions of activated complement system in inflammation are as follows:

- C3a, C5a, C4a, it activates mast cells basophils to release histamine and causes increased vascular permeability causing edema is tissues.
- C3b is an opsonin.
- C5a acts as a chemotactic for leucocytes.

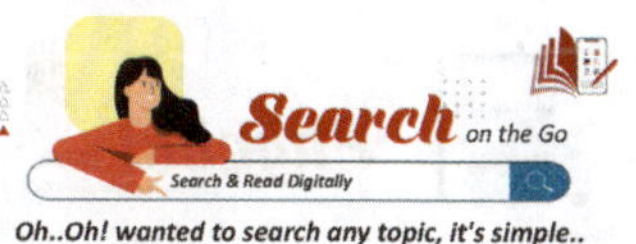

Morphological Patterns of Acute Inflammation

Acute inflammation is essentially a response which is morphologically characterized by a predominance of neutrophils. However, variations of morphological features are noted when such tissue is examined microscopically. These include:

- **Suppurative inflammation:** This is the most common presentation and is associated with the formation of pus or purulent exudate. Pus is composed of neutrophils, pyogenic organisms (bacteria/fungi) and damaged tissue debris. Suppurative inflammation may be a localized collection of purulent material in tissue (abscess)/widespread when associated with sepsis. It is also referred to as empyema when the inflammation is confined to hollow viscera, e.g., gallbladder.
- **Necrotizing inflammation:** When the inflammatory process is associated with necrosis leading to widespread tissue destruction. This is also called *gangrenous inflammation* when tissue damage is also associated with a reduction in vascular supply which, in turn, leads to necrosis, e.g., gangrenous inflammation of the intestine/appendix.
- **Serous inflammation:** Associated with the formation of thin watery (serous) fluid which is protein-rich but cell poor, e.g., synovial inflammation in early arthritis. When such fluid accumulates in the body cavities, e.g., pericardial/pleural, it is called an effusion.
- **Fibrinous:** Acute inflammation associated with the presence of a thick fibrin-rich exudate formed due to leakage of fibrinogen from blood vessels that are damaged due to inflammation. The leaked out fibrinogen precipitates as dense fibrin which coats the inflammed surface, e.g., fibrinous pericarditis in rheumatic heart disease, immune mediated vasculitis, like polyarteritis nodosa.
- **Serofibrinous:** A pattern in which both serous fluid and fibrinous exudate are observed, e.g., in some cases of viral pericarditis.
- **Catarrhal:** When the acute inflammatory response is accompanied by damage to the mucosal membranes along with abundant mucus secretion. For example, upper respiratory tract infection.
- **Pseudomembranous:** When inflammation is accompanied by an adherent false membrane formed by dead neutrophils, fibrin and damaged tissue, e.g., pseudomembranous colitis associated with clostridum difficile infection, pseudomembrane obstructing the airways in case of diphtheria.
- **Ulcers:** Localized inflammatory defects on the surface of organs is known as ulcers. The stomach, duodenum, intestinal ulcers in typhoid fever, intestinal tuberculosis, bacillary and amoebic dysentery, leg ulcers from varicose veins, etc. are common locations for ulcerations. In the acute stage, polymorphs infiltrate the ulcer and cause vasodilation, whereas lymphocytes, plasma cells, and macrophages infiltrate chronic ulcers and cause scarring and fibroblastic growth.
- **Cellulitis:** It is a diffuse soft tissue inflammation caused by the proliferative effects of compounds, like hyaluronidase which are released by some bacteria.
- **Bacterial infection of Blood:** It includes: Bacteremia, septicemia, pyemia.

Systemic Response to Inflammation

The inflammatory response can lead to a number of changes at the actual site of injury as enumerated in the vascular and cellular events of inflammation. In addition, a number of systemic effects can be seen which include:

- Fever.
- Tachycardia.
- Leukocytosis.
- Release of acute phase reactants such as procalcitonin, C-reactive protein, interleukin-6 (IL-6), fibrinogen, ferritin.

- Reduced appetite and loss of weight (*anorexia*).
- Increased sleep.

EXTRA EDGE

Systemic Inflammatory response syndrome (SIRS) is an exaggerated response to injurious stimuli defined by **any two of:**
1. Body temperature >38°C
2. Heart rate >90 beats/min
3. Respiratory rate >20 breaths/min
4. Total leukocyte count >12000 or <4000/μL or >10% immature forms

SIRS with a suspected source of infection: **Sepsis**

Altered organ function in acutely ill septic patients, requiring intervention to maintain vital functions: **Multiple Organ Dysfunction Syndrome (MODS)**

Biomarkers: Serum procalcitonin, IL-6 when elevated help predicting an infectious origin of sepsis.

Acute Inflammation–Fates/Outcomes

The major sequelae of acute inflammation include:

- **Resolution:** Restoration of the inflammed tissue to its original state—both anatomical and functional. With resolution, the exudate associated with inflammation has been absorbed and evidence of tissue destruction is not present.
- **Healing by fibrosis and the formation of a scar:** When the inflammatory exudate is organized, the damaged tissue is subsequently replaced by fibroblasts and collagen leading to the development of a scar.
- **Chronic inflammation:** Persistence of the injurious stimuli leads to failure of the resolution/healing by organization. Subsequently chronic inflammation ensues.
- **Abscess formation:** Localized collection of the inflammatory exudate leading to the formation of an abscess, which is a localized collection of pus in the affected tissue.
- **Empyema:** Collection of acute inflammatory exudate (pus) in the body cavities, especially the pleural space.
- **Subcutaneous spread:** When inflammatory exudate spreads throughout the subcutaneous portion of the skin, this pattern is referred to as *cellulitis*.
- **Systemic spread:** Spread through the blood stream of causative micro-organisms can lead to *sepsis and septic shock*.

CHRONIC INFLAMMATION

In this type of inflammation the inflammatory process persists for an increased duration (weeks to months) due to a persisting injurious agent or failure of the resolution of acute inflammation. In chronic inflammation, attempts to repair the tissue, i.e., healing and destructive events leading to tissue damage, occur together.

Cells of Chronic Inflammation

Key cells involved in chronic inflammation are:

Lymphocytes

Lymphocytes are an important part of the hematopoietic system and are small round cells with scant cytoplasm. These are produced in the bone marrow and are of two major subsets:

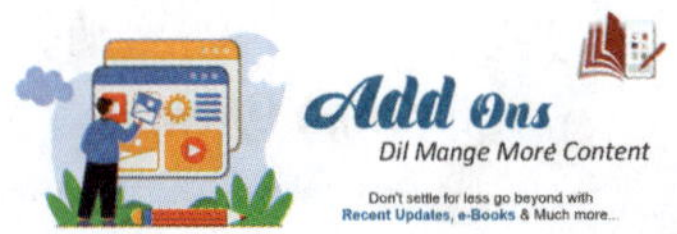

1. **B lymphocytes:** Differentiate to produce antibodies and are involved in antibody mediated responses in inflammation.
2. **T lymphocytes** are involved in cell mediated immune response and have cytotoxic effects, i.e., help in killing the offending agent. Important T cell subsets involved in inflammation are CD4 positive and CD8 positive. Subsets of CD4 positive T cells include:

Subset of CD 4 T cell	Key molecule produced	Cell targeted by these key molecules	Destructive action on
Helper T cell-1 (TH1)	Interferon-γ, Interleukin-2	Macrophages	Intracellular bacteria/fungi
TH 17	IL-17	Neutrophils	Fungi/extracellular bacteria
Helper T cell-2 (TH2)	Interleukin-4 (IL-4)	Eosinophils	Parasites

Macrophages

Macrophages play a key role in:

- Destroying the causative agent.
- Recruitment of inflammatory cells.
- Regulating the host response when the injurious stimulus persists.
- Eventual phagocytosis or "clean-up" phase.

They are a part of the monocyte-macrophage (reticuloendothelial) system. Macrophages circulate in the bloodstream as monocytes and have a limited lifespan of 2–3 days. They interact with lymphocytes during the process of chronic inflammation and on activation or modification, liberate various cytokines, important ones being IL-1, IL-2, TNF-α, which in turn, liberate other types of cytokines to regulate inflammation. Normal macrophages can be seen at specific sites in the body as follows:

Macrophage	Specific site
Liver	Kupffer cells
Brain	Microglial cells
Alveoli	Alveolar macrophages
Bone	Osteoclasts
Connective tissue/lymph node sinuses	Histiocytes

Various modified macrophages include:

- **Epithelioid cells:** Seen in granulomas of tuberculosis, sarcoidosis, Crohn's disease.
- **Lipophages:** Seen in cases of traumatic fat necrosis.
- **Melanophages:** Seen in cases of chronic dermatitis.
- **Hemosiderin laden macrophages (Siderophages):** Seen in hemosiderosis, chronic venous congestion of the lung, where they are also called **"heart failure cells"**.

Mast Cells

Mast cells characteristically liberate preformed mediators, e.g., histamine by release of their granules, a process called "degranulation". Mast cells are usually seen in the connective tissues after release from the bone

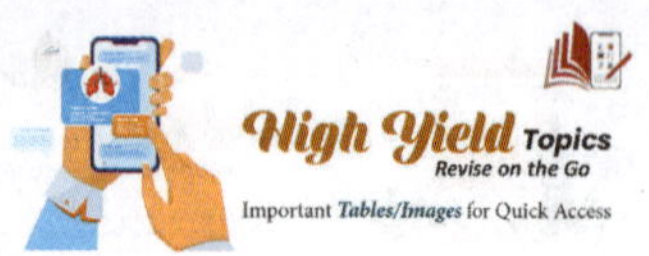

marrow and the release of granules is triggered by an IgE mediated reaction to an inciting antigen. Mast cells are recognized in tissues by their characteristic deep purple color, ovoid to spindle shape, obscuring granules and are highlighted by special stains such as *toluidine blue, tryptase, CD117 (c-kit).*

Eosinophils

Eosinophils play an important role in parasitic infections, atopic (IgE-mediated) hypersensitivity response as seen in allergies and asthma. They also may be seen in certain forms of acute on chronic inflammation where the process of healing has started, e.g., resolving appendicitis.

Eosinophils characteristically have numerous granules which harbor a protein called the major basic protein which helps in destroying parasites and damages the tissue in allergic response.

Plasma Cells

Plasma cells represent a differentiated subset of B-cells and produce immunoglobulins or antibodies in response to the injurious antigens. Morphologically, plasma cells are characterized by abundant basophilic cytoplasm and an eccentrically placed nucleus which displays "clock-face" or "cartwheel" chromatin. Reactive plasma cells can also show binucleation. Plasma cells are typically seen along with lymphocytes in various chronic inflammatory conditions of immune origin, i.e., autoimmune disease, in a special group of disease called IgG4-related disorders and uncontrolled proliferation of the plasma cells occurs in malignant disease such as multiple myeloma.

Causes of Chronic Inflammation

- Failure to remove the offending agent-microorganism.
- Recurrent episodes of acute inflammation.
- Autoimmune disease involving inflammatory response directed against self.
- When the body is unable to remove or phagocytose foreign bodies/inert material, like sutures, talc fibers, etc.

Morphological Features

The hallmark of chronic inflammation is:

- The presence of **tissue mononuclear inflammatory infiltrate** comprising cells with a single nucleus, such as lymphocytes, macrophages and plasma cells.
- **Altered tissue architecture** due to the persistence of the injurious stimuli. The tissue is eventually destroyed or disrupted by the inflammatory cells, proliferating vessels and/or accompanying necrosis.
- Laying down of fibroblasts and collagen **(Healing by fibrosis).**
- **Formation of a scar:** This can eventually with time heal with regaining of tensile strength or it may eventually lead to the development of deformities.

Types of Chronic Inflammation

Chronic inflammation is associated with the following systemic features:

- **Non-specific:** An irritant causes a non-specific chronic inflammatory response that results in the formation of granulation tissue and fibrosis-induced healing, such as in the case of chronic ulcers or osteomyelitis.
- **Specific:** When the harmful agent causes a typical histologic tissue reaction, such as syphilis, leprosy, or TB.

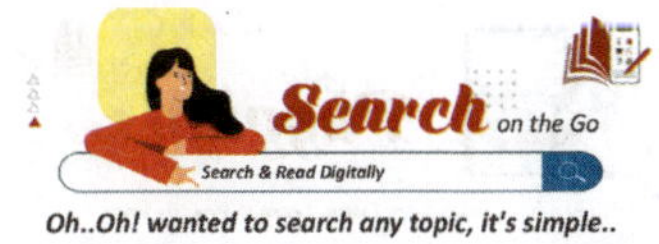

On the basis of the histological features, chronic inflammation can be divided into:

- **Chronic non-specific:** It is characterized by a non-specific infiltration of inflammatory cells, such as in lung abscesses and chronic osteomyelitis.
- **Chronic granulomatous inflammation:** It is characterized by the formation of granuloma. For example, tuberculosis, leprosy, syphilis.

Granulomatous Inflammation

It is a type of chronic inflammation characterized by the collection of circumscribed, tiny lesion about 1 mm, composed predominantly of:

- Modified macrophages.
- Frequently admixed with T lymphocyte cells.
- With or without central necrosis.
- With or without giant cells.

Granulomas are usually formed when the inciting agent is difficult to eradicate either due to increased virulence or a weakened host immune system. Granulomas can further be due to the host mounting an immune response to a persisting infectious agent ***(immune granuloma)*** or due to the presence of a foreign substance (foreign body) in the host, e.g., surgical sutures/talc/inhaled environmental pollutants. Granulomas in such a setting are referred to as ***foreign body granulomas***.

Examples of granulomatous inflammation due to infectious agents include:

- Tuberculosis
- Leprosy
- Sarcoidosis
- Syphilis
- Fungal infections

It is important to recognize the presence of granulomatous inflammation as it points to a few distinct diseases.

Morphology

Microscopically noted features include (Fig. 4.8):

- Aggregation of **macrophages** that are transformed into **epithelioid cells**. Epithelioid cells refer to modified macrophages which have a characteristic "slipper-shaped" nucleus displaying vesicular chromatin and ill-defined pale staining cytoplasm. Because of their resemblance to epithelial cells, hence the term "epithelioid".
- Fusion of these modified macrophages form **giant cells**. In tuberculosis, the giant cells show a peculiar arrangement of nuclei in a horse-shoe arrangement. These types of giant cells are called *Langhans giant cells*.
- The macrophages and giant cells are surrounded by a collar of mononuclear leukocytes, principally **lymphocytes** and occasionally plasma cells.
- A peripheral rim of **fibroblasts** may also be seen as the disease persists.
- Long-standing granulomas which eventually heal show dense hyaline tissue with subsequent collagen deposition (hyalinized scar). Secondary calcification deposits/bone formation may also be noted in granulomas of increased duration.

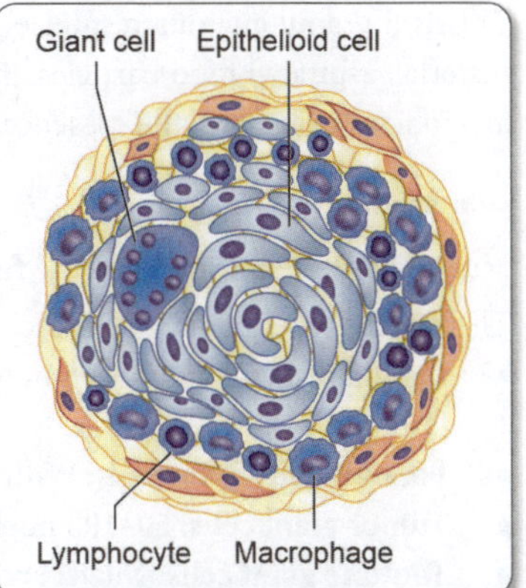

Figure 4.8: Microscopic appearance of granulomatous inflammation

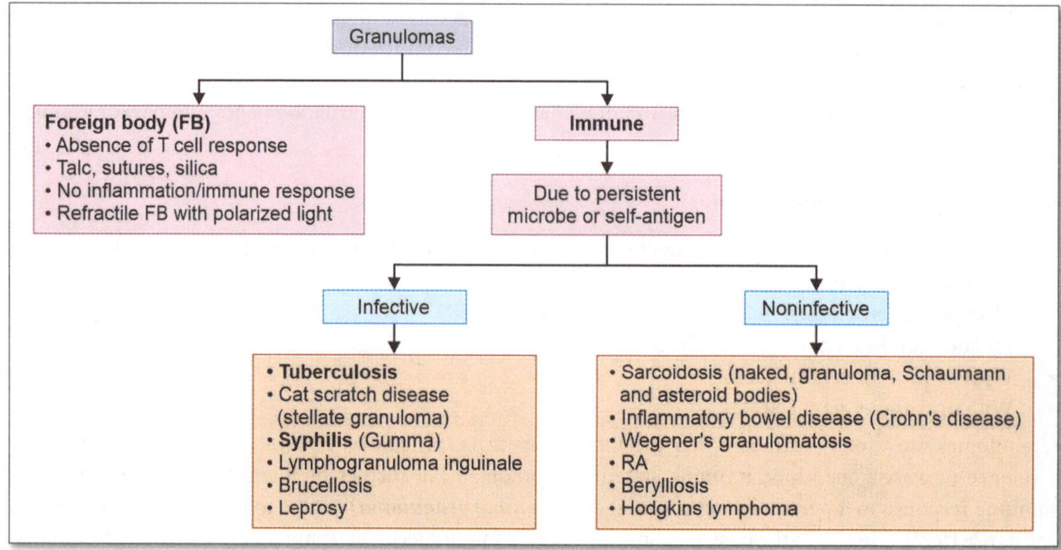

Figure 4.9: Types of granuloma

Types of Granuloma

There are two types of granuloma (Fig. 4.9):

1. Immune Granuloma

These are caused by the agents which are capable of inducing immune response that produces granuloma when the inducing agent is poorly particulate.

2. Foreign Body Granuloma

This is a granulomatous response to the presence of any material that is foreign to the body, e.g., suture material, aspirated food particles, inert substances, drugs. The granulomas are of varying sizes and typically are noncaseating, with the presence of foreign body giant cells.

Giant Cells

Multinucleate cells formed by the fusion of activated macrophages are called **giant cells**.

The various types of giant cells include (Fig. 4.10):

- **Langhans giant cells:** Seen in tuberculosis,10–20 nuclei arranged peripherally in the cell in a horse-shoe fashion.
- **Foreign body giant cells:** With 10–15 nuclei arranged haphazardly in a cell in response to a foreign body.
- **Tumor giant cells:** 50–100 nuclei displaying pleomorphism, seen in various types of malignant tumors.
- **Touton's giant cells:** Nuclei arranged at both poles of the cell, seen in xanthomatous inflammation.
- **Reed Sternberg cells:** Large cell with binucleate "owl eye" nuclei, seen in Hodgkin's lymphoma.
- **Aschoff giant cells:** Multinucleated giant cells seen in cases of rheumatic heart disease.
- **Osteoclastic giant cell:** Large multinucleated giant cells with 10–15 nuclei, involved in bone resorption.

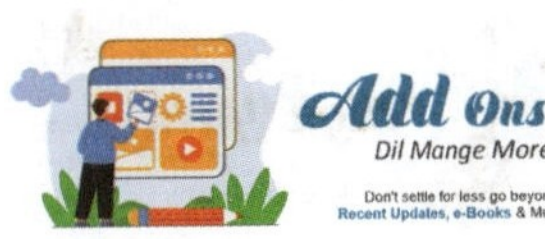

Giant cells

- Pathological
  - Foreign body giant cell (haphazardly arranged nuclei shown by arrow)
  - Langerhans giant cells (nuclei arranged horseshoe-shaped shown by arrow) → Seen in TB
  - Touton giant cell (ring of nuclei surrounded by foamy cytoplasm) → Seen in xanthomas
- Physiological
  - Osteoclasts, syncytiotrophoblas, megakaryocytes (*Note:* Megakaryocytes have multilobulated nuclei)

Special type of giant cells

- Warthin-Finkeldey syncytial giant cell may have 50 nuclei, many with intra-nuclear inclusions
- Reed sternberg cells with eosinophilic nucleoli
- Aschoff giant cells-Rheumatic heart disease

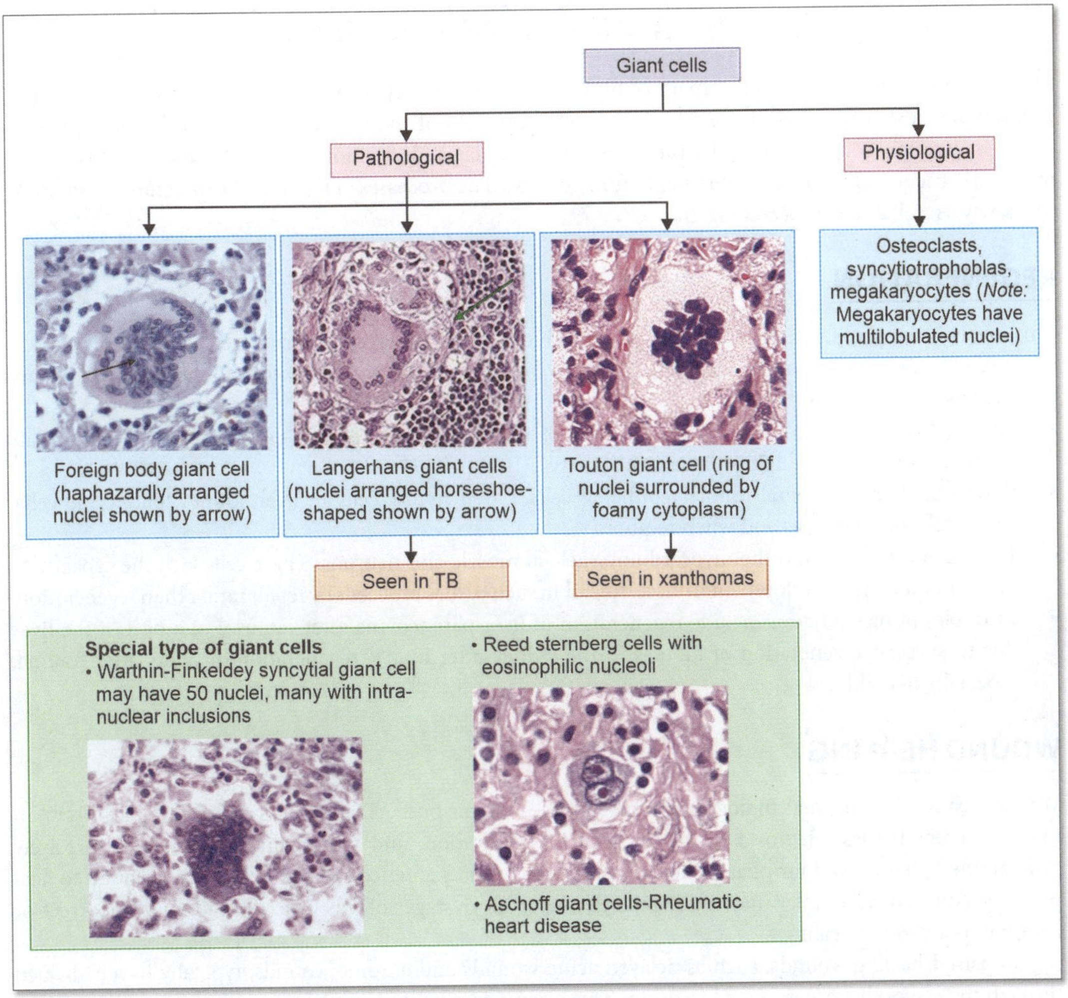

Figure 4.10: Types of giant cell

Granuloma versus Granulation Tissue

A ***granuloma*** represents a unique form of the chronic inflammatory response as described above, *granulation tissue* represents proliferating tissue comprised of fibroblasts, newly-formed vessels and inflammatory cells in a backdrop of edema.

Granulation tissue is often seen in the setting of wound healing or when the body attempts to repair damage at an injured site. Exuberant granulation tissue formation may sometimes be seen in complicated cases of wound healing. Granulation tissue is also called **"proud flesh"** (Fig. 4.11).

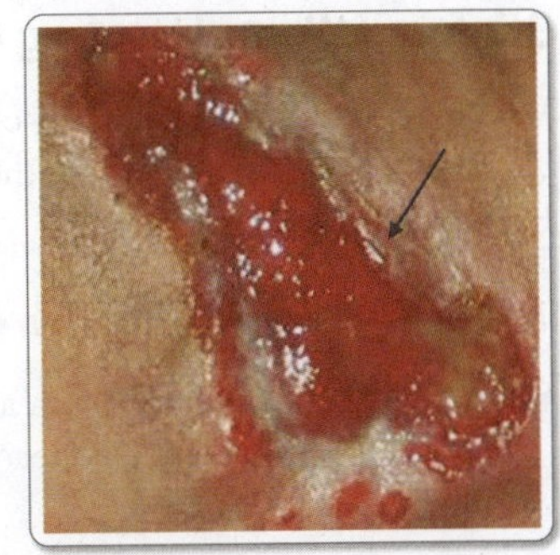

Figure 4.11: Proud flesh

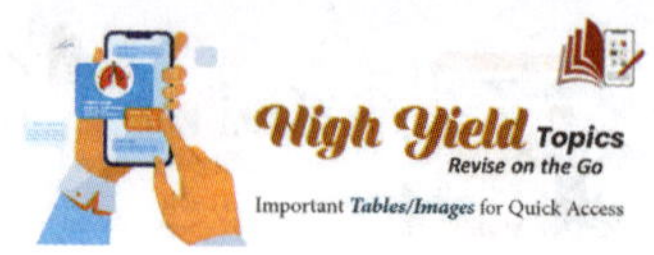

REGENERATION AND WOUND HEALING

The healing process can be broadly separated into regeneration and repair. *Regeneration* results in the complete restoration of lost or damaged tissue. This includes both structural and functional restoration after any injury. *Repair* may restore some original structures but involves collagen deposition and scar formation. This may or may not, subsequently lead to a reduction in functionality. The processes of repair and regeneration can occur separately as well as can proceed together.

REGENERATION

This involves the proliferation of specialized cells and tissue to replace lost structure. The extent to which a damaged tissue can regenerate depends on its *proliferative capacity*. Cells within tissues accordingly are classified as:

- **Labile:** Intestinal enterocytes, epithelial cells of the skin, hematopoietic cells. These cells proliferate continuously and have high proliferative activity.
- **Quiescent (stable):** Renal tubular epithelial cells, parenchymal cells in liver, kidney, endocrine cells. These cells proliferate as and when required.
- **Permanent:** Cells within the myocardium, skeletal muscle and neurons. These cells lack the capacity to proliferate after the developmental phase. Repair in such tissues proceeds by repair rather than regeneration.
- Examples of regeneration include regeneration of liver parenchyma after removal of a part of the liver due to surgery, regeneration of tubules in the kidney after injury, regeneration of digits after trauma, especially in children.

WOUND HEALING

Wound healing is a normal biological process in the human body. The process of healing can occur in many different tissues. Hemostasis, inflammation, proliferation, and remodelling are the four precisely programmed phases. All four phases should occur in the right sequence and timeframe for a wound to heal properly. Numerous variables may interfere with one or more stages of this process, leading to incorrect or compromised wound healing.

Impaired-healing wounds, such as delayed acute wounds and chronic wounds, typically haven't healed through the stages that are expected to occur. These wounds often progress into a pathologic inflammatory state as a result of a delayed, insufficient, or disorganized healing process.

Stages of Wound Healing in Skin Wounds

Wounds in the skin are primarily of two types—the first with clean margins that are close to each other (incised wound) and the second where the margins of the wound show a gap (open/excised wound). Accordingly, healing is of two types:

1. Healing by First Intention (Primary Union)

- Primary union, also known as first-intention healing, is the process by which tissues approximated by surgical sutures or tapes recover with the least amount of tissue loss. Such injuries heal with a neat, little scar.

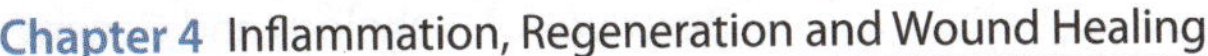

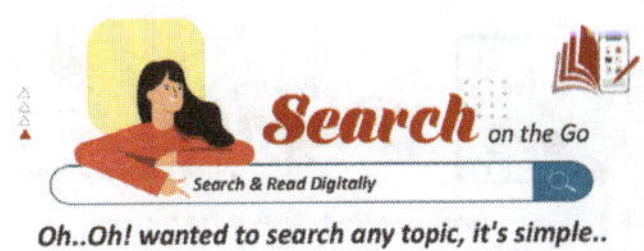

- This is described as the healing of a wound with the following characteristics:
  - Clean and uninfected.
  - Surgically incised.
  - Minimal loss of cells and tissue.
  - Surgical sutures approximately approximate the wound's edges.
- **Initial hemorrhagic phase:** As soon as the wound is formed, in the minimum space of a clean wound, blood oozes out due to hemorrhage and the blood clots to form a fibrin-rich hematoma. This also protects the wound from dehydration and infection.
- **Acute inflammatory reponse:** Within 24 hours, polymorphs start to appear from the incisional edges. On the third day, macrophages replaces polymorphs.
- **Epithelial changes:** Epithelial cells lining the margins migrate and proliferate and ultimately fuse to cover the surface of the clotted blood. Epithelial spurs, or basal cells of the epidermis from both cut borders, begin to proliferate and migrate toward the incisional cavity. An epithelial layer covers a well-approximated wound in 48 hours. The migrating epidermal cells produce a scab that is shed once they separate the underlying viable dermis from the necrotic debris and clot above. The margin-derived basal cells keep dividing. On the fifth day, a new, multilayered epidermis that is divided into deeper and superficial layers forms.
- **Organization:** By the third day, the wound area is also invaded by fibroblasts. On the fifth day, new collagen fibers begin to form and continue to grow until the healing process is finished. In four weeks, the scar tissue forms, exhibiting a scant cellular and vascular elements, a few inflammatory cells, and an epithelialized surface.
- **Suture tracks:** Due to the close apposition of the wound borders, a sutured wound forms a clean scar; the use of adhesive tapes avoids removal of stitches and the associated complications.

2. Healing by Second Intention (Secondary Union)

This is the type of healing which occurs in wounds which have a large gap between wound margins and the inciting agent is either due to trauma or other injurious stimuli. In such wounds, bacterial superinfection or accompanying ulceration of the lining epithelium or the presence of necrotic debris is also seen (unclean/dirty wounds) (Fig. 4.12).

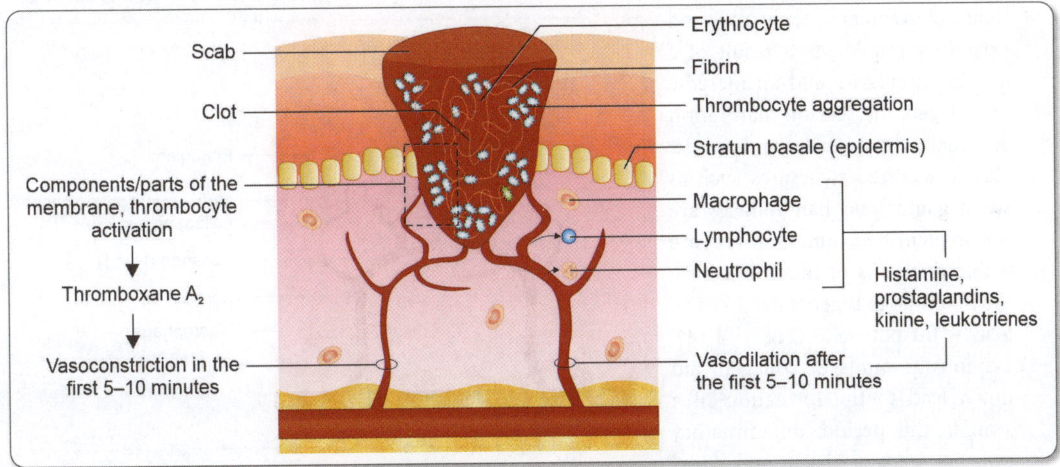

Figure 4.12: Wound immediately after injury showing hemostasis and inflammation

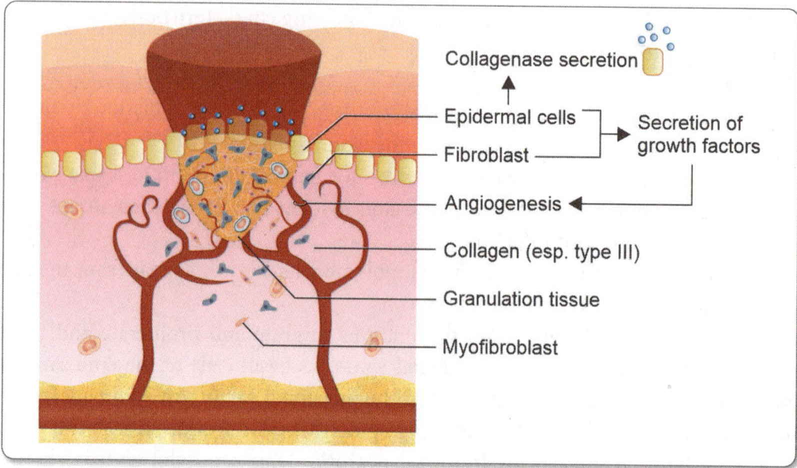

Figure 4.13: Granulation phase

This is described as the healing of a wound that has the following characteristics: (i) It is open with a significant tissue defect that may occasionally be infected; (ii) It has a significant loss of cells and tissues; and (iii) It is not closed with surgical sutures but is left open.

- **Initial hemorrhage:** As soon as the wound is formed, in-between the margins of the open wound, blood oozes out due to hemorrhage and the blood clots forming as in cases of primary intention, a fibrin-rich hematoma.
- **Inflammatory phase:** On day 1 (first 24 hours), neutrophils collect at the junction of the wound with the surrounding tissue, edema is also present. Later on, macrophages clear off the debris as in primary union.
- **Epithelial changes:** Similar to primary healing, the proliferating epidermal cells from both wound margins migrate into the wound as epithelial spurs, eventually meeting in the center to fully re-epithelialize the gap.
- **Formation of granulation tissue (Fig. 4.13):** The granulation tissue formed completely bridges the space between the mound margins, collagen is laid down extensively. The newly-formed granulation tissue is granular, deeply red, and extremely fragile. As a result of a loss in vascularity and an increase in collagen, the scar on maturation eventually turns pale and white. Skin specialized structures such as sweat glands and hair follicles are not replenished unless there are viable remnants of them that have the potential to regenerate.
- **Scar formation (Fig. 4.14):** Copious amounts of collagen laid down lead to the formation of a scar. In this period, inflammatory cells are scant or absent and vessel

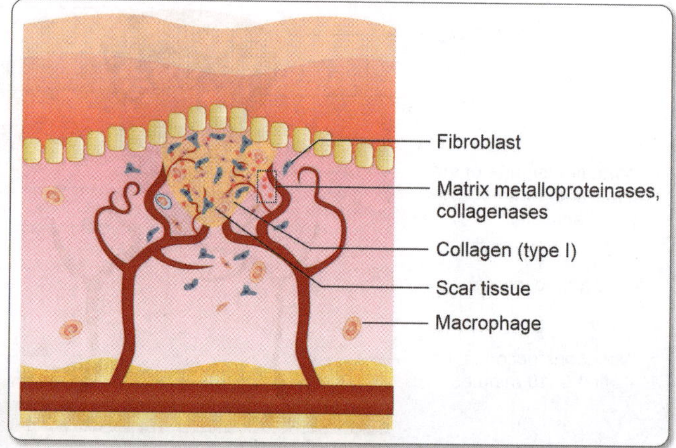

Figure 4.14: Formation of scar tissue

density decreases. In healing by second intention, the scarring is extensive and it takes a longer duration for the wound area to regain original tensile strength.

- **Wound contraction:** The granulation tissue's myofibroblasts cause the wound to shrink to a third to a quarter of its initial size. Contraction of the wound occurs when active granulation tissue is developing.
- **Wound infection:** When bacteria infect an open wound, they emit toxins that cause necrosis, suppuration, and thrombosis, which slow down the healing process. Debridement, the surgical removal of dead and necrosed tissue, aids in keeping open wounds free from bacterial infection.

MUST KNOW

Healing by Primary, Secondary and Tertiary Intention

After four to six days, primary wound healing is delayed to tertiary healing (third intention). This occurs when the wound is mechanically closed and the secondary intention process is intentionally interrupted. This usually happens following the formation of granulation tissue. The following illustration shows healing by primary, secondary and tertiary intention.

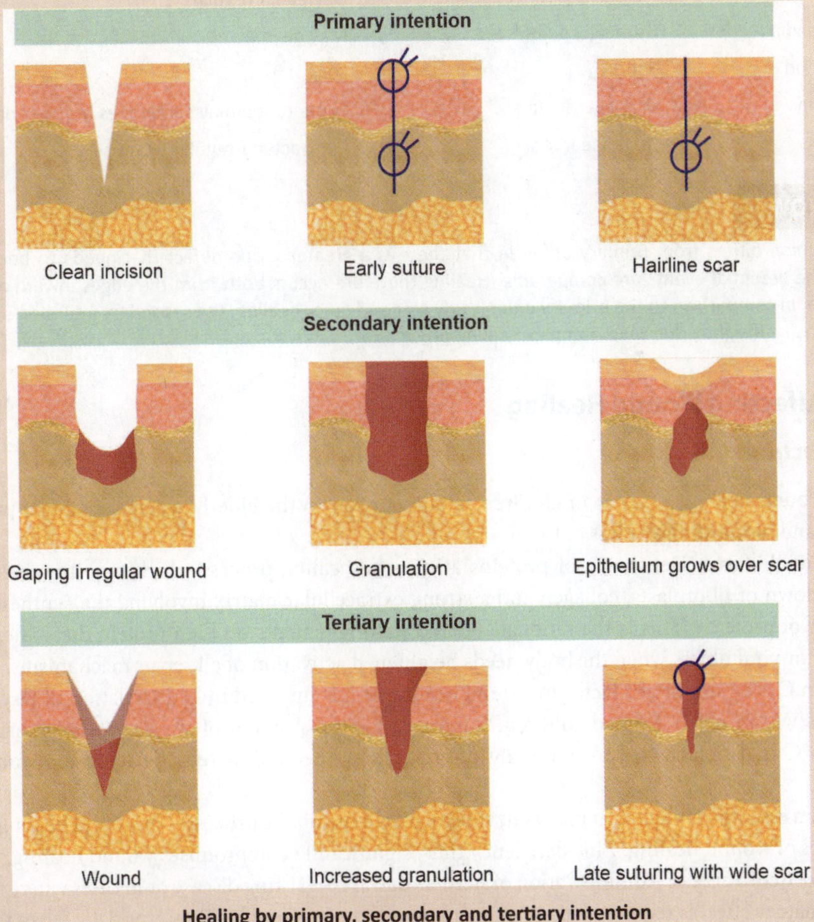

Healing by primary, secondary and tertiary intention

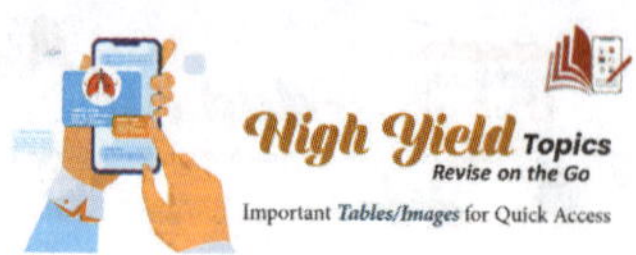

Comparative features of primary and secondary healing intention have been depicted in Table 4.3.

Table 4.3: Comparative between healing by primary and secondary intention

Feature	Primary intention	Secondary intention
Tissue loss/defect	Less	More
Inflammation	Less intense	More
Granulation tissue	Less	More
Scar tissue mass	Less	More
Connective tissue deposition	Less	More
Wound contraction (myofibroblast activity)	Less	Much more
Margins	Surgically clean, apposed	Unclean, irregular
Superimposed infection	Generally uninfected	May be infected
Healing period	Short	Long
Complications	Infrequent	Suppuration may sometimes requires debridement
Outcome	Neat linear scar	Contracted irregular wound

MUST KNOW

Secondary union differs from primary union in that there is a greater tissue defect that needs to be bridged, but otherwise the essential events are comparable. Healing therefore occurs both from the edges inward and from the base upward. In comparison to the primary union's tidy scar and quick healing, the secondary intention's scar is larger and occasionally unsightly due to its complex healing process.

Factors Affecting Wound Healing

General Factors

- **Age:** Wound healing is faster in children in comparison to the elderly where metabolic processes are slower and blood supply is less optimal.
- **Nutritional status:** Deficiency of proteins affects the healing process which requires the presence of laying down of fibroblasts, collagen and a strong extracellular matrix involving the synthesis of a large number of proteins. This is the rationale behind putting patients on high protein diets after any major surgery or viral illness when the body needs heightened activation of all repair mechanisms.
- **Vitamin C** is an important factor in wound healing as it is involved in hydroxylation of lysyl and prolyl residues within newly-formed collagen, important for the strength of the extracellular matrix. When vitamin C is deficient, the cross linking of collagen is affected, thereby delaying the wound-healing process.
- **Zinc** is an essential co-factor in many enzyme mediated metabolic processes in wound healing and affects all stages of wound healing. Zinc deficiency thus, significantly compromises wound healing.
- **Glucocorticoid excess:** Administration of steroids due to co-existing disease or in cases where a rapid anti-inflammatory effect is required has an antagonistic effect on wound healing, especially when the steroid is given just after injury. Steroid administration affects cross linking of collagen and delays the recruitment of inflammatory cells as well as laying down of fibroblasts, all adversely affecting wound healing.

- **Diabetes mellitus:** Diabetics have poor blood supply leading to less vascular perfusion of wounds. In addition, persistently high levels of blood glucose affect neutrophil recruitment, alter immune response and increases catabolic processes. This adversely affects the healing of the wound.
- **Uremia:** Uremia represents the accumulation of nitrogenous and toxic waste in the bloodstream. Toxemia, in turn, impairs the hemostatic function of platelets and the formation of granulation tissue. Patients of uremia also have high levels of interleukin -6 (IL-6) which leads to increased inflammatory cell recruitment, preventing the progress of the healing process to laying down of fibroblasts and subsequent stages.

Factors Accelerating Healing

- **Ultraviolet light:** UV therapy is believed to have a beneficial effect on wound healing by increasing blood flow, increasing growth factor levels and promoting epidermal cell proliferation, important for giving the wound a new skin cover.
- **Rise in temperature:** Wound healing is promoted under conditions of higher temperature. On the contrary, decreased temperature as seen in winters delays healing as vasoconstriction further decreases blood supply to the affected region.

Specific Factors Affecting Healing

- **Extent of injury:** Localized smaller injuries are more likely to heal faster rather than extensive, deep wounds.
- **Type of wound injury:** When the wound has irregular margins and a large wound gap, poor apposition or alignment occurs increasing the wound time.
- **Infection:** Presence of superadded infection can delay or hamper the healing process.
- **Poor blood supply:** A good continuous perfusion of the wound by blood is critical to ensure timely healing. Whenever the blood supply is compromised due to local or systemic factors, the wound takes more time to heal.
- **Excessive movement:** Movement interferes with the stabilization of the fibrin clot and apposition of the wound margins preventing narrowing of the wound gap.
- **Presence of foreign body material:** In wounds which are seen in road traffic accidents or military operations, wounds despite surgical intervention may have residual entrapped suture material or splinters and shrapnel. This promotes persistent inflammation (foreign body giant cell reaction) at the wound site adversely affecting healing time.

Complications of Wound Healing

- **Wound rupture (dehiscence):** After abdominal or pelvic surgeries, persistent coughing, sneezing or other factors causing an increased intra-abdominal pressure, may pronote rupture of a healed wound. The patient can present with "burst abdomen" which is a surgical emergency and can even be life threatening.
- **Infection:** During the course of healing and just after, the newly-laid down skin cover is delicate and prone to being penetrated by bacterial micro-organisms. Superadded infection is a major cause of morbidity and can even affect the ultimate strength of the healed area as well as its appearance.
- **Excess granulation tissue formation:** When granulation tissue formation is exuberant, a lesion called "pyogenic granuloma" (a misnomer) develops. This is also known as "proud flesh". Granulation tissue formation beyond the normal prevents the wound gap to close properly delaying healing.

- **Persisting hypertrophied scars:** Seen due to excessive laying down of collagen during wound healing. Raised scar-like areas are usually seen a few months after the injury and is usually confined within the margins of the wound.
- **Contractures and deformities:** Excessive wound contraction can lead to restricted joint mobility and deformities affecting the muscles, tendons and ligaments of the affected area. Treatment incudes physiotherapy, analgesics to relieve pain and in severe contractures surgical procedures to release the contracture.
- **Keloid formation:** When the collagenous deposition in the scar is markedly exuberant extending beyond the wound margins or the site of injury. It is seen more frequently in African and Asian populations and is characterized by markedly increased fibroblastic activity with upregulation of TGF-B and platelet-derived growth factor (PDGF). It has a tendency for recurrence.
- **Malignant change:** Malignant transformation of scars has a reported incidence of 2–6% of cases. The most common type of malignancy associated with chronic wounds is squamous cell carcinoma. **Marjolin's ulcer** refers to an ulcerative squamous cell carcinoma seen in long standing wounds or burn ulcers.

CLINICAL CORRELATION

- A type III or type V collagen deficit causes **Ehlers-Danlos syndrome**. Hyperextensible skin is a common presentation for patients with this disease.
- Type I collagen deficit known as **osteogenesis imperfecta** is characterized by blue sclera and numerous fractures, which are common presenting features for patients with this disease.

HEALING IN VARIOUS ORGANS

- **Kidney:** The tubular epithelium is the component of renal tissue that regenerates after injury. Chronic kidney disease usually irreversibly damages the glomeruli leading to glomerulosclerosis.
- **Heart:** Cardiac muscle after ischaemic injury does not show regeneration. In myocardial infarction (heart attack), loss of cardiac muscle is accompanied by laying down of fibrous tissue and scarring from the tenth day onward.
- **Liver:** Injury to hepatocytes due to acute viral hepatitis, toxins or drugs usually resolves with the liver tissue regenerating after damage. Chronic liver disease is associated with expansion of portal tracts by fibrous tissue and scarring, in advanced cases leading to nodule formation or cirrhosis. Recent studies have shown cirrhosis can be reversed to varying degrees if the inciting stimulus, e.g., alcohol intake is completely stopped.
- **Mucosal surfaces:** Superficially ulcerated tissue may be covered with regenerating epithelium that covers the ulcerated area. However metaplastic change of the regenerated epithelium may be noted.
  More extensive and deeper ulcerations heal by laying down of collagen, fibrosis and scarring.
- **CNS:** Injury to glial astrocytes is often accompanied by liquefactive necrosis. The tissue subsequently heals by reactive gliosis forming a glial scar.
- **Skeletal muscle:** Shows a limited capacity to regenerate after injury. The healing process after a fracture shall be discussed in the subsequent section on bone pathology.

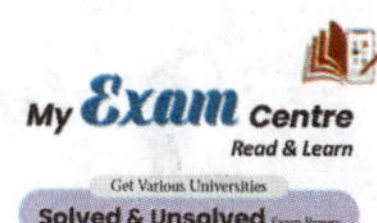

SUMMARY

- The local reaction of living mammalian tissues to damage caused by any agent is known as inflammation.
- Four cardinal signs of inflammation as named by a Roman writer Celsus include: Rubor (Redness), tumor (Swelling), calor (Heat) and, dolor (Pain) and functio laesa (loss of function).
- Acute inflammation is usually characterized by early resolution and repair.
- The formation of edema fluid in the interstitial compartment within and around the inflammatory tissue.
- The primary characteristic of the inflammatory reaction is the leucocytes' escape from the microvasculature lumen into the interstitial tissue.
- Chemical mediators of inflammation are substances produced during inflammation inducing and regulating specific events in the inflammatory response.
- Chemical mediators may be cell-derived or plasma derived.
- The term "chemokines" refers to a group of substances that are released by activated macrophages and platelets, including interleukin-8 and platelet factor-4.
- Interferon-γ causes activation of macrophages and neutrophils and is important in the development of granulomatous inflammation.
- Acute inflammation is essentially a response which is morphologically characterized by a predominance of neutrophils.
- Suppurative inflammation may be a localized collection of purulent material in tissue (abscess)/widespread when associated with sepsis.
- *Regeneration* results in the complete restoration of lost or damaged tissue.
- *Repair* may restore some original structures but involves collagen deposition and scar formation.
- Hemostasis, inflammation, proliferation, and remodelling are the four precisely programmed phases of wound healing.
- Primary union, also known as first intention healing, is the process by which tissues approximated by surgical sutures or tapes recover with the least amount of tissue loss.
- Healing by second intention occurs in wounds which have a large gap between wound margins and the inciting agent is either due to trauma or other injurious stimuli.
- Keloid formation occurs when the collagenous deposition in the scar is markedly exuberant extending beyond the wound margins or the site of injury.
- Marjolin's ulcer refers to an ulcerative squamous cell carcinoma seen in long-standing wounds or burn ulcers.

ASSESS YOURSELF

Long Answer Questions

1. Explain various events in the process of acute inflammation.
2. Discuss various stages of wound healing.

Short Answer Questions

1. Define acute inflammation.
2. Define wound healing.
3. Write about the difference between acute and chronic inflammation.
4. Write short notes on:
   i. Granulomatous inflammation
   ii. Mediators of inflammation

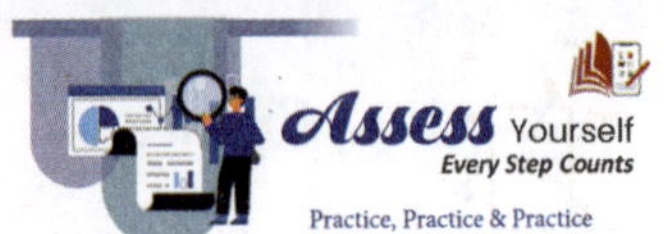

Multiple Choice Questions

1. **Which of the following is not a function of inflammation?**
   a. Delivery of leucocytes
   b. Concentration of toxins
   c. Initiate repair processes
   d. Vasodilation
2. **Which of the following is not the classic sign of acute inflammation?**
   a. Rubor
   b. Dolor
   c. Collagen deposition
   d. loss of function
3. **Cytotoxic T lymphocyte infiltrate of tissue is a sign of?**
   a. Acute inflammation
   b. Chronic inflammation
   c. Ischaemic foci
   d. Caseous necrosis
4. **A patient with insidious fever, hemoptysis and recurrent URTI has a lung parenchyma granuloma pathologically assessed. What will the outer ring of the granuloma show?**
   a. Eosinophil
   b. Lymphocytes
   c. Necrosis
   d. Basophils
5. **A granuloma has formed on the skin surface post laceration. What is the inner collar about the necrotic tissue?**
   a. T cell
   b. B cell
   c. NK cell
   d. Macrophage
6. **The first event in the primary wound healing is:**
   a. Formation of blood clot
   b. Acute inflammatory response
   c. Epithelial changes
   d. Organization of vascular and inflammatory cells
7. **Healing by second intention is characterized by all; except:**
   a. Wound contraction
   b. Abundant granulation tissue
   c. Thin scar
   d. More common complications
8. **Complications of wound healing include all; except:**
   a. Ulcer
   b. Keloid
   c. Sinus
   d. Wart

Answer Key

1. b **2.** c **3.** b **4.** c **5.** d **6.** a
7. c **8.** d

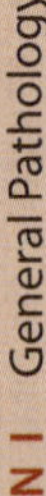

Chapter 5

Neoplasia

LEARNING OBJECTIVES

After the completion of the chapter, the readers will be able to:

- Explain neoplasia and its types.
- Differentiate between normal and cancerous cells.
- Distinguish between benign and malignant tumors.
- Describe epidemiology and incidence of cancer.
- Elaborate characteristics of cancer.
- Identify clinical features of cancerous conditions.
- Understand gross and microscopic features of cancerous cells.
- Explain route of spread of cancer such as local spread, hematogenous spread and spread through cavities.
- Understand grading and staging of cancer.
- Know about the nomenclature of cancer.

CHAPTER OUTLINE

- Introduction
- Components of Neoplasia or Tumor
- Epidemiology of Cancer
- Cancer Incidence
- Characteristics of Tumor
- Cancer Phenotype and Stem Cells
- Clinical Features
- Gross and Microscopic Features
- Metastasis or Distant Spread
- Grading and Staging of Cancer
- Nomenclature
- Laboratory Diagnosis of Cancer

KEY TERMS

Anaplasia: A condition where cells lose the mature cell's morphological traits and orientation toward endothelial cells and each other.

Benign tumors: They are encapsulated, localized or well-circumscribed, freely mobile, and typically hard and uniform.

Differentiation: The degree of morphological and functional similarity between parenchymal cancer cells and corresponding normal cells.

Hamartoma: It is a benign tumor-like malformation composed of abnormal arrangement of cells and tissues, which can grow anywhere on the body.

Malignant tumors: They typically have an irregular shape, are poorly contained, and invade nearby tissues.

Metastasis: Refers to the spread of a tumor by invasion in which a discontinuous secondary tumor mass or masses form at the site of lodgement.

Neoplasia: A mass of tissue formed as a result of abnormal, excessive, uncontrollably proliferating cells.

Teratomas: Tumor containing mature or immature cells or tissues representative of more than one germ layer, sometimes all the three layers.

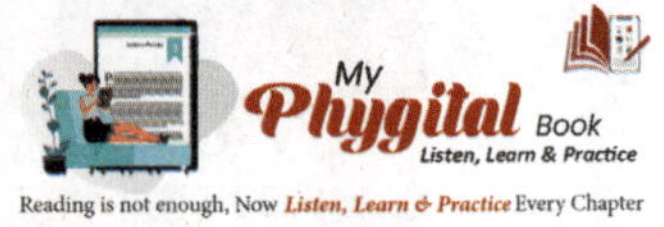

INTRODUCTION

Neoplasia, referred to as "new growth", is sometimes known as a "neoplasm" or "tumor" but not every "new growth" is a tumor because there are also instances of fresh tissue and cell proliferation in the procedures related to regeneration, repair, and embryogenesis, both hormonal stimulation and hyperplasia.

Certain adult normal cells grow throughout life due to regulation over their proliferation and maturation. These cells are known as labile cells. While some have stable cells with minimal growth, others do not replicate (permanent cells). But conversely, neoplastic cells are unable to regulate and control their multiplication, and generate an atypical tissue mass.

Definition: Neoplasia can be defined as "a mass of tissue formed as a result of abnormal, excessive, uncontrollably proliferating cells—even after the growth stimulus that initially triggered them, has stopped."

COMPONENTS OF NEOPLASIA OR TUMOR

Both benign and malignant tumors have two fundamental components:

1. The "parenchyma", which is made up of proliferating tumor cells, dictates the kind and course of the tumor.
2. The "supportive stroma", which is made up of blood vessels and fibrous connective tissue, serves as the foundation for the growth of parenchymal tumor cells.

   The parenchymal component that makes up the tumors determines their name. It adds the suffix "-oma" to indicate benign tumors. Cancerous tumors carcinomas are epithelial-derived growths, whereas malignant sarcomas are the term for mesenchymal tumors (sarcos means meaty). Nonetheless, certain tumors are made up of cells that lack differentiation and are regarded as cancerous tumors.

> **MUST KNOW**
>
> While most cases support the broad generalization about the nomenclature of tumors, there are some exceptions to it, such as melanoma, which is for carcinoma of the melanocytes, hepatoma, which is for carcinoma of the hepatocytes, lymphoma, which is for malignant tumor of the lymphoid tissue, and seminoma, which is for malignant tumor of the testis.

EPIDEMIOLOGY OF CANCER

In the discipline of oncology, numerous clinical, experimental, and epidemiological investigations have been conducted in order to understand the potential causes of cancer as well as the mechanisms by which a normal cell might transform into a neoplastic cell. It is commonly acknowledged that multiple factors contribute to the growth of tumors. The pattern and incidence of cancer depend upon the following:

Predisposing Factors

- **Familial and genetic factors:** Multiple factors contribute to the growth of tumors. Certain factors have a proven involvement in the development of neoplasia. The risk of developing cancer in relatives of known cancer patient is almost three times higher as compared to those having no family history.

  Melanoma, cancers of colon, breast, brain, and ovary are among the cancers that run in families. Familial malignancies affect two or more close relatives, manifest in several sites, and occur at a relatively young age.

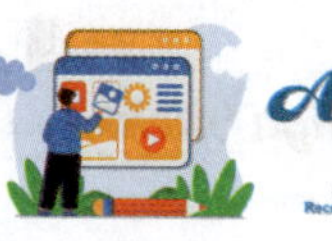

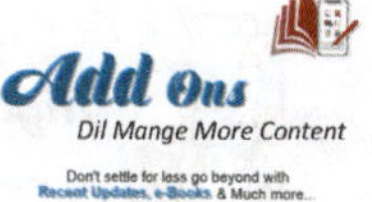

- **Racial factors:** There may be a genetic component to the variations in the racial incidence of certain malignancies.
- **Geographic factors:** Geographic factors such as climate, soil, water, habits, customs, etc., are some of the determining factors, which can predispose an individual for developing cancer. For example, white Europeans and Americans develop common malignancies of lung, breast and colon, Japanese have higher incidence of carcinoma of stomach as compared to Americans; Indian males have higher incidence of carcinoma of oral cavity and Indian females have higher incidence of carcinoma cervix and carcinoma breast.
- **Environmental and cultural factors:** Some of the carcinogens include:
  - Cigarette smoking, alcohol abuse.
  - Industrial and environmental substances, such as benzene, asbestos, vinyl chloride, arsenic, etc.
  - **Dietary constituents:** Deficiency of vitamin-A, low fiber and high fat diet predispose an individual for colonic cancer. Diet rich in vitamin-E has some protective influence by its anti-oxidant action.
  - Cervical cancer is associated with several factors such as parity, frequency of coitus, age at first coitus, etc. Compared to partners of uncircumcised males, sexual partners of circumcised males have a decreased risk of cervical cancer.
- **Age:** Generally, cancer occurs in older individuals, usually above 65 years of age. Some cancers have two peak incidence, e.g., acute leukemia which occurs in children and elderly. Some cancers are more commonly seen in infancy and childhood period, it includes neuroblastoma, nephroblastoma, Ewing's sarcoma, etc.
- **Gender:** The existence of particular sex hormones may be linked to the variations in the occurrence of some malignancies between the sexes. For example, breast cancer is the most common cancer in females throughout the world, while lung cancer is the most common cancer in men.

Non-neoplastic Premalignant Conditions

Premalignant lesions are group of condition predisposes an individual to the subsequent development of invasive cancer. These conditions include:

- **Carcinoma in situ:** Carcinoma in situ, sometimes known as cervical intraepithelial neoplasia (CIN), is the term used to describe a condition in which the cytological characteristics of malignancy are present but the malignant cells are limited to the epithelium and do not invade beyond the basement membrane.
- **Benign tumors and inflammatory conditions:** There are some benign cancer which can become cancerous, such as: Neurofibromatosis, multiple villous adenomas. Also, patients with certain inflammatory condition are more prone for developing certain cancerous conditions. For example: patients with persistent ulcerative colitis may predispose them for colorectal cancer.

Hormonal Factors

Hormones and cancer: Cancer is more prone to arise in tissues and organs that proliferate as a result of high levels of hormone stimulation. The thyroid, liver, prostate, testis, endometrium, myometrium, breast, and vagina are hormone-sensitive tissues that can develop into tumors.

Example: Adenocarcinoma of vagina is seen in adolescent daughters of those mothers who have received estrogen therapy during pregnancy.

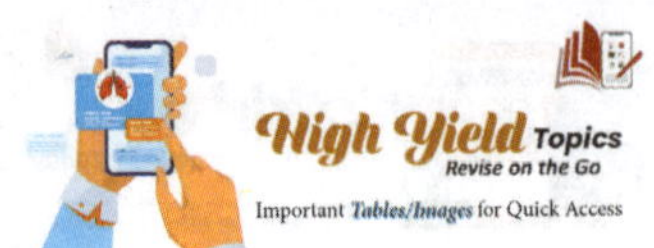

CANCER INCIDENCE

In India, the incidence of cancer is still rising. Planning initiatives for early detection, risk reduction, and management of cancer will be made easier with the aid of these updated estimations.

- The estimated number of incident cases of cancer in India for the year 2022 was 14,61,427 (crude rate: 100.4 per 100,000).
- In India, one in nine person is likely to develop cancer in his/her lifetime.
- Lung and breast cancers are the leading sites of cancer in males and females, respectively. Among the childhood (0–14 years) cancers, lymphoid leukemia (boys: 29.2% and girls: 24.2%) is the leading type of cancer.
- The incidence of cancer cases is estimated to increase by 12.8% in 2025 as compared to 2020.
- According to the Global Cancer Observatory (GLOBOCAN) estimates, there were 19.3 million incident cancer cases worldwide for the year 2020· India ranked third after China and the United States of America·
- GLOBOCAN predicted that cancer cases in India would increase to 2.08 million, accounting for a rise of 57.5% in 2040 from 2020.

CHARACTERISTICS OF TUMOR

- **Rate of growth:** Generally speaking, cancer cells multiply faster than normal cells. Benign tumors typically grow more slowly than malignant ones. There are, nevertheless, several exceptions to this broad statement. There are two primary determinants of the tumor growth rate:
    1. **The rate of cell division, growth fraction, and cell loss:** Malignant tumor cells often exhibit an increased rate of mitosis (doubling time) and a slower rate of death, meaning that they are immortal and do not adhere to normal cell cycle controls. It is possible that cancer cells in the tumor's core undergo ischemic necrosis due to inadequate nutrition if the rate of cell division is high. Ultimately, malignant tumors grow in size because the cell production exceeds the cell loss.
    2. **The tumor's level of differentiation:** Secondly, the rate of growth of malignant tumor is directly proportionate to the degree of differentiation. Poorly differentiated tumors show aggressive growth pattern as compared to better differentiated tumors. The regulation of tumor growth is under the control of growth factors secreted by the tumor cells.

CANCER PHENOTYPE AND STEM CELLS

In an organ, normally developing cells are related to nearby cells; they carry out their designated functions, grow in accordance with normal growth controls, and the rate of cell proliferation and cell death is balanced.

Single cell's progeny is clonally reproduced to create cancer cells (monoclonality). These stem cells are capable of transdifferentiation, or plasticity, asymmetric replication, and prolonged self-renewal.

Cancer cells exhibit characteristics which are as follows:

- Cancer cells multiply quickly because they are unresponsive toward the body's growth-controlling signals.
- Cancer cells become immortal by escaping death signals.
- An imbalance between the rate of cell division and death of cells leads to overgrowth.
- Cancer cells lose their ability to differentiate, and as a result carry out minimal or no tasks.
- Cancer cells are genetically altered because they lack growth regulators.
- Cancer cells infiltrate into the nearby tissue.
- The capacity to spread from the site of origin to different parts of the body allows cancer cells to colonize and create distant metastases.

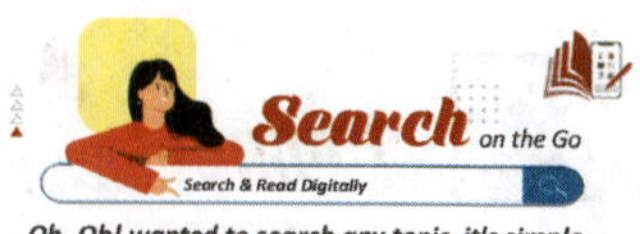

CLINICAL FEATURES

Clinically, benign tumors typically grow slowly, and depending upon the location, can remain asymptomatic (subcutaneous lipoma, for example) or manifest more severe symptoms (meningioma in the nerve system, for example). Malignant tumors, on the other hand, have a fast rate of growth, the ability to ulcerate on the surface, penetrate deeper tissues locally, spread to distant locations (metastasis), and cause systemic symptoms such as anemia, anorexia, and weight loss (Fig. 5.1).

Table 5.1 shows the differences between benign and malignant tumors.

- **Benign:** These tumors are characterized by a usually indolent nature, i.e., the growth is usually localized, does not invade the surrounding tissues, does not spread to other organs and are microscopically typified by bland nuclear characteristics and low proliferative activity, reflected by a low mitotic count.
- **Malignant:** Malignant lesions on the other hand are characterized by the tendency to invade surrounding tissue, the tendency to metastasize, microscopically features of nuclear hyperchromasia and atypia and a worse prognosis as compared to benign lesions. The differences between benign and malignant tumors are enumerated in the Table 5.1.

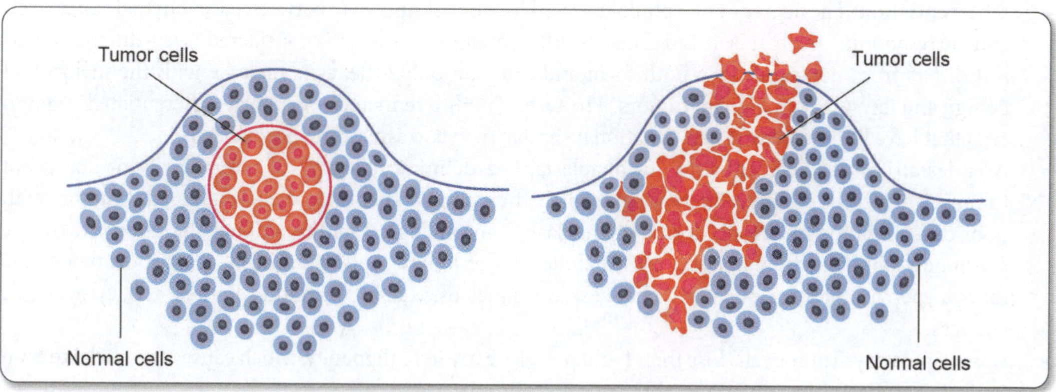

Figure 5.1: Benign tumor versus malignant tumor

Table 5.1: Differentiation between benign and malignant tumors

Benign tumors	Malignant tumor
Slowly growing mass	Rapidly growing mass
Regular surface, capsulated, not attached to deep structures	Irregular surfaces, noncapsulated attached to deep structures
Noninvasive to another organ or tissues	Invasive to other organs
No spread or metastasis	Spread and metastasis
Well differentiated	Poorly differentiated, moderately or well-differentiated
No recurrence after surgery	Recurrence after surgery
No bleeding in cut surfaces	Bleeding from cut surfaces is common
Named by adding suffix-oma	Named by adding suffix sarcoma or carcinoma
Slight pressure effect on the neighboring organ	Remarkable pressure effect on neighboring tissue

GROSS AND MICROSCOPIC FEATURES

Gross Features

Benign and malignant tumors can have quite different gross appearances, and characteristics may not be diagnostic based just on appearance. Nonetheless, nearly all tumors differ in color, texture, and consistency from the surrounding normal tissue of origin due to a few unique characteristics. Macroscopic words used to characterize the tumors' appearance include papillary, fungating, infiltrating, hemorrhagic, ulcerative, and cystic.

- Benign tumors typically have an oval or spherical form. They are encapsulated or well-circumscribed, freely mobile, and typically hard and uniform.
- Malignant tumors typically have an irregular shape, are poorly contained, and invade nearby tissues. It is more common to observe secondary alterations such as ulceration, bleeding, and infarction.

Microscopic Features

Neoplastic cell shows functional and morphological alterations called differentiation and anaplasia.

- **Differentiation:** The degree of morphological and functional similarity between parenchymal cancer cells and corresponding normal cells is defined as differentiation. A tumor is considered "well-differentiated" if it differs from normal cells in both form and function only little, as is the case with the majority of benign and low-grade malignant tumors. The terms "undifferentiated" or "poorly differentiated" refer to cells that have little structural and functional similarity to corresponding normal cells.
- **Anaplasia:** Lack of differentiation, or anaplasia, is a defining hallmark of the majority of malignant tumors. The degree of differentiation determines the extent of anaplasia, such as malignant tumors with poor differentiation have high degree of anaplasia. Morphological and functional alterations which are commonly observed in anaplastic cells include loss of polarity, pleomorphism, disproportionate N:C ratio, hyperchromatism, nucleolar changes, anisonucleosis, atypical mitotic figures and cytoplasmic changes.
- **Loss of polarity:** Tumor cells lose their basal polarity early in malignancy, which causes the nuclei to tend to lie away from the basement membrane.
- **Pleomorphism:** It refers to differences in the tumor cells' dimensions and morphology. Although tumor cells are frequently larger than normal, they can also be smaller than usual in certain types of tumors.
- **N:C ratio:** Nuclei enlarge in proportion to the size of the cell, increasing the nucleocytoplasmic ratio from the normal 1:5 to 1:1.
- **Hyperchromatism:** Malignant cells are characterized by enlarged and coarsely clustered nuclear chromatin. This is caused by an increase in nucleoprotein, which causes dark-staining nuclei, also known as hyperchromatism.
- **Nucleolar changes:** A conspicuous nucleolus or nucleoli in the nucleus of malignant cells usually indicates enhanced nucleoprotein production.
- **Anisonucleosis:** Similar to cellular pleomorphism, malignant tumor cells exhibit size and form diversity in their nucleus.
- **Mitotic figures:** In contrast to benign tumors and well-differentiated malignant tumors, the parenchymal cells of poorly differentiated tumors frequently exhibit a high number of mitoses. Malignant tumor cells have tripolar, quadripolar, and multipolar spindles.
- **Tumor giant cells:** Anaplasia in malignant tumors is also characterized by multinucleate tumor giant cells, or giant cells with a single large and bizarre nucleus.

The salient features of neoplastic and normal cells are displayed in Figure 5.2.

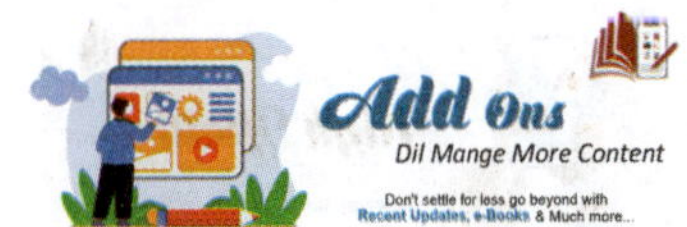

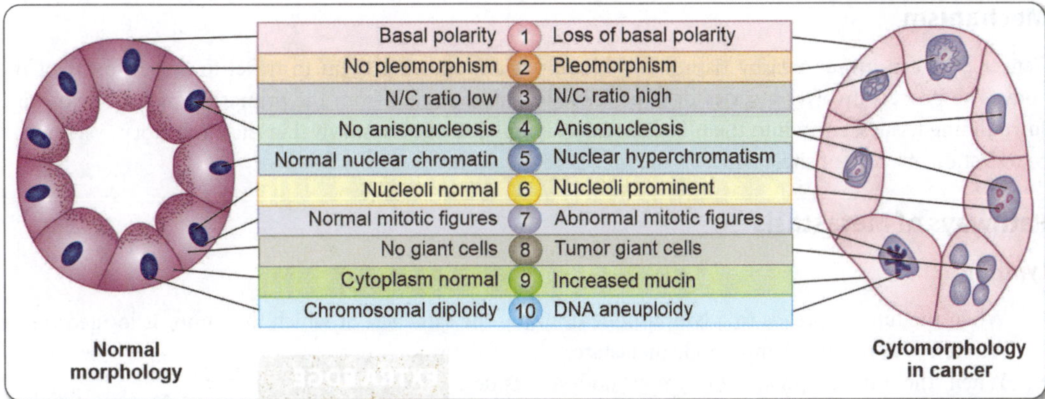

Figure 5.2: Features of neoplastic cell versus normal cell

Arrangement of Tumor Cells

Tumor cells may be arranged in various pattern such as:

- Epithelial tumors can be arranged in papillary and solid pattern.
- Mesenchymal tumors have intercellular matrix such as hyaline material.
- Teratomas, fibroadenoma of breast show mixed pattern.

Tumor Angiogenesis

The vascular network and connective tissue provide a framework that allows parenchymal tumor cells to proliferate and receive nourishment. Angiogenesis is the process by which new blood vessels originate from pre-existing ones to nourish a growing tumor.

Inflammatory Reactions

There can occasionally be a noticeable an inflammatory reaction inside and around the tumors. It can be the outcome of the cancer's ulceration when there is a subsequent infection. In these situations, the inflammatory response may be transient or persistent.

METASTASIS OR DISTANT SPREAD

Definition: The term "metastasis" refers to the spread of a tumor by invasion in which a discontinuous secondary tumor mass or masses are formed at the site of lodgement. Metastasis is defined as "meta means transformation, stasis = residence".

Pathology of Tumor

- **Gross:** Blood-borne metastases in an organ manifest as multiple rounded nodules scattered throughout the organ that vary in size.
- **Histological:** Different sites of metastasis from the same source tumor may exhibit varying levels of differentiation, presumably because the surrounding environment affects the tumor's growth.

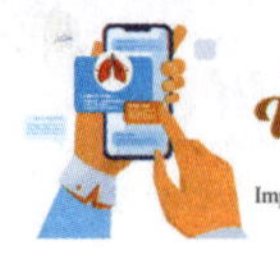
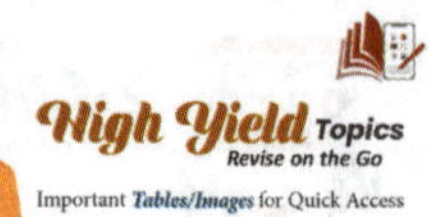

Mechanism

Cancer cells can invade nearby tissues and blood vessels, allowing them to travel to distant parts of the body. The process involves a series of steps, including detachment from the primary tumor, invasion into surrounding tissues, entry into the bloodstream or lymphatic vessels, survival in the circulatory system, and colonization at a distant site.

Pathways of Metastasis

Lymphatic

- When the tumor spreads to a lymph node draining the same site at which the tumor is located this is referred to as regional lymph node metastases.
- When the tumor spreads to lymph nodes outside the regional draining area, this refers to as distant metastases.
- In terms of type specific spread, carcinomas (tumors of epithelial origin) usually spread by the lymphatic route and sarcomas (tumors of mesenchymal origin) usually favor the hematogenous pathway (mnemonic: CL: Carcinomas through lymphatics)
- **Virchow's node:** Metastasis to the left supraclavicular lymph node (Fig. 5.3)
- **Sister Mary Joseph's nodule:** Metastasis to the umbilicus
- **Clinical relevance:** Enlarged lymph nodes in a patient of malignancy should always be viewed with suspicion with FNAC samples being sent for cytological evaluation for a quick diagnosis.

EXTRA EDGE

Virchow's Lymph Node

When malignancies of the stomach, colon, and gallbladder spread to the supraclavicular lymph node, it is known as Virchow's lymph node.

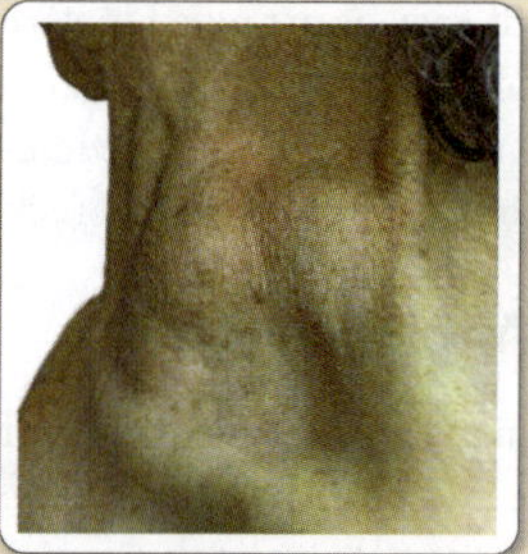

Figure 5.3: Virchow's lymph node

Hematogenous Spread

This refers to the spread of malignancy through blood. This is the common route of spread for sarcomas (tumors of mesenchymal tissue). In the later stage, carcinomas may also adopt this route.

MUST KNOW

- **Spread along natural body cavities and passages:** Some cancers may spread by seeding across body cavities and natural passages. The routes of distant spread are as follows:
  - **Transcoelomic spread:** In which cancer spreads through serosal wall of coelomic cavity. For example, carcinoma of stomach, ovary.
  - **Spread *via* CSF:** Tumor fragments of leptomeninges, ependymal may spread *via* CSF to other sites in central nervous system.

Common Sites of Metastasis

- **Lung:** A common site for metastasis from various primary tumors.
- **Liver:** Frequently affected by metastases, especially from colorectal, pancreatic, and breast cancers.
- **Bone:** Some cancers, such as breast and prostate cancer, often metastasize to bones.
- **Brain:** Metastasis to the brain can occur from various primary tumors.

Factors Favoring Metastasis

- **Tumor type:** Different cancers have varying tendencies to metastasize.
- **Tumor stage:** Advanced stages of cancer are more likely to metastasize.
- **Genetic factors:** Some individuals may have a genetic predisposition to metastatic spread.
- **Tumor microenvironment:** The surrounding tissues and immune response can influence metastatic potential.

Steps Involved in Metastasis

All the steps are highly regulated and involves a complex interplay of genetic, molecular, and micro-environmental factors, nevertheless not all cancer cells that enter the circulation successfully complete all steps of the metastatic process, and many are eliminated by the immune system (Fig. 5.4).

- **Local invasion:**
  - **Cellular changes:** Cancer cells undergo genetic and molecular changes that enable them to break away from the primary tumor.
  - **Invasion of surrounding tissues:** Cancer cells invade the nearby tissues, breaking through the normal tissue boundaries.
- **Intravasation:**
  - **Entry into blood vessels or lymphatics:** Cancer cells enter either blood vessels (hematogenous spread) or lymphatic vessels, gaining access to the circulatory system.
- **Survival in circulation:**
  - **Avoidance of immune system:** Cancer cells must evade the immune system's surveillance as they travel through the bloodstream or lymphatic system.
  - **Anchorage-independent survival:** Ability of cancer cells to survive in the circulation without being attached to a solid surface.

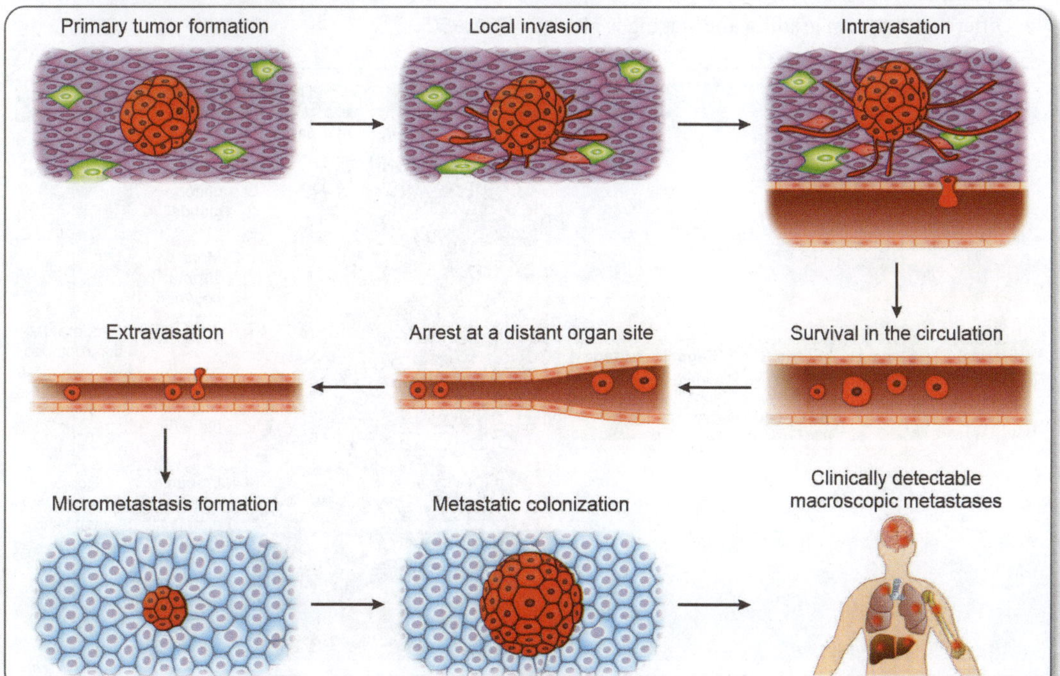

Figure 5.4: Steps involved in metastasis

- **Transportation:**
  - **Circulation:** Cancer cells are carried by the bloodstream or lymphatic system to distant parts of the body.
- **Arrest and extravasation:**
  - **Arrest in capillaries:** Cancer cells lodge in small blood vessels (capillaries) at a distant site.
  - **Exit from blood vessels or lymphatics:** Cancer cells exit the bloodstream or lymphatic system and invade the tissue at the distant site.
- **Formation of micrometastasis:**
  - **Proliferation at distant site:** Cancer cells undergo division and form micrometastases, small clusters of cells at the secondary site.
- **Angiogenesis:**
  - **Formation of new blood vessels:** Cancer cells stimulate the growth of new blood vessels to supply nutrients and oxygen to the developing metastatic tumor.
- **Colonization:**
  - **Establishment of macroscopic metastasis:** The micrometastasis develops into a macroscopic metastatic tumor, establishing itself in the distant organ.

GRADING AND STAGING OF CANCER

"Grading" and "staging" are the two systems to predict tumor behaviour and guide therapy after a malignant tumor is detected.

- Grading is defined as the gross and microscopic degree of differentiation of the tumor.
- Staging means extent of spread of the tumor within the patient. Thus, grading is histologic while staging is clinical.
- Difference between grading and staging is given in Figure 5.5.

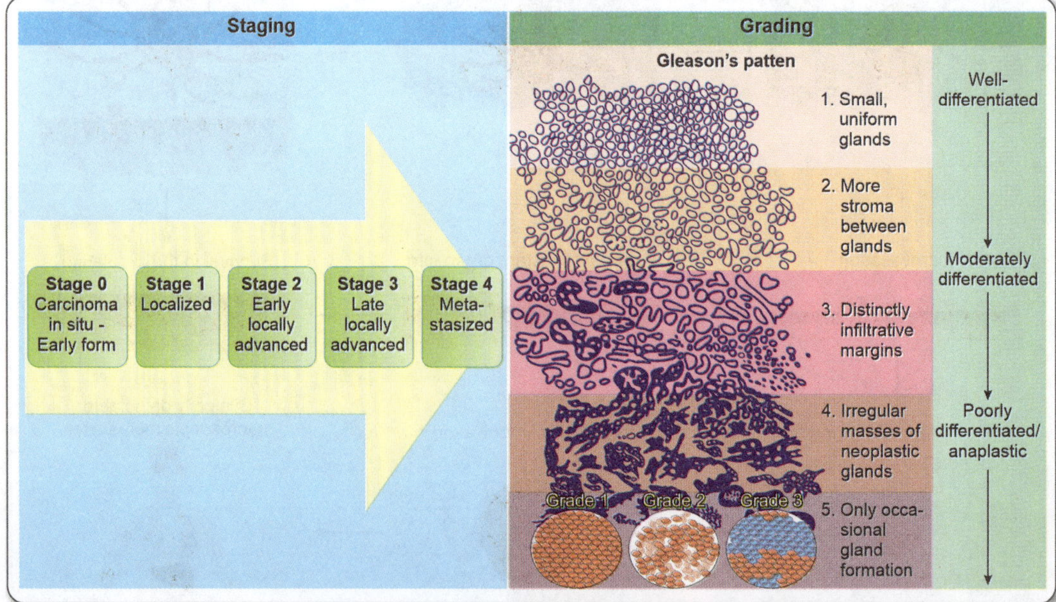

Figure 5.5: Grading and staging of cancer

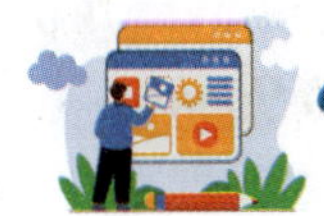
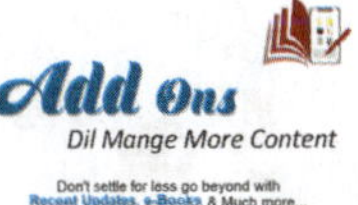

Grading

Cancer grading can be done grossly or microscopically. Cancer can be categorized from grade-I (most differentiated), to grade-III, IV (most undifferentiated or anaplastic). Broders' grading is as follows:

- **Grade-I:** Well differentiated (<25% anaplastic cells)
- **Grade-II:** Moderately differentiated (25–50% anaplastic cells)
- **Grade-III:** Moderately differentiated (50–75% anaplastic cells
- **Grade-IV:** Poorly differentiated or anaplastic (>75% anaplastic cells)

Staging

The extent of cancer spread can be assessed by the following three ways:

1. By clinical examination
2. By investigations
3. By pathologic examination

TNM Staging

T for primary tumor, N for regional nodal involvement and M for metastasis. For each of the three components, i.e., T, N and M, numbers are added to indicate the extent of involvement such as:

- **Tumor (T):** It is used to characterize the primary tumor's size and the extent of its invasion of nearby tissues. T0 denotes the absence of any tumor evidence, while T1–T4 are used to determine the tumor's size and extent, with T1–T4 shows progressive growth and invasiveness.
- **Node (N):** It is used to indicate a tumor's involvement of regional lymph nodes. While N1–N3 show some degree of nodal spread with a progressively distal spread from N1 to N3, N0 indicates no regional nodal spread.

EXTRA EDGE

Clinical Significance

The TNM system helps to establish the anatomic extent of the disease. The following is a brief overview of cancer staging and how it's related to the TNM classification.

- **Stage 0:** Indicates carcinoma in situ. Tis, N0, M0.
- **Stage I:** Localized cancer. T1–T2, N0, M0.
- **Stage II:** Locally advanced cancer, early stages. T2–T4, N0, M0.
- **Stage III:** Locally advanced cancer, late stages. T1–T4, N1–N3, M0.
- **Stage IV:** Metastatic cancer. T1–T4, N1–N3, M1

NOMENCLATURE

Benign tumors are generally identified by attaching the suffix -oma to the original cell. Mesenchymal cell tumors typically adhere to this guideline. For instance, an osteoblast tumor is referred to as an osteoma, a chondroma is a cartilaginous tumor, and a fibroma is a benign tumor originating from fibroblastic cells.

The word "adenoma" refers to both benign epithelial neoplasms that exhibit glandular patterns and tumors that are derived from glands but do not always exhibit glandular patterns.

Naming of Benign Tumors

Naming can be done by attaching the suffix "-oma" to the type of cell (glandular, muscular, stromal, etc.) plus the name of the organ (Table 5.2).

Example: Adenoma of thyroid.

Naming of Malignant Tumors

- **Carcinoma:** Malignant tumor of epithelial cell origin. The name of organ and derived tissue/cell + carcinoma = renal cell carcinoma.

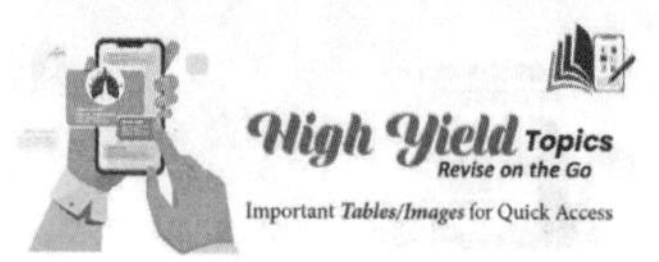

Table 5.2: Nomenclature of tumors

Tissue of origin	Benign tumom	Malignant tumors
Composed of one parenchymal cell		
Type		
• Mesenchymal tumors	• Fibroma • Lipoma	• Fibrosarcoma • Liposarcoma
• Connective tissue and derivatives	• Chondroma • Osteoma	• Chondrosarcoma • Osteogenic sarcoma
Endothelial and related tissues		
• Blood vessels	• Hemangioma	• Angiosarcoma
• Lymph vessels	• Lymphangioma	• lymphangiosarcoma
• Synovium	• Synovial chondromatosis	• Synovial sarcoma
• Mesothelium	• Benign mesothelioma	• Malignant mesothelioma
• Brain coverings	• Meningioma	• Invasive meningioma
Blood cells and related cells • Hematopoietic cels • Lymphoid tissue		• Leukemia • Lymphoma
Muscle • Smooth • Striated	• Leiomyoma • Rhabdomyoma	• Leiomyosarcoma • Rhabdomyosarcoma
Epithelial tumors • Squamous lining • Basal cells of skin or adnexa • Glands or ducts • Ovarian cyst epithelial lining	• Squamous papilloma • Basal cell adenoma • Adenoma • Cystadenoma	• Squamous cell carcinoma • Basal cell carcinoma • Adenocarcinoma • Cystadenocarcinoma
Respiratory passages	Bronchial adenoma (carcinoid)	Bronchogenic carcinoma
Neuroectoderm	Neyus	Malignant melanoma
Others		
• Renal epithelium	• Renal tubular adenoma	• Renal cell carcinoma
• Liver cells	• Hepatic adenoma	• Hepatocellular carcinoma
Urinary tract epithelium (transitional)	Transitional cell papilloma	Transitional cell carcinoma
• Placental epithelium (trophoblast • Testicular epithelium (germ cells	• Hydatidform moe • Germ cell neoplasia in situ	• Choriocarcinoma • Seminoma embryonal carcinoma
• Salivary gland	• Pleomorphic adenoma (mixed tumor of salivary origin	• Malignant mixed tumor of salivary gland origin
• Breast	Fibroadenoma	Malignant cystosarcoma phyllodes

- **Sarcoma:** Malignant tumor developing from mesenchymal or its derivatives. The name of the organ and derived tissue/cell+ sarcoma.
  Example: Leiomyosarcoma of uterus.

- Special nomenclature:
  - **Blastoma:** Tumors developing from immature tissue or nervous tissue, most of them are malignant. For example, medulloblastoma, retinoblastoma, nephroblastoma
  - Some tumors have the suffix-oma, but are malignant. For example, seminoma, lymphoma, melanoma, endodermal sinus tumor.
  - **Mixed tumors:** Tumors which are derived from one germ layer may undergo divergent differentiation creating, e.g., mixed tumor of salivary gland.
  - **Teratomas:** Tumor containing mature or immature cells or tissues representative of more than one germ layer, sometimes all the three layers.
  - **Hamartoma:** It is a benign tumor-like malformation composed of abnormal arrangement of cells and tissues found in areas of body where growth occurs.

LABORATORY DIAGNOSIS OF CANCER

Step 1

Clinical evaluation leading to suspicion

- **Symptoms:** Refers to the patient's complaints
- **Signs:** Refers to features the clinician finds when he examines the patient
- **Malaise:** Lethargy/listlessness
- **Hepatomegaly:** Enlarged liver
- **Splenomegaly:** Enlarged spleen
- **Hepatosplenomegaly:** when both the liver and the spleen are enlarged.
- **Lymphadenopathy:** Enlarged lymph nodes
- **Hemoptysis:** Coughing up bloody sputum
- **Hematemesis:** Vomiting blood
- **Melaena:** Passing blood through the stool
- **Hematopoietic:** Of the blood and/or bone marrow
- **Nonhematopoietic:** Of other systems/organs

  Clinical suspicion of a case of malignancy is arrived at by a number of clinical features including weight loss, anorexia, loss of appetite, lethargy, any rapidly enlarging mass or persistently increasing abdominal distention, unexplained bleeding episodes or persisting fever of unknown origin. Examination may reveal persisting and enlarging masses, lymph nodes or palpable liver and spleen This by no means represents the entire list of symptoms and signs as organ specific cancers can have additional signs and symptoms not enlisted above.

Step 2

- **Routine investigations and radiological evaluation:** Ordering for a complete blood count [CBC] (blood sample collected in purple/EDTA vacutainers) gives the baseline status of hemoglobin levels, platelet count, white blood cell count, red blood cell count. In hematopoietic malignancy (blood cancers), the white blood cell count may show an exponential increase leading to a definite suspicion for malignancy, hemoglobin levels may be reduced, platelet count may be reduced or sometimes increased and most importantly.
- **Radiological evaluation:** Radiology is a good means of identifying lesions that are likely to be malignant. Its advantage is its non-invasiveness. However, radiation exposure is a definite pitfall with techniques like the X-ray and computed tomography (CT) scan.

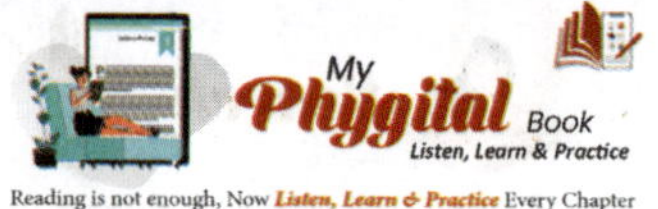

Commonly used techniques include:

- X-ray
- CT scan
- Ultrasound (USG)
- Magnetic resonance imaging (MRI)

Pathological confirmation however remains essential to confirm a malignant tumor.

Cytological Evaluation

Cytology is the study of cells. This can be performed by analyzing material which is obtained from a fine needle aspiration cytology (FNAC) procedure or by analyzing cells which are shed off from the body cavities into the body fluids which is called as effusion cytology.

The FNAC procedure is most suitable for superficially located palpable lumps, aspirated material is stained with stains such as Giemsa and Papanicolaou to highlight cellular features under the microscope. It is commonly used to diagnose tuberculosis of the lymph nodes, lymphomas involving lymph nodes, metastatic tumors in lymph nodes, benign and malignant breast tumors, etc.

Advantages of FNAC

- Easy to perform
- Performed at minimal/no cost
- Report turnaround time is less
- Can be repeated

Disadvantages of FNAC

- Only a limited plane of the lesion is sampled, hence material obtained may be nonrepresentative.
- Deep seated lesions may be completely missed in the absence of image guidance.
- Distinguishing in-situ carcinoma from invasive tumors is challenging on FNAC.
- In certain sites, e.g., thyroid distinguishing benign lesions from malignant (follicular adenoma versus carcinoma) is unsatisfactory.

Histopathology

- Histopathological evaluation of tissue is the gold standard for arriving at a diagnosis of malignancy.
- Tissue is obtained either through an incisional biopsy in which only a part of the lesion is removed for analysis or an excisional biopsy in which the lesion is removed in toto.
- Tissue removed is processed, embedded in paraffin wax and stained for evaluation. The morphological features of malignancy as described earlier include an infiltrative growth pattern, nuclear pleomorphism, nuclear hyperchromasia, an increased nucleocytoplasmic ratio and irregular nuclear chromatin. Further sub typing of the malignant tumor is aided by the use of immunohistochemical markers.
- *Immunohistochemistry (IHC)* involves the usage of monoclonal antibodies directed against specific antigens which are expressed by the cells in the tissue. They are commonly used for diagnostic purpose. IHC can also be used to prognosticate tumors, e.g., HER-2/neu, ER, PR in breast cancer.

Common immunohistochemical markers used for analysis include:

IHC marker	Detects	Corresponding tumor diagnosis which is aided by the marker
LCA	Lymphocytes	Lymphoma
CD 20	B-lymphocytes	Lymphoma
CD 3, CD 5	T-lymphocytes	Lymphoma
CK	Epithelial cells	Carcinoma
Vimentin	Mesenchymal cells	Sarcoma
Desmin	Muscle	Rhabdomyosarcoma
Smooth muscle antigen (SMA)	Smooth muscle	Leiomyosarcoma
S-100	Neural tissue, adipocytes	Neural tumors
HMB-45	Melanocytes	Melanoma

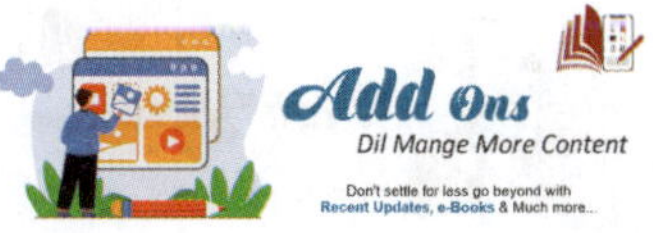

Frozen Section

This a rapid diagnostic method in which tissue is frozen at –20°C in a special equipment called cryostat or frozen section machine. The tissue becomes hard because of this extreme cooling and is sectioned and stained.

This is a frequently used method to guide surgeons during the course of an operative procedure.

- **Applications:** To diagnose whether surgical margins resected are positive/negative. If positive for malignancy the surgeon further extends his surgery.
  - To give a preliminary diagnosis in ovarian tumors, other solid tumors, i.e., whether the lesion is benign or malignant.
  - To confirm the presence of metastatic malignancy in a tissue distant from tumor, e.g., metastatic adenocarcinoma in omental tissue.
- **Tumor markers:** Tumor markers are substances found in an increased amount in the body. These substances are liberated either by the tumor itself or by the host in response to the presence of tumor.
  - Tumor markers can be detected in the tissue, body fluids or serum of the patient.
  - Tumor markers help both in diagnosis of malignancy as well as to determine the prognosis, i.e., likelihood of cure.

Commonly used tumor markers include:

Name of the tumor marker	Organ involved	Type of carcinoma
Alpha fetoprotein	Liver	Hepatocellular
Prostate specific antigen	Prostate	Carcinoma prostate
Human chorionic gonadotropin (hCG)	Placenta	Choriocarcinoma
CA–125	Ovary	Ovarian carcinoma
CA 15–3	Breast	Carcinoma breast
Calcitonin	Thyroid	Medullary carcinoma thyroid
Carcinoembryonic antigen	Intestine, pancreas	Colonic carcinoma, pancreatic carcinoma

Flow Cytometry

Flow cytometry is an modality in the diagnosis of cancer, especially in the case of hematological malignancies. In this technique, cells move in an isotonic fluid under pressure. The cells move singly and after encountering a laser beam of light are scattered. On the basis of their scatter properties, the cell type can be made out and neoplastic cells which are usually larger and heavier, having different scatter properties can also be picked up. The cells are also treated with monoclonal antibodies against cell surface/nuclear antigens and coupled with a dye for visible detection of the antigen-antibody reaction.

Important markers helping us to diagnose the types of cells are:

Lineage of cells	Marker
B-lymphocytes	CD19, CD 20
T-lymphocytes	CD 3, 5, 7, 4, 8
Myeloid cells	CD 13, CD 33
Monocytes and their precursors	CD 11b, CD 14, CD 11c

Flow cytometry can also be used in the **diagnosis of solid tumors** by analyzing the DNA content.

Another application of flow cytometry is **detecting the presence of residual tumor after chemotherapy.**

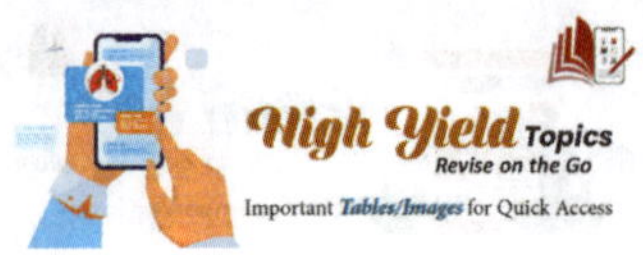

Molecular Diagnostics

- **Fluorescence in situ hybridization:** This is a molecular technique used to identify specific DNA sequences at a tissue level. The tissue is treated with a probe which has DNA sequence complementary to the target DNA sequence of interest. This probe is labelled with a fluorescent dye. If the target has the particular DNA sequence one is looking for, hybridization occurs which is observed under a fluorescence microscope that picks up the fluorescent signal generated indicating hybridization.
- **Applications:** Used to detect gene amplification, translocation and deletions. E.g., detection of BCR-ABL translocation in the diagnosis of chronic myeloid leukemia (CML)
  Diagnosis of various soft tissue tumors which are characterized by specific translocations, e.g., Ewings sarcoma-EWS-FLI1 translocation, synovial sarcoma-SYT-SSX translocation.
  Detection of HER-2/neu amplification in cases of breast carcinoma where immunohistochemistry results are 2+ (equivocal).
- **Polymerase chain reaction:** This technique selectively amplifies the target sequence of interest which can be either a DNA/RNA sequence using oligonucleotide primers complementary to this sequence. This amplification process enables the detection of a few circulating malignant cells (1 in 10^5). This technique is very sensitive.
- **DNA microarray analysis:** A tumor of one patient may be completely identical to the same type of tumor in another patient in terms of microscopic features. Despite that, the two patients have a different biological behavior, one doing well with chemotherapy while the other not having a favorable outcome. This difference is possibly due to difference in the molecular profile of the tumor. DNA microarrays detect the expression of thousands of genes simultaneously and help in identifying the molecular signatures of a tumor which helps to prognosticate.

SUMMARY

- Neoplasia, refers to "new growth", sometimes known as a "neoplasm" or "tumor".
- Melanoma, colon, breast, ovarian, brain, and ovarian cancers are among the cancers that run in families.
- Cancer is more prone to arise in tissues and organs that proliferate as a result of high levels of hormone stimulation.
- Benign tumors typically have an oval or spherical form. They are encapsulated or well-circumscribed, freely mobile, and typically hard and uniform.
- The degree of morphological and functional similarity between parenchymal cancer cells and corresponding normal cells is defined as differentiation.
- Lack of differentiation, or anaplasia, is a defining hallmark of the majority of malignant tumors.
- Pleomorphism refers to differences in the tumor cells' dimensions and morphology.
- The term "metastasis" refers to the spread of a tumor by invasion in which a discontinuous secondary tumor mass or masses form at the site of lodgement.
- Blood-borne metastasis is a common route of spread for sarcomas, but certain carcinomas also spread through lung, breast, thyroid, liver, prostate and ovary.
- Grading is defined as the gross and microscopic degree of differentiation of the tumor, while staging means extent of spread of the tumor within the patient.
- Benign tumors are generally identified by attaching the suffix -oma to the original cell.
- Teratomas are the tumor containing mature or immature cells or tissues representative of more than one germ layer, sometimes all the three layers.
- Benign tumors proliferate but do not spread to nearby tissue.
- Malignant tumors multiply, spread to nearby tissues, and/or metastasis.

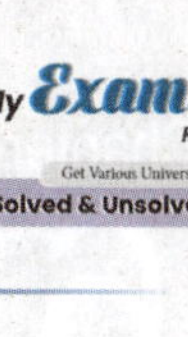

ASSESS YOURSELF

Long Answer Questions

1. Define neoplasia and explain grading and staging of cancers.
2. Explain epidemiology of cancer. Differentiate between benign and malignant cancers.

Short Answer Questions

1. Define carcinoma in situ.
2. Define metastasis.
3. What is TNM classification?
4. Write short notes on:
   i. Grading
   ii. Pathology of tumor

Multiple Choice Questions

1. **Which of the following is property of a benign neoplasm?**
   a. Marked aneuploidy
   b. Lymph node metastasis
   c. Invasion
   d. Surrounding capsule
2. **Which of the following is benign?**
   a. Seminoma
   b. Melanoma
   c. Teratoma
   d. Lymphoma
3. **All of the following characterize familial tumors; except:**
   a. Earlier age at onset
   b. Close relatives with the same tumors
   c. Specific marker phenotypes
   d. Increased relative risk in siblings
4. **Malignant tumors**
   a. When arising from epithelial cells are called sarcomas
   b. Are well differentiated
   c. When arising from glandular cells are called adenocarcinoma
   d. Rarely metastasize
5. **Hamartoma refers to:**
   a. Tumor differentiating towards more than one cell line
   b. Tumors arising from totipotent cells
   c. Mass of disorganized but mature cells indigenous to the part
   d. Mass of ectopic rests of normal tissue

Answer Key

1. d **2.** c **3.** c **4.** c **5.** c

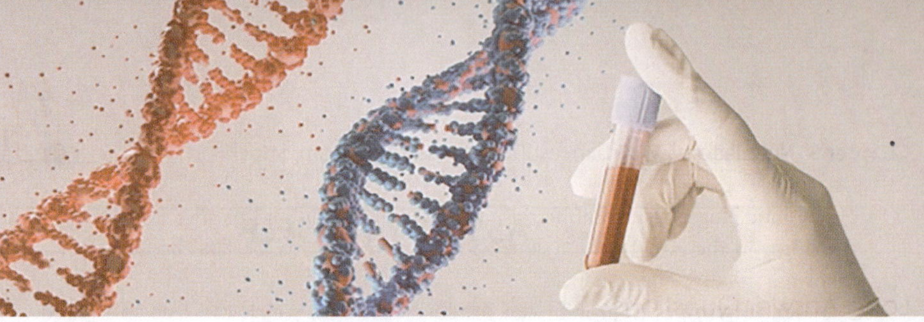

Chapter 6

Circulatory Disturbances: Thrombosis, Embolism, Shock

LEARNING OBJECTIVES

After the completion of the chapter, the readers will be able to:

- Define thrombosis and understand its pathogenetic mechanisms.
- Discuss embolism and know about its different types.
- Diagnose shock and be aware of its pathogenetic mechanisms as well as types.
- Know the morphological features of shock in different organs.

CHAPTER OUTLINE

- Thrombosis
- Embolism
- Ischemia
- Infarction
- Shock

KEY TERMS

Embolism: An *embolism* is the lodging of an embolus, a blockage—caused by fragment of material, inside a blood vessel.

Hematoma: A hematoma is an extravascular thrombus that has accumulated within tissues.

Infarction: Localized area of tissue necrosis occurring due to a reduced blood supply (ischemia) leading to decreased perfusion.

Ischemia: The phenomenon in which tissue receives insufficient blood supply.

Thrombosis: The formation of a solid or semi-solid mass within the lumen of a blood vessel is called thrombosis.

THROMBOSIS

- The formation of a solid or semi-solid mass within the lumen of a blood vessel is called thrombosis. A thrombus is an aggregate of blood constituents, i.e., red blood cells, white blood cells and fibrin.
- The normal bodily steady state or homeostasis is established by a balance between factors favoring thrombosis (prothrombotic) and factors preventing thrombosis (antithrombotic).
- A hematoma is an extravascular thrombus that has accumulated, e.g., within tissues. Blood clots known as hemostatic plugs occur near the site of bleeding, such as a blood vessel injury, in healthy persons. The most basic type of thrombosis could be a hemostatic plug at the severed end of a blood vessel.

- Hemostatic plugs are helpful because they prevent blood and plasma from escaping, however thrombi that form in the circulatory system without a rupture can be fatal because they can have any of the following negative consequences:
  - **Ischemic injury:** Thrombi can produce ischemia, which can lead to infarction, by reducing or stopping the blood supply to a portion of an organ or tissue.
  - **Thromboembolism:** A portion of the thrombus or the entire clot may get dislodged and travel through the bloodstream as an embolus to lodge in a distant vessel.

Classification

According to location: Cortex of TG Notch 3 mice.

- **Cardiac thrombus:**
  - Valvular thrombus in valves-arteries
  - Mural thrombus in wall of heart-arteries
- **Arterial thrombus:** Strongylus vulgaris in arteries.
- **Venous thrombus:** More common in veins.
- Capillary thrombus.
- Lymphatic thrombus.

According to location within the blood vessel:

- Lateral thrombus one side of BV.
- Occluding thrombus-entire circumference of BV.
- Saddle thrombus at bifurcation of BV.
- Canalized thrombus new blood channels through the clot.

According to infective agent:

- Septic thrombus contains bacteria.
- Parasitic thrombus contains parasites.
- Aseptic thrombus no bacteria or parasites.

According to color:

- **Pale or white thrombus:** In rapid blood flow, only platelets.
- **Red thrombus:** In slow blood flow, fibrin attach to platelets.
- **Mixed thrombus:** Most common.
- **Laminated thrombus:** Alternate layers of white and red.

Factors Causing Thrombosis

Thrombosis is dependent on three factors as enumerated by Virchow in 1856, also called the *Virchow's triad* (Fig. 6.1):

- Altered blood flow (stasis/turbulence)
- Hypercoagulability
- Vascular endothelial injury

Altered Blood Flow (Stasis/Turbulence)

Normal blood flow is referred to as *laminar* which is streamlined and orderly. Alteration in the laminar blood flow could be of two types (Fig. 6.2):

1. **Stasis:** When the blood flow slows down, leading to blood stagnation. Clinical scenarios where stasis occurs include right-sided heart failure where the blood does not reach the left side of the heart and

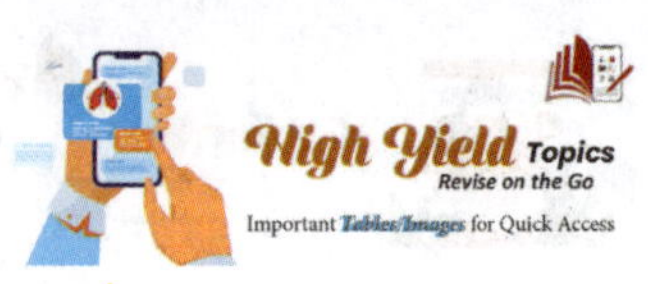

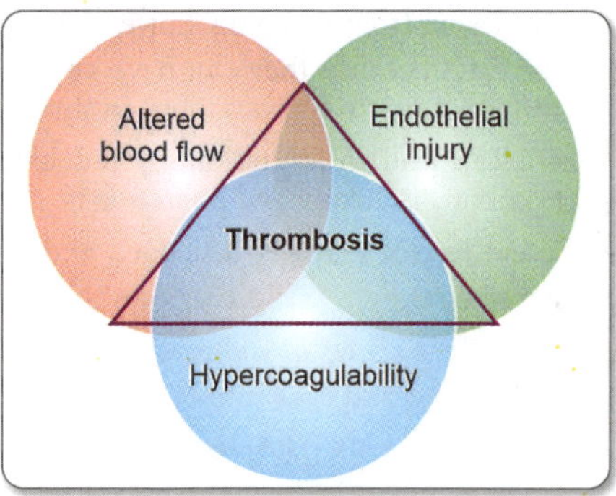

Figure 6.1: Factors causing thrombosis

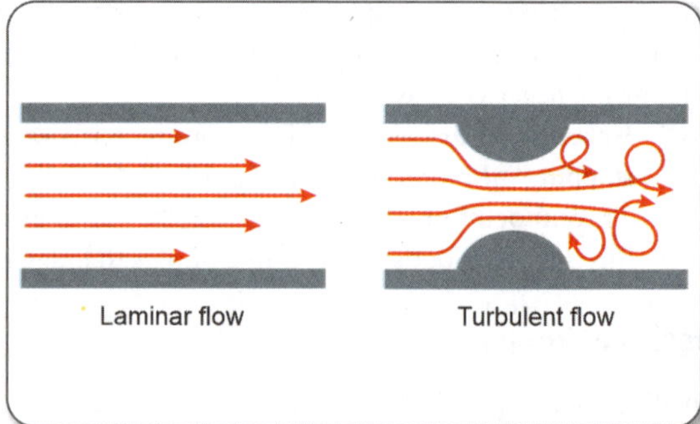

Figure 6.2: Laminar and turbulent flow

stagnates in the right ventricle. Another example is mitral stenosis or narrowing of the mitral valve leading to stagnation of blood in the left atrium. Slowing down of the blood flow increases the contact time between the platelets and endothelial cell lining.

2. **Turbulence:** When the blood flow instead of being orderly, becomes disorderly with numerous currents of flow and at times with an increased flow. Examples include hypertension in which blood flows at an increased pressure, acute myocardial infarction.

Hypercoagulability of Blood

The blood is more prone to coagulation in certain hereditary and acquired states. Such states predispose to the formation of thrombi (thrombophilic states).

Inherited hypercoagulable states include:

- Protein C and S deficiency.
- Deficiency of anti-thrombin III.
- Factor V mutation (Leiden mutation).
- Prothrombin factor mutation.

Acquired conditions leading to hypercoagulability include:

- Pregnancy.
- Intake of oral contraceptive pills.
- Chronic smokers.
- Disseminated intravascular coagulation.
- Prolonged bed rest.
- Malignancies such as leukemias and lymphomas.

Endothelial Injury

Any injury caused to the vessels exposes the subendothelial extracellular matrix comprised of elastin, collagen and laminin. These substances are prothrombotic, that is favor the development of a thrombus.

Endothelial injury may be seen in cases of:

- Myocardial pathology—myocardial infarction, myocarditis.
- Valvular pathology—due to the presence of vegetations on the valves as seen in endocarditis.
- The presence of prosthetic valves.
- Rupture of atherosclerotic plaques.
- Chemical injury—due to nicotine, bacterial toxins.
- Diseases which have dyslipidemia (abnormal lipid profiles) diabetes, hypercholesterolemia.

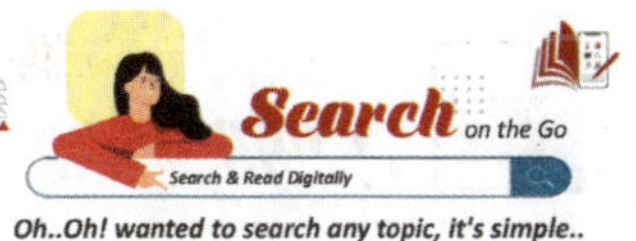

Morphological Features of Thrombus

Thrombosis can occur in the capillaries, arteries, veins, and heart. In addition to the variations in thrombus formation mechanisms at these locations, these sites also differ in terms of their clinical outcomes. Venous and cardiac thrombi result in embolism, whereas arterial thrombi generate ischemia and infarction.

Gross Appearance

Thrombi are friable and dry and show alternating pale and dark areas, called **lines of Zahn**, which comprise red cells that form the dark layer and fibrin that forms the pale area (Figs 6.3 and 6.4A and B).

Venous thrombi are typically red and occlusive, whereas arterial thrombi are typically white and mural. White thrombi are firm and pale, while red thrombi are soft, red, and pale.

Microscopically

Microscopically, the rate of blood flow determines the composition of thrombus, i.e., whether it forms in the slow-moving veins or the rapid arterial and cardiac circulation. Alternating layers of dark-staining red cells and light-staining aggregated platelets combined with fibrin meshwork generate the Zahn lines. More red cells, leucocytes, and platelets get trapped in fibrin meshwork in red (venous) thrombi. Consequently, red thrombi *in vitro* closely resemble blood clots.

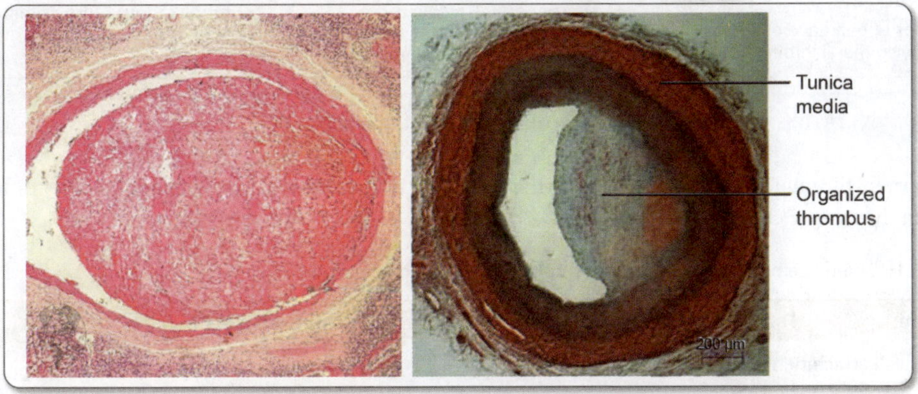

Figure 6.3: Thrombus—microscopic pathology

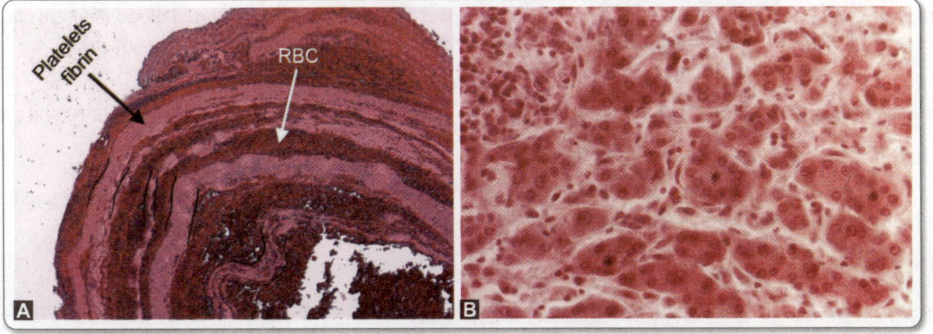

Figures 6.4A and B: **A.** Line of Zahn composed of granular looking platelets and fibrin meshwork; **B.** Microscopic appearance

Types

There are three types of thrombosis have been depicted in Figure 6.5.

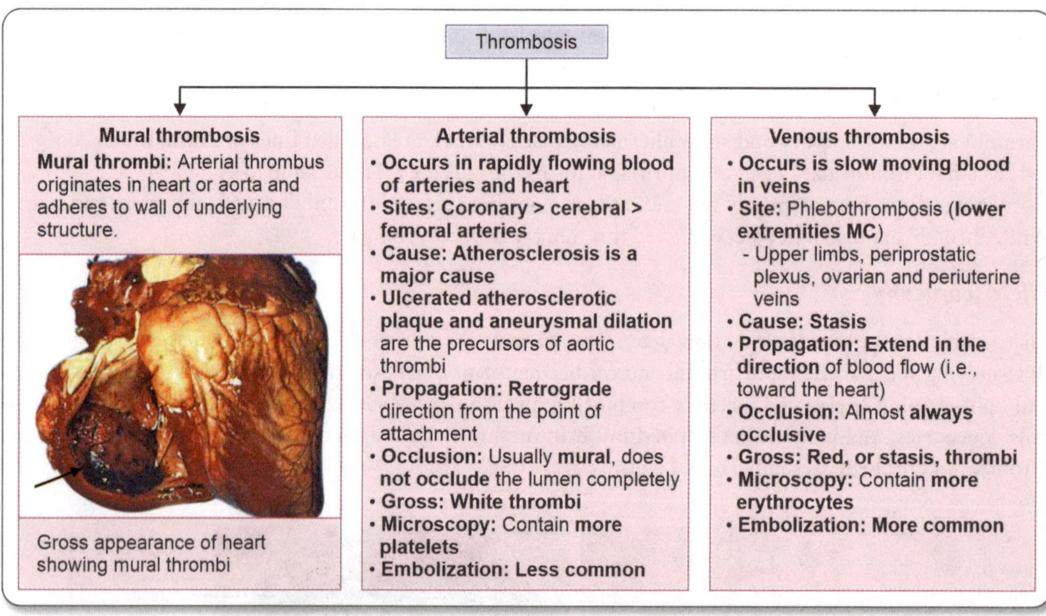

Figure 6.5: Types of thrombosis

Antemortem thrombi are strongly attached to the vessel wall in contrast to postmortem clots. Other differences between the two are enumerated in Table 6.1.

Table 6.1: Difference between antemortem thrombi and postmortem clots

Feature	Antemortem thrombi	Postmortem clots
Vessel wall attachment	Firm	Weak
Site	Any location	At dependent sites, where the blood components settle down
Pathogenesis	In response to hemostatic processes/ hypercoagulability, endothelial cell injury and altered blood flow	Due to settling down of blood elements as a gravitational effect
Gross appearance	Firm/friable	Upper layers are relatively cell poor and give a *"chicken fat"* appearance Lower layers are red cell rich due to sedimentation effect giving a *"currant jelly"* appearance
Lines of Zahn	Present	Absent
Shape	May adapt to vessel size or fragment leading to emboli	Usually takes the shape of the vessel involved

Thrombi in addition may be of arterial or venous origin.

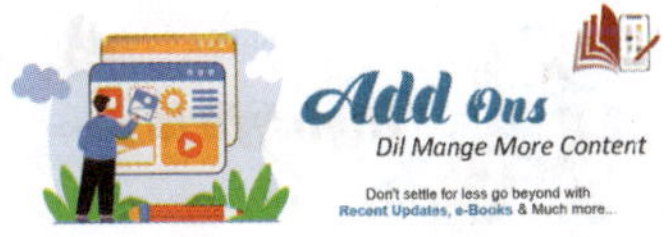

The comparison between these two types is also listed in Table 6.2.

Table 6.2: Difference between arterial and venous thrombi

Feature	Arterial thrombi	Venous thrombi
Pathogenesis	Endothelial injury	Slowing of venous blood
Site	Heart, arteries	Lower limb veins
Direction	Against blood flow	In the direction of blood flow
Color	Gray white	Reddish
Consistency	Friable	Firm
Lines of Zahn	More prominent	Less prominent
Composition	RBCs, fibrin, leukocytes	Mainly red blood cells

Fate of Thrombus

Fate of thrombus is given as mnemonic—ROPE (Figs 6.6A and B)

- **Resolution:** Smaller thrombi can completely dissolve by the action of fibrinolytic agents and spontaneous fibrinolysis mediated by plasminogen activator. The superadded action of macrophages aid in scavenging the thrombi.

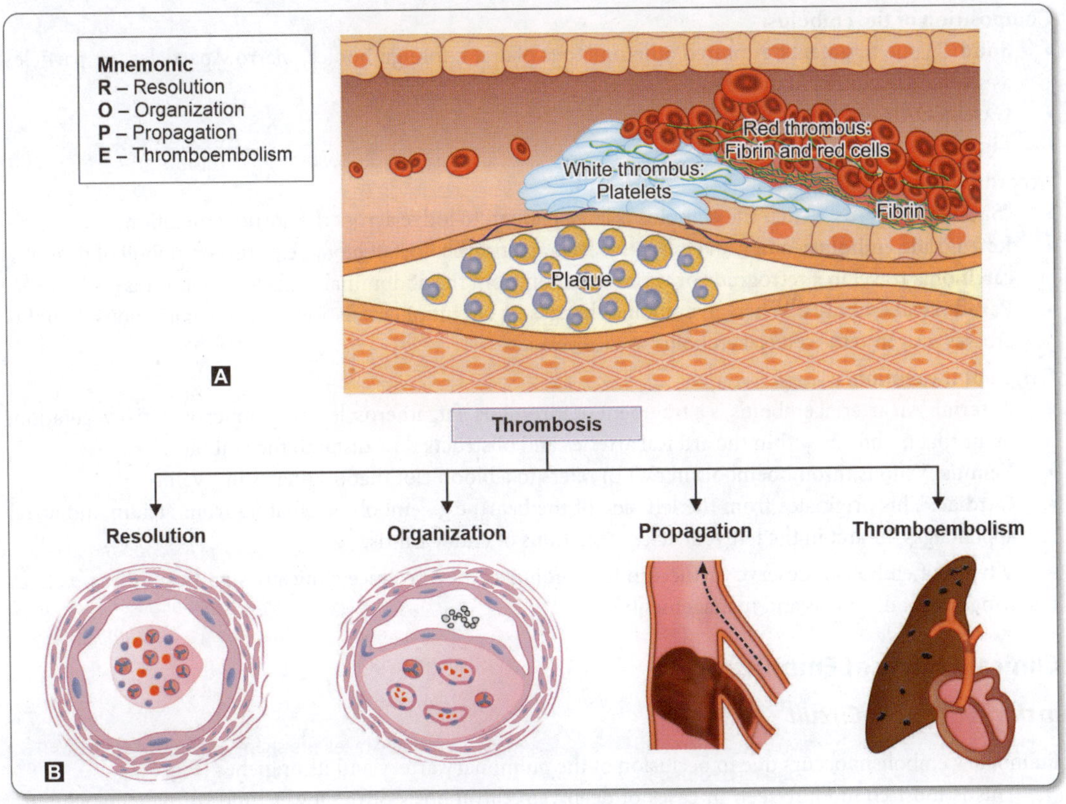

Figures 6.6A and B: Fate of thrombus

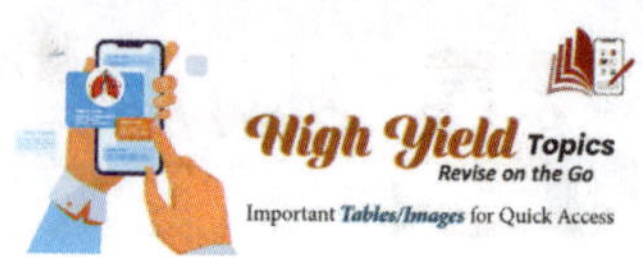

- **Organization:** Persistence of the thrombus is followed by the process of organization in which fibroblasts and capillaries proliferate forming granulation tissue overlayed by endothelial cells, giving an altered lumen referred to as "recanalization". This organized thrombus may also show secondary changes of hyalinization and calcification.
- **Propagation:** Expansion of size of the thrombus due to increasing deposition of fibrin and blood elements primarily red blood cells and platelets, leading to obstruction of the vessel lumen.
- **Embolism:** Fragments of the thrombus may break off to move to a distant site, also known as "embolization".

EMBOLISM

Definition

Partial or complete obstruction by any mass in the lumen of a vessel, carried by the blood stream to a site distant from the origin of the abnormal material. Thromboemboli, or emboli originating from thrombi or their parts get detached from the vessel wall, which accounts for 90% of usual form of emboli.

Types of Embolism

Whether infected or not:

- Septic embolism—shows the presence of infection.
- Bland embolism—superadded infection is absent.

Composition of the embolus:

- **Solid:** Tissue fragments, ruptured atheromatous plaques, foreign bodies, marrow particles, fat particles as seen in fracture of long bones.
- **Gaseous:** Air embolism.
- **Liquid:** Amniotic fluid embolism.

According to the blood flow:

- **"Saddle" embolus:** When the embolus is large enough to lodge across the aortic bifurcation.
- **Retrograde embolus:** When an embolus travels against the flow of blood, e.g., tumor emboli of prostatic carcinoma travel in a retrograde or reverse fashion from the abdominal veins to spinal veins.
- **Paradoxical embolus:** When an embolus changes its circuit of circulation, e.g., when a venous embolus crosses over into the arterial embolus or vice versa.

Origin of the embolus:

- **Arterial:** An arterial embolus is a fragment of thrombus, fat, atherosclerotic plaque, bacterial vegetation, or air that mobilizes within the arterial arteries and obstructs flow distal to the embolus.
- **Venous:** Venous thromboembolism (VTE) refers to a blood clot that originates in a vein.
- **Cardiac:** This originates from the left side of the heart, e.g., emboli originating from atrium and atrial appendages, infarct in the left ventricle, vegetations of endocarditis.

A few types of embolism deserve further understanding as they produce clinically significant disease states requiring urgent diagnosis and management.

Clinical Effects of Embolism

In the Pulmonary Circuit

Pulmonary embolism occurs due to occlusion of the pulmonary artery and its branches (Fig. 6.7).

This is most commonly seen in cases of deep vein thrombosis of the lower limbs of patients who are immobilized on bed for a long time or those who are hospitalized.

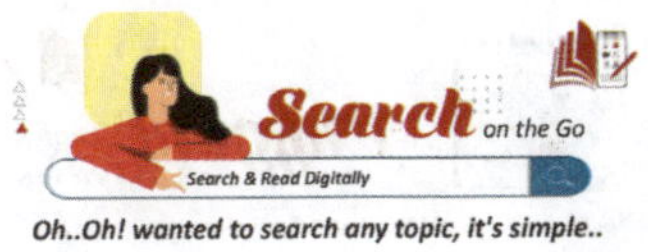

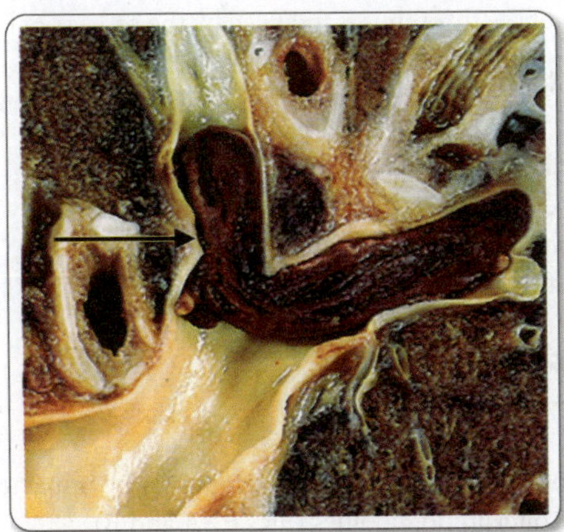

Figure 6.7: Pulmonary emboli: Gross appearance

- Smaller emboli enter the right side of the heart and then subsequently enter the pulmonary vessels blocking them.
- Larger emboli can occlude the vessels completely and when they block the pulmonary artery bifurcation due to size, they are referred to as **"saddle"** embolus.
- Sequelae of pulmonary emboli:
  - Pulmonary hypertension-due to occlusion of pulmonary vessels.
  - Hypoxic injury.
  - Red infarct of the lung.
  - Massive embolism can cause cardiovascular collapse and death.

In the Systemic Circuit

- Heart-Occlusion of the coronary vessels leads to myocardial infarction.
- Renal vessels-renal infarction.
- Brain (cerebral) vessels-stroke.
- Lower limbs-gangrene.
- Intestine-gangrene.

Thromboembolism

When a thrombus detaches from the vessel wall and moves in the circulation, it is called thromboembolism. They may arise in arterial or venous circulation.

Arterial Thromboembolism

- These include vegetations on the mitral or aortic valves, prosthetic heart valves, mural thrombi in the left atrium or ventricle, and cardiomyopathy.
  - 80–58% of the thrombus originates from inside the heart and include cardiomyopathy, vegetations on the aortic or mitral valves, and mural thrombi in the left atrium or ventricle.
  - Causes within the arteries include paradoxical arterial emboli from the systemic venous circulation, aortic aneurysms, pulmonary veins, and emboli forming in relation to atherosclerotic plaques.

Venous Thromboembolism

Venous emboli can originate from the subsequent sources:
- The most frequent cause of venous emboli is thrombus in the lower leg veins.
- Venous thrombi in the pelvic veins.
- Venous thrombi in the upper extremities.
- Brain thrombosis in the cavernous sinus.
- Thrombi in the right side of the heart.

Special Types of Embolism

Fat Embolism

This refers to the partial or complete obstruction of vessel lumina by impacted fat globules. Fat may exist as fibrofatty fragments or as semi-solid/liquid globules (Figs 6.8A and B).

Causes of Fat Embolism

- Fractures of long bones due to trauma.
- Surgical intervention involving musculoskeletal system which involves trauma to the bones.
- Extensive soft tissue or abdominopelvic injury.
- Severe burns.
- Trauma to a liver showing marked fatty change.
- Acute/chronic pancreatitis, leading to leakage of pancreatic enzymes and fat.

Pathogenesis of Fat Embolism

- Mechanical obstruction of the vessel lumen by fibrofatty fragments leads to occlusion and a reduced blood supply.
- **Chemical injury:** Free fatty acids released after the breakdown of fat after traumatic injury have a toxic effect on the vascular endothelial lining due to the liberation of free radicals.
- **Altered emulsion effect:** According to this theory, alteration of emulsion stability of circulating blood lipids, i.e., chylomicrons lead to the formation of composite aggregates of fat globules.

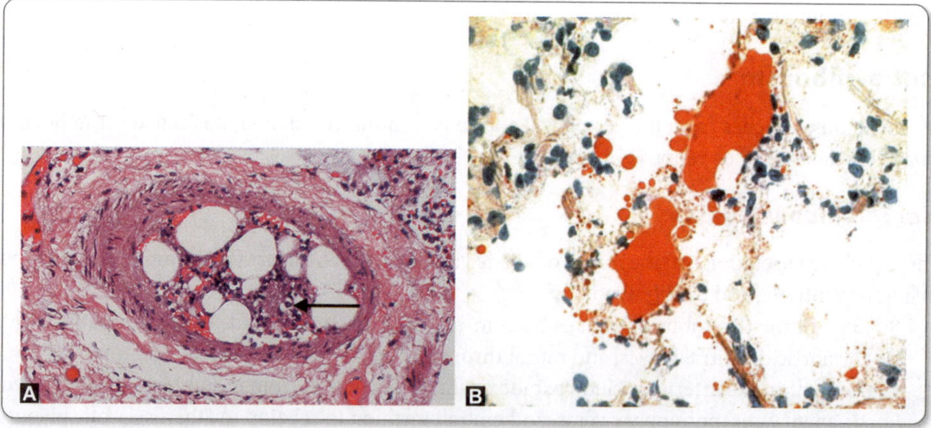

Figures 6.8A and B: **A.** Minimum inhibitory concentration (MIC) showing fat and hematopoietic elements; **B.** Fat emboli highlighted by oil red O

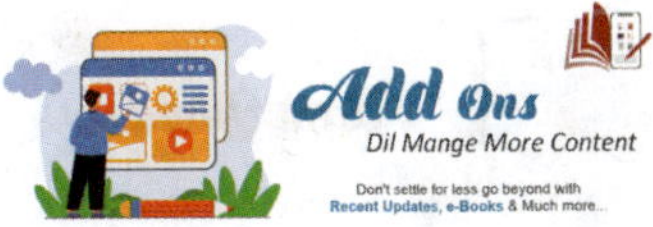

Clinical Presentation

The patient presents with shortness of breath, fever, nausea, increased heart rate (tachycardia), increased respiratory rate (tachypnea), altered sensorium and petechial hemorrhages due to thrombocytopenia.

- Hemorrhages due to thrombocytopenia. Occlusion of the pulmonary microvasculature.
- Shortness of breath and occlusion of the cerebral microvasculature leads to altered sensorium.

Site-wise Effects

Fat embolism presents either as pulmonary embolism, when the obstruction is confined to the pulmonary vessels or systemic embolism when the fat emboli obstruct any of the vessels in the systemic circulation.

Amniotic Fluid Embolism

This type of embolism is caused when amniotic fluid enters the maternal circulation along with fetal tissue including fetal fat, lanugo hair, squamous epithelial cells, fetal respiratory/gastrointestinal lining epithelium and debris (Fig. 6.9).

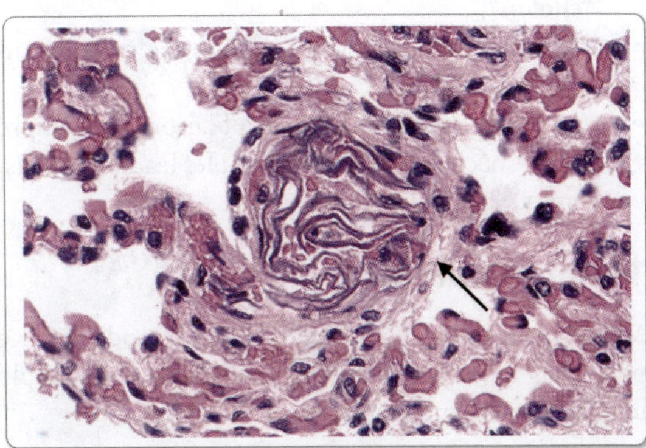

Figure 6.9: Photomicrograph showing amniotic membranes s/o amniotic fluid embolism in lung alveoli

Causes

This can occur in cases of complicated labor or due to intrauterine surgical instrumentation which lead to the development of a tear in the placental membranes. It may even occur within the post-partum period without any causative factors.

Clinical Presentation

The patient presents with sudden onset of shortness of breath (dyspnea), cyanosis, reduced blood pressure (hypotension), seizures, coma, shock and even death.

The nursing professional on duty must be aware of this presentation for the timely management of this condition.

Pathogenesis

- Fetal tissue and fluid can mechanically obstruct the vessels leading to secondary changes of ischemia.
- The fetal cells act as foreign antigens in the circulation and in addition, have thrombogenic action promoting.

Morphological Features

- Sections from the maternal lung show the presence of *fetal squames and debris in the alveolar spaces.*
- Diffuse alveolar damage may be seen which is represented by the presence of *hyaline membranes* lining the alveolar spaces.
- Pulmonary edema may be present.

Air Embolism/Decompression Sickness

The presence of air in the circulation is called air embolism. This may be due to trauma to the chest-either after a surgery or due to an accident. Other causes include introduction of air during intravenous infusion or injecting contrast for radiological techniques/angiography.

When a subject is exposed to changes in atmospheric pressure which are sudden and marked during underwater diving, then air may enter the circulation and this air in the form of gas bubbles can obstruct the circulation. This represents a special form of air embolism called ***decompression sickness***.

A chronic form of decompression sickness seen in deep sea divers who are exposed to sudden alterations in pressure is called ***Caisson's disease***.

The effects of air embolism in decompression sickness include:

- **The "bends":** Occlusion of vessels in the musculoskeletal system lead to muscle and joint pain called the **"bends"** which is taken from the term called Grecian bends, a stooped posture adopted as a fashion trend by Greek women in the late 19th century.
- **The "chokes":** Occlusion of vessels in the pulmonary circulation leads to shortness of breath, called the **"chokes"**.
- **Delirium:** Occlusion of vessels in the cerebral circulation leads to altered mental status (*delirium*) and even seizures.
- **Avascular necrosis:** In cases of chronic decompression sickness (Caisson's disease), vessels of the bone may be occluded by the gas bubbles leading to avascular necrosis of the bones, commonly the long bones-femur, tibia and humerus.

Tumor Embolism

Malignant tumor cells invade the local blood vessels and may form tumor emboli to be lodged elsewhere, producing metastatic tumor deposits. Notable examples are clear cell carcinoma of kidney, carcinoma of the lung, malignant melanoma, etc.

Atheroembolism

Small and medium-sized arteries can become home to atherosclerotic emboli, which are eroded from atheromatous plaques, particularly those originating from the aorta. These emboli can cause a foreign body reaction at the site of lodgement and are composed of calcified material, hyaline debris, and cholesterol crystals.

ISCHEMIA

Ischemia is a phenomenon in which tissue receives insufficient blood supply. The cessation of blood supply may be complete (complete ischemia) or partial (partial ischemia).

The adverse effects of ischemia may result from three ways:

1. **Hypoxia:** Due to lack of oxygen to the tissues. It can be due to low level of oxygen, hemoglobin in the blood or may be due to inadequate blood supply or low oxygen uptake.
2. **Malnourishment of cells:** Commonly due to inadequate supply of nutrients to the tissues (glucose, amino acids).
3. Inadequate clearance of metabolites, which results in accumulation of metabolic waste products in the affected tissue.

Etiology

- **Heart-related factors:**
  - Inadequate cardiac output due to heart block, ventricular arrest and fibrillation.

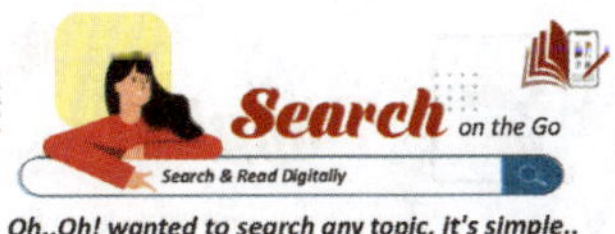

- **Arteries or circulation-related factors:**
  - **Occlusion of artery:** Thrombosis, embolism.
  - **Causes in the arterial wall:** Vasospasm, hypothermia, arteriosclerosis, polyarteritis nodosa.
  - **External pressure on arteries:**
    - Tourniquet
    - Tight plasters, bandages
- **Venous causes:** Blockage of venous drainage may lead to engorgement or obstruction to arterial blood supply causing ischemia. Examples include: Occlusion of vein, varicose veins of leg, strangulated hernia, volvulus, etc.
- **Microcirculation-related factors:** Occlusion or arterioles, venules and capillaries may result in ischemia. Examples include: Sickle cell anemia, fat embolism, bedsores, vasculitis, frost-bite.

Effect of Ischemia

The effect of ischemia can vary, which may include:

- If the collateral channels sufficiently develop to prevent the effects of ischemia from occurring, no effect can be seen over tissues.
- Functional disturbances can occur when blood can flow through collateral channels during regular activity, but not enough to survive the effects of exercise. Intermittent claudication and angina pectoris are the two instances.
- Cellular alterations such as cloudy swelling, fatty changes, ischemic atrophy, and replacement fibrosis can result from partial or progressive ischemia. When the blood supply is entirely deprived, the damaged tissue necrotizes and an infarction occurs.
- Sudden death can result from ischemia, such as myocardial and cerebral infarction.

INFARCTION

Definition

- Localized area of tissue necrosis occurring due to a reduced blood supply (ischemia) leading to decreased perfusion.
- The infarcts may be either red (hemorrhagic) or white (anemic) and may be either septic or bland.
- This may either be due to occlusion of arterial blood supply to a tissue or obstruction to the venous drainage of the affected area. This kind of necrosis when superadded with bacterial infection, is referred to as *gangrene*.
- **Examples:** myocardial infarction (commonly referred to as heart attack), cerebral infarction (clinically manifesting as stroke) and intestinal gangrene.

Causes of Infarction

- **Arterial:** These include all causes of arterial occlusion in which either due to factors within or outside of the artery, blood supply to an organ is compromised. The main factors are:
  - **Atherosclerosis:** Atherosclerotic plaques comprising lipids and foamy macrophages can narrow vessel lumen, also known as *stenosis*.
  - **Thromboembolism:** Both the formation of a thrombus within an artery or its migration to a distant site in the circulation (embolism) can lead to a reduced blood supply.
  - Compression due to a tumor pressing the artery from the outside.

- **Venous:**
  - Obstruction to venous drainage as is seen in cases of *torsion (twisting) of the testis and ovary.*
  - Twisting of an intestinal loop can also lead to reduced venous outflow. This condition is called *volvulus.*

Classification of Infarcts

From a pathological standpoint, the two commonly discussed entities are the red and white infarct (Table 6.3).

Table 6.3: Classification of infarcts

Color	Superadded infection +/–	Time since infarction
Red infarct	Bland infarct	Fresh infarct
White infarct	Septic infarct	Healed infarct

Red Infarct

This type of infarct is also called hemorrhagic infarct and is typically seen in organs with (Figs 6.10A and B):

- A loose spongy parenchyma such as the lung or which can allow percolation of blood into an already infarcted area such as the intestine.
- A double blood supply like the lung and intestine. These organs as described above are already prone to hemorrhagic infarction due to their loose texture. In addition, in these organs, when one blood vessel is obstructed, an infarct develops and the other vessel tries to compensate. The result is percolation of red blood cells in an already infarcted area, hence leading to the red color of the infarct.
- **Venous occlusion** also predisposes to the development of a red infarct.

White Infarct

This type of infarct is also called a pale or anemic infarct and is seen in the following settings (Figs 6.11A and B):

- When the organ is solid, compact and has firm texture.
- When the organ has a single/end arterial blood supply.

Hence, the type and extent of infarction depends on the following factors:

- Rate of occlusion of blood supply.
- Extent of occlusion.
- Type of organ-solid/spongy.
- Type of blood supply to the organ.

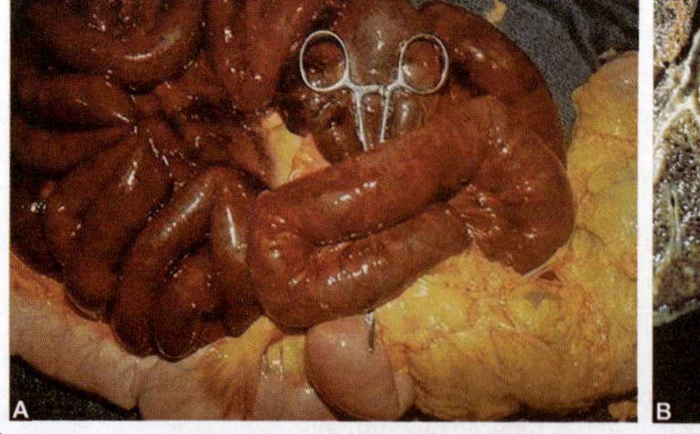

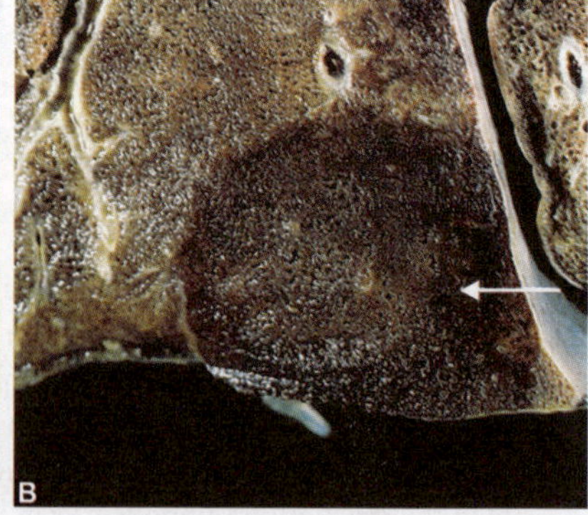

Figures 6.10A and B: Gross appearance **A.** Red infarct in intestine; **B.** Red infarct in lung

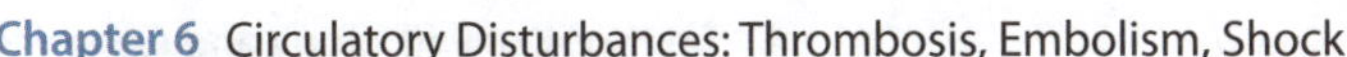

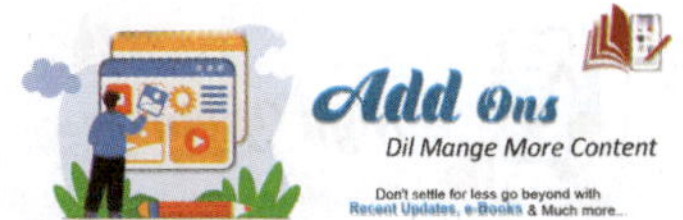

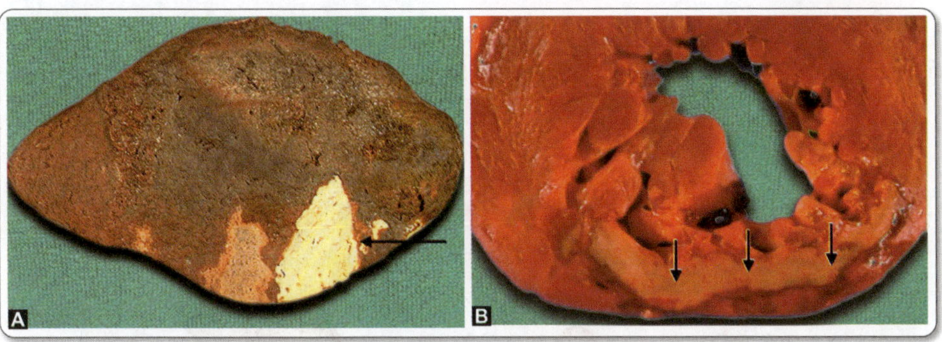

Figures 6.11A and B: Gross appearance **A.** White infarct in spleen; **B.** White infarct in myocardium

Morphological Features

Gross Examination

- **Shape:** Triangular *(wedge)-shaped* with the base at the peripheral surface of the organ and the apex at the occluded vessel.
  Myocardial infarcts and cerebral infarcts are more *irregular* in shape.
- **Consistency:** Soft to firm.
- **Color:** Pale in the case of anemic/white infarct. Anemic infarcts are pale due to destruction of red blood cells. Hemorrhagic infarcts on account of a collateral blood supply show a red color.
- **Margins:** Pale infarcts are well-demarcated and delineated from the uninvolved parenchyma. Hemorrhagic infarcts are distinct but the margins are comparatively less well defined.

Microscopic Examination

- Microscopically, all infarcts are characterized by **coagulative (ischemic) necrosis** in which cell outlines are barely preserved giving a "tombstone" appearance (Fig. 6.12).
- Cerebral infarcts are slightly different morphologically and are characterized by the presence of liquefactive necrosis, characterized by areas of loss of glial cells, inflammation, debris, lipidaceous substance and compensatory areas of reactive gliosis.
- Hemorrhagic infarcts show a preponderance of **hemosiderin laden macrophages** which is lacking in the pale infarcts.
- The boundary of the infarct shows the presence of **inflammatory infiltrate** comprising neutrophils and subsequently, lymphocytes and macrophages.
- Long standing infarcts, with time are replaced by proliferating fibroblasts to form a **scar**, e.g., Healed myocardial infarcts show a loss of cardiac myocytes with intervening areas of collagenous tissue.

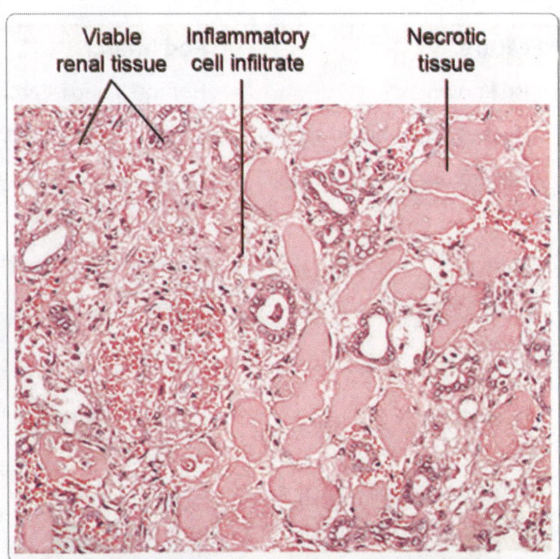

Figure 6.12: Microscopic view of renal infarct, note typical coagulative necrosis of renal tubules and glomeruli

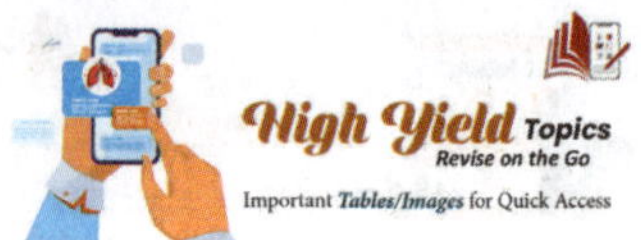

Sites

Various sites of infarcts have been shown in Figure 6.13.

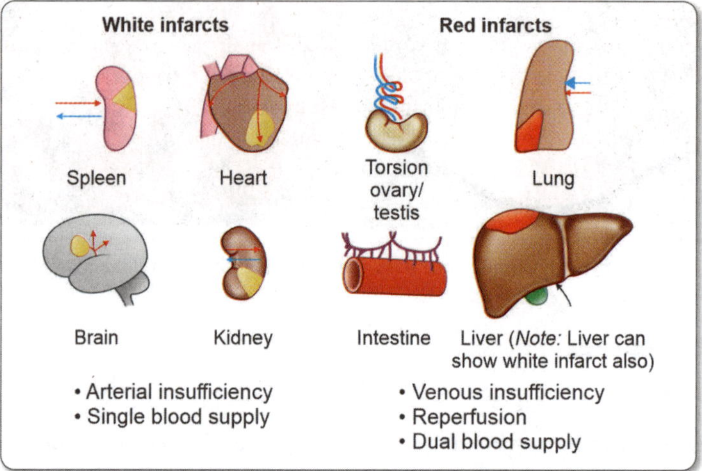

Figure 6.13: White and red infarct sites in different body organs

EXTRA EDGE

Infarct of Zahn: It is a pseudo-infarct (nonischemic infarct) of the liver in which actual ischemic necrosis does not occur. There is obstruction to the portal blood supply leading to atrophy of hepatocytes and accompanying parenchymal collapse.

Table 6.4 does a comparative analysis of red infarct and white infarct.

Table 6.4: Comparative table: Red infarct versus white infarct

Feature	Red infarct	White infarct
Also known as	Hemorrhagic infarct	Pale infarct
Affected organ blood supply	Organs with dual blood supply	Organs with end arterial blood supply
Affected organ texture	Organs with a spongy texture	Organs with a solid texture
Color	Red, hemorrhagic	Pale, white
Cause	Arterial/venous occlusion	Usually arterial occlusion
Shape	No specific shape	Wedge-shaped, apex at the occlusion site, marked demarcation from surrounding parenchyma
Margins	Not very sharply defined	Sharply-defined, well-circumscribed lesion distinct from surrounding parenchyma
Microscopic appearance	Coagulative necrosis	Coagulative necrosis with inflammation at the boundary
	Hemosiderin laden macrophages present	Hemosiderin laden macrophages absent
Example:	Lung infarction	Splenic, renal infarct

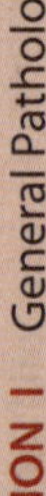

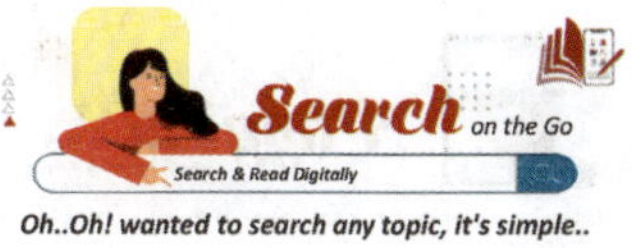

SHOCK

Definition

It can be defined as a clinicopathological state resulting from inadequate tissue perfusion. The key feature is *reduced blood circulation* leading to *hypoxic damage* of the cells and tissues. These pathways have the potential to cause cellular death and decreased metabolism, if uncompensated.

When a transient, benign vasovagal attack occurs due to a sudden reduction in venous return to the heart, neurogenic vasodilation causes peripheral blood pooling. This can happen immediately after trauma, severe pain, or an emotional overreaction such as grief, surprise, or fear. This condition is referred to as "initial (or primary) shock".

"True (or secondary) shock", also known as circulatory shock, is a circulatory imbalance between the supply and needs of oxygen at the cellular level.

Inadequate blood supply to key organs of the body such as the heart, brain and kidneys can even lead to death, hence timely recognition of shock and understanding its pathogenesis is extremely important.

Clinical Features

The patient presents with low blood pressure (hypotension)

- Increased pulse rate (tachycardia).
- Feeble/weakly felt pulse.
- Increased respiratory rate (tachypnea).
- Shallow respiration.
- Cold clammy extremities.
- Reduced urinary output (oliguria).
- Drowsiness/confusion.

In addition, *specific features* may be seen according to the type of shock present, e.g., Urticaria (hives), wheezing, edema in anaphylactic shock, elevated jugular venous pressure in cardiogenic shock, fever/cellulitis (skin infection) in septic shock, urinary incontinence in neurogenic shock.

Clinical complications include acute renal failure, disseminated intravascular coagulation, multiorgan dysfunctional syndrome and acute respiratory distress syndrome.

Types of Shock

Shock is of four types as per recent classification systems:

1. **Cardiogenic:** This type of shock is characterized by a sudden reduction in cardiac output because of cardiac pathology (pump failure) leading to hypoperfusion of multiple organs.
2. **Hypovolemic:** In hypovolemic shock, reduction of cardiac output occurs due to marked decrease of effective circulating blood volume. This could either be due to hemorrhage/burns/severe gastroenteritis with profuse diarrhea or vomiting. The result is reduced perfusion affecting tissue metabolism. A special form of shock is the *traumatic hemorrhagic shock* in which fractures to multiple bones aggravates inflammatory response, worsening shock.
3. **Distributive shock:** This type of shock arises from relative hypovolemia, which occurs due to excessive dilation of blood vessels leading to an abnormal redistribution of the intravascular volume, i.e., vessels dilate to the extent where normal blood pressure required for circulation is not maintained.

   Distributive shock is further of three types:

   i. **Septic:** This occurs in the setting of severe, often life-threatening bacterial infections, more commonly due to gram positive rather than gram negative bacteria. It is characterized by a markedly abnormal or dysregulated response to bacterial infection involving vasodilation and increased

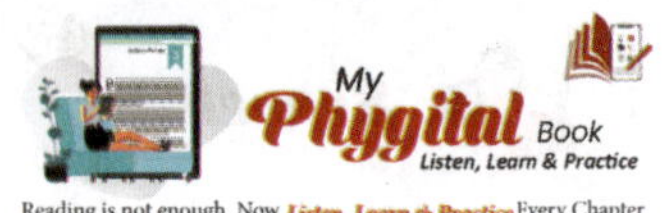

capillary permeability leading to loss of intravascular fluid (Sepsis-3 criteria). The three criteria used to define septic shock include:

- Reduced blood pressure (hypotension) requiring usage of vasopressors.
- An elevated serum lactate (>2 mmol/L).
- Persisting shock despite IV fluids.

ii. **Neurogenic:** Loss of vasomotor tone of blood vessels leads to pooling/stagnation of blood in the large vessels. Circulation of blood is reduced again leading to decreased tissue perfusion. This is seen in cases where there is an injury to the spinal cord.

iii. **Anaphylactic shock:** IgE mediated hypersensitivity reactions can lead to pronounced vasodilatation.

4. **Obstructive shock:** Obstruction to the flow of the blood itself leads to a reduced venous return. This can occur in causes such as cardiac tamponade and tension pneumothorax.

Stages of Shock

- **Compensated phase:** This is reversible. To maintain adequate tissue perfusion, a number of compensatory neurohormonal mechanisms are activated. This includes:
  - Constriction of blood vessels which increases the heart rate and cardiac output.
  - Release of catecholamines such as epinephrine and norepinephrine from the adrenal gland which have a vasopressor action, i.e., increase the heart rate, blood pressure and thus cardiac output.
  - **Retention of fluid by kidneys:** In the early phase of shock, renin-angiotensin -aldosterone mechanism is activated. This causes sodium retention which leads to conservation of fluid by osmosis.
- **Progressive decompensated:** The second phase is characterized by progressive clinical deterioration, persisting hypoperfusion of the tissues leading to hypoxic/ischemic injury and switch from aerobic to anaerobic metabolism leading to lactic acidosis. In this stage, the vessel tone starts diminishing (vasodilation) leading to pooling of blood compromising circulation and perfusion.
- **Irreversible phase:** This is the stage when all compensatory mechanisms have failed and the patient clinically deteriorates further. There is increased vascular permeability and release of cytokines.

Morphological Findings in Shock

- **Lung:** Diffuse alveolar damage with the presence of thickened hyaline membranes lining the alveoli, congestion of alveolar capillaries, pulmonary edema in cases of left-sided heart failure.
- **Hematological/hemodynamic manifestations:** Disseminated intravascular coagulation (DIC) widespread microthrombi, vessel thrombi.
- **Renal:** Acute tubular necrosis.
- **Liver:** Fatty change, centrilobular necrosis.
- **Heart:** Fatty change, subendocardial hemorrhage.
- **Brain:** Hypoxic encephalopathy.
- **Pituitary:** Hypoxia leads to necrosis.
- **Gastrointestinal tract:** Ulceration with burns (curling ulcer), hemorrhage in the intestinal mucosa.
- **Adrenals:** Adrenal cortical cell depletion, necrosis, hemorrhage.

EXTRA EDGE

Morphologic Features

Hypoxic encephalopathy: A changed state of consciousness may result from cerebral ischemia in compensated shock. The region that is supplied by the cerebral arteries' most distal branches—typically the area separating the anterior and middle cerebral arteries—generally experiences significant ischemic necrosis. Changes become apparent at the microscopic level when ischemia persists for a full day or more. Purkinje cells in particular are more vulnerable to the effects of ischemia in neurons. The impacted neurons have a tiny, pyknotic nucleus and highly eosinophilic cytoplasm. Gliosis replaces dead and dying nerve cells.

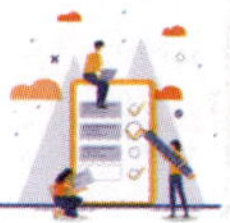

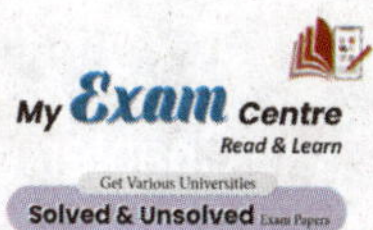

SUMMARY

- The formation of a solid or semi-solid mass within the lumen of a blood vessel is called **thrombosis**.
- Embolism is the partial or complete obstruction by any mass in the lumen of a vessel, carried by the blood stream to a site distant from the origin of the abnormal material.
- When a thrombus detaches from the vessel wall and moves in the circulation, it is called thromboembolism.
- The presence of air in the circulation is called air embolism.
- Infarction is localized area of tissue necrosis occurring due to a reduced blood supply (ischemia) leading to decreased perfusion.
- Shock can be defined as a clinicopathological state resulting from inadequate tissue perfusion.

ASSESS YOURSELF

Long Answer Questions

1. Define shock and explain its stages and morphological features.
2. Explain infarction and various morphological factors seen in infarction.

Short Answer Questions

1. Define Thromboembolism.
2. What is fat embolism?
3. Write short notes on:
   i. Red infarct and white infarct
   ii. Types of shock

Multiple Choice Questions

1. **What is the most common site of origin of thrombotic pulmonary emboli?**
   a. Lumen of left ventricle
   b. Deep leg veins
   c. Lumen of right ventricle
   d. Mesenteric veins
2. **Line of Zahn is seen in:**
   a. Venous thrombi
   b. Pulmonary congestion
   c. Postmortum clot
   d. Arterial thrombi
3. **The most common site of venous thrombosis is:**
   a. Brain
   b. Kidney
   c. Legs
   d. Liver
4. **Mural thrombi is the term used to define thrombi of:**
   a. Thrombi of heart valve
   b. Venous thrombi of the legs
   c. Thrombi of atherosclerotic coronary arteries
   d. Thrombi occurring in the heart chambers
5. **Endothelial cell injury is the principal mechanism for production of thrombosis in case of:**
   a. Thrombosis occurring in postpartum women
   b. Thrombosis associated with pancreatic cancer
   c. Thrombosis of atherosclerotic coronary arteries
   d. Protein C deficiency

Answer Key

1. b **2.** d **3.** c **4.** c **5.** c

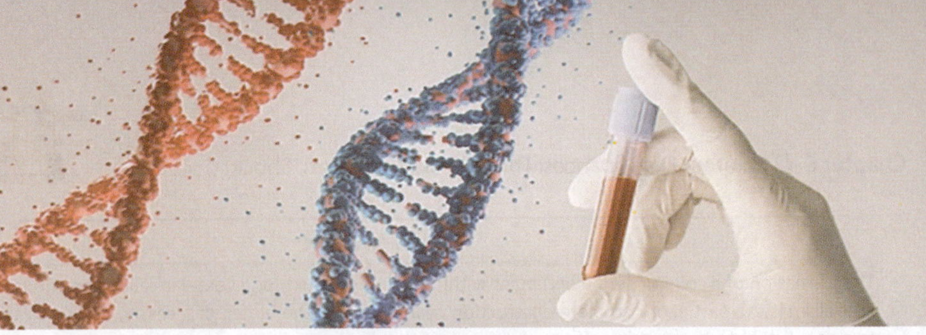

Chapter 7

Disturbances of Body Fluids and Electrolytes

LEARNING OBJECTIVES

After the completion of the chapter, the readers will be able to:

- Understand the normal fluid balance.
- Discuss edema and its types.
- Explain the pathogenetic mechanisms of the type of edema.
- Understand the different types of electrolyte imbalance and how to calculate anion gap.
- Know the types of hemodynamic derangements and their morphological features.

CHAPTER OUTLINE

- Introduction
- Disturbances in Body Fluid
- Electrolyte Disturbances
- Acid-Base Imbalances
- Derangements in Blood Flow (Circulatory/ Hemodynamic Disturbances)

KEY TERMS

Anasarca: Severe generalized accumulation of fluid or edema in the interstitial space.

Congestion: Poor venous outflow is referred to as congestion of the veins or passive hyperemia.

Edema: Edema is swelling of soft tissues due to increased interstitial fluid.

Exudates: Exudates are usually unilateral and result from increased capillary permeability or decreased lymphatic resorption associated with infection, connective tissue disease, pancreatitis or cancer.

Hyperemia: The increased volume from arterial and arteriolar dilatation, is referred to as hyperaemia.

Respiratory alkalosis: A decrease in the blood's bicarbonate level and an excess of H^+ ions cause the blood pH to drop as a result of metabolic processes.

Transudates: Transudates are usually bilateral and arise from either increased capillary hydrostatic pressure or decreased oncotic pressure secondary to congestive heart failure, fluid overload, cirrhosis or hypoalbuminemia.

INTRODUCTION

The internal environment, also known as the "milieu interieur", was first described by Claude Bernard in 1949 to document the environment in which the tissues and cells of the body retain their normal morphology and function due to the interstitial fluid that surrounds them and the plasma. Homeostasis is the process by which the consistency of interior environment is preserved and guaranteed.

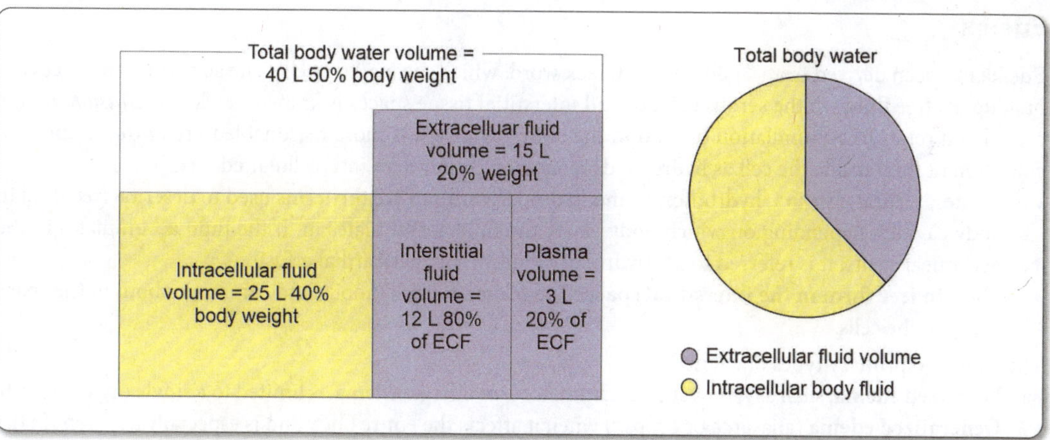

Figure 7.1: Distribution of body fluid

The following elements make up a typical interior environment composition:

- **Water:** The primary and most important component of the body is water. In a typical adult male, total body water makes up 50–70% (on average 60%) of body weight; in a typical adult female, total body water makes up roughly 10% less (on average 50%). As a result, a typical male 65 kg body has about 40 liters of water in it. There are two primary compartments of bodily fluids, separated from one another by freely permeable membranes, which hold 60% of the total body water in average (Fig. 7.1):
    1. **Intracellular fluid compartment:** It is the fluid compartment inside cells. This makes up roughly 40% of the body weight, the majority of which is made up of muscles.
    2. **The extracellular fluid compartment:** This is the remaining 20% of body weight that is made up of water. This includes the four extracellular fluid (ECF) subdivisions listed here:
        i. Interstitial fluid including lymph fluid.
        ii. Intravascular fluid or blood plasma.
        iii. Mesenchymal tissues.
        iv. Transcellular fluid.
- **Electrolytes:** The concentration of negatively-charged anions to positively-charged cations varies in intracellular and extracellular fluids.
- The primary anions in intracellular fluid are proteins and phosphates, whereas the primary cations are potassium and magnesium. Its sodium and chloride concentrations are lowest.
- Sodium is the main cation and chloride and bicarbonate are the main anions in the extracellular fluid. In addition to these, the ECF contains a negligible amount of nondiffusible proteins as well as some diffusible nutrients and metabolites including glucose and urea.

DISTURBANCES IN BODY FLUID

The common dearangements in body include:

- Edema.
- Dehydration.
- Over-hydration.

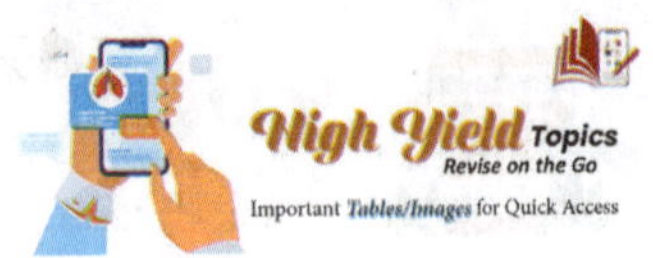

Edema

Edema has been derived from, "Oidein" is a Greek word, which means "to swell". The abnormal and excessive buildup of "free fluid" in the serous cavities and interstitial tissue spaces is known as edema. *Effusion*, on the other hand refers to accumulation of fluid in the body cavities. It is more reasonable to refer to the aberrant collection of fluid inside the cell as hydropic degeneration rather than intracellular edema:

- Ascites, pleural effusion, hydrothorax, and hydropericardium are the terms used to describe free fluid in body cavities, depending on which body cavity the fluid accumulates in. If the fluid accumulates in the peritoneal cavity, it is referred to as "hydropericardium" or "pericardial effusion".
- **Fluid in free form in the interstitial space:** The edema fluid is mobile and can move about in the space between the cells.

There are two primary types of edema:

1. **Localized edema**, such as lymphatic, inflammatory, or allergic edema, is limited to a single organ or limb.
2. **Generalized edema** (anasarca or dropsy) when it affects the entire body and is especially apparent in the subcutaneous tissues, such as in the case of renal, cardiac, or nutritional edema.

MUST KNOW

Examples of effusions include:

- **Ascites:** Fluid in the peritoneal cavity (Fig. 7.2).
- **Pleural effusion:** Fluid in the pleural cavity (Fig. 7.2).
- **Hydrothorax:** Fluid in the thoracic cavity (Fig. 7.2).
- **Pericardial effusion:** Fluid in the pericardial cavity.

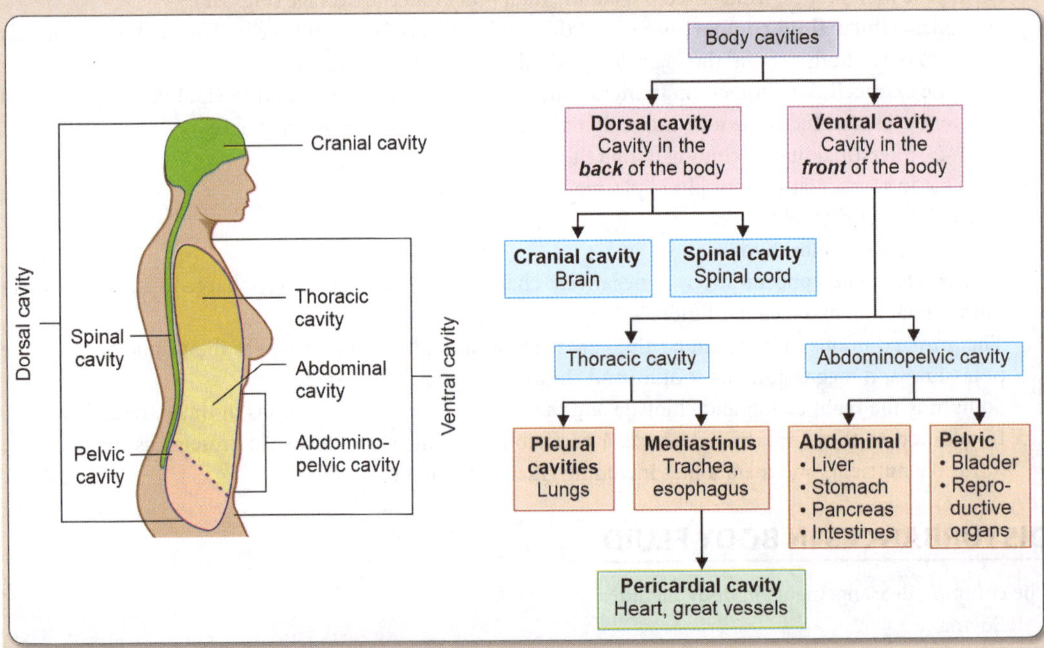

Figure 7.2: Body cavities

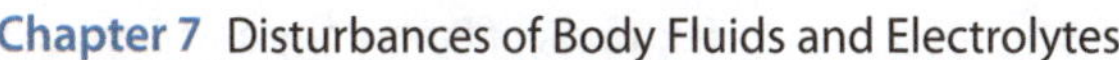

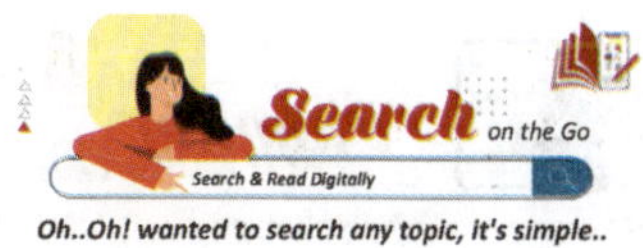

Table 7.1: Characteristic features of transudate and exudate

Characteristics	Transudate	Exudate
Mechanism	Due to increased hydrostatic pressure with normal vascular permeability	Due to increase in vascular permeability caused by inflammatory mediators
Gross appearance of fluid	Clear	Cloudy/turbid, sometimes hemorrhagic
Color	Colorless/Straw yellow	Yellow/red
Specific gravity	<1.018	>1.018
Protein content	Low	High
Formation of clot	Absent	Clots spontaneously due to the presence of fibrinogen
Cell count	Low	High
Cell type	Occasional lymphocytes	Neutrophils (acute), lymphocytes (chronic)
Bacterial growth	Absent	Usually present
Examples	Congestive heart failure	Bacterial infection

Types of Edema

- **Depending on association with inflammation-Inflammatory (exudative) and non-inflammatory (transudative):** Edema may be secondary to an inflammatory process associated with infection or other disease(s). It may also be free of an inflammatory exudate, as seen in conditions of hemodynamic derangement, e.g., cardiac edema. Differences between the transudate and exudate seen in both these types of edema are enumerated in Table 7.1.
- **Depending on extent-localized/generalized:** When edema is confined to a restricted area in the body, it is referred to as being localized. Examples include varicose veins, thrombophlebitis, lymphatic obstruction due to trauma and myxedema in hypothyroid patients which is seen in the shins of the patient (pretibial myxedema).

  Generalized edema is usually seen in patients of cardiac disease, renal disease.
- **Depending on the clinical presentation—pitting/nonpitting:** When after applying pressure on the edematous area, if the skin shows a "pit" or indentation, it is called pitting type of edema, e.g., cardiac failure. On the other hand, lack of any skin changes on applying pressure is seen in the case of non-pitting edema, e.g., myxedema.

  Fluid accumulated in the interstitial space/body cavities may be protein-poor (transudate) or protein-rich (exudate) (Table 7.1 or Fig. 7.3).

Pathogenesis of Edema

Mechanisms that disrupt the regular balance of plasma, interstitial fluid, and lymph flow are the root cause of edema. The following processes could be operating alone or in combination to cause edema. Edema develops when the net rate of fluid movement is greater than the rate of lymphatic drainage.

Five factors can contribute to the formation of edema. There are various factors in the development of edema discussed as follows:

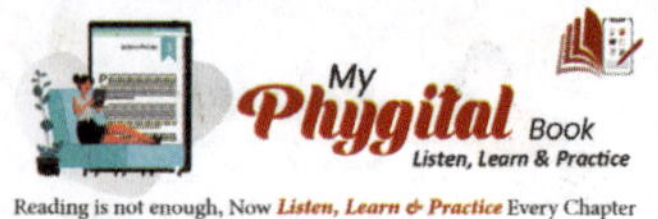

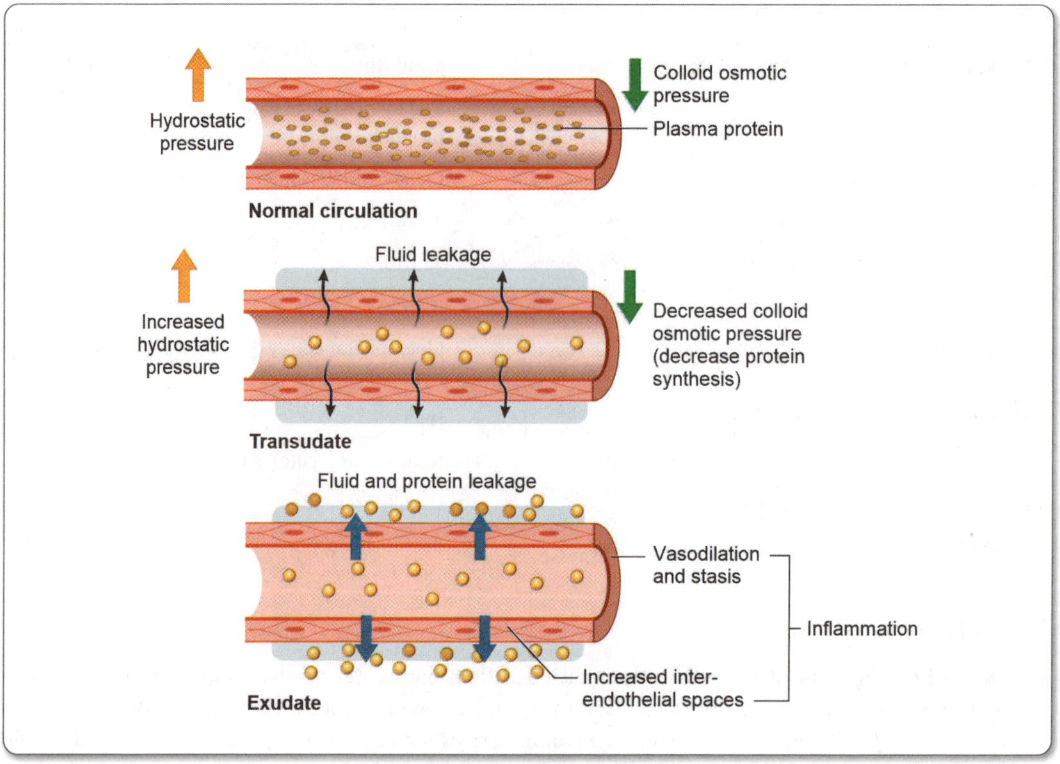

Figure 7.3: Transudate and exudate

Increased Capillary Hydrostatic Pressure (Fig. 7.4)

When the force pushing fluid out of small blood vessels (capillaries) is stronger than the force pulling it back in, it causes swelling called edema. This happens when the pressure is too high at the end of these vessels, preventing proper fluid reabsorption.

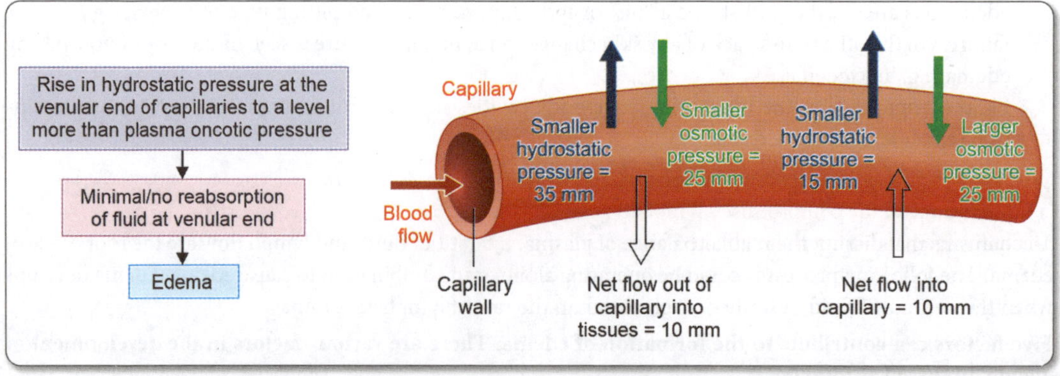

Figure 7.4: Mechanism of edema formation due to increased capillary hydrostatic pressure

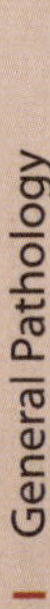

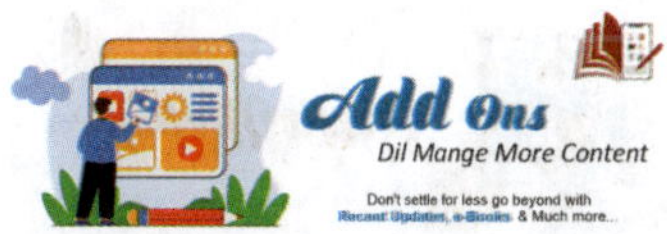

Examples

- Impaired venous return.
- Congestive heart failure.
- Constrictive pericarditis.
- Ascites (liver cirrhosis).
- Venous obstruction or compression.
- Thrombosis.
- External pressure (e.g., mass).
- Lower extremity inactivity with prolonged dependency.
- Arteriolar dilation.
- Heat.
- Neurohumoral dysregulation.

Reduced albumin synthesis in liver/protein malnutrition → Fall in plasma oncotic pressure → Net movement of fluid into interstitial tissues → Edema

Figure 7.5: Mechanism of edema formation due to reduced plasma oncotic pressure

Reduced Plasma Oncotic Pressure

When the liver produces less albumin (a type of protein) or when the body lacks enough protein due to malnutrition, the oncotic pressure in the blood drops. This reduction in oncotic pressure disrupts the balance, causing fluid to move from blood vessels into the surrounding tissues. This imbalance results in edema (Fig. 7.5).

Example

All conditions causing protein loss/reduced levels of body protein include:

- Cirrhosis.
- Malnutrition.
- Protein losing enteropathy.
- Protein losing nephropathy (nephrotic syndrome).

Inflammation

Capillary endothelial injury, triggered by toxins, histamine, anoxia, or drugs, induces gaps in the endothelial layer which allows plasma proteins to escape into the interstitial spaces. Consequently, there is a decline in plasma oncotic pressure due to the loss of proteins. This imbalance leads to the movement of fluid from the blood vessels into the interstitial spaces, resulting in edema accumulation of fluid in the tissues (Fig. 7.6).

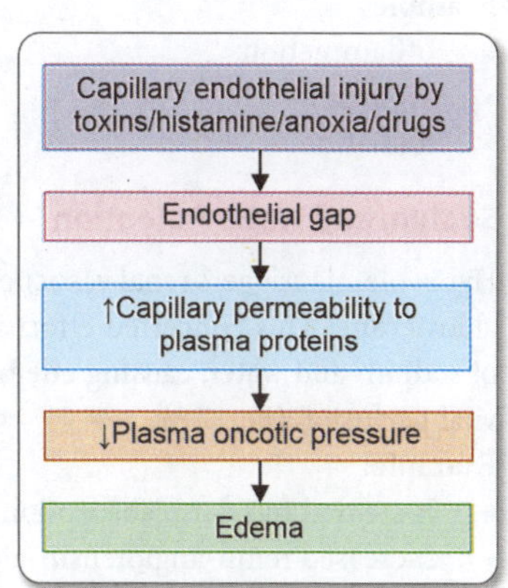

Figure 7.6: Mechanism of edema formation due to capillary endothelial injury

Examples

- Inflammation.
- Angiogenesis.

Impaired Lymphatic Drainage

Impaired lymphatic drainage leads to localized lymphedema. In these instances, the compromised lymphatic system fails to efficiently drain fluid from the affected area, resulting in the accumulation of lymph and subsequent swelling. Conditions that impede lymphatic flow contribute to the development of lymphedema, which often manifests as persistent localized swelling in the affected region (Fig. 7.7).

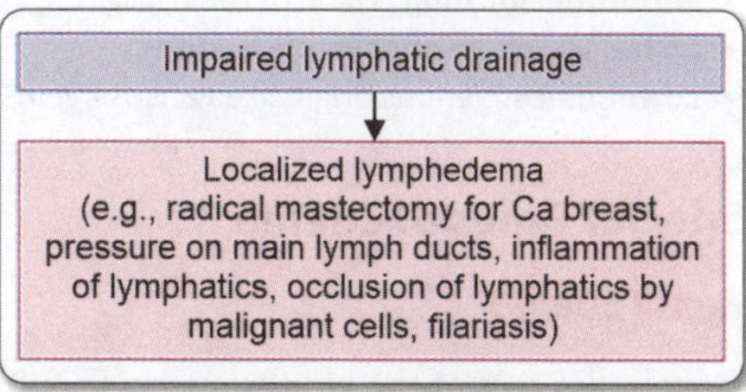

Figure 7.7: Mechanism of edema formation due to impaired lymphatic drainage

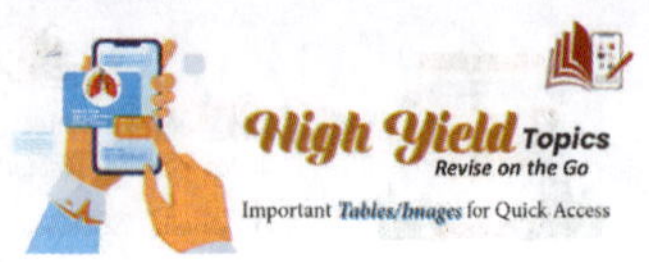

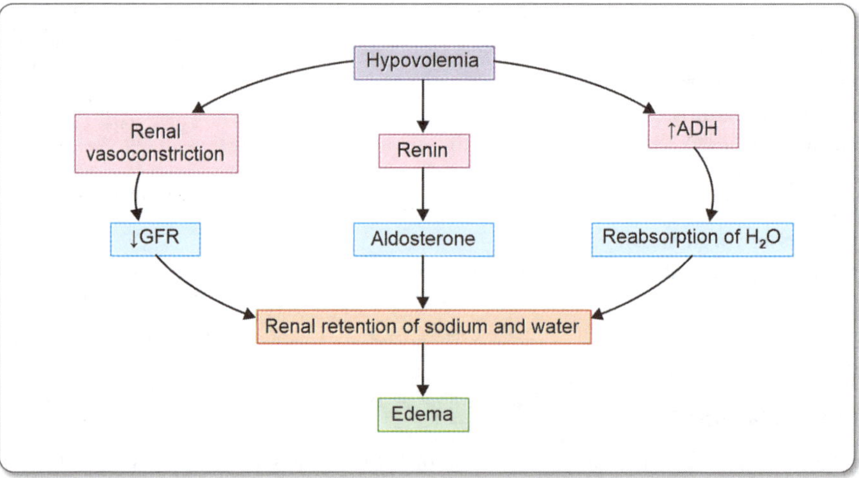

Figure 7.8: Mechanism of edema formation due to sodium and water retention

Examples

- Inflammation.
- Trauma.
- Radiation.
- Parasitic infection.
- Malignancy.

Sodium and Water Retention

Hypovolemia triggers renal vasoconstriction, stimulating renin release and subsequent activation of ADH and aldosterone. This concerted effort increases water reabsorption, lowers GFR, and promotes renal retention of sodium and water, causing edema. The coordinated response aims to restore blood volume and maintain vital perfusion (Fig. 7.8).

Example:

- Increased tubular reabsorption of sodium.
- Increased renin-angiotensin-aldosterone secretion.
- Increased salt intake but poor renal function.
- Decreased blood supply to kidney because of CVS disease.

NURSING CONSIDERATIONS

- **Periorbital location:** Think of renal origin.
- **Shins:** Myxedema of hypothyroidism.
- **Lower limbs:** Venous origin like varicose veins.

Special Types of Edema

Renal Edema

Certain diseases of the kidney, such as nephrotic syndrome, various forms of glomerulonephritis, and acute tubular injury-induced renal failure, can cause generalized edema. It often appears initially in parts of the body containing loose connective tissue such as eyelids.

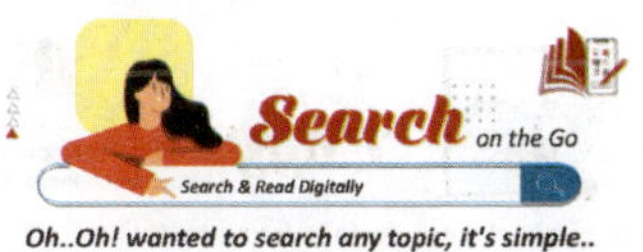

Heavy proteinuria (albuminuria) in nephrotic syndrome causes decreased oncotic pressure resulting in severe generalized edema. Nephritic edema differs from nephrotic edema in that hypoproteinemia is not the cause. But is mostly caused by the renal tubules' increased reabsorption of water and salt through the renin-angiotensin-aldosterone pathway.

Microscopically, the edema fluid divides the subcutaneous tissues' connective tissue fibers under a microscope. The edema fluid can appear homogenous, pale, and eosinophilic or it can be profoundly eosinophilic and granular, depending on the protein concentration.

Cardiac Edema

When a patient has both congestive and right-sided heart failure, generalized edema occurs. The following theories provide an explanation for the pathogenesis of cardiac edema.

Cardiac edema is a type of edema that is typically reliant on gravity; in an ambulatory patient, it affects the lower extremities, whereas in a bedridden patient, it affects the sacrum and genital areas. Serous cavities might also experience fluid buildup.

Cerebral Edema

- Swollen brain exhibits narrowed sulci and distended gyri, compressed by unyielding skull.
- It is life-threatening, if severe, it can lead to herniation of brain substance through foramen magnum or compression of brain stem vascular supply.

Pulmonary Edema

- Acute pulmonary edema has unique characteristics. It produces significant functional impairment and is the most significant type of local edema. It varies from edema elsewhere in that the pulmonary alveoli are also affected by the fluid buildup in addition to the tissue space.
- In the pulmonary capillaries, the hydrostatic pressure is substantially lower (average 10 mm Hg). Normally, there is no edema in the lungs because the plasma oncotic pressure is sufficient to stop fluid from escaping into the interstitial space. Either an increase in pulmonary hydrostatic pressure or a rise in capillary permeability can cause pulmonary edema.
- Pulmonary edema is characterized by heavy, moist and sub-crepitant lungs. Frothy fluid (a combination of fluid and air) is exuded from the cut surface.
- The alveolar capillaries are clogged at the microscopic level.
- Initially excess fluid collects in the interstitial between the lungs (interstitial edema).

Cerebral Edema

Edema that poses the greatest concern is cerebral edema, or swelling of the brain. The brain's fluid exchange system is different from that of other parts of the body because the brain lacks draining lymphatics. Instead, the blood-brain barrier, which is found at the endothelial cells of the capillaries, is responsible for fluid-electrolyte exchange.

Cerebral edema can be of three types:

1. Vasogenic edema.
2. Cytotoxic edema.
3. Interstitial edema.

Microscopically, the white matter is soft, swollen and characterized by restricted sulci and flattened gyri. The surface is gelatinous and softly divided.

On a microscopic level, astrocyte swelling and tissue element separation caused by edema fluid are visible. There is an enlargement of the perivascular (Virchow-Robin) space and the small blood vessels are surrounded by transparent halos.

Dehydration

It is the state in which body gets deprived of water. Excessive loss of water from body is called dehydratin.
Examples: Vomiting, diarrhea.

Overhydration

It is the state in which the body is deprived of water, usually due to excessive loss of water from the body.
Examples: Renal dysfunction, cirrhosis, etc.

ELECTROLYTE DISTURBANCES

The balance of electrolytes in the body is essential to maintain normal bodily functions. Clinical knowledge of electrolyte imbalance is essential for all nursing personnel as in various clinical settings rapid decline in clinical outcomes is seen due to acid-base derangements.

The normal distribution of ions in the body:

- **Cations/positively charged ions involved in acid base balance:** Na^+, K^+, Mg^{2+}, Ca^{2+}
- **Anions or negatively charged ions involved in acid base balance:** HCO_3^-, Cl^- and organic acids in the bloodstream. The compartment-wise distribution of ions is:
  - **Intravascular compartment:** This shows a predominance of calcium, potassium and magnesium ions (Mnemonic: K-IN (potassium, calcium-IN)
  - **Extravascular compartment (extracellular fluid):** This has a higher concentration of sodium, chloride and bicarbonate

EXTRA EDGE

The normal reference ranges for electrolytes

Electrolyte	Normal
Na^+	135–145 mEq/L
K^+	3.5–5.2 mEq/L
Cl^-	96–106 mEq/L
HCO_3^-	22–30 mEq/L

The net sum of all positively- and negatively-charged species in the body in the normal state should be equal.

- One or more conditions may be the cause of an electrolyte imbalance in a particular instance.
- The abnormal serum levels of multiple electrolytes could be related to one another. For example, anomalous serum levels of sodium, potassium, calcium, and phosphate, for instance.
- Rather than morphological signs in organs, metabolic syndrome and clinical symptoms are typically the reflection of biochemical serum electrolyte levels.

The clinical manifestations of a specific electrolyte imbalance in particular organ or tissue is associated to its clinical symptoms.

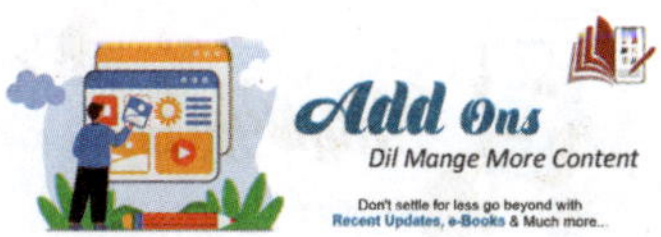

Major electrolyte imbalances are as follows:

Sodium

Imbalance in sodium causes the following two major conditions:

Hyponatremia	Hypernatremia
Gain of relatively more water than loss of sodium: • Overuse of diuretics • Excessive IV infusion of 5% dextrose • Addison's disease • Hypotonic fluid irrigation	Gain of relatively more salt than loss of water: • IV infusion of hypertonic solution • Excessive sweating
Loss of relatively more salt than water: • Renal failure • Excessive use of diuretics	Loss of relatively more water than salt: • Diabetes insipidus

Potassium

Imbalance in potassium gives rise to major conditions which are as follows:

Hypokalemia	Hyperkalemia
Decreased potassium intake: • Anorexia • Fasting • Diet low in potassium	Excessive potassium intake: • Rapid infusion containing potassium • Large volume of transfusion of stored blood
Excessive potassium excretion: • Loss from GI tract (vomiting, diarrhea, laxative) • Loss from kidneys (corticosteroid therapy, cushing syndrome, etc.)	Decreased potassium excretion: • Oliguric phase of ARF • Addison's disease
Excessive mobilization from extracellular to intracellular compartment: • Alkalosis • Excess insulin therapy	Excessive mobilization from intracellular into extracellular compartment: • Hemolysis • Insufficient insulin

Calcium

Imbalance of calcium in the body can manifest in two forms:

Hypocalcemia	Hypercalcemia
• Vitamin D deficiency • Hypoparathyroidism	• Hyperparathyroidism • Carcinoma breast • Carcinoma lung

ACID-BASE IMBALANCES

Carbon dioxide and metabolic acids are produced during cell metabolism. Carbon dioxide reacts with water to form carbonic acid. The bicarbonate buffering system plays a role in the extracellular compartment.

In order to achieve acid-base homeostasis to maintain blood pH of 7.4, both carbonic acid and metabolic acids must be expelled from the body *via* lungs (for CO_2) and kidneys (for metabolic acids). The pH of blood depends upon two principal factors:

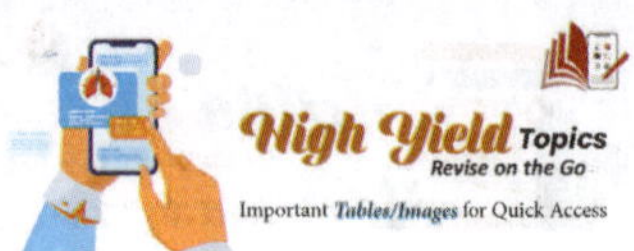

1. Serum concentration of bicarbonate.
2. Partial pressure of CO_2 that determines the concentration of carbonic acid.

MUST KNOW

If pCO_2 is increased and pH is less (that is as per expected lines)—Respiratory acidosis.
If HCO_3^- is decreased and pH is less—Metabolic acidosis.
If pCO_2 is decreased and pH is increased—Respiratory alkalosis.
If HCO_3^- is increased and pH is increased—Metabolic alkalosis.

Respiratory Alkalosis

A decrease in the bicarbonate level of blood and an excess of H^+ ions cause the blood pH to drop as a result of metabolic processes. This happens in the subsequent circumstances:

Hyperventilation of the lungs leads to low pCO_2 levels elevating the blood pH

- Anxiety
- High altitude
- CNS infection
- Drug induced hyperventilation
- Meningitis

Respiratory Acidosis

Respiratory acidosis is a drop in blood pH caused by elevated pCO_2 as a result of inadequate lung ventilation (CO_2 retention).

A reduced breathing rate or hypoventilation leads to pCO_2 elevation and a dip in pH, causing respiratory acidosis.

- Chronic obstructive pulmonary disease (COPD).
- Impairment in the neuromuscular function, e.g., Parkinson's disease.
- Restricted mobility because of kyphoscoliosis/thoracic deformity.

Metabolic Alkalosis

Metabolic alkalosis is characterized by rise in blood pH, caused by decrease in H^+ ions and an increase in plasma bicarbonate levels.

Clinically, metabolic alkalosis is characterized by depression of respiration, depressed renal function with uremia and increased bicarbonate excretion in the urine. The blood level of bicarbonate is elevated:

- Excessive vomiting.
- Cushing's syndrome.

Metabolic Acidosis

Metabolic acidosis occurs due to build up of acid in the body because of kidney failure. A reduced blood pH occurs due to a reduction in bicarbonate levels and an excess of H^+ ions. Elevated blood H^+ ion levels in metabolic acidosis activate the respiratory center, causing deep, fast breathing (also known as Kussmaul's respiration or "air hunger"):

- Lactic acidosis, e.g., shock, vigorous exercise.
- Starvation.
- Diabetic ketoacidosis.
- Chronic renal failure.

Table 7.2: Distinction between hyperemia or congestion

Feature	Hyperemia	Congestion
Type of process	Active	Passive
Color of affected organ	Red	Bluish
Pathogenesis	Dilation of arterioles leading to an increased blood flow to the affected organ	Engorgement of tissue by blood due to impaired venous drainage
Blood flow	Increased inflow	Decreased outflow
Type of blood involved	Arterial, oxygenated	Venous, deoxygenated
Examples	Fever, exercise	Chronic venous congestion spleen, liver

DERANGEMENTS IN BLOOD FLOW (CIRCULATORY/HEMODYNAMIC DISTURBANCES)

Hyperemia and congestion represent altered states of blood flow to organs leading to a net increase in the blood volume within an organ.

"Hyperemia" and "congestion" refer to the localized increase in blood volume within an organ or tissue's dilated vessels. The increased volume from arterial and arteriolar dilatation, is referred to as hyperemia, while the poor venous outflow is referred to as congestion of the veins or passive hyperemia. If the condition develops quickly, it's referred to as acute, but more extended and chronic reaction is a slow one.

The difference between hyperemia and congestion is tabulated as follows (Table 7.2):

Chronic venous congestion is more common and afflicts a number of organs such as the spleen, liver and kidneys with varied presentations. Venous outflow obstruction may be local or systemic. It is of two types:

1. Local venous congestion results from the obstruction to the venous outflow from an organ or part of a body, such as a portal venous obstruction in cirrhosis of the liver, venous blockage due to external pressure from tight bandage, plasters, etc.
2. Systemic venous congestion results from engorgement of the systemic veins occurs in conditions such as left- and right-sided heart failure and lung disorders, like pulmonary fibrosis and emphysema that impede the flow of blood through the lungs. This condition is known as systemic (general) venous congestion. Typically, the fluid builds up upstream to the particular heart chamber that is originally impacted.

Morphology of Chronic Venous Congestion

Chronic Venous Congestion Liver

Chronic venous congestion of the liver can result from hepatic vein and inferior vena cava blockage as well as right heart failure.

Gross Features

Enlarged liver, increased weight of the liver, stretched capsule, "Nutmeg" appearance or mottled appearance of the liver which is a result of congestion in zone 3 (centrilobular) and yellow areas corresponding to fatty change in zone 1 (peripheral, periportal) which occurs due to hypoxic injury (Fig. 7.9).

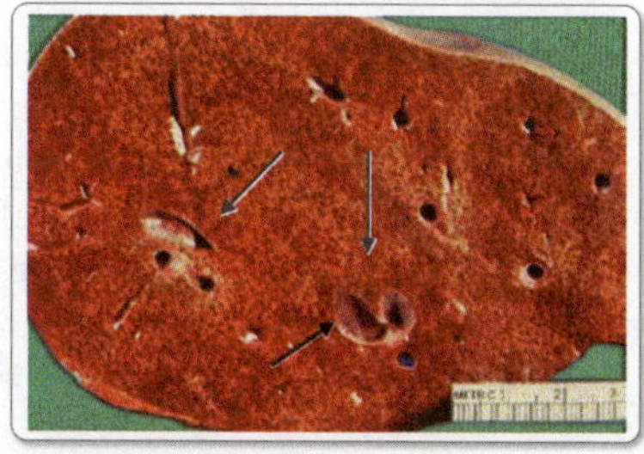

Figure 7.9: Nutmeg liver

Microscopic Examination

- **Zone 3 (centrilobular):** Central vein and sinusoids are markedly dilated and congested. The zone 3 hepatocytes show eventual necrosis accompanied by hemorrhage (centrilobular hemorrhagic necrosis) (Fig. 7.10).
- **Zone 1 (periportal):** Hepatocytes in the periportal zone undergo fatty change.
- In long-standing cases, fibrotic bands extend from one central vein to the other, this venovenal bridging and subsequent nodule formation is also called *reverse cirrhosis or cardiac cirrhosis.*

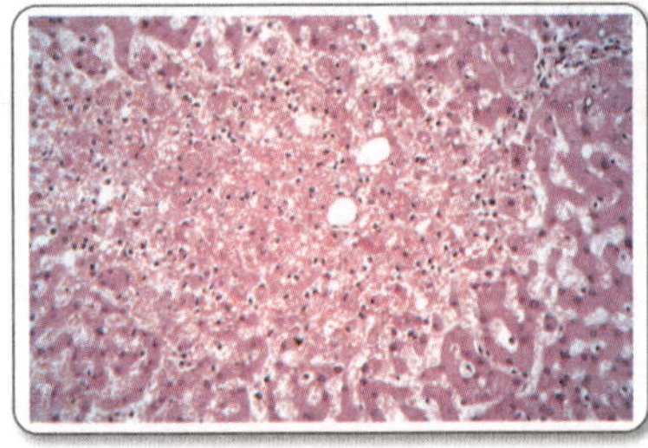

Figure 7.10: Microscopic appearance shows centrilobular hepatic necrosis

Chronic Venous Congestion of Spleen

Chronic venous congestion of the spleen is associated with portal hypertension resulting from liver cirrhosis and right-heart failure.

- **Gross:** Spleen is enlarged in dimensions and shows an increase in weight (250–750 g) (Fig. 7.11).
- Mild to moderate enlargement is usual.
- **Cut surface:** Congested, fleshy with whitish specks in the case of fibrocongestive splenomegaly. Cut surface appears tan and gray.

Figure 7.11: Chronic venous congestion of spleen. Note the heavy and enlarged appearance of spleen and gray-tan appearance of the cut surface

Microscopic Features

- Thickened capsule.
- Thickened indipping trabeculae.
- Plump splenic macrophages.
- Congested red pulp—represented by dilated sinusoids which are congested.
- Obliteration of the white pulp.
- Presence of Gamna Gandy bodies fibrosis coupled with hemosiderin pigment and hemosiderin laden macrophages, calcium deposits forming a sidero fibrotic nodule (Fig. 7.12).

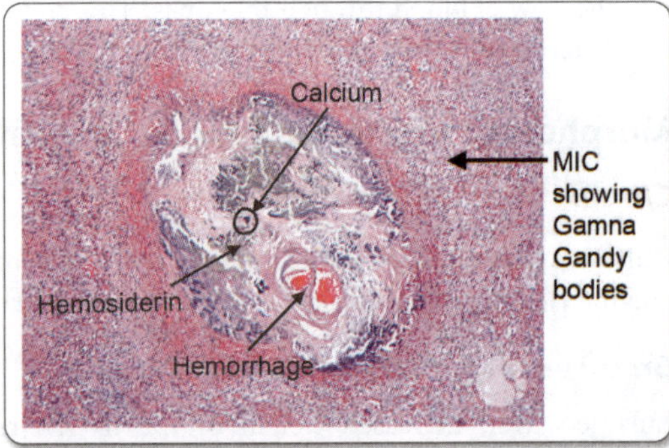

Figure 7.12: Chronic venous congestion of spleen showing Gamna Gandy bodies

Chronic Venous Congestion Lung

Cause of venous congestion of the lung is *left-sided heart failure* which results in pooling or congestion of blood in the pulmonary circuit. Pulmonary venous pressure rises as a result of chronic lung venous congestion in left heart failure, particularly in rheumatic mitral stenosis.

Gross Findings

Lungs are enlarged, heavy, boggy with an increased weight, brown in color, also called **brown induration.**

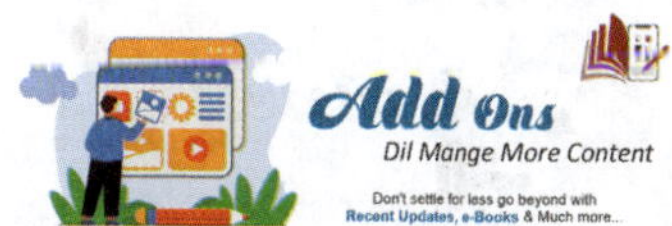

Microscopy

- Alveolar spaces are of varying sizes.
- Alveolar septa are thickened and congested.
- Many of the alveoli are distended with red blood cells (*intraalveolar hemorrhage*).
- With the breakdown of the red blood cells, hemosiderin pigment is liberated ingested by alveolar macrophages, also known as **heart failure cells** (Figs 7.13A and B).
- These brown pigment laden macrophages elicit a fibrogenic response causing the gross appearance of the brown indurated lung.

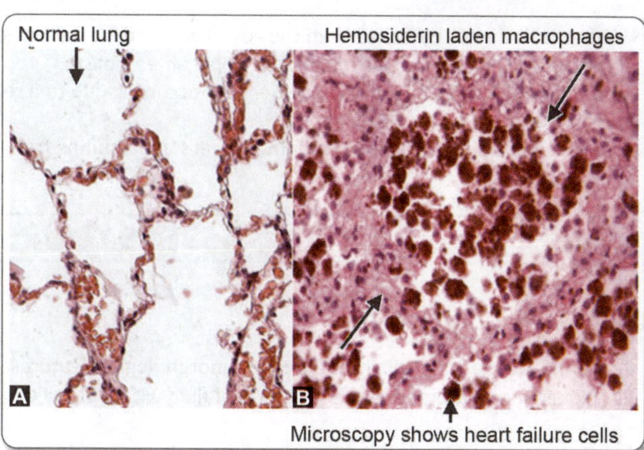

Figures 7.13A and B: **A.** Normal lung; **B.** CVC of Lung. Note the thickened alveolar septa due to congestion, edema and fibrosis. Heart failure cells are also visible in the alveolar lumina

Chronic Venous Congestion Kidney

Venous congestion of the kidney is caused due to *right-sided heart failure* which results in pooling or congestion of blood in the systemic circuit.

Gross Findings

Kidneys are enlarged, heavy with congested medulla and an increased weight. Corticomedullary differentiation is lost as the medulla and subsequently the cortex becomes congested.

Microscopic Findings

Microscopically, the changes are rather mild. Degenerative alterations such as cloudy swelling and fatty changes may be seen in the tubules. Mesangial proliferation may be seen in the glomeruli.

SUMMARY

- Homeostasis is the process by which the interior environment's consistency is preserved and guaranteed.
- Sodium is the main cation and chloride and bicarbonate are the main anions in the extracellular fluid.
- The abnormal and excessive buildup of "free fluid" in the serous cavities and interstitial tissue spaces is known as edema.
- Edema develops when the net rate of fluid movement is greater than the rate of lymphatic drainage.
- Heavy proteinuria (albuminuria) in nephrotic syndrome causes decreased oncotic pressure resulting in severe generalized edema.
- Pulmonary edema is characterized by heavy, moist and subcrepitant lungs.
- Metabolic alkalosis is characterized by rise in blood pH, caused by decrease in H^+ ions and an increase in plasma bicarbonate levels.
- *Hyperemia and congestion* represent altered states of blood flow to organs leading to a net increase in the blood volume within an organ.
- The formation of a solid or semi-solid mass within the lumen of a blood vessel is called **thrombosis**.
- Embolism is the partial or complete obstruction by any mass in the lumen of a vessel, carried by the blood stream to a site distant from the origin of the abnormal material.

Contd...

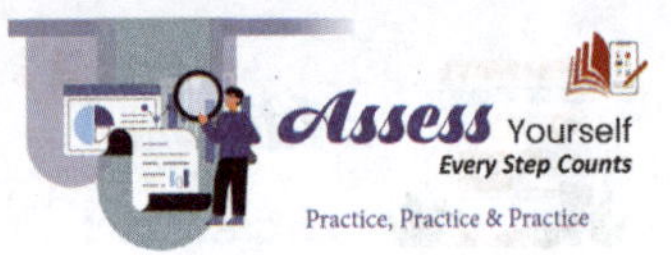

- When a thrombus detaches from the vessel wall and moves in the circulation, it is called thromboembolism.
- The presence of air in the circulation is called air embolism.
- Infarction is localized area of tissue necrosis occurring due to a reduced blood supply (ischemia) leading to decreased perfusion.
- Shock can be defined as a clinicopathological state resulting from inadequate tissue perfusion.

ASSESS YOURSELF

Long Answer Questions

1. Define Edema and explain its types and morphological features.
2. Explain forces promoting the retention of fluid within blood vessels.

Short Answer Questions

1. State about acid-base imbalances.
2. Define hyperemia and congestion.
3. Write short notes on:
   i. Types of edema
   ii. Dehydration

Multiple Choice Questions

1. **Difference in transudate & exudate is that the former has a ____________________.**
   a. Low protein
   b. Cloudy appearance
   c. Increased specific gravity
   d. High protein
2. **Generalized edema results from all the following; except:**
   a. Systemic hypertension
   b. Congestive heart failure
   c. Liver cirrhosis
   d. Nephrotic syndrome
3. **"Nutmeg Liver" is seen in:**
   a. Liver cirrhosis
   b. Liver necrosis
   c. Chronic passive congestion
   d. Thrombosis of the portal veins
4. **Which of the followings is the mechanism of edema in patients with congestive heart failure?**
   a. Decreased plasma oncotic pressure
   b. Endothelial damage
   c. Increase hydrostatic pressure
   d. Increase vascular permeability

Answer Key

1. a **2.** a **3.** c **4.** c

SECTION II

Systemic Pathology

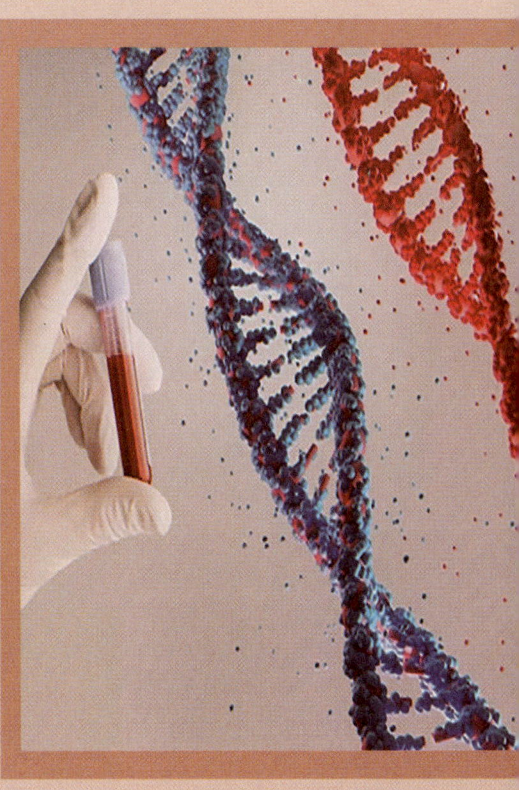

SECTION OUTLINE

Chapter 8

Respiratory System Diseases

LEARNING OBJECTIVES

After the completion of the chapter, the readers will be able to:

- Understand the overview of respiratory system.
- Pathological changes in disease conditions of the respiratory system.
- Know about pulmonary infection.
- Describe chronic obstructive pulmonary diseases.
- Explain the tumors of the lung.

CHAPTER OUTLINE

- Overview of Respiratory System
- Pulmonary Tuberculosis
- Pneumonia
- Chronic Obstructive Pulmonary Disease
- Lung Abscess
- Pleural Effusion
- Lung Tumors

KEY TERMS

Atelectasis: Failure of the lung to expand (inflate) completely.
Bronchiectasis: Abnormal dilatation of the bronchi.
Bronchodilators: A type of drug that causes small airways in the lungs to open up.
Bronchoscopy: A procedure involving a bronchoscope to examine the inside of the trachea, bronchi, and lungs.
Carcinogen: Any substance that causes cancer.
Cyanotic: Pertaining to abnormal color of blue (bluish color, lips and nail beds) caused by deoxygenation.
Dyspnea: Shortness of breath.
Hilum of the lung: A concave region where blood vessels, lymphatic vessels, and nerves also enter the lungs.
Mucus: A thick, viscous fluid made by the membranes that line certain organs of the body especially respiratory tract.
Pleural effusion: An abnormal collection of fluid between the thin layers of tissue (pleura) lining the lung and the wall of the chest cavity.

OVERVIEW OF RESPIRATORY SYSTEM

The respiratory system (Fig. 8.1) is entrusted with the function of ensuring adequate oxygenation of the blood as well as defence against microorganisms. It comprises:

- **The upper respiratory tract**, i.e., the portion of the respiratory system above the cricoid cartilage (nasal cavity, paranasal sinuses and pharynx).

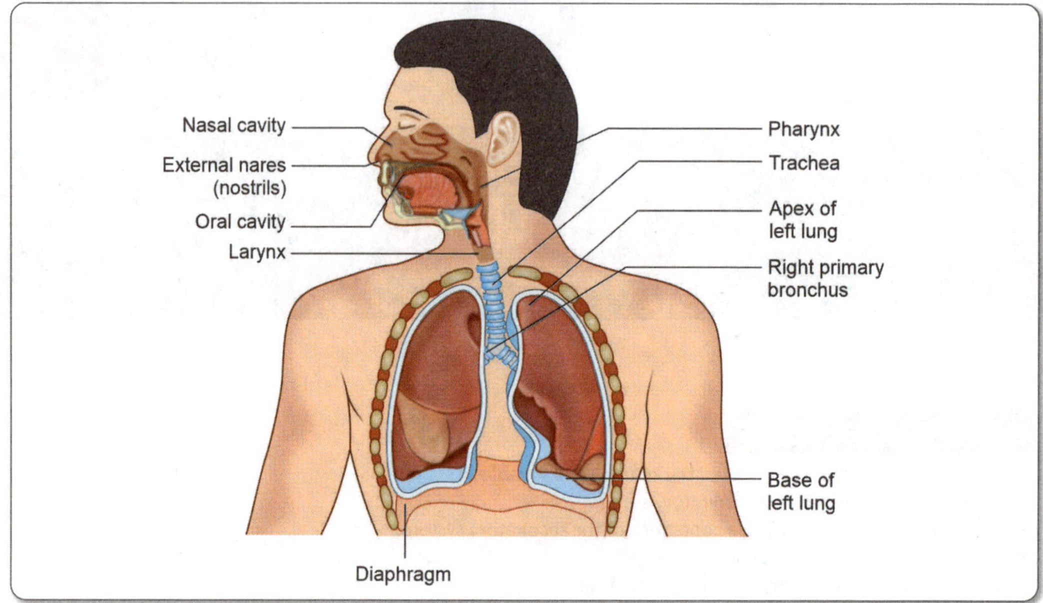

Figure 8.1: Respiratory system

- **The lower respiratory tract** (below the cricoid cartilage)—larynx, trachea, lungs and bronchial tree.
  - The trachea bifurcates into the right and left bronchi, which further branches into bronchioles. The bronchioles further undergo three/four sequential divisions with the end division being at the level of the terminal bronchiole.
  - Distal to the terminal bronchiole is the acinus, comprising the bronchioles, alveolar ducts and alveoli.
  - A group of 3–5 acini is called a pulmonary lobule.
  - The respiratory tract is characteristically lined by pseudostratified ciliated columnar epithelium.
  - The lungs comprise the alveoli (alveolar spaces) separated by interstitium. The alveoli are lined by two types of cells- Type 1 and type 2 pneumocytes. The interstitium shows the presence of capillaries lined by endothelial cells.

Pleura

The pleura refers to membranes of serous nature lining both the surface of the lungs (visceral pleura) as well the thoracic cavity (parietal pleura) which harbors the lungs. It is lined by a lining of cells called as mesothelial cells.

Functions:

- The pleural cavity is the space between the visceral and parietal pleural and normally has only a small (<10 mL) amount of fluid.
- This serves to lubricate this space which helps in coordinated movement along with the lung during the phases of inspiration and expiration.
- Another function of pleural fluid is to create surface tension which in turn pulls both layers of the pleura together during inspiration facilitating easy respiration.
- Numerous diseases can afflict the human lung. These include those of infectious etiology/chronic obstructive pulmonary diseases and neoplasias. Common infections are tuberculosis (TB) and pneumonia.

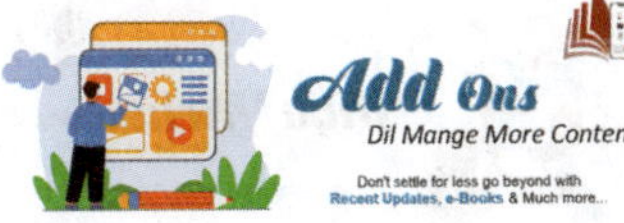

PULMONARY TUBERCULOSIS

Clinical Features

The classic symptom complex of pulmonary tuberculosis is represented by the following clinical features:

- Shortness of breath
- Blood in sputum (hemoptysis)
- Chronic cough with sputum production
- Loss of appetite and weight
- Low grade fever with evening rise in temperature
- Fatigue

Etiology

Tuberculosis is a chronic granulomatous disease caused by:

- *Mycobacterium tuberculosis hominis.*
- *Mycobacterium bovis* (in the past, when unpasteurized milk was consumed).
- *Mycobacterium avium intracellulare* (in immunocompromised patients).

Mycobacterium tuberculosis is an acid-fact aerobic bacterium. Mycobacteria have a lipid-rich cell wall which has a high quantity of lipids and mycolic acids. This makes it resistant to staining by usual methods. When stained by Ziehl-Neelsen (ZN) stain, mycobacteria are not decolorized by acid alcohol and retain the carbol fuchsin part of ZN stain giving a magenta color to the bacilli that are easily picked up on a blue background.

Atypical mycobacteria: Infection usually spreads through the environment and incudes other species, like *M. scrofulaceum, M. avium intracellulare, M. kansasii, M. marinum, M. chelonae.*

Mode of Transmission

- **Inhalation:** Through organisms transmitted by air (droplet infection).
- **Ingestion:** Consumption of unpasteurized milk/ingestion of infected sputum.
- **Transplacental:** Transmission from an infected mother through the placenta, leads to the development of congenital tuberculosis.
- Inoculation into the skin-rarely seen.

Risk Factors

Lower socioeconomic social groups, poor hygiene.

Immunosuppressed individuals: Those on long-term steroids/other immunosuppressants, diabetics, patients of malignancy and those being treated by chemotherapeutic agents.

Pathogenesis

Tuberculosis infection develops due to the persistence of *Mycobacterium tuberculosis* bacilli in the body (Fig. 8.2). This in turn is due to the inability of macrophages to destroy/phagocytose the bacteria. Persistence of the organism leads to a delayed (type IV) hypersensitivity reaction.

The inability of the macrophages to remove *M. tuberculosis* bacilli is central to the pathogenesis of tuberculosis.

M. tuberculosis has a different cell wall composition in comparison to other bacteria. The cell wall typically has glycolipids and mycolic acids. One such compound, the cord factor is also responsible for the low cell wall permeability of the mycobacterium, thus preventing the entry of drugs easily and also rendering the destruction of the bacilli by macrophages, difficult. *M. tuberculosis* bacilli also inhibit the formation of the phagolysosome, thereby inhibiting the destructive effect of the lysosomes on the bacilli.

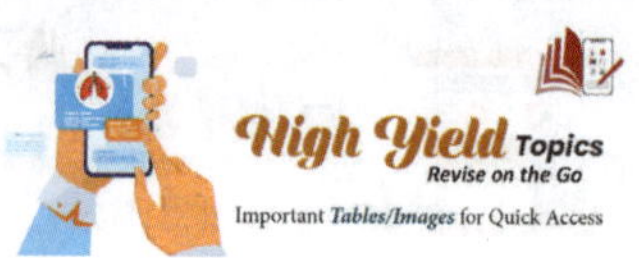

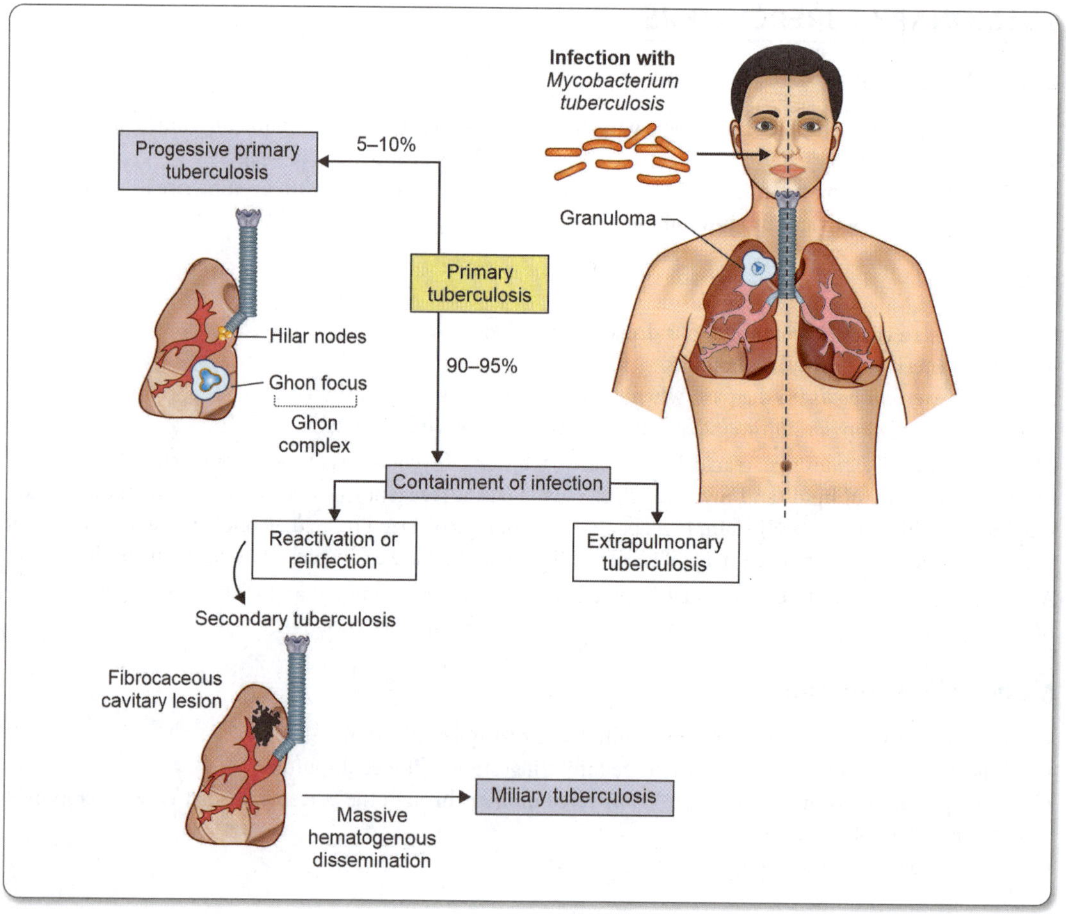

Figure 8.2: Pathogenesis of tuberculosis

- Once the bacilli reach the lungs through aerosol droplets (the most common mode of transmission), by the third week of exposure, CD4 + T cells (T-helper cells) are activated. This activation is in response to cytokine IL-12 which is liberated by the antigen presenting cells that first interact with the tubercular bacilli.
- Activated T cells in turn activate macrophages by the liberation of the cytokine interferon-gamma (IFN-γ) and tumor necrosis factor-α (TNF-α).
- Interferon-gamma which is released, promotes the formation of the phagolysosome which exposes the bacilli to an acidic environment unfavorable for their existence.
- Interferon-gamma also produces nitric oxide which has a bactericidal action.
- The T-helper cells (Th1) that liberate IFN-γ also result in the conversion of the activated macrophages into epithelioid cells and also the formation of granulomas, which are the key histological features for the diagnosis of tuberculosis. TNF-α helps in recruitment of monocytes, macrophages thus intensifying the granulomatous response.

Types of Tuberculosis

Tubercular infection (Fig. 8.3) of the lung is mainly of two types:

1. Primary Tuberculosis

Primary tuberculosis refers to infection in individuals who have no past history of infection/immunization against tuberculosis. The most common site of involvement in TB is the lung (primary pulmonary tuberculosis). Other sites in which a primary focus of infection is common include lymph nodes, intestine, and skin. Primary pulmonary tuberculosis is represented by the lesion called primary complex or Ghon's complex. The primary complex is composed of:

- **Ghon's focus/primary focus:** The lung lesion which is frequently solitary, subpleural and situated at the lower part of the upper lobe/upper part of lower lobe.

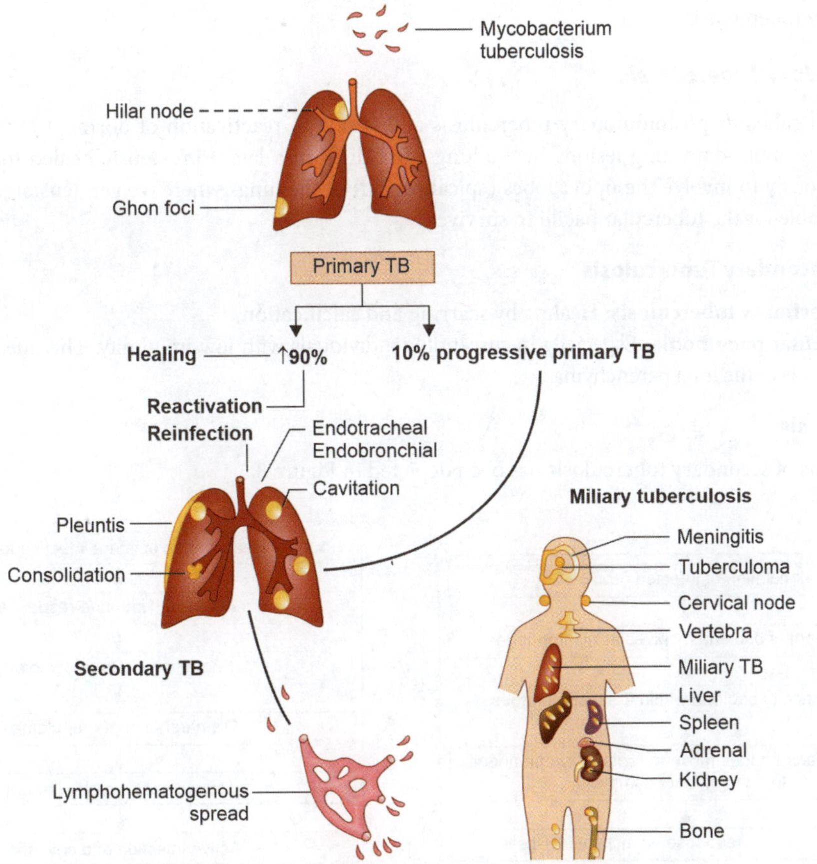

Figure 8.3: Types of tuberculosis

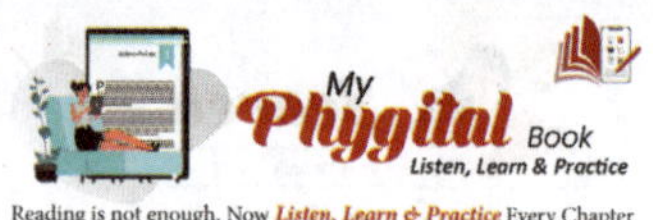

- **Hilar lymph nodes:** The bacilli in the lungs are transported to the regional hilar lymph nodes. These nodes enlarge, become matted and along with tracheobronchial lymph nodes are affected by the tubercular infection. Macrophages laden with tubercular bacilli are also present.
- **Lymphatic vessels:** Draining the area of the Ghon's focus are also involved and form the third component of the Ghon's complex.

Pathogenesis

Pathogenesis of primary tuberculosis have been depicted in Figure 8.4.

Fates of the Primary Focus

- Healing by fibrosis (causing scarring)
- Calcification/rarely ossification
- Persisting primary infection with enlarging primary focus, spread to the other lung
- Secondary tuberculosis
- Miliary tuberculosis

2. *Secondary Tuberculosis*

This is also called as postpulmonary tuberculosis and is due to reactivation of dormant foci of infection. This leads to more damaging lesions in the lungs. Bacilli from a latent/previously healed focus is spread hematogenously to involve the upper lobes (apical region) of the lungs where oxygen tension is higher and more favorable for the tubercular bacilli to survive.

Fates of Secondary Tuberculosis

- **As in primary tuberculosis:** Healing by scarring and calcification.
- **Tubercular pneumonia:** Especially in susceptible individuals with low immunity. The infection involves large areas of the lung parenchyma.

Pathogenesis

Pathogenesis of secondary tuberculosis has been depicted in Figure 8.5.

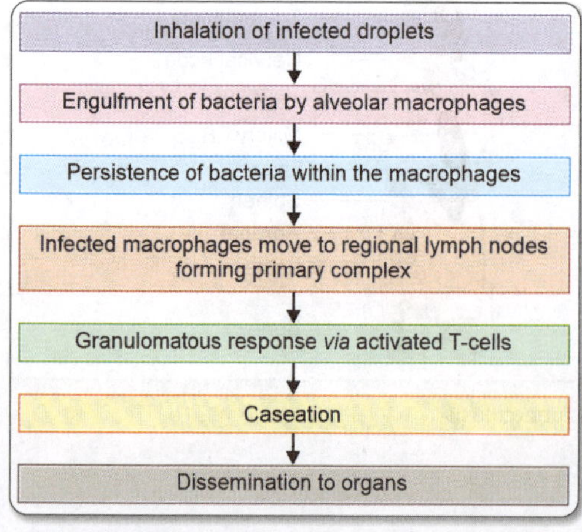

Figure 8.4: Pathogenesis of primary tuberculosis

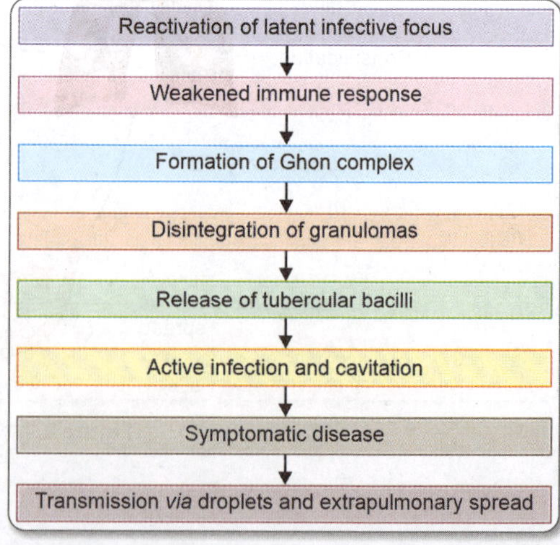

Figure 8.5: Pathogenesis of secondary tuberculosis

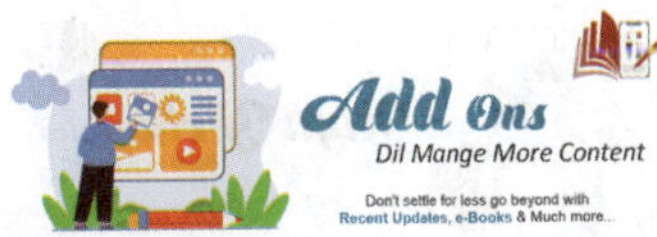

Miliary Tuberculosis

When lungs show multiple tiny millet-like lesions, it is called miliary tuberculosis (Fig. 8.6). This is due to hematogenous spread of the bacilli in primary infection. It also may be a consequence of reactivation of old disseminated foci. A single organ or multiple organs may be affected.

- Spread through pulmonary artery leads to lung involvement.
- Spread through pulmonary veins leads to multiple organ (spleen, kidney, liver, etc.) involvement.

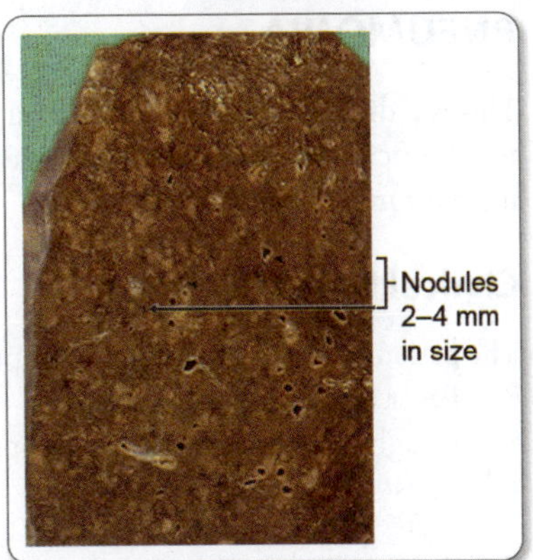

Figure 8.6: Miliary tuberculosis

Pathological Changes

- **Gross appearance (Fig. 8.7A):** The lesions are small (1–2 mm) in size, i.e., millet-like, yellow, firm, devoid of visible necrosis.
- **Histological changes (Figs 8.7B and C):** Epithelioid cell granulomas. Foci of caseous necrosis may be present microscopically.

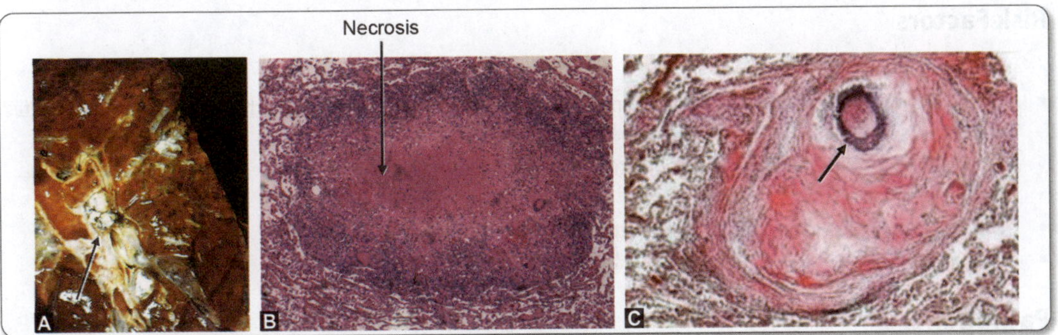

Figures 8.7A to C: **A.** TB granuloma (gross); **B.** Ghon complex; **C.** Ghon focus (histology)

Diagnosis of Tuberculosis

- Screening—Mantoux test.
- Sputum for AFB by microscopy (Fig. 8.8).
- Sputum culture/culture of aspirated lymph node material- on Lowenstein-Jensen medium.
- Hemogram (complete blood counts showing lymphocytosis, raised ESR).
- Chest X-ray/high resolution CT chest (HRCT).
- If lymphadenopathy is present—FNAC of the affected lymph nodes.
- GeneXpert test (PCR based test) to detect the presence of infection.
- Drug sensitivity testing (DST)—PCR based assays.
  - CBNAAT/GeneXpert test (cartridge-based nucleic acid amplification test).
  - Rifampicin resistance detected by mutations in RNA polymerase rpoB.
  - Line probe assay (LPA)—for detection of isoniazid and rifampicin resistance.

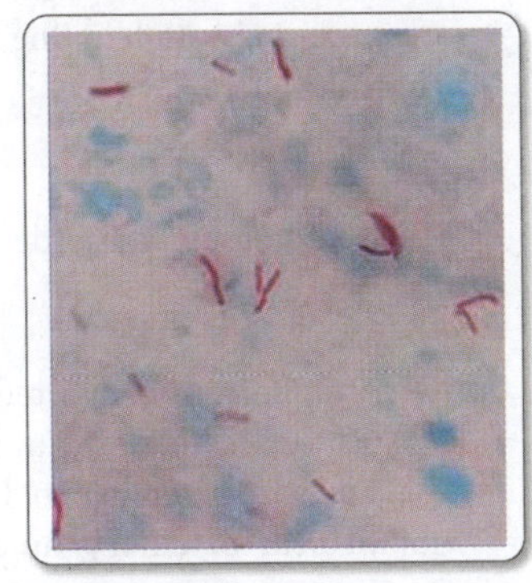

Figure 8.8: AFB staining showing mycobacteria

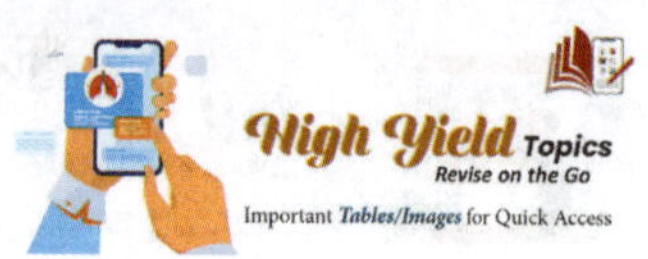

PNEUMONIA

This is a disease which involves inflammation of the lung parenchyma of the lower respiratory tract leading to solidification (consolidation) of the lung tissue. The inflammation may be within the alveolar spaces or the interstitium. The term "pneumonitis" also refers to such an inflammatory process.

Clinical Features

The patient of pneumonia usually appears sick and is lethargic. Patients commonly present with:

- Fever (with or without chills)
- Cough, expectoration and hemoptysis
- Chest pain (Pleuritic)
- Breathlessness
- Wheezing
- Altered sensorium

Etiology

Hemophilus influenzae, Moraxella catarrhalis, Streptococcus pneumoniae, Mycoplasma pneumoniae. Chlamydia species, Pneumocystis, Staphylococci (in newborn).

Risk Factors

- Smoking.
- Weak immune system, such as from immunosuppressive drugs, or a health problems, like diabetes, cancer, or HIV.
- Lung problems such as chronic obstructive pulmonary disease.
- Health problems such as kidney failure.
- Use of certain medicines, including proton-pump inhibitors.
- Heavy alcohol use.

Pathogenesis

- **Impairment of local defence mechanisms (Fig. 8.9)**
  Loss/suppression of the cough reflex: Certain states/conditions are associated with blunting of the protective cough reflex. These include:
  - Coma.
  - Anesthesia.
  - Neuromuscular disorders.
  - Intake of drugs.
  - Chest pain.
  - A diminished cough reflex promotes accumulation of pent-up secretions within the respiratory tract making a person susceptible to develop infections.
- **Impairment of ciliary function/loss of epithelial cilia:** Destruction of the normal ciliated epithelium lining the respiratory tract may be seen in the following conditions:
  - Persistent exposure to cigarette smoke.
  - Inhalation of hot/corrosive gases.
  - Viral diseases.
  - Genetic defects of ciliary function (immotile cilia syndrome).

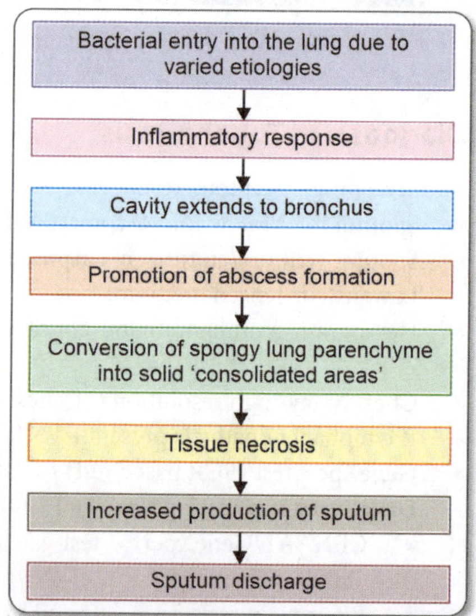

Figure 8.9: Pathogenesis of pneumonia

- Similar to the conditions in which the cough reflex diminishes:
  - In states where the normal ciliated lining epithelium is destroyed, an increased tendency of respiratory secretions and mucus to accumulate is seen (Fig. 8.9). This also predisposes to an enhanced chance of infection or pneumonia.
  - **Other disease states associated with accumulation of secretions:** Cystic fibrosis and bronchial obstruction.
- **Defective functionality of alveolar macrophages:** Seen in chronic alcoholics and smokers.
- **Diminished host resistance:** When a person is immunodeficient and has defects either in the innate/humoral/cell mediated immune defence mechanisms, the chances of developing pneumonia are more.

Classification of Pneumonia

Based on the anatomical involvement:

- Lobar pneumonia—involvement of a lobe of the lung.
- Bronchopneumonia—involvement which is centered on the bronchi and bronchioles.
- Interstitial pneumonia (atypical pneumonia)—involvement of the lung interstitium.

Differences between lobar pneumonia, bronchopneumonia and interstitial pneumonia are tabulated in Table 8.1.

Table 8.1: Differences in lobar pneumonia, bronchopneumonia and interstitial pneumonia

Pneumonia	Lobar pneumonia	Bronchopneumonia	Atypical (interstitial pneumonia)
Age group	Any age group	Infancy and old age common	Any age group
Predisposing factors	Highly virulent organisms	Immuncompromised disseminated malignancy, pre-existing bronchitis, bronchiolitis	Malnutrition, alcoholism, underlying debilitating illnesses
Etiologic agents	90–95% of cases caused by pneumococci (Strep. pneumoniae)	• *Staphylococci* • *Streptococci* • *Pneumococci* • *H. Influenzae* • Pseudomonas aeruginosa • Coliform bacteria	Mycoplasma pneumoniae Chlamydia Coxiella burnetti viral infection
Distribution	Consolidation of large areas of one lobe or the whole lobe	Patchy consolidation of more than one lobe of the lung	Involvement maybe patchy or involve whole lobes unilaterally or bilaterally
Microscopic features	Involvement of all alveoli of one lobe by inflammatory exudate; the 4 classical stages of consolidation are best seen in lobar pneumonia. Right upper lobe consolidation Lobar denisty At bronchogram No singnificant less of lung volume	Patchy involvement of alveoli around the bronchioles in more than one lobe by inflammatory exudate.	Interstitial inflammation composed of lymphocytes, virtually localized within alveolar walls.

Based on the onset of symptoms:

- Acute
- Chronic

Based on the etiology:

- Infectious—bacterial, viral, parasitic, fungal.
- Drug/toxin associated (chemical pneumonitis).
- Persistent inhalation of foreign bodies/environmental pollutants/allergens.

Lobar Pneumonia

This type of pneumonia involves a significant part of or an entire lung lobe. Inflammation is usually fibrinosuppurative in nature, leading to solidification or consolidation which is apparent grossly. Classically, four stages of lobar pneumonia have been described, though with modern day medical practice and the institution of high efficacy antibiotic therapy, these phases are seldom seen in antemortem cases.

Stages of Lobar Pneumonia

The four stages/phases of lobar pneumonia are as follows:

1. Congestion
2. Red hepatization
3. Gray hepatization
4. Resolution phase

1. Congestion

This represents the initial response to infection/other injurious stimuli and is seen from day 1 to 2.

- **Gross appearance:** The lung weight is increased and the lung itself is enlarged. The appearance of the lung is reddish brown, congested.
- **Cut section**: Reddish pink (blood-stained) frothy fluid is seen when the lung is sliced. Alveoli are variably sized and distended with fluid which is pink (eosinophilic). Within the fluid numerous neutrophils are seen admixed with red blood cells, clusters and singly lying bacteria. The alveolar septae show numerous congested blood vessels.

2. Red Hepatization

This phase occurs for the next 2–3 days (day 2–5). This clinically represents a phase of consolidation on imaging. Consolidation refers to the loss of the normal spongy texture of the lung parenchyma. Instead, the lung becomes firm and liver-like.

- **Gross appearance:** The lung is enlarged firm and the affected lobe is reddish brown in color (Fig. 8.10A)
- **Cut section:** Solid, firm and the affected area has a liver like texture, thus giving the name of this phase as "red hepatization".
- **Histological changes:** The alveoli are variably sized and the edema fluid seen in the congestive phase is replaced by fibrin. The alveolar exudate showed neutrophils, red blood cells and macrophages. Numerous bacterial colonies also may be present (Fig. 8.10B).

3. Gray Hepatization

This stage marks a phase of further consolidation (day 5–9)

- **Gross appearance (Fig. 8.10C):** The lung parenchyma in this phase shows a grayish color and is dull.
- **Cut section:** Solid, firm with persistence of the liver like texture.
- **Histological changes:** Progressive disintegration of red cells. Neutrophils are replaced by macrophages. The alveoli contain fibrinous material. There is a clear space between the alveoli and exudate. The colonies of bacteria also undergo degeneration.

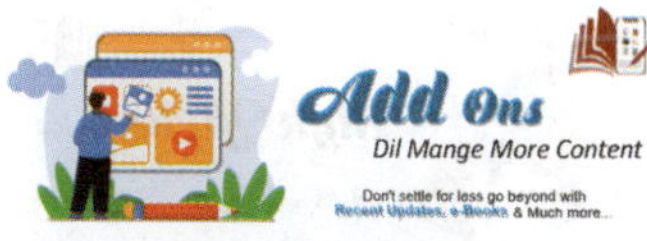

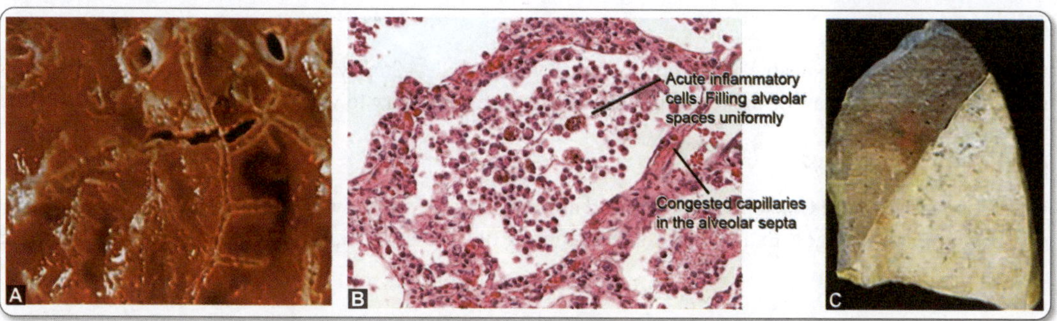

Figures 8.10A to C: **A.** Red hepatization (gross); **B.** Red hepatization (histology); **C.** Gray hepatization (gross)

4. Resolution Phase

(Day 9 – week 2/3): This represents the final stage of healing. With the administration of improved antibiotics cases rarely show these features unless they are refractory to treatment or the host immunity is markedly diminished.

- **Gross appearance:** The alveolar contents undergo liquefaction due to enzymatic action.
- **Cut section:** Shows a creamy yellowish and dirty exudate.
- **Histological changes:** The exudate in the alveolar spaces undergoes progressive enzymatic digestion and is resorbed and digested by macrophages. Alveolar spaces are hence full of macrophages but devoid of edema fluid or red blood cells. Residual fibrin remains.

Bronchopneumonia

This is also known as lobular (Table 8.2) pneumonia but unlike lobar pneumonia where the inflammatory process is confined to a lobe of the lung, in bronchopneumonia, inflammation is patchy. The ensuing consolidation may be restricted to patches within a single lobe or may involve multiple lobes of the lungs. It frequently involves both the lungs.

- Bronchopneumonia is usually seen in patients at both extremes of age, i.e., the young and the elderly.
- Prior history of upper respiratory tract infection, long standing illness or immunocompromise may also be present. As the name suggests, inflammation is significantly centered around the main bronchi and its subsequent branches (bronchioles). Further it subsequently extends to the alveolar spaces resulting in the typical patchy distribution.
- X-ray findings also show patchy consolidation.

Table 8.2: Stages of lobar pneumonia

Stage	Characteristics
Congestion (1–2 days)	• **Grossly:** Lung is heavy, boggy and red. • **Microscopically: Vascular engorgement,** intra-alveolar fluid with **neutrophils** and bacteria
Red hepatization (2–4 days)	• **Grossly: Red,** firm and **airless,** with a **liver-like consistency,** hence, the term **hepatization** • **Microscopically:** Confluent **exudation** with neutrophils, **RBCs, fibrin** filling alveoli
Gray hepatization (5–8 days)	• **Grossly: Grayish brown,** dry surface • **Microscopically: Disintegration of RBCs** and persistence of a **fibrinosuppurative exudate**
Resolution (8–9 days)	• Exudates within alveoli broken down by enzymatic digestion to produce **granular debris** • Debris may be reabsorbed/ingested by macrophages/expectorated/**organized by fibroblasts.**

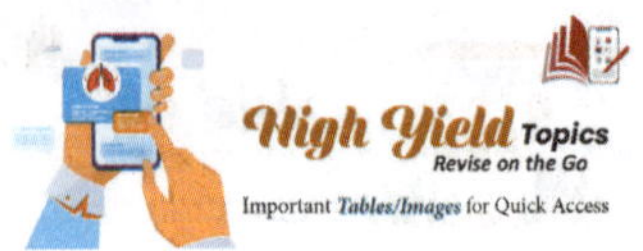

Etiology

Common bacteria responsible for bronchopneumonia include—Staphylococci, Streptococci, Hemophilus influenzae, Pseudomonas. Bronchopneumonia may also be secondary to viral infections.

Pathological Changes

- **Gross appearance:** Consolidation localized around airways in the lower lung.
- **Histological changes:** Exudate rich in neutrophils fills the bronchi, bronchioles and adjacent alveolar spaces.

Interstitial Pneumonia

Interstitial pneumonia is a group of diseases where inflammation and fibrosis damage the spaces between the alveoli, i.e., the interstitium. The damage further causes scarring and restricts the lungs from working properly.

Scarring caused can be seen on imaging such as a CT scan and under the microscope.

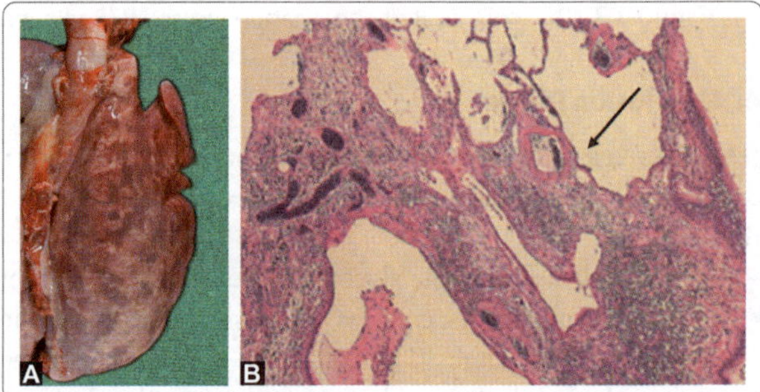

Figures 8.11A and B: Interstitial pneumonia: **A.** Gross; **B.** Histology (arrow showing enlarged air spaces)

- **Gross appearnce (Fig. 8.11A):** Severe scarring (fibrosis), worse at the periphery and bases of the lungs—"honeycomb change".
- **Histological changes (Fig. 8.11B):** Foci of relatively normal lung alternating with areas of prominent interstitial fibrosis. Enlarged airspaces are surrounded by fibrosis and chronic inflammation. The spaces are focally lined by bronchiolar type epithelium.

Complications of Pneumonia

- Lung abscess
- Empyema formation
- Spread of infection to the pleural cavity (pleuritis)
- Bacteremic dissemination causing sepsis
- Organization

Differences between lobar pneumonia and bronchopneumonia are given in Table 8.3.

Table 8.3: Differences between lobar pneumonia and bronchopneumonia

Feature	Lobar pneumonia	Bronchopneumonia
Involvement of	Nearly all of the entire lobe	Patchy involvement of multiple lobes
Site predilection	Any lobe may be affected	The basal/lower lobes are affected more
Age predilection	Adults	Extremes of age-children and elderly
Stages/phases of inflammation	Four phases described	No such description
Bronchial/bronchiolar involvement	Usually, absent	Present
Exudate formation	More	Less
Resolution	Depends on timely treatment, completely resolved in early cases	Through fibrosis, complications more

CHRONIC OBSTRUCTIVE PULMONARY DISEASE

Lung disease can clinically be categorized as restrictive and obstructive. The major differences between these two categories are enumerated in the Table 8.4.

Chronic obstructive pulmonary disease (COPD) is a more frequent clinical entity, its clinical and pathological features being relevant to nursing professionals and is discussed below.

Definition of COPD as per the WHO

A common, preventable, treatable disease characterized by persistent respiratory symptoms and airflow limitation due to airway and/or alveolar abnormalities caused by exposure to noxious particles or gases.

The four major clinical entities described under this entity include:

1. Emphysema
2. Bronchiectasis
3. Chronic bronchitis
4. Bronchial asthma

Table 8.4: Differences between restrictive and obstructive lung disease

Restrictive lung disease	Obstructive lung disease
Increased in interstitial fibrotic tissue	Destruction of interstitial tissue
Collapse of alveoli	Increased air-spaces
Stiff lung parenchyma	Hyperinflated lung (soft lung)
Lung function test: • PEFR is normal • FEV1/FVC ratio is normal	• PEFR is decreased • FEV1/FVC ratio is low
Characterized by progressive breathlessness with or without cough and wheezing	Characterized by cough and expectoration, wheezing and breathlessness

1. Emphysema

This lung disease is characterized by dilatation of the airspaces which is:

- Permanent.
- Distal to the terminal bronchiole.
- Accompanied by destruction of the alveolar walls.

Types of Emphysema

This classification is based on the part of the acinus involved by emphysematous change:

- **Centriacinar:** Involvement of the central portion of the acinus, i.e., changes are more frequently seen around the bronchiole. The upper zones of the lung show this type of emphysema more frequently (Fig. 8.12A).
- **Panacinar:** The entire acinus is involved. The lower lobes of the lung are more commonly involved. It is commonly associated with $\alpha 1$ antitrypsin deficiency (Fig. 8.12B).
- **Paraseptal:** This type is also known as distal acinar as the distal parts of the acini are dilated. This is frequently seen along the pleural surface of the lung (Fig. 8.12C).
- **Irregular:** The acini are involved in an irregular/patchy distribution with the lungs frequently showing scarring (Fig. 8.12D).

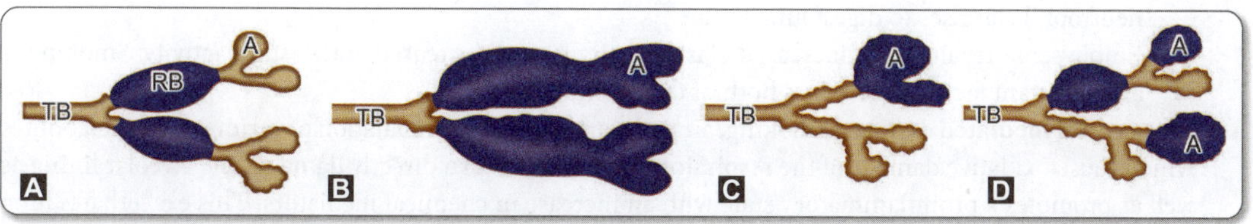

Figures 8.12A to D: Types of emphysema: **A.** Centriacinar; **B.** Panacinar; **C.** Paraseptal; **D.** Irregular

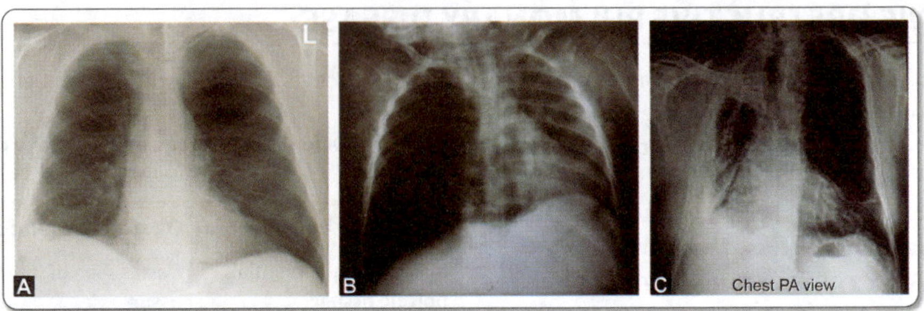

Figures 8.13A to C: Forms of emphysema: **A.** Bullous; **B.** Obstructive; **C.** Compensatory

Uncommon Forms of Emphysema

- **Bullous emphysema:** Characterized by the presence of large subpleural blebs/bullae. Usually involving the apex of the lung with bleb/bulla rupture causing potential pneumothorax (Fig. 8.13A).
- **Obstructive:** Any obstruction caused by a tumor/embolus/foreign body causes trapping of air and subsequent expansion of the lung (Fig. 8.13B).
- **Compensatory:** When the lung parenchyma hyperinflates in cases where a surgery is performed to remove a lobe or part of the lung parenchyma (Fig. 8.13C).

Clinical Features

- Shortness of breath—gradually increasing with time, worse on exertion.
- Increased respiratory rate (tachypnea), effort to breathe (*laboured breathing*).
- Barrel shaped chest.
- Cough with scant sputum.
- Patients are usually well-oxygenated despite respiratory difficulty, hence are called "pink puffers".
- Weight loss.
- X-ray chest classically shows hyperinflated lungs with a small heart.

Pathogenesis

- **Protease antiprotease theory** (Fig. 8.14) is the main causative theory. In normal health, protease activity is perfectly counteracted by antiprotease activity.
  - **Protease aspect:** The main protease in the body is neutrophil elastase. Elastase activity can be increased by any condition resulting in an increase in neutrophils. Smoking is a prime factor increasing free radicals and elastase activity leading to breakdown of extracellular matrix including elastin molecule, leading to a loss of elastic recoil causing overinflated lungs. In a normal individual, neutrophil elastase is inhibited by protease inhibitors.
  - **Antiprotease aspect:** The main protease inhibitor is alpha-1-antitrypsin. This molecule prevents neutrophil elastases to digest lung tissue.
  - Emphysema results from increased elastase activity and decreased antielastase activity. Smoking is an important factor which does both of these actions.
- **Free radical mediated damage:** Smoking, air pollutants lead to the inhalation of various toxic metabolites which cause oxidative damage of the respiratory tree. This in turn directly damages the alveolar lining as well as promotes a proinflammatory state with an increase in chemical mediators. This exacerbates lung parenchymal damage.

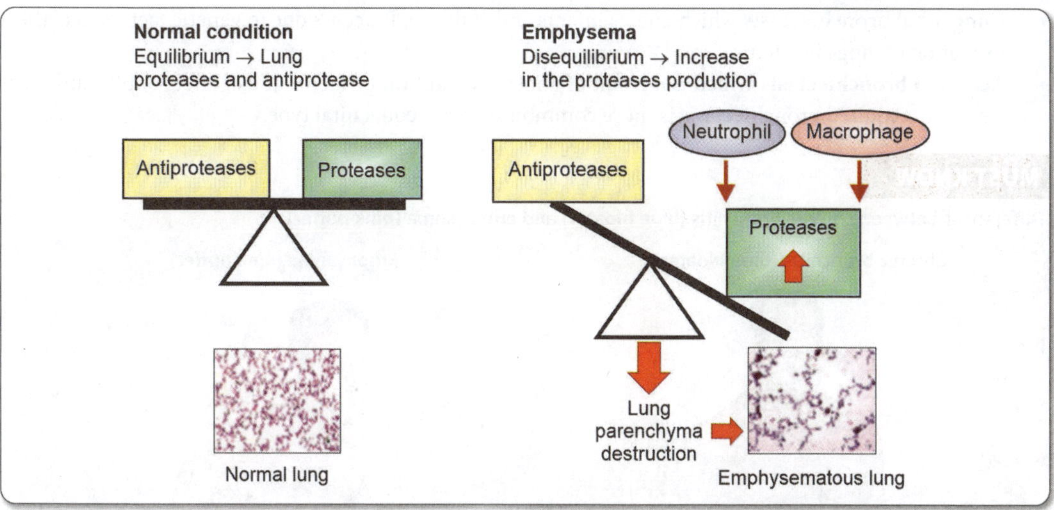

Figure 8.14: Protease antiprotease theory of emphysema occurrence

Pathological Changes

Gross appearance: Destruction of the air sacs or the alveoli (Fig. 8.15A).

Histological changes:

- Abnormally large, distended alveoli, with large pores of Kohn.
- Alveoli are separated by thin septa.
- Alveolar wall destroyed, septal spurs protruding into the alveoli with club shaped ends (Incomplete free-floating septa) (Fig. 8.15B).
- Focal centriacinar fibrosis.
- Inflammatory changes-small airways.
- **Vascular changes:** Capillaries may be thin and stretched out.
- Loss of elastin can be demonstrated by VGE stain.

2. Bronchiectasis

Bronchiectasis is an irreversible and abnormal dilatation of the bronchi and bronchioles secondary to the destruction of the bronchial wall (muscle and elastic fibers) due to any etiology. It may be a diffuse or localized process. Bronchiectasis can be:

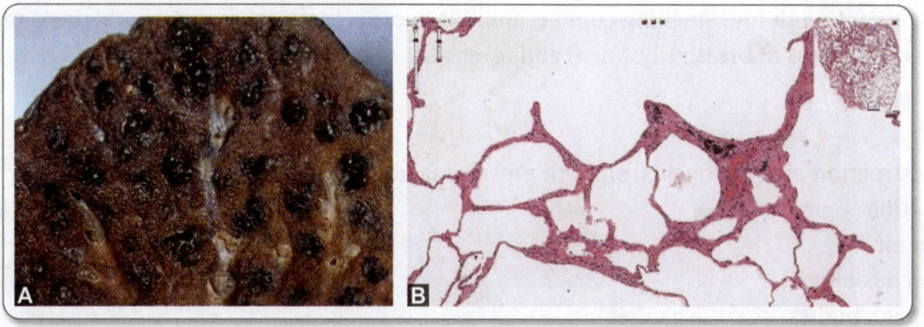

Figures 8.15A and B: Emphysema: **A.** Gross appearance; **B.** Microscopic appearance

- **Congenital bronchiectasis** which affects infants and children. It occurs due to genetic factors that affect formation of lungs in a fetus.
- **Acquired bronchiectasis** which is a result of another condition or factor. It can affect adults and older children. Acquired bronchiectasis is more common than the congenital type.

MUST KNOW

Differences between chronic bronchitis (blue bloater) and emphysema (pink puffer)

Chronic bronchitis (blue bloater)	Emphysema (pink puffer)
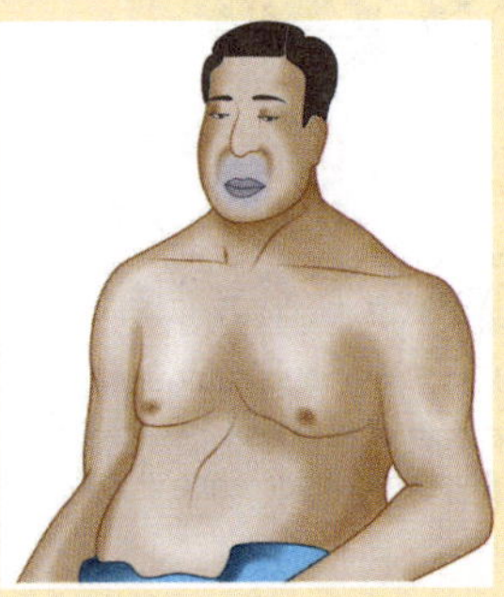	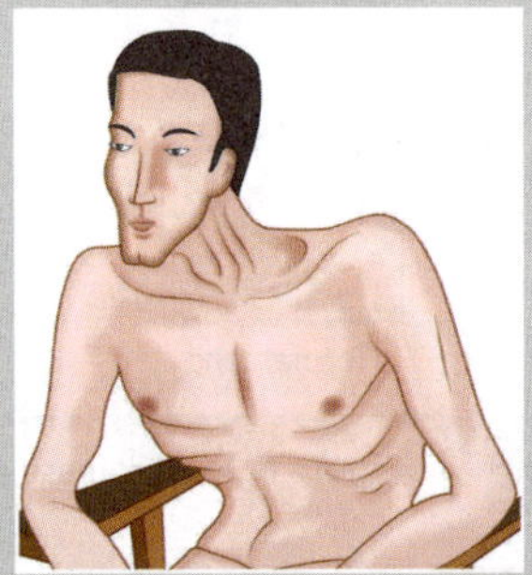
Symptoms • Chronic, productive cough • Purulent sputum • Hemoptysis • Mild dyspnea initially • Cyanosis (due to hypoxemia) • Peripheral edema (due to cor pulmonale) • Crackles, wheezes • Prolonged expiration • Obese	**Symptoms** • Dyspnea • Minimal cough • Increased minute ventilation • Pink skin, pursed-lip breathing • Accessory muscle use • Cachexia • Hyperinflation, barrel chest • Decreased breath sounds • Tachypnea
Complications • Secondary polycythemia vera due to hypoxemia • Pulmonary hypertension due to reactive vasoconstriction from hypoxemia • Cor pulmonale from chronic pulmonary hypertension	**Complications** • Pneumothorax due to bullae • Weight loss due to work of breathing

Clinical Features

The patient presents with foul smelling copious amount of expectoration. Sputum sometimes may be bloody (hemoptysis). Shortness of breath (dyspnea) and fever may also be observed.

Etiology

Causes of destruction of the bronchial smooth muscle include:

- Obstruction
  - Tumor
  - Mucous plugs
  - Foreign bodies

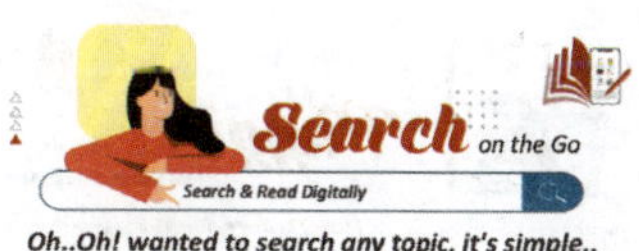

- Inflammation: Viral/bacterial/immune mediated causes
- Congenital anomalies impairing mucociliary apparatus
- Cystic fibrosis

Risk Factors

In adults, disorders that can increase the risk of bronchiectasis include COPD, asthma, GERD (gastroesophageal reflux disease, rheumatoid arthritis, and inflammatory bowel disease. Bronchiectasis may also be caused by infections from nontuberculous mycobacteria (NTM).

Pathogenesis

The combined processes of airway obstruction and inflammation in the presence of a susceptible host with weakened defence (immunity) lead to destruction, fibrosis and dilatation of the airways seen in this disease (Fig. 8.16).

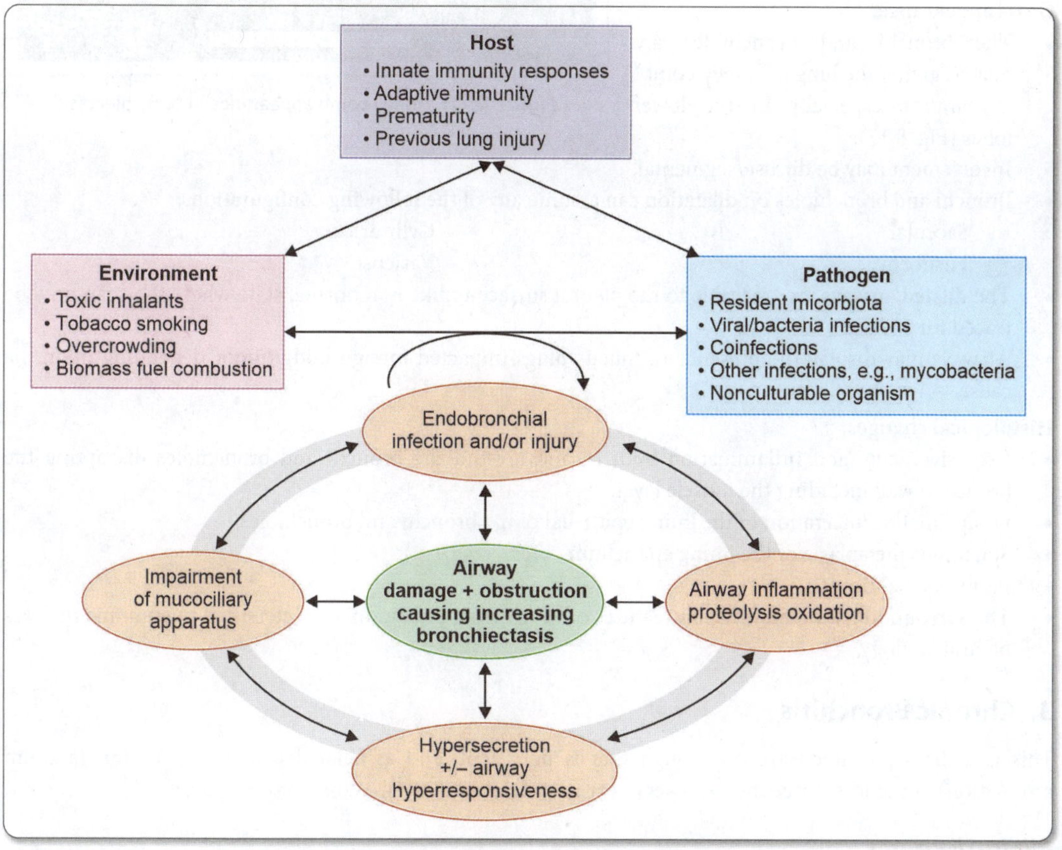

Host
- Innate immunity responses
- Adaptive immunity
- Prematurity
- Previous lung injury

Environment
- Toxic inhalants
- Tobacco smoking
- Overcrowding
- Biomass fuel combustion

Pathogen
- Resident micorbiota
- Viral/bacteria infections
- Coinfections
- Other infections, e.g., mycobacteria
- Nonculturable organism

Endobronchial infection and/or injury

Impairment of mucociliary apparatus

Airway damage + obstruction causing increasing bronchiectasis

Airway inflammation proteolysis oxidation

Hypersecretion +/– airway hyperresponsiveness

Figure 8.16: Pathogenesis of bronchiectasis

Complications

- **General:**
  - Hemoptysis
  - Amyloidosis
  - Septicemia
    - Septic shock
- **Chest:**
  - Lung abscess
  - Pneumonia (aspiration)
  - Pleurisy and empyema
  - Fibrosis
  - Cor pulrnonale

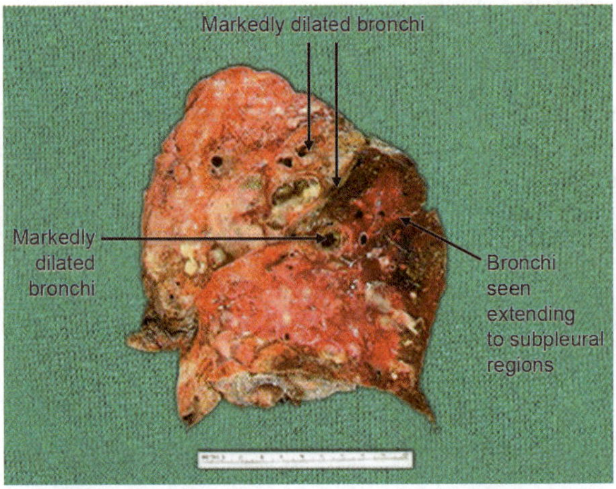

Pathological Changes

Gross appearance:

- The bronchi and bronchioles are dilated giving the lung a "honey comb" appearance, especially in the lower lobes (Fig. 8.17).
- Involvement may be diffuse/segmental.
- Bronchi and bronchioles on dilatation can assume any of the following configurations:
  - Saccular
  - Cylindrical
  - Fusiform
  - Varicose
- The dilated airways are traceable to the pleural surface unlike in a normal state where they can only be traced for 1–2 cm.
- Airways may display the presence of mucus plugs/impacted foreign body/tumor depending upon the cause.

Figure 8.17: Honey comb appearance in bronchiectasis

Histological changes:

- Extensive acute and inflammation both in and around the bronchi and bronchioles disrupting the bronchial wall including the muscle layer.
- Desquamation/ulceration of the lining epithelial of the bronchi and bronchioles.
- Squamous metaplasia of the lining epithelium.
- Peribronchial fibrosis.
- The surrounding lung may display features of necrotizing pneumonia or interstitial pneumonia in cases of viral etiology.

3. Chronic Bronchitis

This is a disease characterized by cough that is persistent, and associated with expectoration (sputum production), for at least three months every year for a minimum of two consecutive years.

Clinical Features

Persistent cough with expectoration, worse in the morning due to accumulation of secretions overnight and exacerbated in cold weather. The patient often has shortness of breath. Pulmonary function is usually within normal limits initially but with time, declines.

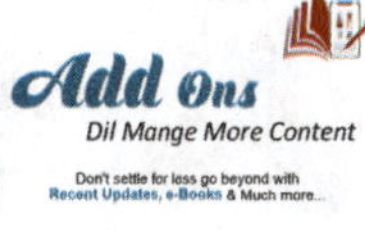

Etiology

By inflammation of the bronchi:

- Short-term bronchitis is usually triggered by an infection.
- Long-term bronchitis is caused by recurrent inflammation of the bronchi, usually as a result of smoking or other inhaled irritants.

Risk Factors

- Pollution.
- Older age.
- Smoking is the leading cause of chronic bronchitis.
- Close and frequent exposure to concentrated inhaled chemicals.
- Respiratory disease as a child.

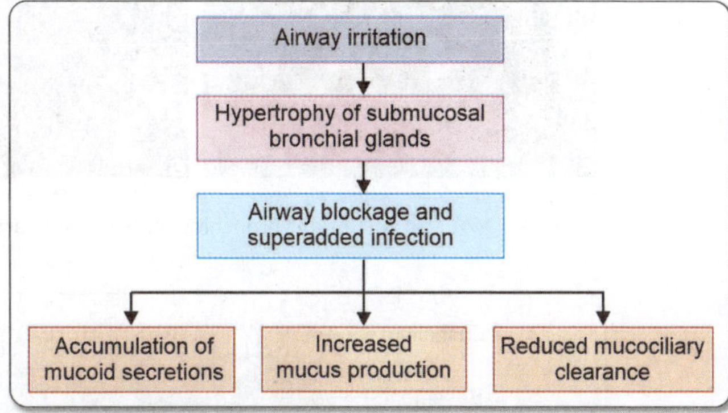

Figure 8.18: Pathogenesis of chronic bronchitis

Pathogenesis

The pathogenesis of chronic bronchitis (Fig. 8.18) is based on the two triggers that are irritation and infection. Both these factors lead to airway inflammation.

1. **Airway irritation:** This is caused by chronic exposure to dust, environmental pollutants and various noxious substances such as smog, tobacco smoke, vehicular emissions and industrial pollutants.
2. **Infections:** This is usually a consequence of the airway being blocked by inspissated secretions, acting as a nidus of superadded infection.

Complications

- Frequent bacterial infections
- Cor pulmonale
- Heart failure

Pathological Changes

Gross appearance (Fig. 8.19A): Viscid secretions in the airway, bronchial casts obstructing the bronchi and bronchioles.

Histological changes (Fig. 8.19B):

- Denudation of the lining respiratory type epithelium with loss of cilia.
- Squamous metaplasia and dysplasia of the lining epithelium.
- Submucosal edema.
- Hypertrophy of bronchial submucosal glands with goblet cell hyperplasia.
- Peribronchial fibrosis.
- Inflammation: Chronic, comprising lymphocytes admixed with few histiocytes, occasional plasma cells.
- Reid index (Fig. 8.20) is an important histological index to diagnose chronic bronchitis.

It is ratio of the thickness of the mucous gland layer to the thickness of the bronchial wall between the epithelium and cartilage (b-c/a-d) is Reid index.

= >0.5 in chronic bronchitis (normal—0.4)

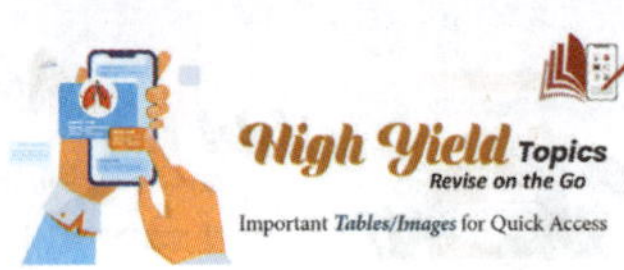

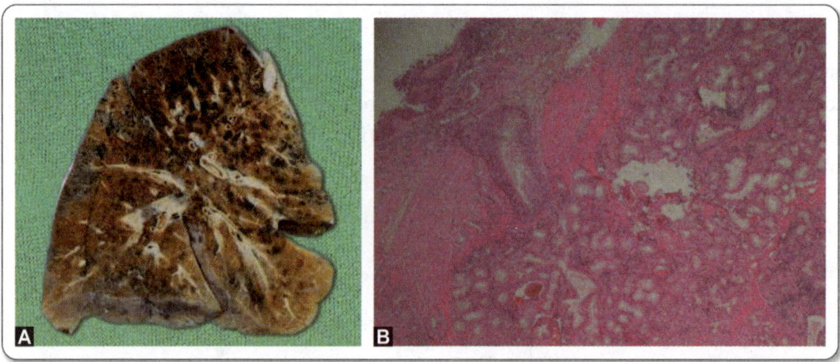

Figures 8.19A and B: Chronic bronchitis: **A.** Gross appearance; **B.** Microscopic appearance

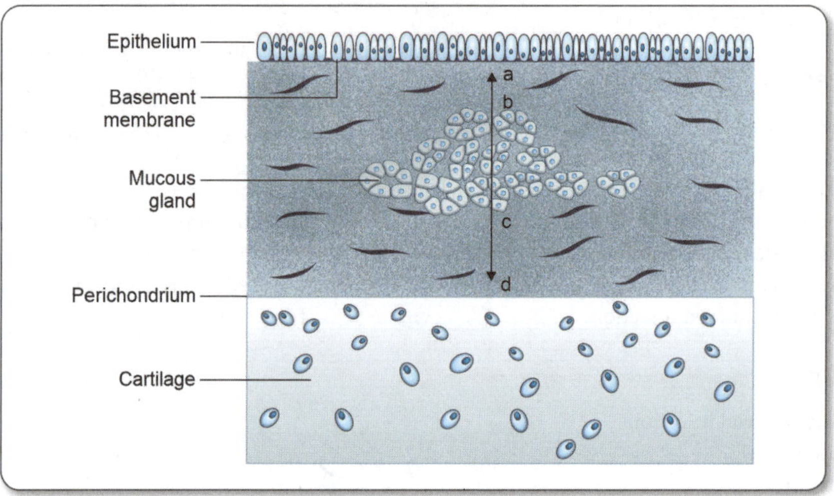

Figure 8.20: Reid index

4. Bronchial Asthma

This is a reversible and intermittent chronic obstructive pulmonary disease caused due to increased irritation of the bronchi and variable expiratory outflow obstruction.

Clinical Features

Cough, shortness of breath, chest wheeze.

Etiology

Pollen, air pollutants, noxious chemicals and irritants, viral infections of the upper respiratory tract, stress, exercise.

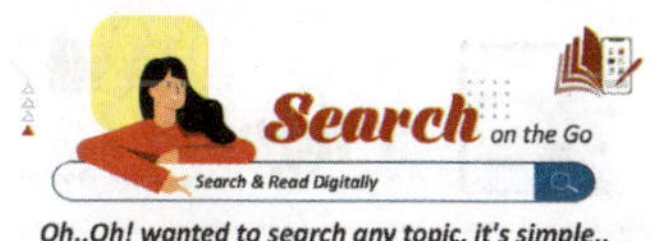

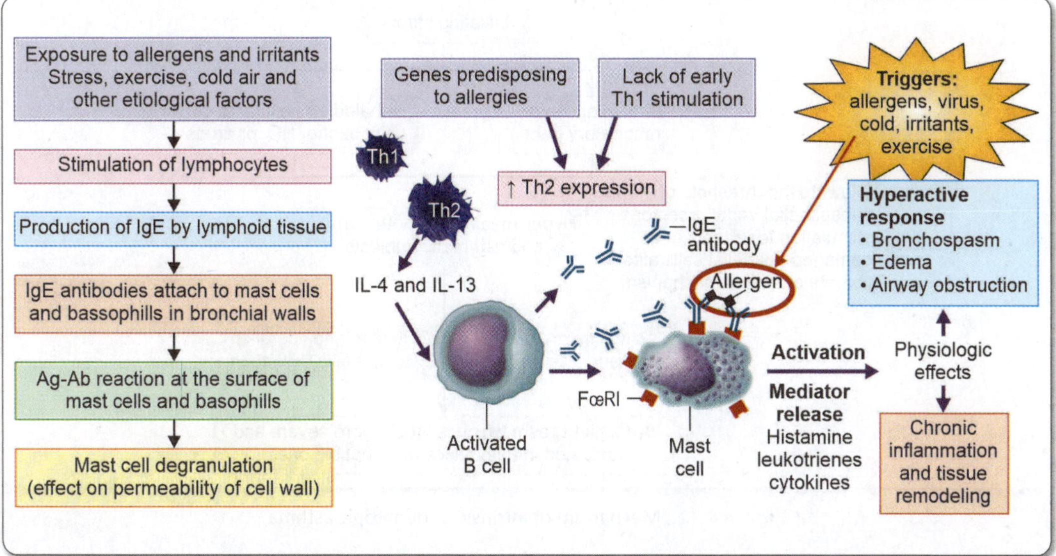

Figure 8.21: Mechanism of pathogenesis extrinsic or atopic asthma

Pathogenesis

The two broad types of asthma according to etiopathogenetic pathways are:

1. Extrinsic asthma or atopic asthma
2. Intrinsic or nonatopic asthma

Extrinsic Asthma or Atopic Asthma

Extrinsic or atopic asthma (Fig. 8.21) is based on a type 1 hypersensitivity reaction involving the following steps:

- **Sensitization phase:** All extrinsic allergens stimulate the Th2 type of lymphocytes which in turn release IL-4 and IL-5. This stimulates the production of antibodies by B lymphocytes, specifically IgE which coats the bronchial subepithelial mast cells.
- **Re-exposure phase:** On reintroduction of the allergen, the sensitized mast cells are activated to produce chemical mediators, primarily histamine.
  - Early phase of this reaction is driven by the production of histamine and other mediators leading to bronchoconstriction, vasodilation, increased mucus production.
  - Late phase is characterized by recruitment of leukocytes, especially eosinophils. These in turn liberate eotoxin causing inflammation and destruction of bronchial lining epithelial.

Intrinsic or Nonatopic Asthma

Unlike atopic or extrinsic asthma where the IgE production is increased, in nonatopic asthma, serum IgE levels remain normal (Fig. 8.22). Lowered threshold of the subepithelial vagal receptors leads to an increased susceptibility of the airways to irritants. This is triggered by viral infections, or pollutants.

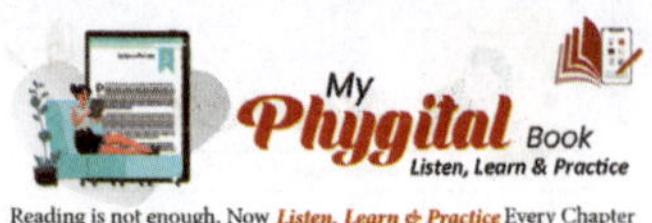

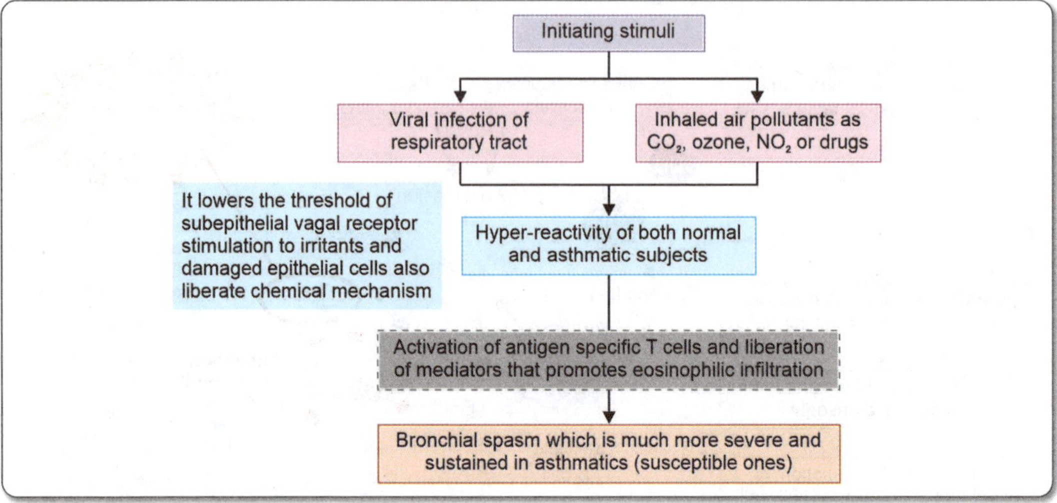

Figure 8.22: Mechanism of intrinsic or nonatopic asthma

Drug Induced Asthma

Drug induced asthma is nonatopic type. Certain drugs cause asthma such as aspirin and β-blockers.

- **Clinical features:** Wheezing, sometimes just at night, coughing, shortness of breath, chest tightness.
- **Pathogenesis:** Mechanism of asthma induced by nonsteroidal anti-inflammatory drugs include altered sensitivity to leukotrienes and abnormal release of cytotoxic compounds from platelets.

Complications of Asthma

Progressive overdistension of the lungs can lead to complications such as:

- Emphysema.
- Superadded infection leads to other chronic obstructive pulmonary diseases.

Pathological Changes

Gross appearance:

The lungs are overinflated resulting in an increased weight and size of the lungs. This is interspersed by areas of atelectasis (lung collapse). The walls of the bronchi are thickened and are filled with mucus plugs (Fig. 8.23A).

Histological changes

- Smooth muscle cell hyperplasia.
- Bronchial gland hyperplasia.
- Submucosal edema.
- Inflammation including eosinophils.
- Mucous plugs and mucous gland hyperplasia (Fig. 8.23B).
- Increased vascularity.
- **The presence of Charcot-Leyden crystals:** (eosinophil protein galectin-10) (Fig. 8.24A).
- **Curschmann spirals:** Spiral shaped mucus plugs in the distal airways (Fig. 8.24B).
- **Creola bodies:** Clusters of bronchial epithelial cells showing reactive changes (Fig. 8.24C).

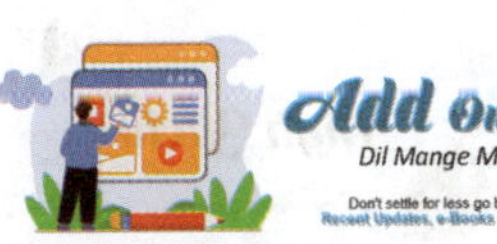

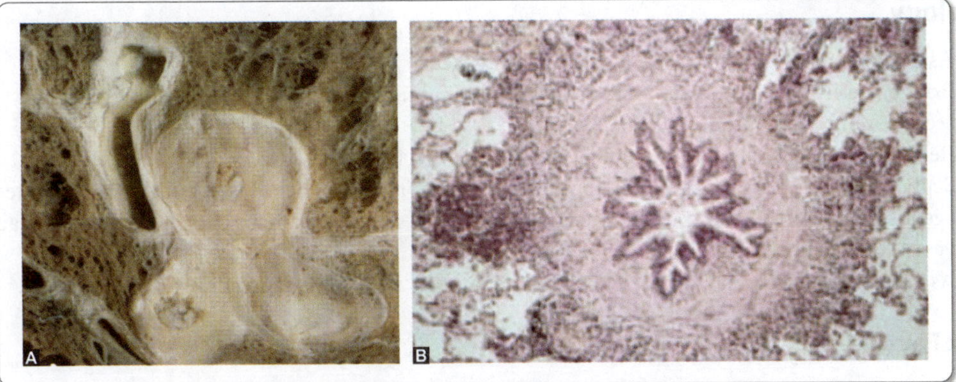

Figures 8.23A and B: Mucus plug: **A.** Gross appearance; **B.** Microscopic appearance

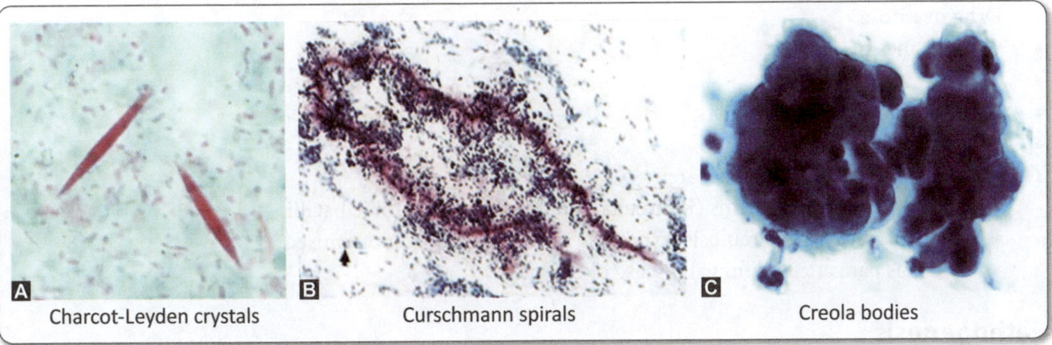

Figures 8.24A to C: Cytological findings in sputum of asthma patient

LUNG ABSCESS

This is a disease characterized by a local suppurative process involving the lung parenchyma resulting in tissue necrosis. It can be primary when the lung is otherwise normal (e.g., in cases of aspiration)/secondary as a complication of pre-existing lung disease or systemic infection.

Clinical Features

Fever, cough, chest pain, loss of appetite, fatigue and abundant expectoration of purulent sputum. Some patients may show clubbing of fingers.

It is important for the clinician to arrive at a timely diagnosis as persistence or spread of a lung abscess leads to complications such as:

- Extension of inflammation to the pleura (pleuritis)/accumulation of pus in the pleural space (empyema).
- Hemorrhage.
- Sepsis and meningitis can especially occur in cases where septic emboli cause the abscess.
- Meningitis.
- Secondary amyloidosis.

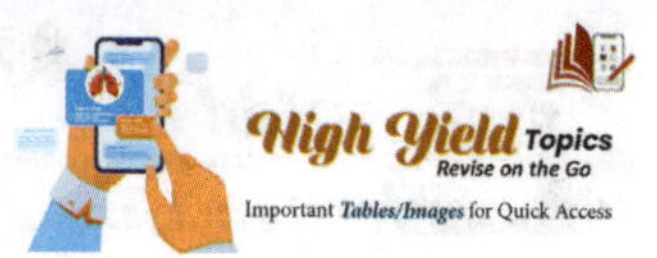

Etiology

- Aspiration of infective material (in coma/neuromuscular disease/epilepsy).
- Prior bacterial infection/pneumonia in the lung, spreading to adjoining areas of the lung. This is typically seen in immunocompromised patients.
- Recurrence of tubercular infection may also present as a walled off abscess.
- Septic embolism: This is a condition in which fragments/masses of debris intermingle with the infectious agent (septic emboli) and travel in the circulation from some other focus outside the lung to reach the vessels of the lung.
- As a complication of malignancy, where the tumor obstructs the airway leading to inflammation.

Risk Factors

- Alcoholism.
- Seizure disorder.
- Neuromuscular disorders.
- Drug overdose.
- General anesthesia.
- Stroke.
- Immunocompnomised patients.
- ICU patients.

The pathogenic organisms involved are:
  - Gram-negative organisms (Klebsiella, *S. aureus*) and anaerobic bacilli.
  - Mycobacterium tuberculosis, expecially in the immunocompnomised.
  - Various parasitic and fungal disease of the lung.

Pathogenesis

Lung abscesses are caused by aspiration of material from the gastrointestinal (GI) tract into the lungs (Fig. 8.25).

Due to etiology (tumor/pnemonia/aspiration)
↓
Mechanical or functional obstruction in airway
↓
Growth of bacteria at site and increased secretion of mucus
↓
Increasing area of infection later becomes necrotic
↓
Forms a cavity filled with purulent mucus material
↓
Lung abscess formation

Figure 8.25: Pathogenesis of lung abscess

Complications

- Chronic abscess as it lingers for >6 weeks.
- **Empyema:** Lungs and chest wall get with pus.
- **Bleeding:** Can destroy a blood vessel and cause serious bleeding.
- **Bronchopleural fistula:** An opening between the tubes in the lungs and layers that cover them.

Pathological Changes

Gross appearance:

- Abscesses vary in size ranging from a few mm to 6 cm and maybe single/multiple (Fig. 8.26A).
- Abscesses (due to aspiration) are more on the right side as the right main bronchus is more vertical, and mostly single.

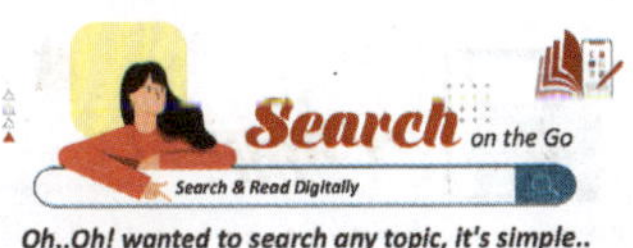

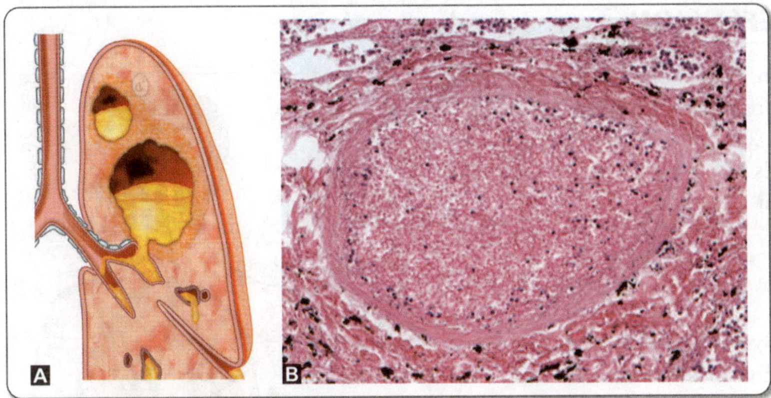

Figures 8.26A and B: Lung abscess: **A.** Gross appearance; **B.** Microscopic appearance

- Abscesses (due to pneumonia/bronchiectasis)—multiple, basal.
- The abscess cavity is usually filled with fibrinopurulent exudate admixed with necrotic material and in long standing cases, it displays a fibrotic wall.

Histological changes:

- Destruction of the alveolar spaces (Fig. 8.26B).
- Extensive acute inflammatory exudate in the abscess wall permeating to the alveolar spaces and interstitium destroying both.
- In chronic cases, fibrosis is present along with a chronic inflammatory infiltrate comprising lymphocytes and macrophages.
- Etiology specific changes:
  - In abscesses of tubercular etiology, epithelioid cell granulomas with caseous necrosis and Langerhans giant cells may be seen.
  - In abscesses of fungal etiology, fungal hyphae and buds of the causative species would be identified with the help of special stains such as PAS and Gomori Methenamine Silver (GMS).
  - In abscesses of amoebic etiology, trophozoites of entamoeba histolytica are noted, highlighted by PAS stain.

Diagnosis

Physical examination:

- Dullness to percussion
- Decreased breath sounds on auscultation over the segment of lung involved
- Crackles

Radiological:

- CT scan
- MRI
- Chest X-ray

Culture:

- Sputum culture or pleural fluid or blood culture
- Bronchoscopy

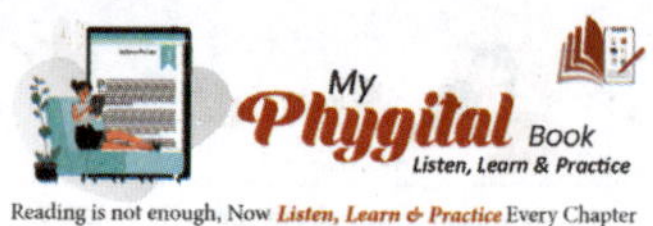

PLEURAL EFFUSION

Pleural effusion is an accumulation of the fluid in the pleural space (Fig. 8.27). Normally the pleural sac contains 5–15 mL of fluid, but if it exceeds to an abnormal amount, it is called pleural effusion. It is secondary to other diseases).

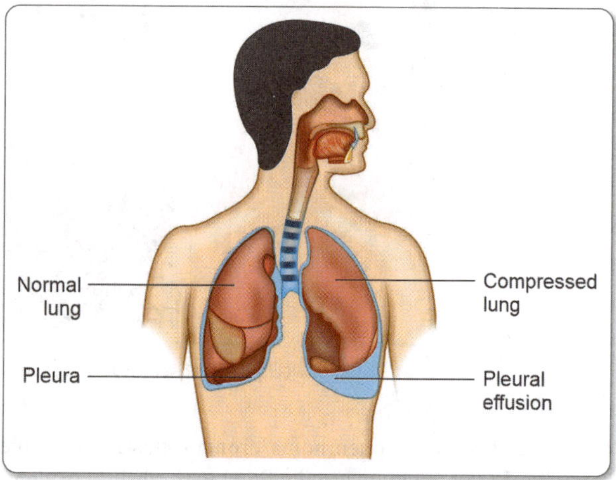

Figure 8.27: Pleural effusion

Types

- **Transudative effusion:** It is caused by non-inflammatory condition which includes an accumulation of poor or low quantity of protein or low cell count fluid.
- **Exudative effusion:** It is caused by inflammatory condition which includes an accumulation of high quantity of protein that occurs due to increased capillary permeability.

Clinical Features

The patient of pleural effusion presents to the physician with complaints of chest pain, cough and shortness of breath.

Causes

The causes of pleural effusion are varied and are enlisted below:

- **Infectious causes:** Any bacterial/viral/fungal/parasitic infection can cause pleural effusion. For example, tuberculosis.
- **Hemodynamic derangements:** Congestive heart failure is a condition that causes disturbance in the normal hemodynamic forces leading to the accumulation of fluid in all the body cavities.
- **Conditions associated with hypoproteinemia:** Any chronic persistent condition leading to loss of protein in the body can cause accumulation of fluid in the pleural space. Examples are cirrhosis, nephrotic syndrome, protein losing enteropathy.
- **Trauma:** Injury to tissues of the chest wall may lead to accumulation of blood in the pleural space (hemothorax). If the thoracic duct is injured in the process it could lead to chylothorax (accumulation of lymph). Accumulation of clear fluid may also occur as a delayed complication to injury, though rarely, as an immune mediated response to residual debris.
- **Malignancy:** Malignant tumors such as lung carcinoma especially adenocarcinoma, breast carcinomas and lymphomas can cause pleural effusions. If the malignant cells have spread to the pleural space it is referred to as a malignant pleural effusion and if the focus of malignancy has not involved the pleural space it is called as paramalignant pleural effusion.
- **Pulmonary embolism/infarction:** This can cause ischemia related injury causing release of cytokines and an increase in interstitial fluid in the lungs as well as pleural effusion.

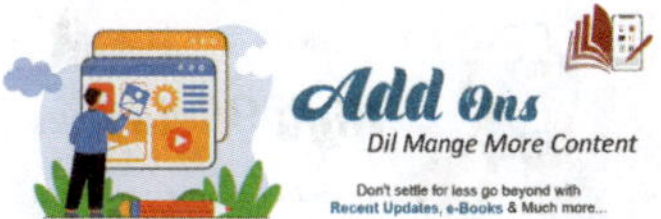

Diagnosis

Indications of performing a pleural tap (thoracocentesis):

- When the fluid accumulated in the pleural space is significant, which is radiologically defined as >10 mm in a lateral decubitus position X-ray/USG.
- **Diagnostic:** When the cause of pleural effusion is to be ascertained, i.e., whether it is of neoplastic or non-neoplastic origin,especially in cases of low volume effusions.
- **Therapeutic:** A pleural tap can also be performed to remove fluid when large volumes are present in the pleural space thereby relieving patient symptoms such as shortness of breath.

The first step in evaluating any fluid including pleural fluid is whether it is a transudate or an exudate.

Gross appearance:

Gross appearance of the fluid is an important indicator of the type of fluid:

- Clear/straw colored/pale colored fluids are usually transudates.
- Turbid/purulent/milky/blood tinged fluids are usually exudates.

Dr Richard Light gave a set of biochemical criteria to differentiate transudates from exudates. These criteria include:

- Pleural fluid protein/serum protein ratio >0.5
- Pleural fluid LDH/Serum LDH ratio >0.6
- Pleural fluid LDH above 2/3 of upper limit of normal for serum LDH

Exudates have at least one of these criteria.

Appearance based diagnosis of pleural fluid

Pleural fluid total leukocyte count: The differentiation of whether a fluid is a transudate or exudate can also be done by analyzing the WBC count of the fluid.

Transudates <1000 cells/cu.mm

Exudates >1000 cells/cu.mm

Lymphocyte predominant effusions include – TB
– Rheumatoid pleuritis
– Lymphoma

Neutrophil predominant effusions include – Empyema
– Pulmonary embolism and infarction

Cytological changes:

Cytological evaluation of a pleural fluid is useful to triage the fluid as benign or malignant. Fluids received are centrifuged and stained with Giemsa (for air dried smears) and Papanicolaou stain (alcohol fixed). In cases of malignancy, further typing of the malignancy can be offered based on morphology and ancillary tests such as cell blocks and immunohistochemistry. Three serial samples can also be evaluated to improve the detection of malignancy.

Microbiological examination:

If purulent exudates/cloudy fluid—suspect an infective etiology viewing the clinical history. Accordingly routine microbiological tests include:

- Gram's smear to assess the absence or presence of bacteria.
- Culture—for an etiological diagnosis and for diagnosing tuberculosis.
- Polymerase chain reaction (PCR) for mycobacterial DNA.

Other tests:

- D-dimer on peripheral blood to confirm pulmonary embolism as a cause.
- NT-proBNP—elevated levels of this biomarker are seen both in serum and pleural fluid in cases of congestive heart failure.

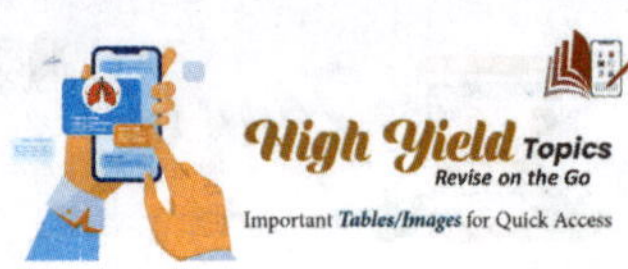

- Flow cytometry—can be used to confirm the absence or presence of a lymphoma
- Rheumatoid factor >1:320 can confirm rheumatoid pleuritis
- Autoimmune profile—ANA, dsDNA to confirm an autoimmune origin of effusion
- Elevated amylase—pancreatitis, esophageal rupture
- Elevated triglyceride >110 mg/dL—chylous effusion in cases of chylothorax
- Elevated ADA >35–40 IU/L in endemic areas has a high predictive value for tuberculosis
- Low glucose-empyema, rheumatoid arthritis, TB.

LUNG TUMORS

Lung cancer constitutes one of the most common cancers worldwide. Most malignant lung tumors are epithelial derived carcinomas (95%). The rest of lung tumors being of neuroendocrine/mesenchymal origin.

Pathogenesis

The pathogenesis of lung tumor is shown in self explanatory Figure 8.28.

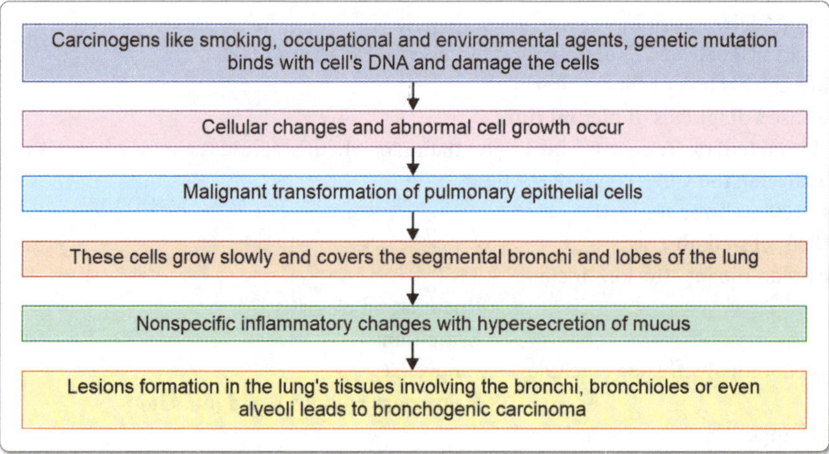

Figure 8.28: Pathogenesis of lung tumor

Classification of Lung Tumors

The lung tumors can be classified as shown in Figure 8.29.

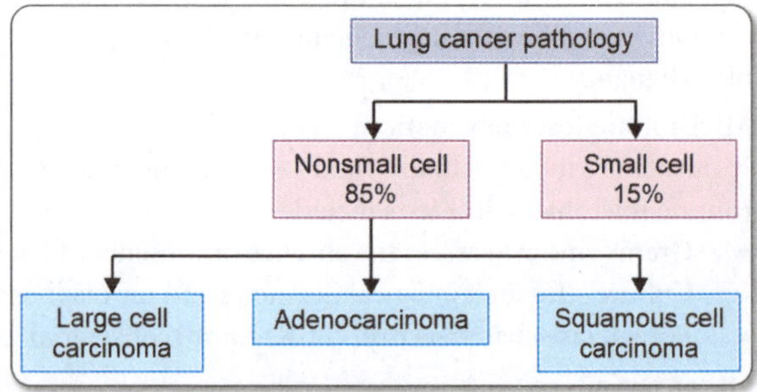

Figure 8.29: Types of lung tumors

Small Cell Tumors

A highly malignant, aggressive tumor which may either be in a central/hilar location. This tumor is associated with cigarette smoking. Small cell tumors may produce ectopic hormones such as ADH, and ACTH.

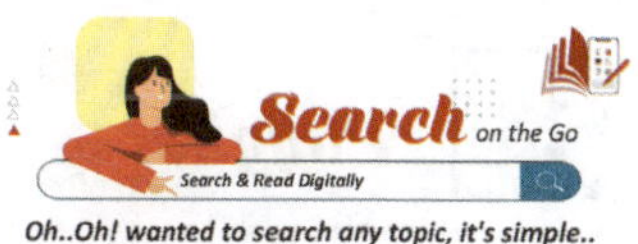

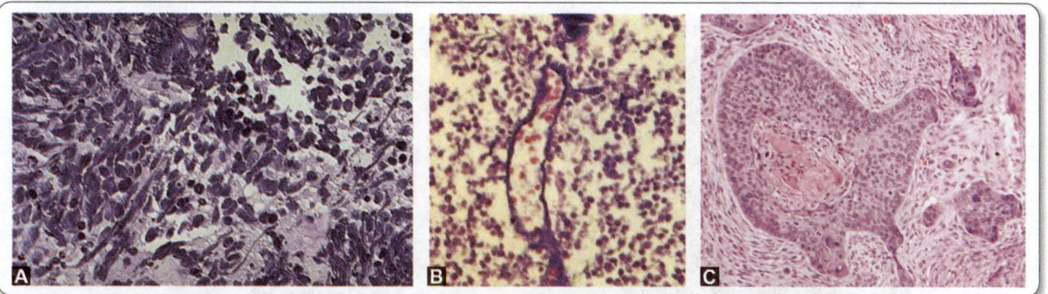

Figures 8.30A and B: Histology of lung carcinoma: **A.** Small cell carcinoma; **B.** Azzopardi effect; **C.** Nonsmall cell carcinoma

Pathological Features

- **Cut surface:** Soft, yellowish white, foci of hemorrhage and necrosis may be seen. The tumor may be friable.
- **Histological changes (Fig. 8.30A):** Sheets, nests and trabeculae of small round/ovoid cells which show scant cytoplasm, mild pleomorphism, nuclear hyperchromasia, smudgy nuclear chromatin. Nuclear moulding is prominent. Nucleoli are inconspicuous.
  - **Necrosis:** Common and extensive
  - Mitoses are frequent.
  - **The Azzopardi effect:** A peculiar morphological feature sees in small cell carcinomas. The vessel walls are highly basophilic due to layering by DNA shed off from the necrotic tumor cells (Fig. 8.30B).

Immunohistochemistry: Synaptophysin, Chromogranin, INSM1 (recent marker).

Electron microscopic findings: Dense core neurosecretory granules are seen.

Nonsmall Cell Tumors

Large Cell Carcinoma (LCC)

The LCC is undifferentiated nonsmall cell malignancy. An uncommon tumor of the lung, this represents an undifferentiated malignant epithelial neoplasm.

Clinical Features

It is usually seen in elderly subjects with a predilection in smokers and is located at the periphery of the lung. Patients present with cough, shortness of breath and sometimes hemoptysis as seen in other types of lung carcinoma.

Pathological changes:

Gross appearance (Fig. 8.31A): Large-sized (>4 cm)

- Have a white to gray or fish-flesh cut appearance.
- Gross tumor necrosis is common.

Histological changes (Figs 8.30C and 8.31B):

- Consists of sheets and nests of large cells with vesicular nuclei, prominent nucleoli, and moderate or abundant cytoplasm.

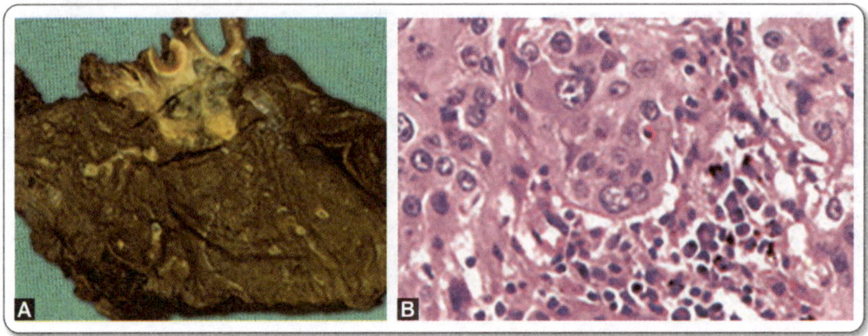

Figures 8.31A and B: Large cell carcinoma: A. Gross; B. Histological depiction

Laboratory Diagnosis

Immunohistochemical markers used to arrive at this diagnosis (which all should be negative for labelling a tumor as large cell) include:

- p40 (squamous differentiation).
- TTF-1 (glandular differentiation).
- Synaptophysin, chromogranin, CD56, INSM1 (neuroendocrine differentiation).

MUST KNOW

The key point is that large cell carcinoma cannot be diagnosed on small biopsy specimens and only on surgical resection specimens where only it is possible to conclusively rule out the lack of differentiation of a tumor.

Squamous Cell Carcinoma

Frequently seen in men and is associated with smoking.

Gross appearance (Fig. 8.32A): Commonly seen in a central/hilar location.

Cut surface: Shows the presence of a gray white, firm tumor mass with foci of necrosis and hemorrhage.

Histological changes (Fig. 8.32B): Tumor cells show varying degrees of squamoid differentiation which are well differentiated and show the presence of keratin pearls and intracellular keratin. Individual cells show intercellular bridges.

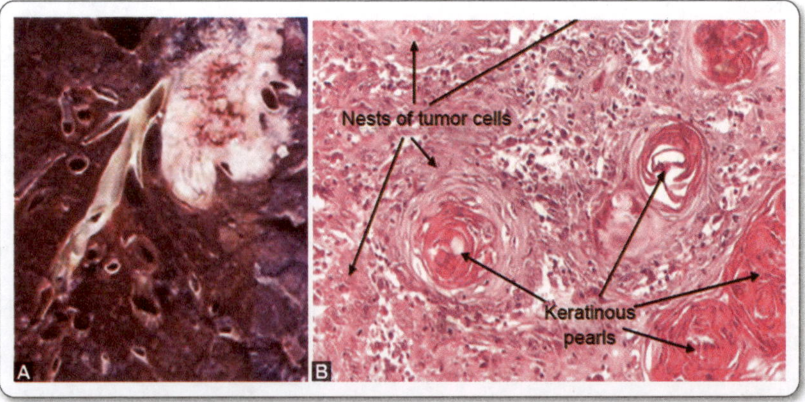

Figures 8.32A and B: Squamous cell carcinoma of lungs: A. Gross appearance; B. Microscopic appearance (keratinizing squamous cell carcinoma)

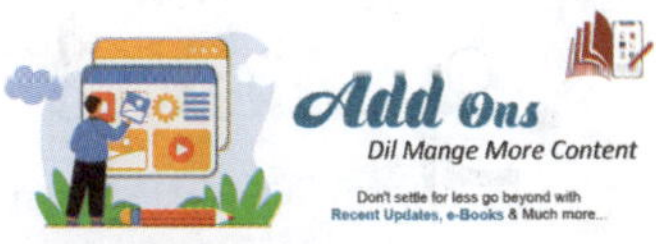

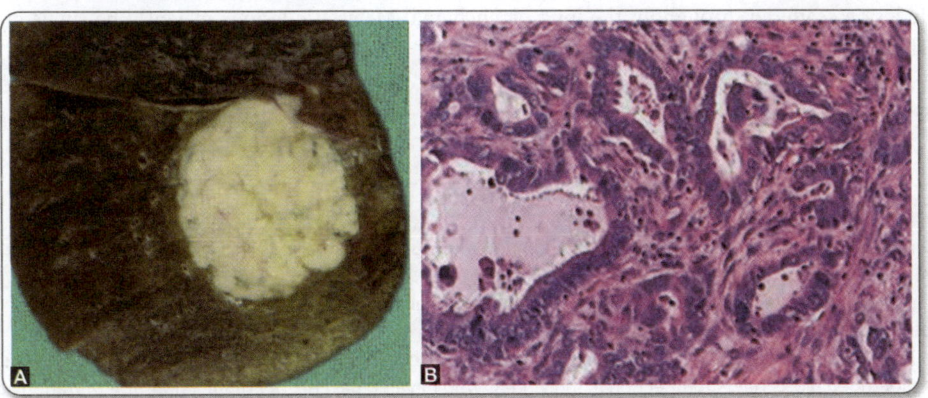

Figures 8.33A and B: Adenocarcinoma of lungs: **A.** Gross; **B.** Histological

- Moderate differentiation shows less keratin while in poorly differentiated cases, identifying a squamoid origin is itself very difficult.
- Mitotic figures are seen. They are usually more frequent in poorly differentiated lesions.
- Tumor islands are surrounded by inflammatory cells and may elicit a desmoplastic reaction.

Adenocarcinoma

This type of lung cancer is seen in up to a third of cases of malignant tumors and is commonly seen in the 5th–6th decades. It is seen frequently in women and nonsmokers and is characteristically seen in a peripheral location of the lung.

Cut surface: Grayish white (Fig. 8.33A)

Histological changes (Fig. 8.33B): Tumor cells are arranged in the form of glands, which may have an infiltrative growth pattern. Some lesions may show the presence of papillae/solid foci/lepidic (butterfly on the fence) arrangement. Evidence of mucin production may be noted.

Molecular/ancillary testing: Lesions may display KRAS, EGFR mutations, ALK rearrangements.

IHC: TTF-1, Napsin A, Beta catenin, CK7 positivity.

Adenocarcinomas typically display a slow rate of growth but ironically have a higher propensity to metastasize.

Metastatic Tumor of Lungs

Tumors present elsewhere can also spread to the lungs (Fig. 8.34). This spread occurs either through the bloodstream or through lymphatic channels. Tumors present in organs close to the lung, such as other mediastinal organs and esophagus are obvious source of metastasis for tumor cells. However, tumors distant from the lung may also reach the lungs such as the kidneys, GI tract and thyroid.

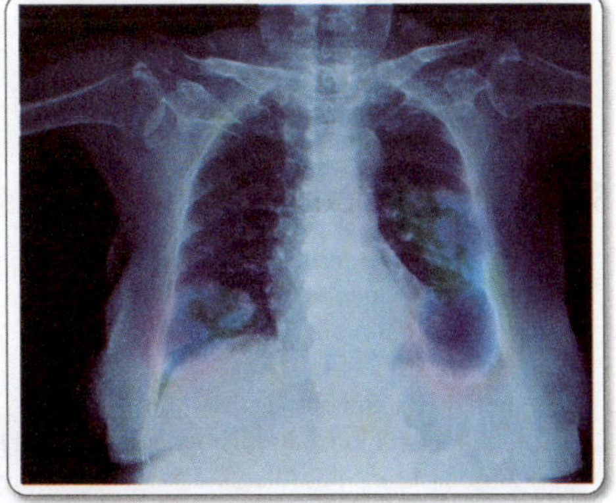

Figure 8.34: Metastatic tumor of lung

Pathological Changes

Gross appearance: Typically, a cannonball appearance is seen on imaging. This refers to the presence of multiple

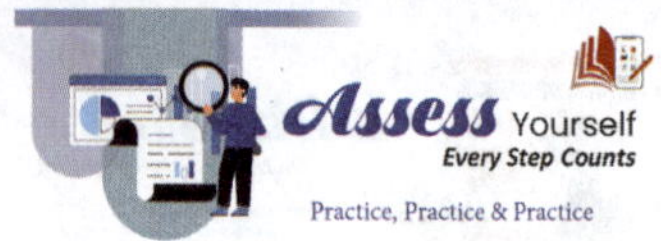

discrete lesion scattered throughout the lung parenchyma. Metastatic lesions may also be single and well-defined or may present as pleural nodules.

Histological changes: Features of the respective tumor would be seen surrounded by lung parenchyma represented by alveolar spaces.

SUMMARY

- The respiratory system is entrusted with the function of ensuring adequate oxygenation of the blood as well as defence against microorganisms.
- Lung disease can clinically be categorized as restrictive and obstructive.
- Tuberculosis is a chronic granulomatous disease.
- The inability of the macrophages to remove *M. tuberculosis* bacilli is central to the pathogenesis of tuberculosis.
- Primary tuberculosis refers to infection in individuals who have no past history of infection/immunization against tuberculosis.
- A diminished cough reflex promotes accumulation of pent-up secretions within the respiratory tract making a person susceptible to develop infections.
- The patient of pneumonia usually appears sick and is lethargic.
- Consolidation refers to the loss of the normal spongy texture of the lung parenchyma.
- Bronchopneumonia is usually seen in patients at both extremes of age, i.e., the young and the elderly.
- Bronchopneumonia may also be secondary to viral infections.

  Interstitial pneumonia is a group of diseases where inflammation and fibrosis damage the small air-filled spaces inside the lungs called alveoli.
- Irreversible and abnormal dilatation of the bronchi and bronchioles secondary to the destruction of the bronchial wall (muscle and elastic fibers) due to any etiology is bronchiectasis.
- Bronchial asthma is a reversible and intermittent chronic obstructive pulmonary disease.
- On reintroduction of the allergen, the sensitized mast cells are activated to produce chemical mediators, primarily histamine.
- Certain drugs cause asthma such as aspirin and β-blockers.
- Progressive overdistension of the lungs can lead to complications.
- Lung abscesses are caused by aspiration of material from the GI tract into the lungs.
- Most malignant lung tumors are epithelial derived carcinomas.
- Adenocarcinomas typically display a slow rate of growth but ironically have a higher propensity to metastasize.

ASSESS YOURSELF

Long Answer Questions

1. Discuss chronic obstructive pulmonary disease.
2. Discuss lung tumors in detail.

Short Answer Questions

1. Write about adenocarcinoma of lungs.
2. What is lobar pneumonia?
3. Write short notes on:
   i. Tuberculosis.
   ii. Restrictive and obstructive lung disease.
   iii. Lobar pneumonia, Bronchopneumonia and Interstitial pneumonia.
   iv. Chronic bronchitis (blue bloater) and emphysema (pink puffer).

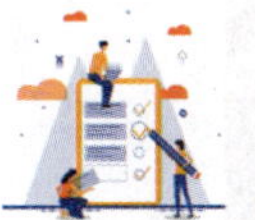
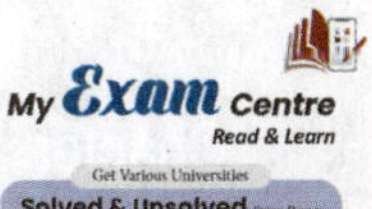

Multiple Choice Questions

1. **Asthma, a respiratory disease, is caused due to:**
   a. Infection of trachea
   b. Infection of lungs
   c. Bleeding into pleural cavity
   d. Spasm in bronchial muscles
2. **Smokers have shorter breath due to:**
   a. Arteriosclerosis
   b. Emphysema
   c. Hypertension
   d. Cough
3. **Complications of bronchiectasis include:**
   a. Amyloidosis
   b. Cor pulmonale
   c. Lung abscess
   d. Metastatic brain abscesses
   e. All of the above
4. **Acute phase reaction of asthma does NOT include:**
   a. Bronchoconstriction
   b. Mucosal edema
   c. Mucus hypersecretion
   d. Epithelial inflammation and damage
   e. All of the above
5. **Site of injury in chronic bronchitis is:**
   a. Main bronchus
   b. Lobar bronchi
   c. Small bronchi and bronchioles
   d. Alveolar wall
   e. All of the above
6. **Risk factors for interstitial emphysema include:**
   a. Positive pressure ventilation
   b. Airway obstruction
   c. Fractured ribs
   d. Cough
   e. All of the above
7. **In emphysema, there is an excess of:**
   a. $\alpha 1$ antitrypsin
   b. Antielastase
   c. Elastase
   d. All of these
   e. None of the above
8. **Cause of pulmonary edema include:**
   a. Left ventricular failure
   b. Massive trauma/shock
   c. Mycoplasmal pneumonia
   d. Drowning
   e. All of the above

Answer Key

1. d **2.** b **3.** e **4.** d **5.** c **6.** e
7. c **8.** e

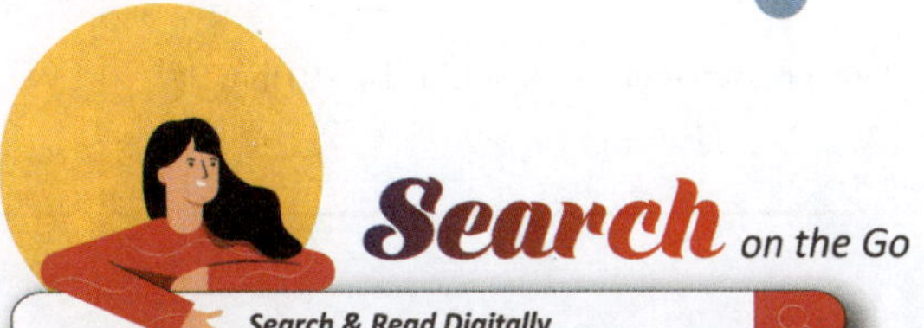

Chapter 9

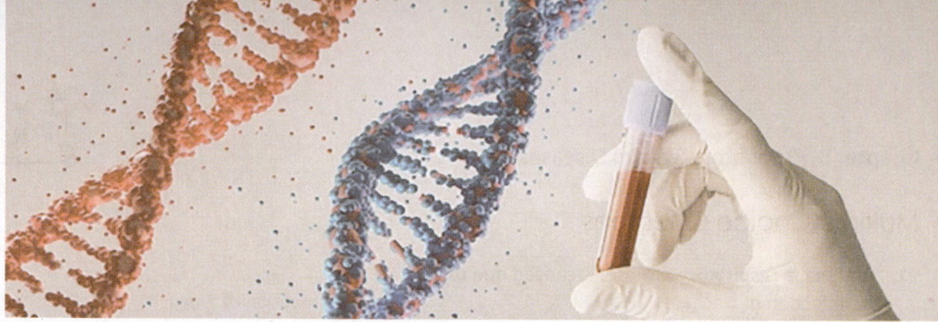

Cardiovascular System Diseases

LEARNING OBJECTIVES

After the completion of the chapter, the readers will be able to:

- Understand pericardial effusion.
- Discuss atherosclerosis.
- Discuss ischemic heart disease.
- Explain aneurysm.
- Understand rheumatic heart disease.
- Explain infections endocarditis.

CHAPTER OUTLINE

- Overview of Cardiovascular System

Diseases of Cardiovascular System

- Pericardial Effusion
- Atherosclerosis
- Ischemic Heart Disease
- Rheumatic Heart Disease
- Infective Endocarditis
- Aneurysm

KEY TERMS

Atheroma: A fatty substance that builds up in arteries over time.

Cardiac biomarkers: Cardiac biomarkers are used to evaluate heart function.

Cardiac tamponade: Pressure on the heart that occurs when blood or fluid builds up in the space between the heart muscle and the outer covering sac (pericardium) of the heart.

Effusion: The escape of a fluid from anatomical vessels by rupture or exudation.

Interstitium: A contiguous fluid-filled space existing between a structural barrier, such as a cell membrane or the skin.

Muffled: Quiet or not clear.

Neoangiogenesis: The development of new blood vessels from a pre-existing vasculature.

Perfusion: The passage of fluid through the circulatory system (blood stream) or lymphatic system to an organ or a tissue.

Pulsus paradoxus: An exaggerated fall in a patient's blood pressure during inspiration by >10 mm Hg.

Syncope: Fainting or passing out.

"Mottled" appearance: Having spots or patches of color.

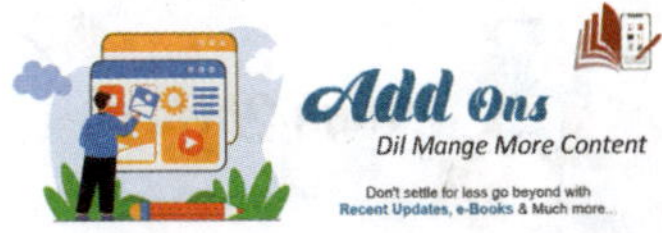

OVERVIEW OF CARDIOVASCULAR SYSTEM

- The cardiovascular system (Fig. 9.1) consists of the heart, veins, arteries, and capillaries. These components make up two circulatory systems–the systemic and pulmonary circulatory systems.
- The heart has four chambers–two atria and two ventricles.
- The left side of the heart is responsible for pumping oxygenated blood to the body, whereas right side receives deoxygenated blood from the body, and sends *via* pulmonary artery to lungs.
- The cardiac cycle consists of two phases–systole (relaxation) and diastole (contraction).
- Some conditions which affect the heart include heart attack, stroke, heart failure, and arrhythmia.
- As the body ages, the heart functions less effectively, especially during periods of high physical activity.
- The arteries also have a higher likelihood of becoming stiff with age, which increases the possibility of high blood pressure and associated cardiovascular issues.

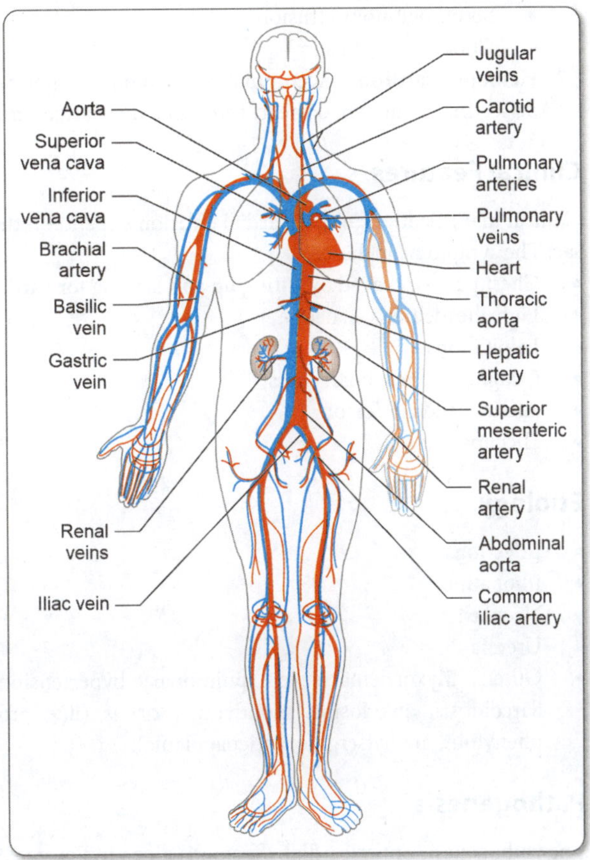

Figure 9.1: Cardiovascular system

DISEASES OF CARDIOVASCULAR SYSTEM

PERICARDIAL EFFUSION

Presence of an abnormal amount of fluid in the pericardial space is called pericardial effusion (Fig. 9.2). The pericardial space normally contains 15–50 mL of fluid. Cardiac tamponade is acute heart failure due to compression of heart by a large or rapidly developing effusion.

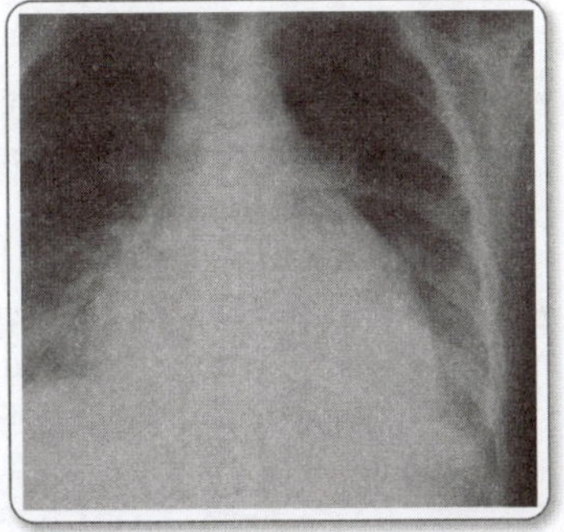

Figure 9.2: Pericardial effusion—An X-ray visual

Types

It is of two types:

1. **Hydropericardium:** Accumulation of fluid due to noninflammatory causes.
   It can be:
   - Serous effusion
   - Chylous effusion

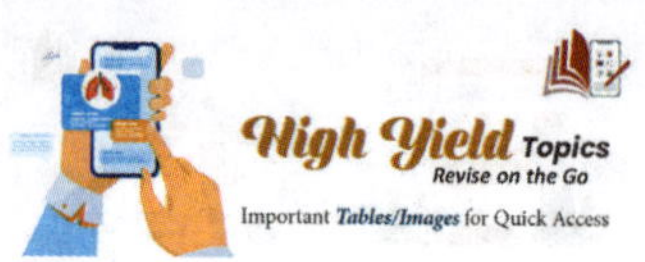

- Serosanguinous effusion
- Cholesterol effusion

2. **Hemopericardium:** Accumulation of blood in pericardial sac. It can be due to trauma, rupture of dissecting aneurysm, or heart through a myocardial infarct.

Clinical Features

Clinical manifestations of pericardial effusion depend on the rate of accumulation of fluid in the pericardial sac. The symptoms include:

- Chest pain—relieved by sitting up and leaning forward, aggravated by lying supine
- Light-headedness, syncope
- Palpitations
- Cough, dyspnea, hoarseness
- Anxiety and confusion
- Hiccups

Etiology

- Infections
- Idiopathic
- Neoplastic
- Uremia
- Hypothyroidism
- Connective tissue diseases
- Postoperative
- Others: Myxoedema, severe pulmonary hypertension, trauma, autoimmune conditions (SLE, RA, Sarcoidosis, ankylosing spondylitis), drugs (like procainamide, hydralazine, isoniazid, minoxidil, phenytoin, methylsergide, anticoagulants).

Pathogenesis

The pathogenesis of pericardial effusion is given in Figure 9.3.

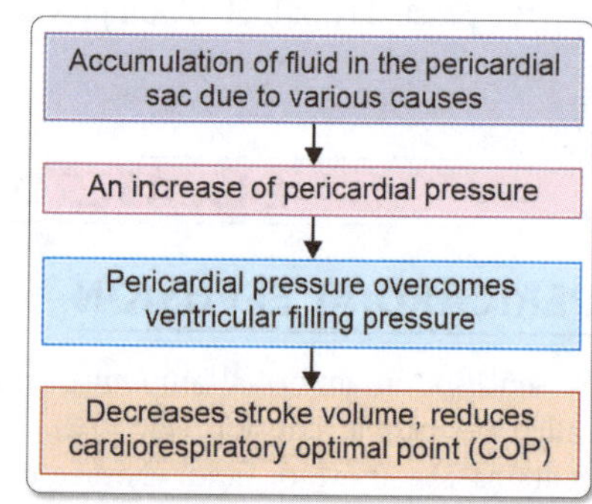

Figure 9.3: Pathogenesis of pericardial effusion

Lab Diagnosis

- Physical examination and complete blood tests.
- Beck's triad (3Ds) seen in cases of cardiac tamponade
  - Decreased blood pressure (hypotension).
  - Decreased/Muffled heart sounds.
  - Distended neck veins (Raised JVP)
- Pulsus paradoxus (An abnormal reduction of patient's systolic BP >10 mm Hg during inspiration).
- Pericardial friction rub.
- Tachycardia and Tachypnea.
- Weakened peripheral pulses, cyanosis and edema.
- Ewart sign—dullness to percussion beneath the angle of left scapula from compression of left lung by pericardial effusion.
- Radiology—ECHO.

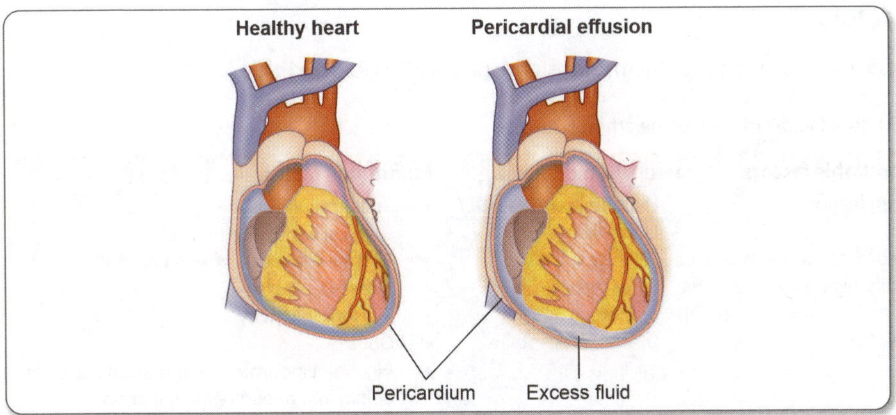

Figure 9.4: Pericardial effusion

Pathological Changes

- **Gross appearance (Fig. 9.4):** Yellow fibrinous exudate on the external surface of the heart.
- **Histological changes:** Mesothelial cells of the pericardium are surrounded by neutrophils.

There is no fibrosis (acute inflammatory response).

ATHEROSCLEROSIS

Atherosclerosis is a disease of the cardiovascular system affecting the vessel wall which includes medium-sized muscular arteries and large elastic arteries. It leads to the narrowing of arteries or complete blockage.

It is characterized by endothelial dysfunction, lipid deposition, inflammatory reaction in the vascular wall and remodeling of vessel wall.

Clinical Features

Symptoms depend on the arteries affected and the percent of blood flow blockage. Generally, chest pain, cold sweats, dizziness, extreme tiredness, heart palpitations, shortness of breath, nausea and weakness are the symptoms.

Etiology

It is caused by a buildup of plaque in the inner lining of an artery. The plaque is made up of deposits of fatty substances, calcium, cholesterol, cellular waste products, and fibrin. Mainly, smoking, intake of unsaturated fat, hyperlipidemia and sedentary lifestyle are responsible for causing atherosclerosis.

- **Smoking:** This increases the risk of developing myocardial infarction by two times. Cigarette smoke has a number of noxious chemicals including polycyclic aromatic hydrocarbons which reduce antioxidant molecules, increase oxidant stress and promote endothelial cell injury which in turn promotes a pro-thrombotic and proatherogenic state.
- **Sedentary lifestyle:** Lack of physical exercise increases the risk of cardiovascular disease and mortality by two times emphasizing the need for a regular form of activity to maintain health.
- **Abnormal lipid profile (dyslipidemia):** This leads to an increased risk of atherosclerosis and subsequent myocardial infarction (MI) both in males and females.

Risk Factors

The risk factors of developing atherosclerosis are tabulated as follows in Table 9.1:

Table 9.1: Risk factors of developing atherosclerosis

Nonmodifiable factors	Potentially modifiable	Modifiable factors
Male predilection Genetic: • Hypercholesterolemia • Family history	• Hyperlipidemia—HDL/LDL ratio • Hypertension • Smoking • Diabetes • Oral contraceptives	• Sedentary lifestyle • High carbohydrate intake • Postmenopausal estrogen deficiency • Stress • Physical inactivity • Obesity • Alcohol, Lipoprotein A and unsaturated fat intake • *Chlamydia pneumoniae* infection

Pathogenesis

The presence of atherosclerosis is directly linked to the development of myocardial infarction (MI) with occlusion due to atheromas being seen in the majority of cases of MI (Fig. 9.5). When occlusion is severe enough to cause symptoms, a 12.5 times risk is documented, whereas in asymptomatic cases, an 8-fold increase has been suggested. The key events are:

The development of myocardial infarction may be due to either of the following mechanisms:

- **Stenosis or occlusion of the coronary blood vessels:** This leads to a reduced blood supply to the heart thereby increasing the chances of infarction. This occurs due to narrowing of atherosclerosis or vasospasm because of drugs or neurohormonal factors.

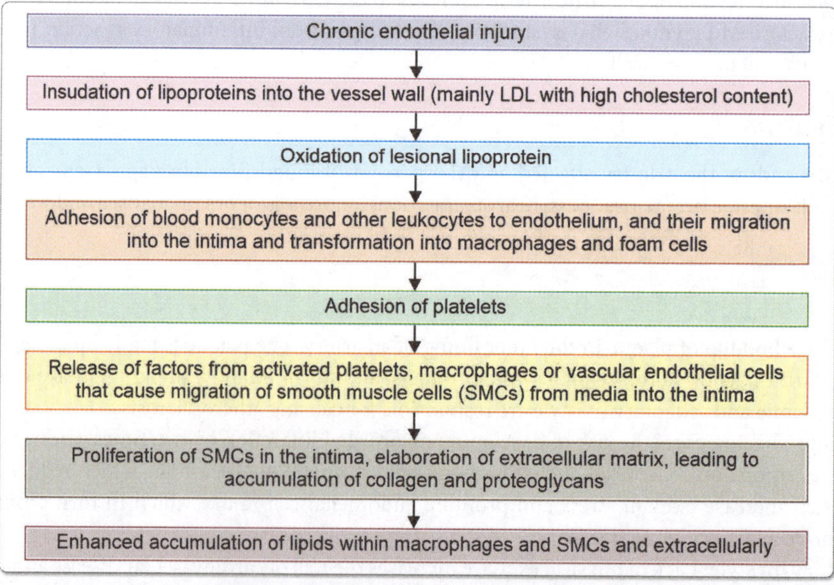

Figure 9.5: Pathogenesis of atherosclerosis

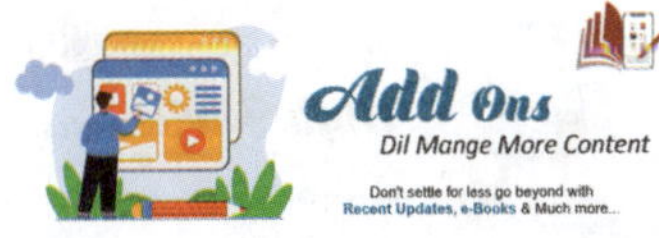

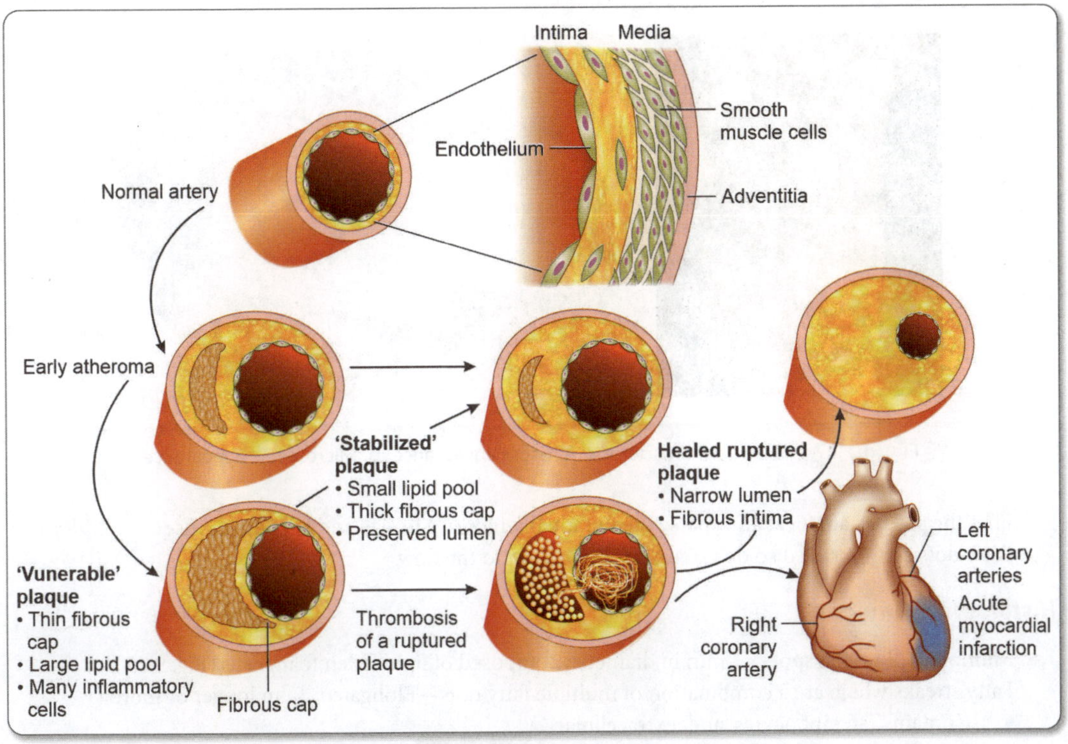

Figure 9.6: Development of atherogenesis

- **An increased demand on the heart:** This is seen in continuous high intensity exercise, fever, thyrotoxicosis and pregnancy. Cardiac hypertrophy is secondary to causes such as hypertension without a corresponding increase in the blood supply to the heart.
- **Rupture of an atherosclerotic plaque:** This leads to endothelial damage and the subendothelial collagen is exposed. This matrix is rich in coagulation factors, especially Von-Willebrand factor. This binds to activated platelets facilitating aggregation and the formation of thrombi (Fig. 9.6).

The net result of all these mechanisms is ischemia. Ischemic-hypoxic injury leads to cell injury of the cardiac myocytes *via* coagulative necrosis.

Irreversible cell injury also leads to a switch from aerobic to anaerobic glycolysis leading to lactic acidosis and impaired muscle contractility leading to loss of myocardial function.

Pathological Changes

Gross Appearance

An atheromatous plaque (Fig. 9.7A) consists of:

- A raised focal lesion, soft, yellow core of lipids (mainly cholesterol and cholesterol esters), covered by a firm, white fibrous cap.
- 0.3–1.5 cm in diameter, sometimes combine to form larger lesions.
- Involves partial circumference of arterial wall (eccentric) with patchy and variable involvement along the length of vessel.

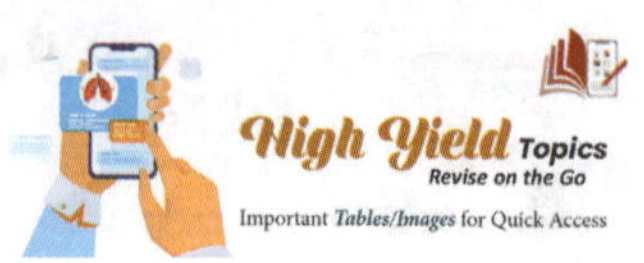

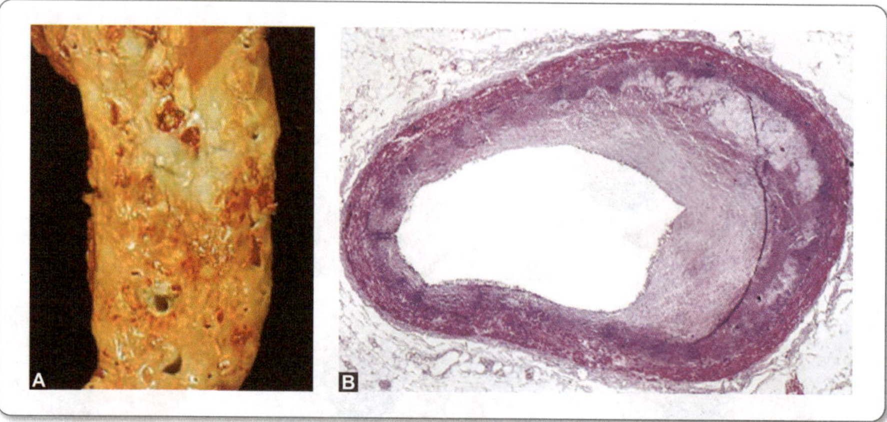

Figures 9.7A and B: Atherosclerosis: **A.** Gross appearance; **B.** Microscopic appearance

- First the patches are focal and sparse then gradually increase in size and become diffuse
- Fatty dots are not raised so do not cause obstruction to the flow.

Histological Changes

- Multiple, yellow, flat spots <1 mm in diameter, composed of lipid laden foam cells (Fig. 9.7B).
- Fatty streaks which are a combination of multiple fatty dots—Elongated, 1 cm longer or more
  - Contain T-lymphocytes and extracellular lipid less than plaques.
  - Appear in aorta in some children younger than 1 year and all children older than 10 years.
  - Histiocytes.
  - Fibrous tissue in advanced lesions.

NOTE

Fatty streaks may be precursor of plaque but not all fatty streaks are converted into fibrous plaque or more advanced lesions.

RECENT UPDATE

New Biomarkers of Atherosclerosis

- hsCRP->2.3 mg/L-adverse prognosis
- SAA, Isoprostane- High levels indicate early mortality
- Pentraxin 3, CD 40 ligand, MMP2, 9-unstable plaques
- Altered fibrinogen, cholesterol efflux capacity—atherosclerosis of the young
- Lp-PLA2-Coronary heart disease
- NT-Pro BNP-Increased in CAD

Lab Diagnosis

- Plasma concentration of lipoproteins (LDL-cholesterol and triacylglycerols)—5.2 mmol/L (200 mg/dL) increases the risk.
- Elevated optimal level of LDL-cholesterol—2.6 mmol/L (100 mg/dL).

ISCHEMIC HEART DISEASE

Clots in any artery block the blood flow and the heart is affected (Fig. 9.8). Ischemia is a diminished blood supply to organs leading to reduced oxygenation or hypoxic injury. Ischemic injury to the heart presents as a spectrum of clinical entities together known as ischemic heart disease (IHD).

This includes four main conditions:

1. Angina pectoris
2. Myocardial infarction
3. Sudden cardiac death
4. Chronic ongoing ischemic heart disease

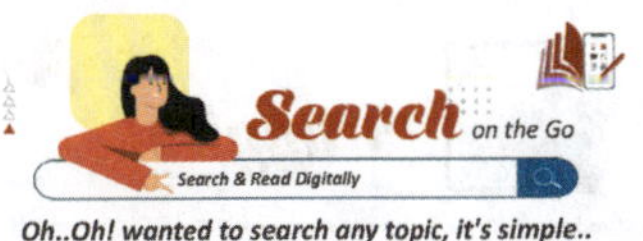

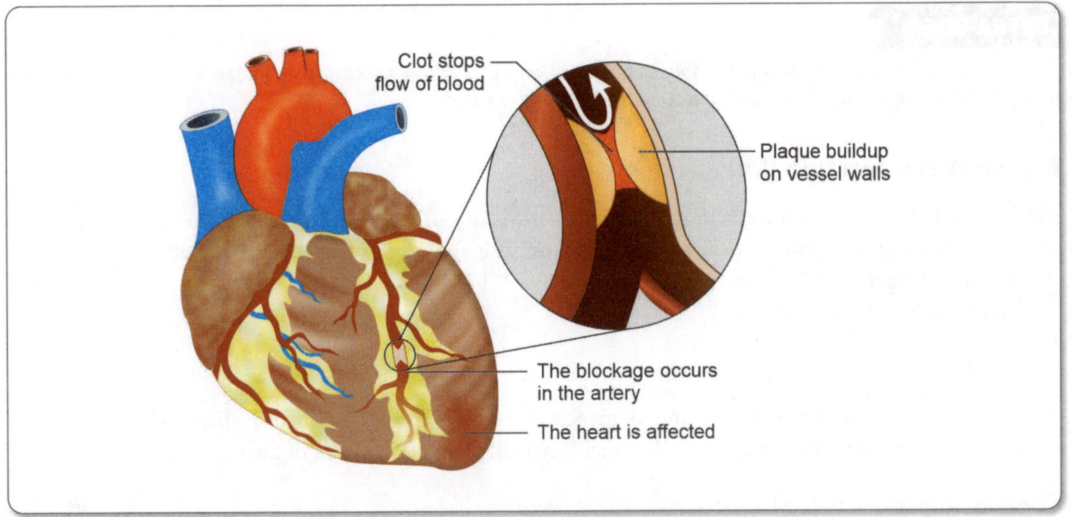

Figure 9.8: Ischemic heart disease

Angina Pectoris

This refers to chest pain which is primarily episodic and is caused by an imbalance between myocardial demand and perfusion.

Types

Angina is further of two types:

1. **Stable,** which is seen on exertion
2. **Unstable,** which is seen even at rest/while sleeping.

Clinical Features

The pain may manifest as tightness or fullness in the chest. The pain usually subsides and lasts not more than half an hour and is caused by ischemia-induced liberation of bradykinin. Patients of angina may also show other symptoms such as sweating, nausea, indigestion, epigastric fullness. When seen in the absence of chest pain this is referred to as "angina equivalent".

Prinzmetal Angina or Vasospastic Angina

Another variant of angina is Prinzmetal angina also called vasospastic angina. It is usually seen in younger patients and is characterized by vasospasm of the coronary arteries leading to narrowing. The patient complains of pain even at rest and this is benefitted by nitroglycerine and calcium channel blockers. β-blockers are contraindicated as they promote vasospasm.

Etiology

Angina is usually caused by atherosclerosis but may also be caused by pressure on the myocardium secondary to left ventricular hypertrophy, in turn secondary to hypertension, and even in patients of hypertrophic obstructive cardiomyopathy. ECG changes noted include ST segment depression.

EXTRA EDGE

It is difficult to distinguish between unstable angina and Non-ST elevation myocardial infarction. Multiple assessments of cardiac troponins may be required to distinguish between the two.

Myocardial Infarction (MI)

Ischemia of the myocardium leads to coagulative necrosis of cardiac myocytes leading to the production of an infarct. In common terms, it is called "heart attack". It is the result of an imbalance between the cardiac demand and oxygen being supplied to the heart. Acute MI is a medical emergency and is a major cause of patient morbidity and mortality.

Types of MI

As per the extent of involvement, two types of myocardial infarction are described: Transmural (involving full thickness of the cardiac wall) and subendocardial (involving half or one third of the ventricular wall).

Complications

- **Rupture of the heart:** The ventricular wall and or even the ventricular septum may rupture within the first week of a myocardial infarction.
- **Cardiac tamponade:** This in turn leads to a sudden filling up of the pericardial space by fluid or blood, also called cardiac tamponade.
- **Arrhythmias:** The normal sinus rhythm may be altered after MI. The patient may show either one or a combination of disturbances in cardiac rhythm (*arrhythmia*) including atrial fibrillation, ventricular fibrillation, sinus tachycardia/bradycardia.
- **Aneurysm formation:** An aneurysm is formed when an artery's wall becomes weak and causes an abnormally large bulge.
- **Thromboembolism:** The inflammatory processes accompanying the process of acute MI result in an increased tendency to the formation of thrombus
- **Shock:** Decreased contractile power of the heart after Acute MI leads to a reduced cardiac output decreasing the effective circulating blood volume affecting tissue perfusion and is leading to shock (cardiogenic type).
- **Sudden cardiac death:** It occurs when the heart stops beating or not beating sufficiently to maintain perfusion.

Clinical Features

The patient presents with chest pain which may or may not radiate to the left arm. In addition, the patient may complain of uneasiness and show profuse sweating. In some cases, the patient may complain of acidity or indigestion rather than chest pain. The complications arise when the myocardial contractility decreases and it leads to death.

Risk Factors of MI

- MI usually occurs in the middle age group to elderly. However, recently a spurt of episodes of MI in the younger generation has also been reported.

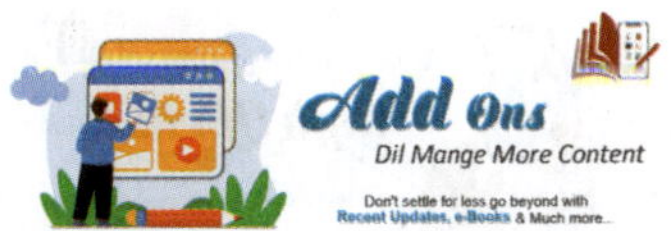

- MI shows a sex predilection for males as it is believed that estrogen hormone in females has a cardioprotective effect. This is also validated by the increased cases of MI in postmenopausal women.
- **Obesity:** The risk of developing myocardial infarction in the obese is approximately 1.5–2.5 times more.
- **Diabetes mellitus:** Patients with diabetes mellitus have a 2–4 fold higher risk of developing MI. Myocardial infarctions in patients of diabetes notoriously may present without symptoms. It is believed that diabetes is associated with neuropathy which alters pain perception, hence the patient becomes unaware of pain. This presentation is called "Silent MI".

Pathogenesis

A myocardial infarct usually begins in the subendocardial zone which is poorly perfused and extends to involve full thickness. Transmural infarcts have a poorer prognosis and are associated with a higher risk of complications. Atherosclerosis, plaque and thrombus formation leads to ischemia and hypoxia. When the thrombus is permanent, it leads to myocardial infarction (Fig. 9.9).

Lab Diagnosis

Myocardial infarction is diagnosed by a combination of clinical features, electrocardiographic findings and serum biomarkers.

- **ECG findings:** ECG is a very important baseline investigation that gives an assessment of the type, site and extent of myocardial infarction.
  - **Transmural infarcts:** ST segment elevation is seen
  - **Subendocardial infarcts:** Non ST segment elevation is seen
  - Additional ECG findings that can be seen include ST depression, inverted T wave, deep Q waves and absence of the R wave.
- **Serum biomarkers:** Cardiac biomarker testing and their analysis is essential to diagnose non-ST elevation MI.

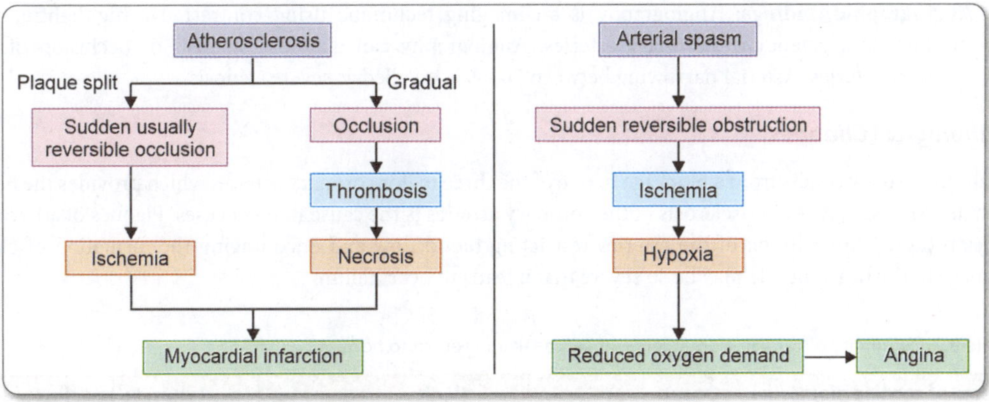

Figure 9.9: Pathogenesis of myocardial infarction

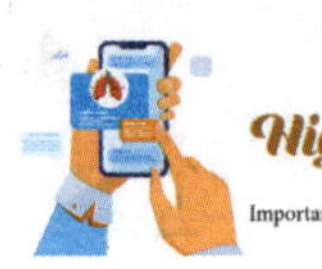
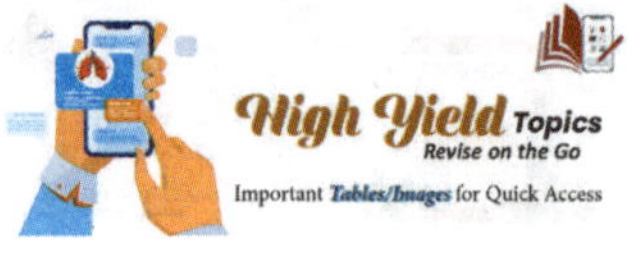

- **Troponins:** Cardiac troponins are sensitive and specific markers of myocardial damage. TnI is used as biochemical markers for the diagnosis of myocardial injury. They appear 3–4 hours after the infarction and may persist till 14 days. Serial estimations are useful to assess early coronary artery reperfusion.
- **CK-MB:** CK-MB is the isoform that is predominantly elevated in patients of acute myocardial infarction. This biomarker increases at 3–5 hours and peaks at 20–24 hours. It reaches baseline normal values between day 2-day 3 post MI. Hence it is unable to detect cases of MI which have presented late for clinical care.
- **Serum LDH:** Lactate dehydrogenase enzyme (LDH) is a non-specific marker of myocardial infarction. LDH however has two isoforms—1 and 2. LDH1 is considered to be specific for myocardial injury and is elevated at Day 1-Day 2 after Acute MI. It persists till Day 14, however CK MB is more specific for cardiac injury and cardiac troponins more sensitive.
- **Myoglobin:** This is the earliest marker to rise after MI and is elevated at 24–48 hours after MI. However, it rapidly disappears from the bloodstream and also lacks specificity.

  The cardiac biomarkers are summarized in Table 9.2.

- **Angiographic findings:** Angiography is an imaging technique using contrast dye highlighting the structure and patency of coronary arteries. Angiography can diagnose stenosis or occlusion of the coronary arteries. Arterial narrowing between 70–99% is called as severe stenosis.

RECENT UPDATE

- High sensitivity cardiac troponins are a latest addition to the panel of cardiac biomarkers. They have the advantage that even very small levels can detect MI.
- A serum value of >14 ng/L in the appropriate setting of symptoms of MI can support the diagnosis.
- Values <14 ng/L can exclude MI.
- The American Heart Association (AHA) guidelines 2021 now recommend high sensitivity cardiac troponin (hs-cTn) as the cardiac biomarker of choice for acute MI.

MUST KNOW

Supply of major coronary arteries:

- **Left anterior descending artery:** This supplies anterior wall of left ventricle and anterior 2/3 of interventricular septum.
- **Left circumflex artery:** Supplies left ventricle (lateral wall)
- **Right coronary artery:** Supplies left ventricle (posterior), posterior 1/3 of interventricular septum Occlusion in any of these arteries affects the blood supply to the corresponding area of the myocardium, causing infarction.

Pathological Changes

Infarction usually results from a blockage in one of the three major coronary arteries which provides the heart with its blood supply. Atherosclerosis of the coronary arteries is the cause in most cases. Plaques of atheroma develop on the inner lining of the arteries restricting blood flow and encouraging the formation of clots. Damage to the heart muscle may be so severe that it leads to heart failure.

Table 9.2: Summary of cardiac biomarkers—onset, peak and return to normal

Name of cardiac biomarker	Onset	Peak	Return to baseline
CK-MB	3–12 hours	18–24 hours	48–72 hours
Troponin I	4–6 hours	24 hours	7–10 days
Troponin T	4–6 hours	12–48 hours	7–14 days
Myoglobin	1–4 hours	8–10 hours	24 hours
LDH	6–10 hours	24–48 hours	10–14 days

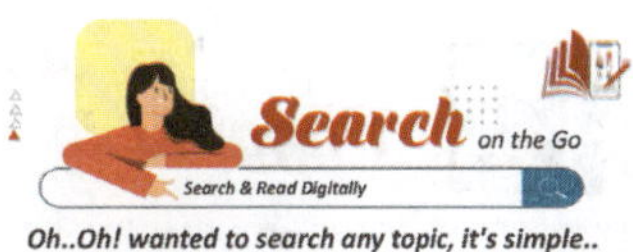

- **Gross appearance (Fig. 9.10A):** An area of myocardial infarction (dark region, bottom left) in the left ventricle. The walls of the ventricle get enlarged (ventricular hypertrophy).
- **Histopathological changes (Fig. 9.10B):** Wavy cardiac muscle cells represent dead or necrotic cells. Inflammation due to necrosis is also evident by the presence of numerous immune cells, especially neutrophils.

The histopathological changes seen in the heart in a case of acute MI vary depending on the number of hours elapsed since the episode. The pathological diagnosis of myocardial infarction though gold standard is usually seen on postmortem analysis. Related to time, the gross and microscopic features of MI are given in Table 9.3.

Figures 9.10A and B: Myocardial infarction: **A.** Gross; **B.** Histology

Sudden Cardiac Death (SCD)

It is a death due to a cardiovascular cause that occurs within 1 hour of the onset of symptoms. A sudden cardiac arrest occurs when the heart stops beating or is not beating sufficiently to maintain perfusion and life.

Warning Signs before SCD

People experience warning symptoms up to 24 hours before a sudden cardiac arrest, but these symptoms vary by sex. Men typically experience chest pain before a cardiac arrest, whereas women typically have shortness of breath. Generally sudden cardiac arrest often occurs without warning.

Clinical Features

The symptoms are immediate and severe, including:
- No breathing
- Sudden collapse
- No pulse
- Loss of consciousness

Table 9.3: Time-based analysis of gross and microscopic changes seen in myocardial infarction

Time	Gross features	Histological changes
0–12 hours	No gross change	• Edema between the myocardial fibers • Myocardial fiber waviness at the margin of infarction
18–24 hours	A pale reddish blue area corresponding to the infarct is seen	• Loss of nuclei of cardiac myocytes/nuclear pyknosis • Foci of coagulative necrosis
First week	Infarcted area shows a heterogenous "mottled" appearance with areas of congestion admixed with necrosis	• Loss of nuclei of cardiac myocytes/nuclear pyknosis • Foci of coagulative necrosis and • neutrophils in the interstitium
Second week	Infarcted area rimmed by a congested area	Foci of coagulative necrosis and congested vessels at the periphery of the infarct + diminished neutrophils and more lymphocytes, histiocytes
After second week	Infarcted area seen as a pale area devoid of necrosis, scarring may be seen grossly	Areas of loss of cardiac myocytes with replacement by scar tissue (collagen)

Chronic Ongoing Ischemic Heart Disease

The patients with chronic ischemic heart disease fall into two general categories:

1. Those with symptoms related to the disease.
2. Those who are asymptomatic.

Etiology

Most patients with chronic ischemic heart disease have coronary atherosclerosis. Consequently, it is easy to become complacent and ignore the fact that other diseases can cause lesions in the coronary arteries. In young people, coronary artery anomalies should be kept in mind; in older individuals, systemic vasculitides are not uncommon. Presently, collagen vascular diseases are the most common vasculitides leading to coronary artery disease, but in the past, infections such as syphilis was a common cause of coronary vasculitis.

Diseases of the ascending aorta, such as aortic dissection, can lead to coronary ostial occlusion. Isolated coronary artery dissection can also occur. Coronary artery emboli may occur as a result of infectious endocarditis or of atrial fibrillation with left atrial thrombus formation. Infiltrative diseases of the heart, such as tumor metastases, may also compromise coronary flow. Therefore, it is essential to keep in mind diagnostic possibilities other than atherosclerosis when managing chronic ischemic heart disease.

RHEUMATIC HEART DISEASE

Rheumatic fever is an acute inflammatory multi-systemic disease involving the heart, joints, skin and blood vessels. The disease affects young children in the age group of 5–15 years. It is usually preceded by an episode of fever and sore throat (i.e., Streptococcal pharyngitis/tonsillitis). Rheumatic heart disease is characterized by both cardiac and extracardiac manifestations. Involvement of the heart involves diffused inflammation of all layers of the heart (pericardium, myocardium and endocardium), also referred "pancarditis".

- **Incubation period:** 1–5 weeks.
- **Causative organism:** Group A β-hemolytic streptococci.

Rheumatic heart disease (RHD) is an immune mediated disease which is triggered by infection in a genetically susceptible host. Group A β-hemolytic streptococci have a carbohydrate antigen resembling the glycoprotein component of cardiac valves (antigenic mimicry). Similarly, the streptococcal M protein resembles the cardiac myocytes. After infection with beta hemolytic streptococci, antibodies develop against the streptococcal proteins. These antibodies cross react against both the valves and the myocardium and cause RHD.

Pathogenesis

Refer to self-explanatory Figure 9.11.

Rheumatic Pericarditis

Gross appearance (Figs 9.12A and B): Grossly, the pericardium appears thick, shaggy and is studded with a dirty fibrinous deposit. The pericardial covering of the heart has a characteristic *"bread and butter"* appearance (Rheumatic pericarditis).

Inflammation of the myocardium in rheumatic heart disease initially causes interstitial edema and a flabby heart (Rheumatic myocarditis).

Later on, the interstitium shows dense inflammation along with Aschoff bodies/nodules. These are granulomatous lesions which may be seen in the myocardium as well as in other layers of the heart.

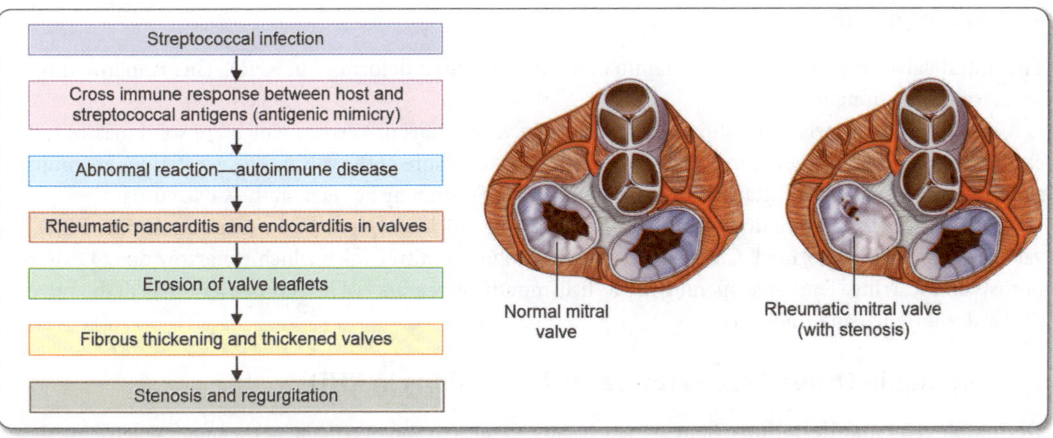

Figure 9.11: Pathogenesis of rheumatic heart disease

These granulomas consist of fibrinoid necrosis, histiocytes, few lymphocytes and Anitschkow cells.

Histological changes (Fig. 9.12C): On microscopy, the pericardium shows fibrin admixed with lymphocytes and histiocytes and few neutrophils. In long standing cases, fibroblasts may also be seen.

Lab Diagnosis

- Physical examination—presence of a heart murmur.
- Medical history—including evidence of past acute rheumatic fever (ARF) streptococcal infection.
- Chest X-ray—to check for enlargement of the heart or fluid on the lungs.

Figures 9.12A to C: Rheumatic heart disease: **A.** Gross showing vegetation; **B.** Rheumatic pericarditis; **C.** Histology

Rheumatic Endocarditis

Inflammation of the endocardium may involve either the valve (rheumatic valvulitis) or the wall (mural endocarditis).

Pathological Changes

Gross appearance: Inflammation of the wall grossly shows a typical lesion called the MacCallum's patch which is a thickened map-like area or patch, seen in the left atrium.

Histological changes: This on microscopic examination shows the presence of Aschoff bodies, necrosis and edema.

MUST KNOW

Aschoff bodies and Anitschkow cells

Anitschkow cells are macrophages with an owl eye appearance on transverse sectioning. When viewed on a longitudinal section they have a typical "caterpillar" like appearance. Sometimes, these macrophages are multinucleated when they are referred to as Aschoff giant cells.

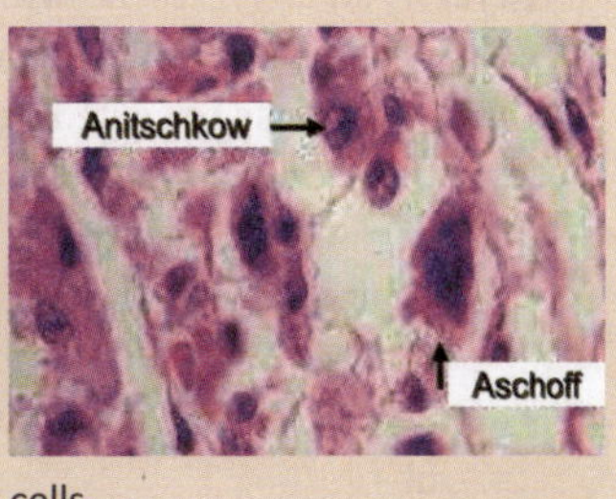

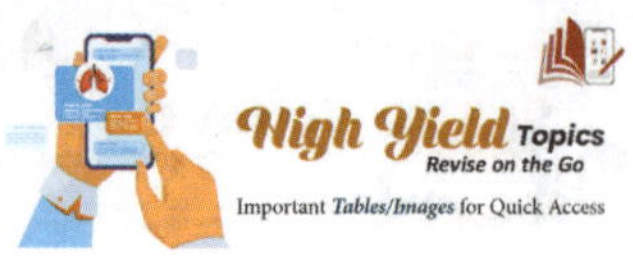

Rheumatic Valvulitis

The mitral valve commonly shows inflammation and structural deformity in RHD. This is followed by the aortic valve inflammation.

Valvulitis characteristically shows the presence of vegetations or verruca which are solid masses lodged on the valves. In RHD, vegetations are seen along the line of closure of the valves. The vegetations are multiple, small, warty and are firmly attached to the valvular cusp. Fibrin may be seen on the valve cusps.

With chronic inflammation, the valves become dull, thick and opaque. In cases of chronic RHD, the valve is structurally deformed. Cases of chronic RHD show a mitral valve which is narrow due to extensive fibrosis and scarring. The valve opening has a "fish-mouth" appearance. The chordae tendinae of the valve get fibrosed, shortened and thickened.

Pathologies in Other Tissues (Extracardiac Lesions in RHD)

Dermatological manifestations: Subcutaneous skin nodules that are small painless palpable nodules can be seen on the extensor surface of joints (Fig. 9.13A).

Neurological manifestations: Syndenham's chorea-purposeless jerky movements seen later in the course of disease and due to inflammation of the central nervous system.

Polyarthritis (Fig. 9.13B): This refers to inflammation of multiple joints and primarily affects the large joints.

Jone's criteria for rheumatic fever: 2 Major/1 Major +2 Minor	
Major criteria: Mnenomic "CASES"	**Minor criteria: Mnenomic "FRAP"**
Carditis	**F**ever
Arthritis	**R**aised ESR, CRP
Sydenham's chorea	**A**rthralgia
Erythema marginatum	**P**rolonged PR interval
Subcutaneous nodule	

Pleuritis: The pleura may be inflammed and show a fibrinous exudate on the surface.

Erythema marginatum: Erythematous rash on the trunk and extremities which gradually fade in the center remaining red at the periphery (Fig. 9.13C).

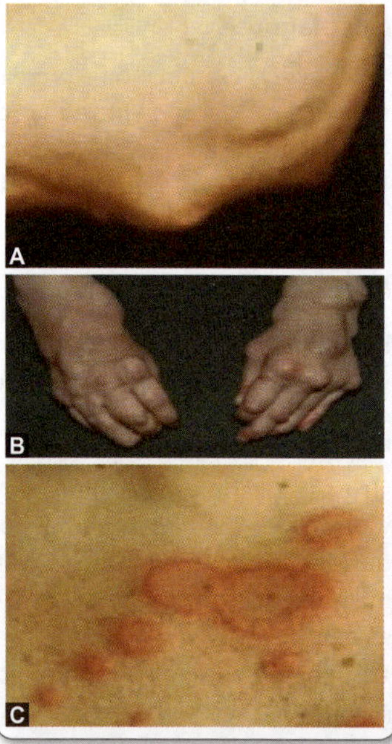

Figures 9.13A to C: **A.** Subcutaneous nodules; **B.** Polyarthritis; **C.** Erythma marginatum

INFECTIVE ENDOCARDITIS

This is also called bacterial endocarditis and is characterized by infection of the valves and endocardium. The microbial nidus along with inflammatory debris constitutes the vegetation of the infective endocarditis. The myocardium is typically spared.

Clinical Features

- **Fever:** Patients present with fever which is high grade when organisms are of high virulence. This may be accompanied by chills in the case of acute infective endocarditis. In subacute cases fever may be low grade/intermittent.
- **Fatigue, muscle/joint pain:**
  - **Subungual hemorrhages:** Pinpoint hemorrhages beneath the nail bed
  - **Cardiac signs:** Cardiac arrhythmias and murmurs, pericardial rub+

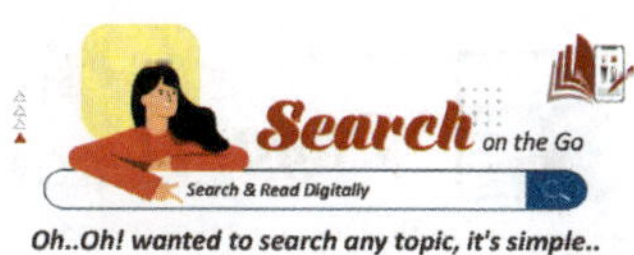

- **Osler nodes:** Tender subcutaneous nodules at the pulp of the fingers
- **Janeway lesions:** Non-tender macules on the hands
- **Roth spots:** Retinal hemorrhages.

Lab Diagnosis

The diagnosis of infective endocarditis is made on the basis of the Duke's criteria. As per revised 2023 Duke's-International society for cardiovascular infectious disease, criteria for infective endocarditis (IE) is as follows:

RECENT UPDATE

Recent updates on diagnosis-infective endocarditis–Revised Duke's Criteria

- **Pathological criteria:** Microorganisms identified either by culture/PCR/In-situ hybridization/genomic sequencing/histopathological features of active endocarditis observed in the clinical setting of active endocarditis from cardiac tissue/prosthetic valve/arterial emboli
- **Clinical criteria:** 2 Major or 1 Major/3 Minor or 5 Minor criteria

  Major criteria
  - Microbiological major—Positive blood cultures for common causative organisms in two or more cultures/PCR positivity for *Coxiella Burnetti, Bartonella, T. Whipplei*
  - Imaging major criteria
    - Echocardiographic and/CT evidence of vegetations, valvular abscess, valvular perforation
    - 18FDG-PET/CT shows abnormal metabolic activity involving a native/prosthetic valve within 3 months

  Surgical major: Evidence of infective endocarditis as seen on direct inspection during cardiac surgery

  Minor criteria
  - Previous history of infective endocarditis/prosthetic valve/congenital heart disease
  - Fever >38°C (100.4°F)
  - Clinical/Radiological evidence of vascular events-intracerebral abscess
  - Positive blood culture consistent with IE but not meeting major criteria
  - Immunological-Roth spots/Osler nodes/Immune complex glomerulonephritis
  - New valvular regurgitation identified on auscultation.

Types of Infective Endocarditis

Acute Infective Endocarditis

This is characterized by a destructive, virulent course and symptoms including aching joints and muscles, chest pain on breathing, murmur, shortness of breath and swelling in the feet, legs or belly.

Fatality is seen, which is caused by highly virulent strains of bacteria, frequently *Staphylococcus aureus* which destroys the involved areas.

Subacute Infective Endocarditis

This shows a relatively less destructive disease course and is caused by less virulent strains. The disease persists for a longer duration.

Etiology

Staphylococcus aureus, *Streptococcus viridans* and the HACEK group of organisms. (Hemophilus, Actinobacillus, Cardiobacterium, Eikenella, Kingella). *Staphylococcus epidermidis* typically infects artificial (prosthetic) valves.

Risk Factors

- Pre-existing diseases of the heart such as rheumatic disease, other valvular diseases, congenital heart disease
- Pre-existing infections at any site of the body which are disseminated *via* the blood stream
- Impaired host immunity (patients taking immunosuppressive drugs, e.g., steroids or patients with comorbid illness such as diabetes/tuberculosis or those having malignant tumors such as leukemias/lymphomas).

Pathogenesis

The vegetations and inflammation in infective endocarditis are induced by bacteremia caused by enhancement of an initially localized infection. The presence of a damaged valvular surface/prosthetic valve/valvular deformity also facilitates the formation of vegetations.

Endothelial injury is usually seen at areas of turbulent blood flow. Platelets aggregate and deposit at the site of injury accumulating both fibrin and clumps of bacteria.

When the causative bacteria are highly virulent, vegetations can develop even in the absence of substantial valvular damage.

MUST KNOW

Comparative of major endocarditis conditions

Feature	Rheumatic heart disease (RHD)	Infective endocarditis (IE)	Libman-Sacks endocarditis (LSE)	nonbacterial thrombotic endocarditis (NBTE)
Vegetations	Small firm	Large, friable	Medium, irregular	Small friable
Site	Along lines of valve closure	Valvular cusps	Both surfaces of the valves	Along lines of valve closure
Organisms	–	+++	–	–
Emboli	Rare	Common	Rare	Common
Association with malignancy	–	–	–	+
Other features	Aschoff bodies seen in surrounding tissue	Bacterial colonies	Hematoxylin bodies with residual nuclear debris	Hypercoagulability

Complications of Infective Endocarditis

Cardiac:

- Valve rupture
- Abscess around the valvular ring
- Myocardial abscess
- Valvular dysfunction stenosis

Extracardiac:

- Septic emboli
- Infarction

Pathological Changes

Gross appearance: The valve appears hemorrhagic and rough (Fig. 9.14A)

- Vegetations in infective endocarditis are either single/multiple and usually center on one side of the valvular cusp
- **Color:** Reddish—brown

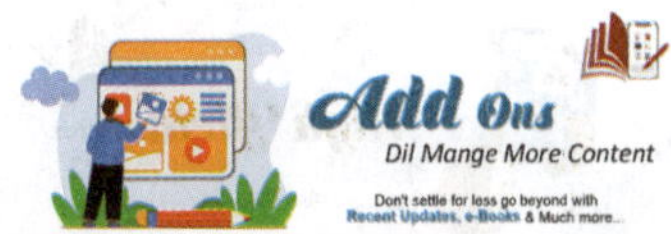

- **Consistency:** Soft, friable
- **Size:** Variable in size but generally large and bulky
- They also have a tendency to break off and embolize elsewhere in the bloodstream (septic emboli).

Histological changes: Microscopic analysis of the cardiac vegetations reveals granulation tissue admixed with fibrin, clumps of bacterial colonies as well as platelet aggregates. When the vegetations are in the healing phase superimposed collagen fibers, i.e, fibrosis and specks of calcification may be seen. Inflammatory changes in valve tissue (Fig. 9.14B).

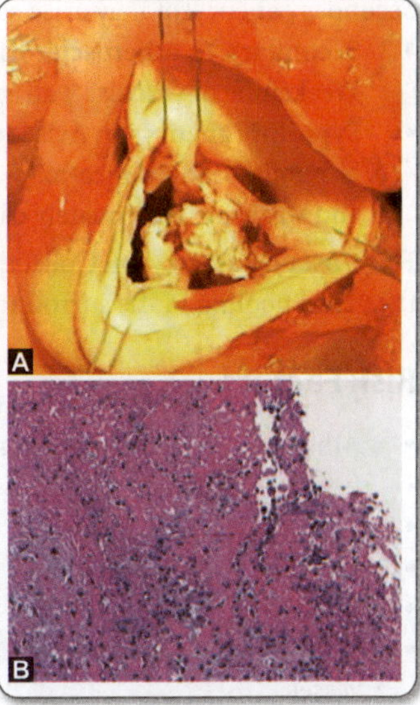

Figures 9.14A and B: Infective endocarditis: **A.** Gross; **B.** Histology

ANEURYSM

An aneurysm is a localized sac or dilation formed at a weak point in the wall of the aorta. Because of the high pressure in the arterial system, aneurysms can enlarge, producing complications by compressing surrounding structures. Aneurysm is the second most frequent disease of the aorta after atherosclerosis.

Types of Aneurysm

The aneurysm is classified (Fig. 9.15) as follows:

True aneurysm: Involves all three layers of the blood vessel wall.

- **Saccular aneurysm:** Spherical in shape and involves only a portion of the vessel wall, they vary in size and are often filled either partially or fully by a thrombus.
  - **Fusiform aneurysm:** A localized dilation of an artery in which the entire circumference of the vessel is distended. The result is an elongated, tubular, or spindle-like swelling.
  - **Berry aneurysm:** Aneurysm, which looks like a berry on a narrow stem, is the most common type of brain aneurysm. Berry aneurysms tend to appear at the base of the brain where the major blood vessels meet, known as the circle of Willis. When a berry aneurysm ruptures, blood from the artery moves into the brain causing subarachnoid hemorrhage.

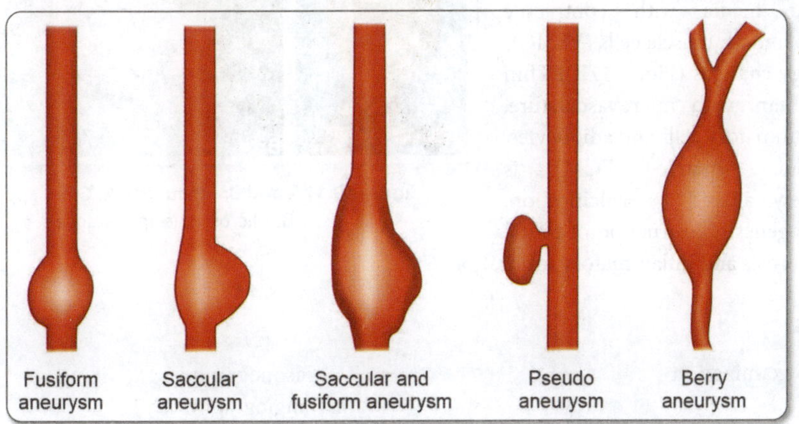

Figure 9.15: Types of aneurysms

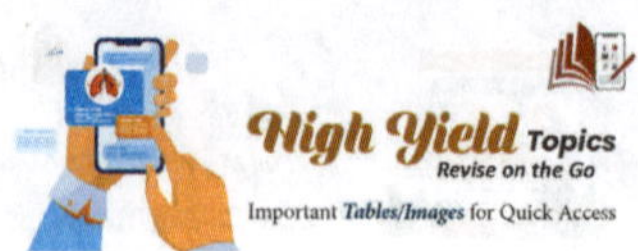

Secondary aneurysm may arise as described ahead:

- **Secondary to atherosclerosis:** Caused by atherosclerosis and typically occurs in the abdominal aorta. Weakening of vascular wall, specifically the tunica media, which leads to aneurysmal dilation of the vessel.
- **Syphilitic aneurysm:** Arises during tertiary syphilis due to chronic inflammation in the tunica adventitia. Ischemia of the tunica media, combined with further syphilitic invasion, results in medial destruction and weakening, ultimately causing dilation and aneurysm formation.

False/pseudo aneurysm: Collection of blood leaking completely out of an artery or vein but confined next to the vessel pooling in the surrounding tissue.

Risk Factors

- Atherosclerosis may contribute to weakening of blood vessel
- Infection which affects the arterial wall
- Syphilis
- Marfan's syndrome
- Penetrating or blunt trauma
- High blood pressure it may enlarge or weaken the blood vessel
- Older age (>60)
- Male sex
- Smoking
- Family history of aneurysmal disease

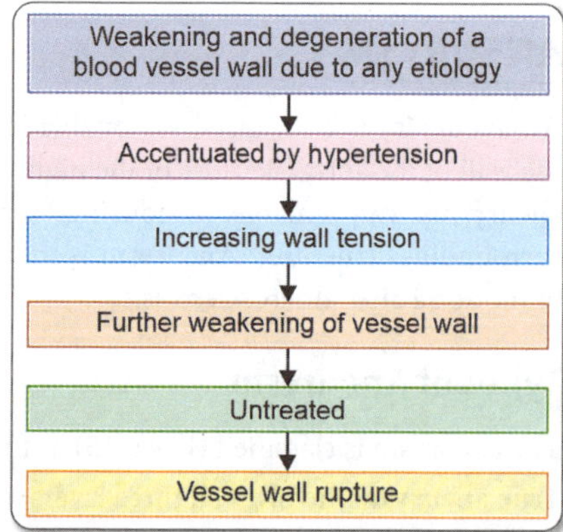

Figure 9.16: Pathogenesis of aneurysm

Pathogenesis

Refer self-explanatory Figure 9.16.

Pathological Changes

- **Gross appearance (Fig. 9.17A):** Inflammation and fibrosis; further distally, a single inner and outer elastic lamellae make up the margin of the muscular media with contractile vascular smooth muscle cells (VSMC).
- **Histology changes (Fig. 9.17B):** Thin endothelium, with microvasculature, few inflammatory cells and adipocytes. extracellular matrix (ECM) is completely altered by calcification, neoangiogenesis, destruction of elastic fibers, fibrosis and inflammatory infiltration.

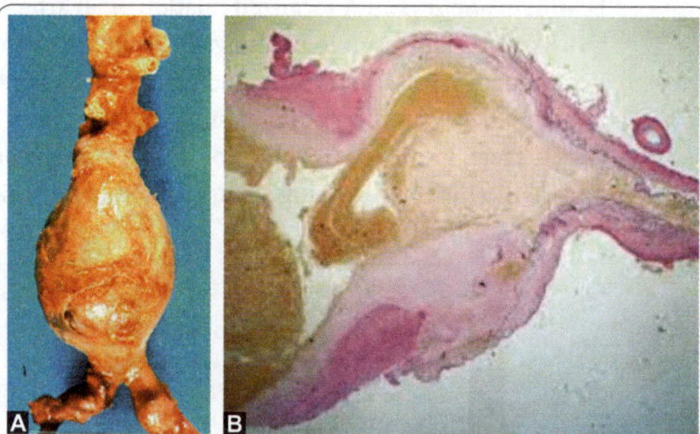

Figures 9.17A and B: Aneurysm **A.** Gross appearance; **B.** Microscopic appearance

Diagnosis

- Physical examination
- X-ray
- Angiography
- Ultrasonography
- CT angiography
- MRI

NURSING CONSIDERATIONS

In case of heart conditions, the nursing considerations are as follows:

- **Rapid triage to appropriate environment for safe clinical care:** Coronary care unit, cardiology ward, general medical ward.
- Objective monitoring for change in signs and symptoms suggestive of response to treatment. Promptly identify and address relevant changes in clinical status.
- Discharge planning and referral to multidisciplinary disease management program.
- Anxiety of the patient should be addressed by promptly answering questions and providing clear information to the patient and family.
- Ensure effective and consistent communication between the patient and/or family and multi-disciplinary team.
- **Objective measurement of dyspnea severity:** Respiratory rate, dyspnea severity scale, tolerance of lying prone, effort of breathing, oxygen saturation.
- **Haemodynamic status:** Systolic and diastolic blood pressure monitoring.
- **Heart rhythm:** Monitor heart rate and rhythm, with 12-lead electrocardiogram.
- **Assess cardiac output:** Body temperature, peripheral perfusion, urine output, mental status.
- **Clinical examination for signs of congestion:** Pulmonary rales, peripheral edema, jugular venous pressure.
- **Laboratory blood tests:** Full blood count, urea, creatinine, electrolytes, glucose, troponin, natriuretic peptide level.
- **Anxiety levels:** Using objective assessment tool.

SUMMARY

- Cardiac tamponade occurs which is acute heart failure due to compression of heart by a large or rapidly developing effusion.
- Atherosclerosis is a disease of cardiovascular system affecting vessel wall which include medium-sized muscular arteries and large elastic arteries.
- The presence of atherosclerosis is directly linked to the development of MI with occlusion due to atheromas.
- Stenosis or occlusion of the coronary blood vessels leads to a reduced blood supply to the heart thereby increasing the chances of infarction. Critical stenosis (70–99% occlusion).
- Atheromatous plaque consists of a raised focal lesion, soft, yellow core of lipids (mainly cholesterol and cholesterol esters), covered by a firm, white fibrous cap.
- Ischemic injury to the heart presents as a spectrum of clinical entities together known as ischemic heart disease (IHD).
- Another variant of angina is Prinzmetal angina also called vasospastic angina.
- Ischemia of the myocardium leads to coagulative necrosis of cardiac myocytes leading to the production of an infarct.
- Transmural infarcts have a poorer prognosis and are associated with a higher risk of complications.
- Myocardial infarction is diagnosed by a combination of clinical features, electrocardiographic findings and serum biomarkers.
- Lactate dehydrogenase enzyme is elevated in a number of diseases where inflammation is seen hence nonspecific.
- Angiography can diagnose stenosis or occlusion of the coronary arteries.
- Plaques of atheroma develop on the inner lining of the arteries restricting blood flow and encouraging the formation of clots.
- Rheumatic heart disease (RHD) is an immune mediated disease which is triggered by infection in a genetically susceptible host.
- Inflammation of the myocardium in rheumatic heart disease initially causes interstitial edema and a flabby heart (Rheumatic myocarditis).
- Aschoff bodies/nodules are granulomatous lesions which may be seen in the myocardium as well as in other layers of the heart.
- The diagnosis of infective endocarditis is made on the basis of the Duke's criteria.
- Most patients with chronic ischemic heart disease have coronary atherosclerosis.
- Aneurysm is the second most frequent disease of the aorta after atherosclerosis.

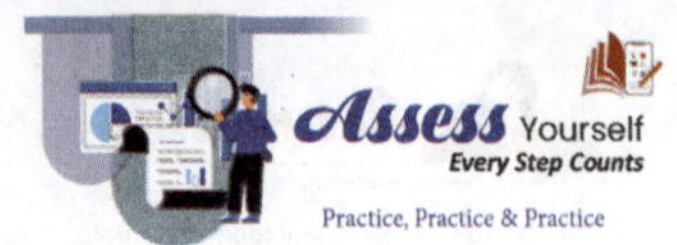

ASSESS YOURSELF

Long Answer Questions

1. Describe etiology and pathophysiology of atherosclerosis.
2. Discuss infective endocarditis in detail.

Short Answer Questions

1. Define aneurysm?
2. What is rheumatic heart disease?
3. Write short notes on:
   i. Ischemia
   ii. Infarction

Multiple Choice Questions

1. **Which of the following is the most common symptom of myocardial infarction?**
   a. Chest pain
   b. Dyspnea
   c. Edema
   d. Palpitations
2. **Rheumatic fever is inflammation of the joints, heart, skin, and nervous system that occurs in children. Which part of the body may be permanently damaged in a small percentage of people?**
   a. Digestive tract
   b. Ears
   c. Heart
   d. Lungs
3. **Which of the following individuals is LEAST likely to develop atherosclerosis?**
   a. Joel, who recently started a weight-loss program.
   b. Rajeev, who struggles to control his diabetes.
   c. Audrena, who is a long-time cigarette smoker.
   d. Carlos, whose father and older sister died from heart attacks.
4. **Is it normal for the pericardial cavity to contain a small amount of fluid?**
   a. Yes, because a small amount of serous fluid prevents the heart tiring.
   b. No, because any fluid can increase the pressure on the heart preventing it functioning efficiently.
   c. Yes, because a small amount of serous fluid protects the heart from infection.
   d. No, because any fluid can result in the stretching of the pericardial cavity deforming the heart.
   e. Yes, because a small amount of serous fluid is necessary to protect the heart during movement.
5. **Which of the following is usually the first symptom of rheumatic fever?**
   a. Chest pain or palpitations
   b. Jerky, uncontrollable movements
   c. Joint pain and fever
   d. Rash
6. **Each of the following drugs is used to treat rheumatic fever in children; except:**
   a. Acetaminophen
   b. Antibiotics
   c. Anti-inflammatory drugs
   d. Corticosteroids
7. **The inadequate supply of blood to a tissue or organ due to obstructed or constricted vasculature is known as ______________.**
   a. An infarct
   b. An ischemia
   c. A blocker
   d. An angina

Answer Key

1. a **2.** c **3.** a **4.** e **5.** c

6. a **7.** b

Chapter 10

Gastrointestinal System Diseases

LEARNING OBJECTIVES

After the completion of the chapter, the readers will be able to:

- To describe the pathogenesis and histological features of peptic ulcer disease.
- To describe the pathological changes in a case of *H. pylori* gastritis.
- To describe the premalignant lesions of the oral cavity and pathogenesis of oral cancer.
- To understand the clinical and pathological features of esophageal and colorectal cancer.
- To differentiate between diffuse and intestinal type of gastric cancer.
- To differentiate between ulcerative colitis and Crohn's disease.

CHAPTER OUTLINE

- Overview of Gastrointestinal System
- Peptic Ulcer Disease
- *H. Pylori* Gastritis
- Typhoid Fever (Ulcer)
- Preneoplastic Lesion of Oral Cavity
- Carcinoma of Gastrointestinal Tract
- Esophageal Cancer
- Gastric Cancer
- Colorectal Cancer
- Inflammatory Bowel Disease

KEY TERMS

Erosion: Superficial breach in the mucosal lining epithelium.

Fungating: Grow like a fungus in its appearance or growth rate.

Goblet cells: Intestinal mucosal epithelial cells that serve as the primary site for nutrient digestion and mucosal absorption.

Linitis Plastica: Leather bottle-like, with diffuse narrowing and loss of pliability.

Ulcer: Breach in the gastrointestinal mucosa through the muscularis mucosa extending to the submucosa/deeper.

OVERVIEW OF GASTROINTESTINAL SYSTEM

The gastrointestinal (GI) system is a complex network of organs and structures responsible for the intake, digestion, absorption, and elimination of waste food (Fig. 10.1).

- **Mouth:** The digestive process begins in the mouth, where both mechanical digestion (chewing) and chemical digestion (enzymatic breakdown of carbohydrates by saliva) take place.
- **Esophagus:** The esophagus is a muscular tube which connects the mouth to the stomach. It facilitates the movement of chewed food (bolus) from the mouth to the stomach through a process called peristalsis.

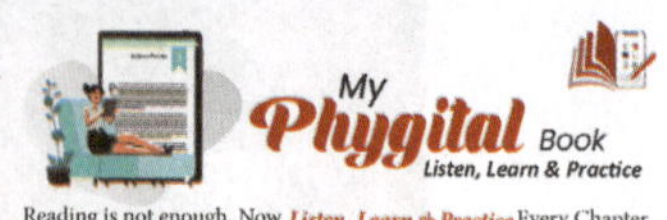

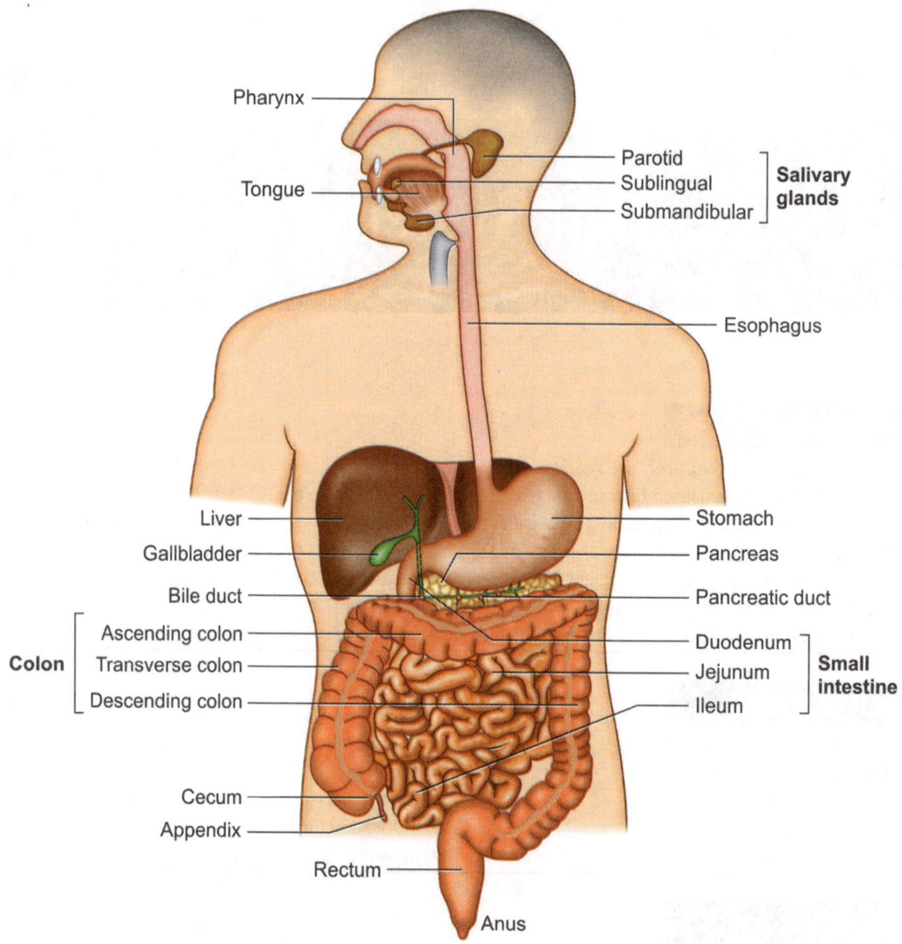

Figure 10.1: Parts of human digestive system

- **Stomach:** The stomach is a muscular organ that further breaks down food through mechanical churning and chemical digestion. Gastric juices, including hydrochloric acid and enzymes, aid in the breakdown of proteins.
  - **Mucosal protective mechanisms:** To withstand the harsh acidic environment of the stomach (extremely low pH around 1), numerous mechanisms protecting the gastric mucosa include:
    - Gastric mucosal lining epithelium—serving as a physical barrier
    - Mucus secreted by gastric foveolar epithelial cells
    - Bicarbonate ions secreted into mucus
    - Prostaglandins
    - Mucosal blood flow which maintains appropriate oxygen supply and washes away excess acid
  - **Mucosal damaging factors:**
    - Infection by *H. pylori*
    - NSAID intake, inhibiting prostaglandin synthesis

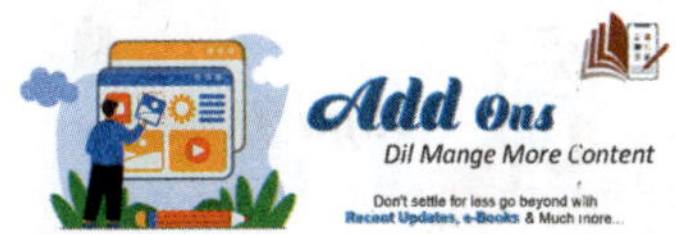

- Reduced oxygen supply due to ischemic injury, high altitude
- Elderly-reduced mucus and bicarbonate secretion
- Ingestion of toxins/chemicals/chemotherapy drugs-cause direct cellular injury by inducing oxidative stress, impair regeneration

- **Small intestine:** The majority of digestion and nutrient absorption occur in the small intestine. It is divided into three parts: duodenum, jejunum, and ileum. Enzymes from the pancreas and bile from the liver and gallbladder assist in breaking down fats, proteins, and carbohydrates.
- **Accessory organs:**
  - **Liver:** The liver produces bile, a substance that emulsifies fats, making them easier to digest. The liver also detoxifies harmful substances and stores and releases glucose as needed.
  - **Gallbladder:** The gallbladder stores and releases bile produced by the liver in response to the ingestion of fatty foods. Bile aids in the emulsification and digestion of fats.
  - **Pancreas:** The pancreas secretes digestive enzymes into the small intestine to further break down carbohydrates, proteins, and fats. It also plays a crucial role in regulating blood sugar levels by producing insulin and glucagon.
- **Large intestine:** The remaining undigested food particles move from the small intestine to the large intestine. The colon absorbs water and electrolytes from the remaining material, forming feces.
- **Rectum:** The rectum stores feces until they are ready to be eliminated.
- **Anus:** Waste is excreted from the body during the process of defecation.

Histology

The GI tract has four layers—mucosa (the innermost layer), submucosa (underneath mucosa), followed by the muscularis propria and the outermost layer—the adventitia. The structure of these layers varies, in different regions of the digestive system, depending on their functions.

PEPTIC ULCER DISEASE

Gastrointestinal ulceration may be defined as mucosal breaches extending beyond the muscularis mucosa. In India, roughly 8–10% of population have or will develop a peptic ulcer. Although the incidence of peptic ulcer disease is on the decline due to the presence of better anti-secretory and antiulcerogenic drugs, it still remains an important cause of morbidity amongst all gastrointestinal diseases. When the protective factors, mentioned before are over weighed by the damaging factors, the net result is injury and the development of peptic ulcer.

Clinical Features

Peptic ulcer disease represents chronic, recurring lesions with significant morbidity. Up to 70% patients are asymptomatic.

Symptomatic patients have:

- Epigastric pain (heartburn): burning/aching (gnawing) nature 1–3 hours after meals during the day, worse at night (11 pm–2 am) relieved by alkali/food.
- With penetrating ulcers, the pain may radiate to the back, the left upper quadrant or the chest, where it may be confused with cardiac pain.
- Nausea, vomiting, bloating, significant weight loss.
- Hemorrhage/Iron deficiency anemia/perforation.

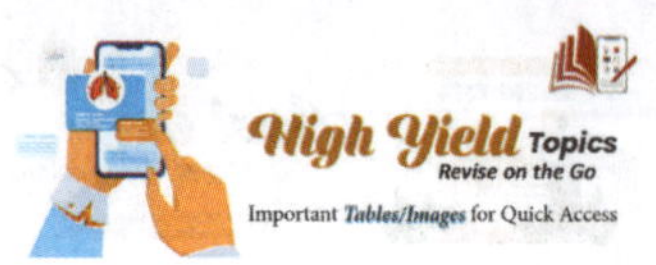

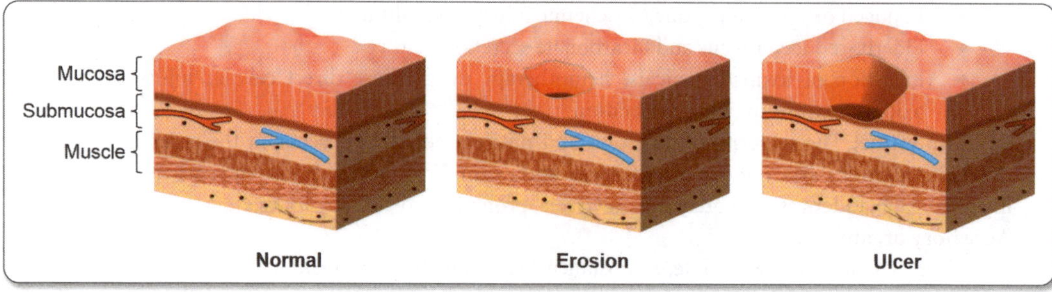

Figure 10.2: Formation of ulcer

Etiology

It is a net result of excessive acid, which in turn, leads to breach and damage of the mucosa producing an ulcer (Fig. 10.2). Peptic ulcer is a usually chronic relapsing lesion characterized by a breach in mucosa >5 mm in size and depth beyond muscularis mucosae.

Risk Factors

The common predisposing factors which favor the development of peptic ulcer include:

- Peptic ulcer disease (usually secondary to *H. pylori* gastritis).
- Chronic gastritis due to any other etiology.
- NSAID use in the elderly.
- Smoking.
- Chronic obstructive pulmonary disease.
- Usage of narcotic drugs which decrease the gut mucosal blood flow.
- Stress.
- Viral infections.

Preferred Sites of Peptic Ulcer

Any part of the gastrointestinal mucosa exposed to the aggressive action of acid/pepsin is predisposed to developing peptic ulcer disease. The two prime sites of involvement are the duodenum and the stomach.

Common sites involved include:

- D1 (1st part of the duodenum) most frequently involved site.
- The gastric antrum.
- Esophagogastric junction and the lower esophagus, especially in cases of gastroesophageal reflux and Barrett's esophagus.
- Margins of a gastrojejunostomy.
- In Meckel's diverticulum, which has ectopic gastric mucosa.
- Any part of the gastrointestinal tract in the Zollinger-Ellison syndrome.

MUST KNOW

Meckel's diverticulum–Rule of Two

- Occurs in about 2% of the population.
- Two times more frequent in males.
- About 2 inches long.
- Within 2 feet of the ileocecal valve.

Pathogenesis

Normally there is a balance between the mucosal protective mechanisms and the mucosal damaging mechanisms. The peptic ulcer ultimately develops due to imbalance between gastroprotective mechanisms and aggressive factors (Fig. 10.3), with external injurious stimuli such as stress and immunological factors acting as triggers.

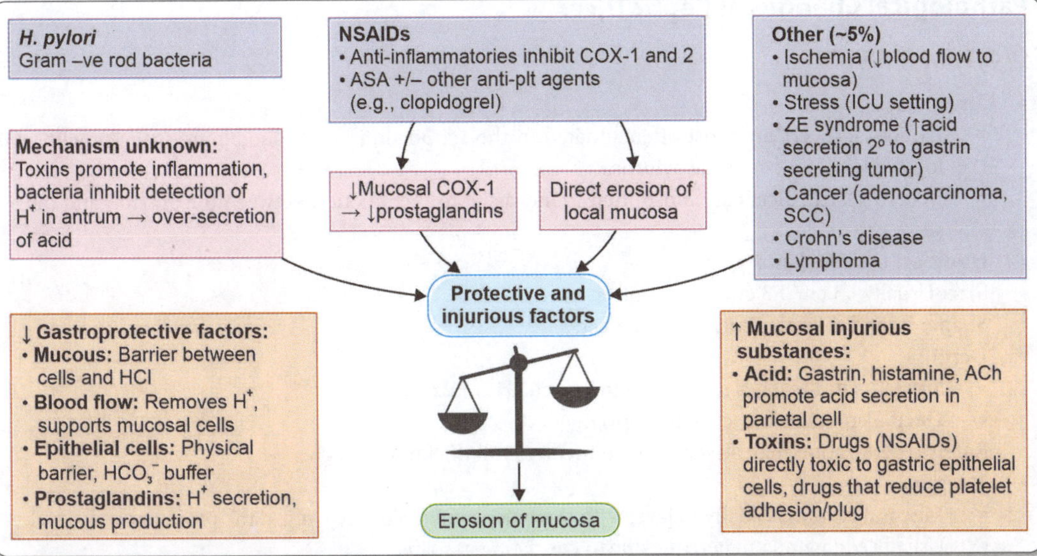

Figure 10.3: Pathogenesis of peptic ulcer

Types of Peptic Ulcers

- Acute
- Chronic

Acute Peptic Ulcer

This is a mucosal defect which is primarily brought about by severe stress.

Predisposing Factors of Acute Peptic Ulcer

The clinical scenarios in which an acute peptic ulcer develops include:

- As a complication of acute gastritis.
- In settings of severe stress:
  - Trauma (stress ulcer)
  - Burns-Curling ulcer
  - Cerebrovascular accident (CVA)—Cushing's ulcer
- When the patient has any other cause of hyperacidity, e.g., Zollinger-Ellison syndrome.

Morphological Features of Acute Peptic Ulcer

- Any site of the stomach may be affected.
- Depth of breach is variable (varies from being superficial to deep breaching the muscularis mucosa).
- When the cause of injury is stopped, the morphological changes are reversed.

Chronic Peptic Ulcer

The chronic gastric ulcer on the other hand is a recurrent, usually solitary lesion which is often secondary to chronic gastritis with no other precipitating condition.

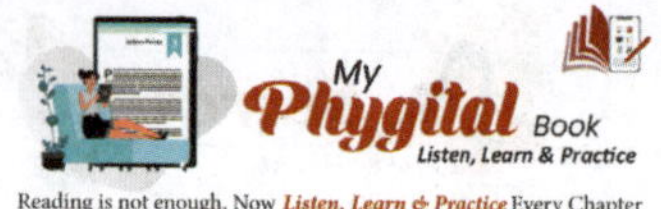

Pathological Changes of Peptic Ulcer

Gross Appearance

- **Site:**
  - Duodenal ulcers are most often situated in the 1st portion of the duodenum (>95%), with ~90% located within 3 cm of the pylorus.
  - Benign gastric ulcers are most often found distal to the junction between the antrum and the acid secretory mucosa.
- **Number:** Usually, solitary.
- **Size:** Usually <3 cm, >3 cm—Giant ulcer.
- **Shape:** Round to oval, punched out defect.
- **Depth:**
  - **Superficial:** Breaches mucosa up to muscularis mucosa.
  - **Deep:** Penetrates muscularis propria.

  Rarely a perforation may be seen, which involves full thickness breach.
- **Margins:**
  - Mucosal margins usually in level with the mucosa/may slightly hang at the proximal end.
  - Usually edematous/hyperemic due to coexisting gastritis.
- **Edge:** Sharp.
- **Base:**
  - Clean/fibrin exudate.
  - Surrounding mucosa—radiating towards the ulcer in a spoke wheel like fashion.
  - The peritoneal surface opposite the ulcer may show fibrinous exudate.

Histological Changes

Four zones of ulcer as described by Askanazy are as shown in Figure 10.4. These are the zones of necrosis, inflammation, granulation and cicatrization (fibrosis).

Figure 10.4: Four zones of peptic ulcer

Complications of Peptic Ulcer

- **Bleeding:** Most frequent, potentially life-threatening, 25% deaths.
- **Perforation:** 2/3 ulcer related deaths, can lead to peritonitis
- **Obstruction:** Crampy abdominal pain, secondary to scarring, common in pylorus (pyloric stenosis) due to fibrous stricture formation
- **Malignant transformation:** Extremely uncommon

Treatment

- Eradicate *H. pylori* by administering antibiotics.
- Suppress gastric acid with proton pump inhibitors, H_2 blockers.
- Withdraw offenders including NSAIDs.

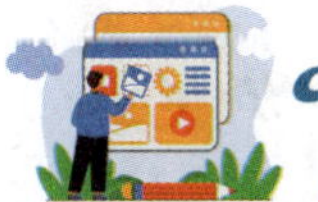
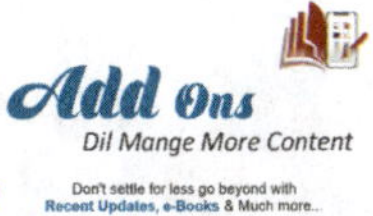

NOTE

Differences between benign and Malignant Ulcers

Feature	Benign ulcer	Malignant ulcer
Age	Younger age	Older age
Site	Lesser curvature	Greater curvature
Ulcer base	Clean	Necrotic
Mucosal folds	Radiating from the ulcer	Discontinuous due to malignant cell invasion
Shape	Punched out lesion	Irregular
Margins	Usually in level with ulcer	Heaped up
Outcome	Usually heal with therapy	Poor response

Differences between Gastric and Duodenal Ulcers

Feature	Gastric ulcer	Duodenal ulcer
Site	Antrum	1st part of duodenum
Age	Peak in 6th decade	30–60 years
M:F	1.5–2:1	3:1
Nausea, weight loss	More	less
Relationship of pain with meal	Aggravated by meal	Relieved by meal. Pain occurs 1.5–3 hours after meal Typically awakes the patient at night
Acid	N/Low	High
Pathogenesis	Decreased mucosal defense	Increased acid production

H. PYLORI GASTRITIS

Clinical Features

The patient usually comes to the clinic with complaints of indigestion, bloating, abdominal pain, dyspepsia and sometimes nausea and vomiting.

Etiology

H. pylori is a common cause of chronic gastritis. *H. pylori* is a gram-negative S-shaped flagellate bacteria, commonly seen in developing countries. The bacterium typically has a large DNA with genes Cag A and Vac A, leading to toxin production.

Pathogenesis

H. pylori is a urea-splitting bacteria and thereby liberates ammonia. Ammonia thus released leads to damage of the mucosa and inflammation. Cag A and Vac A proteins encoded by the respective genes along with the toxins liberated also lead to mucosal damage along with inflammation.

Complications

Long-standing cases of *H. pylori* have an association with:

- Atrophic gastritis
- Gastric lymphoma
- Gastric adenocarcinoma

Some cases of malignancy have even regressed after treatment for *H. pylori* infection. Hence, it is important to make a timely diagnosis.

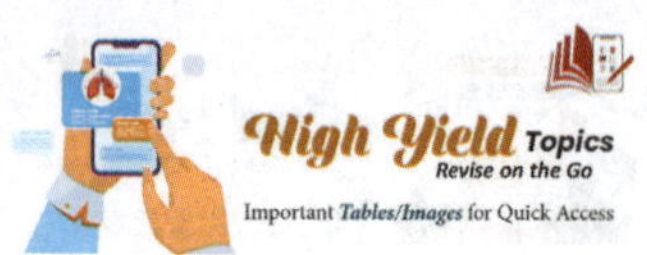

Pathological Changes

Gross Appearance

- *H. pylori* is usually seen on the surface of gastric biopsies, i.e., between the overlying epithelium and the covering mucus layer.

Histological Changes

- The overlying epithelium may be intact or ulcerated.
- The lamina propria shows chronic inflammatory infiltrate comprising lymphocytes and plasma cells. Lymphoid aggregates are frequently found.
  - In chronic cases, mucosal atrophy may also be seen.
  - In some cases, dysplasia may be noted.

MUST KNOW

Ancillary tests: *H. pylori* bacteria can sometimes be missed on evaluation of routine H&E stain. Modified Giemsa stain and silver stains can aid in the diagnosis. Recently, an IHC stain highlighting *H. pylori* has also been developed.

TYPHOID FEVER (ULCER)

The manifestation of typhoid is primarily seen in the gastrointestinal tract.

Clinical Features

The patient presents with fever, lethargy, headache, muscle pain, loss of appetite, nausea, diarrhea and in some cases abdominal distension. On examination, small reddish macules/papules are seen on the skin (Rose spots). Some patients may show a reduced heart rate (bradycardia). On abdominal examination the spleen and liver are enlarged.

Complications of typhoid fever: Severe cases where the causative bacteria are highly virulent or the host is immunosuppressed the following complications can be seen:

- Intestinal perforation
- Peritonitis
- Hemorrhagic inflammation of the intestine with blood loss
- Meningitis
- Coma

Etiology

Typhoid fever, also known as enteric fever is an infectious disease caused by Salmonella species, i.e., *typhi and paratyphi.*

Incubation period: 7–14 days

Pathogenesis

Typhoid is caused by the intake of contaminated food/water or through fomites of infected patients. *Salmonella typhi* bacteria cross the acidic environment in the stomach (Fig. 10.5). The bacilli reach the ileum and penetrate the ileal mucosa reaching the Peyer's patches and lymphoid follicles of the ileum.

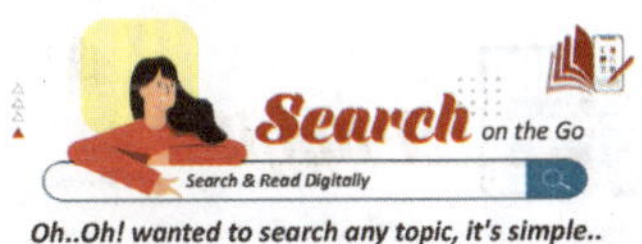

Within the Peyer's patches, the bacteria are phagocytosed by macrophages (microfold M cells). Despite being within the macrophages, they escape destruction by altering their surface protein composition and *via* the monocyte-macrophage system, quietly disseminate subsequently, reach the lymphatics, causing enlargement of the mesenteric lymph nodes. Through the thoracic duct the organisms reach the bloodstream from where they reach the organs of the reticuloendothelial system (liver, spleen) and the gallbladder, causing their enlargement.

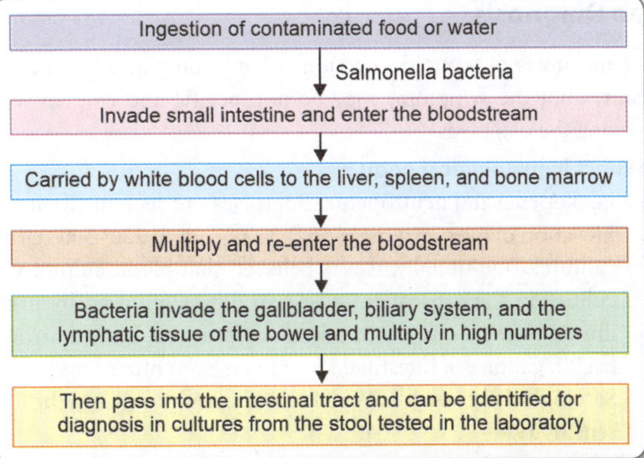

Figure 10.5: Pathogenesis of typhoid fever

Further multiplication leads to the bacilli re-entering the bloodstream and through the bile, the bacilli re-enter the Peyer's patches. In some cases, the bacilli remain within the bile in the gallbladder and do not spread further leading to a chronic carrier state.

Pathological Changes

Reduced white blood cell count (leukopenia) or a normal blood count.

Gross appearance (Fig. 10.6A): Lesions due to typhoid are more frequent in the terminal ileum. However, other segments of the small/large intestine may be seen. Enlarged Peyer's patches cause elevated, well-demarcated lesions.

Histological changes (Fig.10.6B)

- Ulceration of the lining epithelium.
- The lamina propria and submucosa shows edema.
- The lamina propria shows the presence of lymphocytes, plasma cells and histiocytes.
- Histiocytes in typhoid lesions characteristically show ingestion of red cells **(erythrophagocytosis).**
- In cases of ileal involvement, there is marked enlargement of the lymphoid follicles.

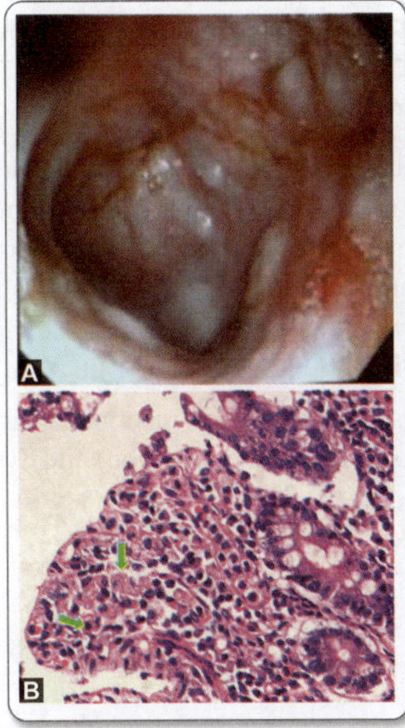

Figures 10.6A and B: Typhoid ulcer: **A.** Gross; **B.** Histology

Morphological changes in other organs:

- **Gallbladder:** Inflammation (**cholecystitis**) is noted.
- **Liver:** Foci of parenchymal necrosis is seen. Hepatocytes are replaced by aggregates of macrophages (**"typhoid nodules"**).
- **Spleen:** The spleen is grossly enlarged and microscopically shows expansion of the white pulp.
- **Bones:** Histopathological features consistent with osteomyelitis may be seen.

NOTE

Typhoid ulcers occur along the long axis of the intestine versus TB ulcer which is transverse. The ulcer is oval, having a necrotic base with a brownish-black appearance and the margins are slightly edematous.

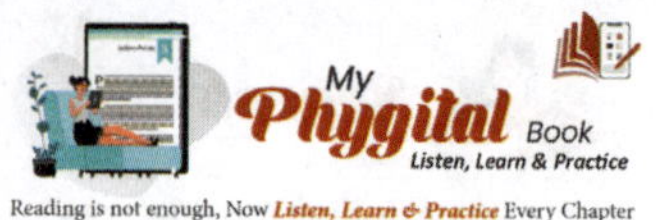

Lab Diagnosis

The diagnosis of typhoid infection is based on clinical suspicion, i.e., observing the characteristic clinical features but the symptoms may be nonspecific and overlap with other gastrointestinal infections thereby delaying the diagnosis.

Indirect hematological pointers:

- Leukopenia and neutropenia. But this is not seen in all cases.
- Elevation of liver enzymes (AST, ALT)—up to 250–300 IU/L
- Culture: Traditionally, it was believed that blood culture yielded positivity in the first week and stool culture in the subsequent weeks of illness followed by urine culture positivity by the fourth week of illness. However, as per modern day practice, bone marrow cultures are more sensitive to pick up the bacilli. Culture of intestinal secretion is even more sensitive.
- Serological tests such as Widal test detect antibodies to the O antigen and flagellar H antigen have limited sensitivity.

With improved antibiotic regimens the rate of complications including intestinal perforation decrease. Histopathology of resected intestinal segments hence, is at best, now a limited diagnostic modality.

PRENEOPLASTIC LESION OF ORAL CAVITY

Oral Leucoplakia

Leucoplakia is a premalignant lesion of the oral cavity. As the name suggests, it is a white patch, defined as measuring >5 mm, which cannot be scraped off and is not due to any specific disease process. Some women may develop leukoplakia on the outside of their genitals in the vulva area. The risk of malignant transformation is 1–10%.

Types of Leucoplakia

Based on the above-mentioned histological features, two main types are described—hyperkeratotic (with more of keratin production) and dysplastic.

Sites of Predilection

Lateral and ventral tongue

- Floor of the mouth
- Alveolar ridge mucosa
- Corner of the mouth
- Less frequently: Soft palate and lip

Risk Factors

- Tobacco consumption
- Chronic alcohol intake
- Fungal/bacterial infections (Candida)
- Chronic irritation, e.g., dentures
- Hormonal imbalance

The candidal leukoplakia occurs when either denture's friction or smoking is accompanied with candida infection. It leads to immune system suppression.

Pathological Changes

Gross appearance (Fig. 10.7A): It is usually well defined and slightly elevated. In the oral cavity, it is usually seen in the oral mucosa or tongue. In addition, it may be smooth/wrinkled. Lesions may be solitary/multiple.

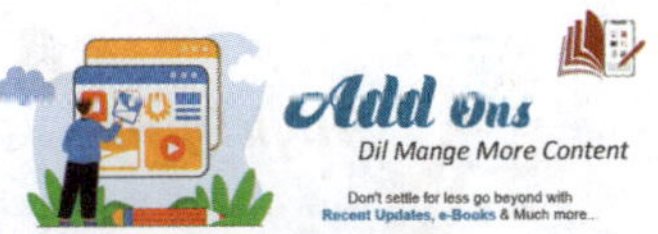

Patches vary in appearance and may have the following features:
White or gray color; thick, hard, raised surface; hairy (hairy leukoplakia only), red spots (rare).

Histological changes (Fig. 10.7B)

- Epidermis is thickened (acanthosis).
- Keratin layer is increased (hyperkeratosis).
- Dysplasia of varying degrees may be present—mild/moderate/severe.
- Mild chronic inflammatory infiltrate is seen in the sub epithelium.
- Cellular pleomorphism.
- Nuclear atypia.
- Increased number of cells seen undergoing mitosis, including both normal and abnormal mitoses.
- The distinction between the epithelial layers may be lost.
- Abnormal keratinization.
- Alteration of the normal epithelial-connective tissue architecture—the rete pegs may become "drop shaped" wider at their base than top, superficially.

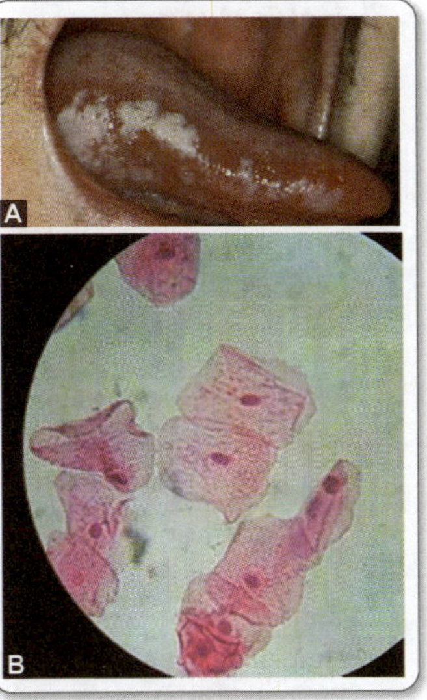

Figures 10.7A and B: **A.** Oral leukoplakia–gross; **B.** Cytological photo

Erythroplakia

This is another premalignant lesion of the oral cavity which has a more ominous prognosis as >90% cases show dysplasia or invasive malignancy.

Histological Features

- Epithelial atrophy.
- Rete pegs may be bullous.
- Subepithelial tissue-increased no of vessels.
- Epithelial dysplasia may be present, if so, modify treatment.

CARCINOMA OF GASTROINTESTINAL TRACT

Gastrointestinal (GI) cancer is the uncontrolled growth of abnormal cells (cancer) in the digestive tract and other abdominal organs. Some important cancers of gastrointestinal tract are discussed ahead.

Buccal Carcinoma

Incidence is increasing in the young with pathogenesis still unclear in nonsmokers and those not infected with human papilloma virus (HPV). The most common sites of involvement in the oral cavity by malignancy are the floor of the mouth, tongue and soft palate.

The broad categories of malignancy involving the oropharyngeal cavity include:

- Epithelial
- Mesenchymal
- Hematolymphoid

Squamous cell carcinoma is an invasive epithelial neoplasm showing varying degrees of squamous differentiation with a tendency of early and extensive lymph node metastases and usually bad prognosis as most cases are detected late. It constitutes 95% of cases of the head and neck.

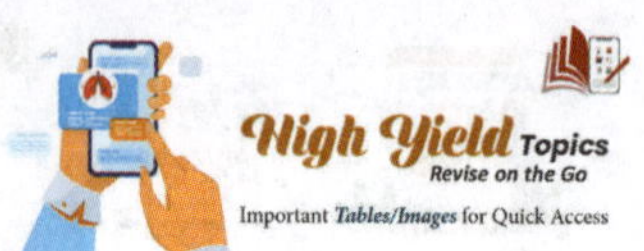

Clinical Features

- Red lesions, mixed red and white lesions, or white plaques.
- Mucosal growth and ulceration.
- Referred pain to the ear.
- Malodor.
- Difficulty while speaking, opening the mouth, or chewing.
- Difficulty and pain with swallowing.
- Bleeding, weight loss, and neck swelling.
- Enlarged neck nodes without any symptoms.

Etiology

- Smoking.
- Alcohol consumption.
- Tobacco (smokeless, chewing/dipping), betel, paan.
- Consumption of areca nut.
- Human papillomavirus 16 infection.
- Prolonged exposure to sunlight, pipe smoking–lip cancers.
- Precancerous lesions:
  - White patches (leukoplakia)—hyperplasia.
  - Red patches (Erythroplakia)—dysplasia higher grade.
  - Erythroleukoplakia—a combination of reddish and white patches.
  - Oral submucous fibrosis.
  - Lichen planus.
  - Syphilitic glossitis.
- Major genetic factors leading to tumor development
  - Mainly mutant genes are responsible for tumor development the epigenetic changes bring alteration of expression and function of tumor suppress or genes.
  - On a genetic level, mutations in proteins such as CDKN2A, PIK3CA accumulate, accompanied with changes in gene expression and inactivation of tumor suppressor genes.

Site

The most common oropharyngeal site of involvement for squamous cell carcinoma is the base of tongue (posterior 1/3rd). Other sites of involvement include the lip, floor of the mouth and palate.

Risk Factors

- Alcohol-based mouthwash.
- Oral mechanical irritation, (ill-fitting dentures and jagged teeth).
- Precancerous conditions—Leukoplakia, erythroplakia.
- Severe iron deficiency (Plummer-Vinson syndrome).
- Oral submucous fibrosis.
- Lichen planus and discoid lupus erythematosis.

Pathogenesis

The HPV 16 infection is believed to have a role in the pathogenesis. Viral infection is followed by integration of viral DNA into host DNA. Transcription of HPV E6, E7 mRNA leads to inactivation of p53 and Rb proteins, which indirectly lead to p16 accumulation. Both the factors contribute to the development of cancer.

Smoking also inactivates p53 protein, leading to tumorigenesis. HPV16 positive oral cavity and oropharyngeal tumors may be associated with a more favorable outcome.

Pathological Changes

Gross Appearance

Lesions are either ulceroproliferative cauliflower-like growths or ulceroinfiltrative type lesions showing mucosal thickening and irregularity. The lesion is irregular and shows a soft to firm white cut surface. In larger ulceroproliferative growths, on cut surface, the lesion may be friable and necrotic (Fig. 10.8A).

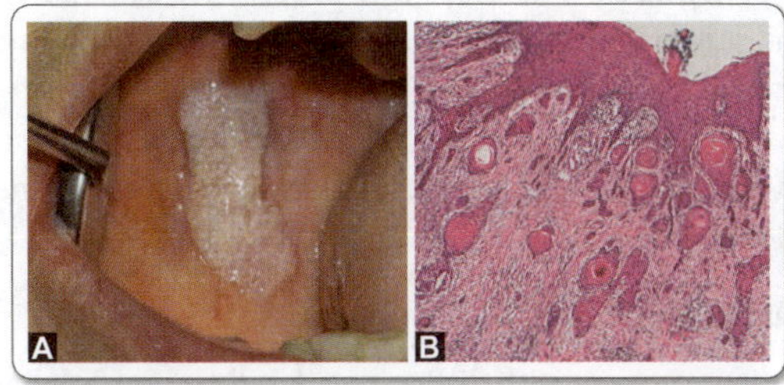

Figures 10.8A and B: Buccal carcinoma: **A.** Gross; **B.** Histology

Histological Changes (Fig. 10.8B)

- Nests and sheets of malignant, infiltrating squamoid cells are seen in varying degrees of differentiation (well/moderate/poor).
- Atypical mitotic figures are often seen.
- The overlying lining squamous epithelium may be intact or ulcerated.
- Accompanying dysplasia may be seen.

ESOPHAGEAL CANCER

Carcinoma of the esophagus is on a recently increasing trend. It is commonly seen among patients in their seventh decade. It shows a predilection for males. Types of esophageal carcinoma are as shown in Figure 10.9.

Risk Factors

- Advanced age.
- Gastroesophageal reflux disease.
- Infection with *H. pylori.*
- Barrett esophagus.
- Smoking/tobacco consumption.
- Chronic alcohol consumption.
- Ingestion of very hot liquids/food.
- Obesity.
- Plummer vinson syndrome (esophageal webs, iron deficiency anemia and dysphagia).

Benign tumors
- Adenomas
- Polyps

Malignant
- Adenocarcinoma
- Squamous cell carcinoma
- Adenosquamous
- Neuroendocrine
- Undifferentiated tumors

Figure 10.9: Types of esophageal cancer

Types of Esophageal Cancers

The two main histological types of esophageal carcinoma are squamous cell carcinoma and adenocarcinoma:

Squamous Cell Carcinoma (SCC)

As per the pathological stage of cancer, SCC can be of the following types:

- **Early stage (superficial) esophageal SCC:** A tumor that is confined to the mucosa/submucosa. This has a good prognosis.
- **Advanced stage esophageal SCC:** This type of SCC shows invasion through the muscularis propria and has a poor prognosis with higher chances of metastatic disease.

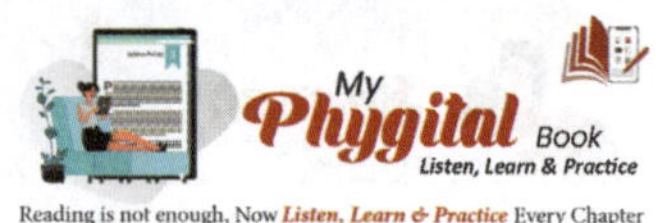

Pathogenesis of SCC

Esophageal SCC develops by a progressive accumulation of genetic alterations. The genetic mutations lead to the conversion of a normal squamous epithelial lining to one that is dysplastic. Dysplasia may further be low or high grade.

The key mutations involved are of p53 (early stage) and p16. EGFR amplification has been described in about 60% cases. Structural rearrangements of genes and copy number variations have also been described in the pathogenesis of this tumor.

Clinical Features

Patients present with difficulty in swallowing (dysphagia), weight loss, acid reflux. Some patients may present with anemia and nausea.

Pathological Changes

Squamous cell carcinoma is the most frequent histological type of esophageal cancer in India and usually involves the upper two-thirds of the esophagus. The middle one-third of the esophagus is the most common site for this tumor.

Gross appearance (Fig. 10.10A): The tumor is gray-white in color and may present as a polypoidal growth/as a fungating exophytic cauliflower-like growth which ulcerates. The lesion may also grow as an infiltrating growth that grows circumferentially leading to stricture formation.

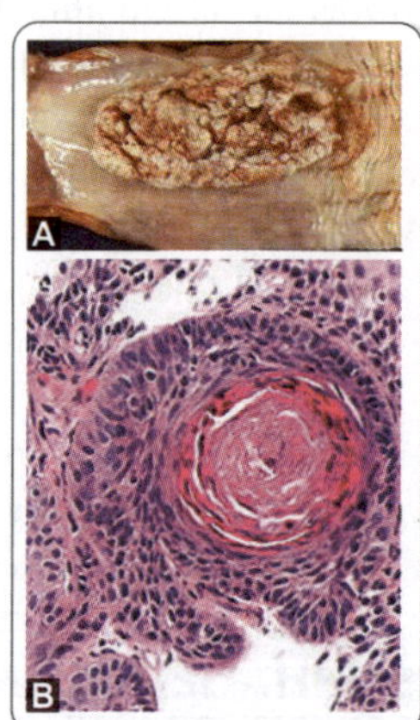

Figures 10.10A and B: Esophageal squamous cell carcinoma: **A.** Gross; **B.** Histology

Histological changes (Fig. 10.10B): Sheets and nests of squamoid cells showing intercellular bridges, and cellular pavementing are seen. Evidence of cytoplasmic keratin production and formation of keratin pearls is seen in well-differentiated squamous cell carcinoma. This is accompanied by other features of malignancy including nuclear hyperchromasia, increased nucleocytoplasmic ratio and irregular nuclear chromatin along with frequent mitoses and necrosis.

Histological variants of SCC are:

- Spindle cell squamous cell carcinoma.
- Basaloid carcinoma.
- Verrucous squamous cell carcinoma.

Immunohistochemical markers: In poorly differentiated cases, immunohistochemistry may be useful to confirm the squamous origin of the tumor (CK5/6, p63, p40).

MUST KNOW

Histological Grades

As per the WHO, squamous cell carcinomas are graded based on nuclear atypia, mitotic activity and keratin production. Accordingly, there are three grades:

Grade 1: Well differentiated (with abundant keratin pearls, low mitotic activity and only mild atypia).

Grade 2: Moderately differentiated (with less keratin production, moderate atypia and more mitoses).

Grade 3: Poorly differentiated (scant if any keratin production, marked atypia and high mitotic activity).

Adenocarcinoma

This is a tumor which is characterized by glandular differentiation and is seen at the lower third of the esophagus or the gastroesophageal junction. Adenocarcinoma is more frequently seen in the western countries while cases of squamous cell carcinoma predominate in Asia, including India. Prognosis is usually poor.

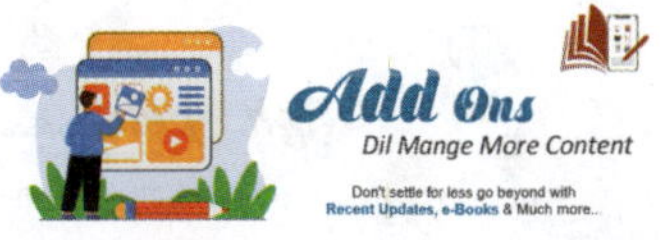

Risk Factors

Long standing cases of gastroesophageal reflux disease, *H. pylori* infection, pre-existing Barrett's esophagus, obesity, smoking and male gender.

Pathogenesis

When exposed to any of the risk factors, the stem cell niche in the lower esophagus is programmed to switch to either gastric cell types or intestinal cell types. Switch to intestinal type lining epithelium with the presence of goblet cells (intestinal metaplasia) is strongly associated with the development of neoplasia (adenocarcinoma). Genetic mutations in p53 gene are also seen in later stages of the disease.

Pathological Changes

Gross appearance (Fig. 10.11A): Esophageal adenocarcinoma usually is detected in an advanced stage where it typically has a varied gross appearance. It could be a fungating ulceroproliferative growth, a firm indurated ulceroinfiltrative growth or it may present an esophageal stricture. Cases detected early usually appear as plaques or even small nodules.

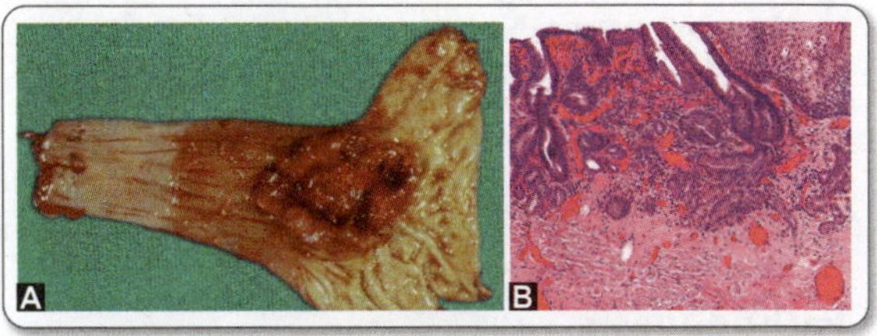

Figures 10.11A and B: Esophageal adenocarcinoma: **A.** Gross; **B.** Histology

Histological changes (Fig. 10.11B): The tumor comprises infiltrating malignant glands, the individual cells of which show nuclear pleomorphism, hyperchromasia, prominent nucleoli and an increased nucleocytoplasmic ratio. The glands may or may not show the presence of mucin. In addition, other patterns may also be seen including the presence of signet rings, small papillae and tumor cells floating within mucin lakes.

A few small groups of cells (1–5 cells) may be seen detached from the main tumor at the invasion front. These are called "tumor buds".

Immunohistochemistry: It can be used to confirm poorly-differentiated cases.

Esophageal adenocarcinomas are characterized by a specific cytokeratin pattern as CK7+, CK19+, and CK20–.

EXTRA EDGE

- Her2Neu stain is used as a therapeutic marker as Trastuzumab a drug developed targeting Her2 protein is approved for treating advanced/metastatic esophageal adenocarcinoma.
- PD-L1 immunostaining is also advocated in advanced esophageal adenocarcinoma.

GASTRIC CANCER

Gastric cancer is known to affect certain geographical sites including Japan and other sites in the Far East. Due to its frequently advanced stage at diagnosis, mortality from gastric cancer is high. The most common histological type of gastric cancer is the adenocarcinoma which is defined as a malignant epithelial neoplasm of the gastric mucosa with glandular differentiation.

Grading of Gastric Carcinoma

The gastric carcinoma is graded as low grade and high grade according to the differentiation:

- Low grade (well/moderately differentiated).
- High grade (poorly differentiated).

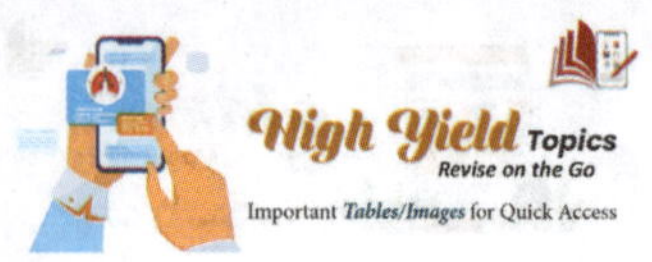

Clinical Features

- Epigastric pain
- Weight loss, anorexia
- Dyspepsia
- Hematemesis
- Lymph node involvement, if advanced

Risk Factors

Many predisposing factors have been described in the context of gastric adenocarcinoma. These include:

- *H. pylori* infection.
- Family history of gastric cancer.
- Barrett's esophagus.
- Partial gastrectomy (removal of part of the stomach)—this leads to atrophy of gastric glands.
- Hypertrophic gastropathy.
- Dietary factors, such as intake of low fiber, lack of intake of fruit and vegetables, lack of antioxidant-rich food, consumption of pickles, highly salty food, processed food.
- Dyspepsia.
- Blood group A.

Pathogenesis

- *Correa's sequence*: Chronic *H. pylori* infection leads to atrophic gastritis and intestinal metaplasia. It causes DNA mutations and epigenetic changes in epithelial cells of the stomach (field cancerization).
- Loss of function in CDH-1[Diffuse] which encodes e-cadherin.
- E-cadherin silencing leads to hypermethylation.
- Mutation of TP53 can be observed in both diffuse and intestinal adenocarcinoma.
- Mutations in APC gene and β-catenin seen in intestinal type of carcinoma.

Classification of Gastric Carcinoma

According to depth of invasion:

- **Early gastric carcinoma (EGC)** limited to mucosa and submucosa irrespective of lymph node status.
- **Advanced gastric carcinoma (AGC)** infiltrates muscularis propria and beyond.

According to gross appearance:

Three types of gross features are described:

1. Exophytic, polypoidal, fungating.
2. Flat/depressed/plaque type (special type—linitis plastica).
3. Ulcerated/excavated lesion.

MUST KNOW

According to histological changes: Two main histological types of gastric carcinoma as are intestinal and diffuse.

1. **Intestinal:** Tumor cells are arranged in the form of glands resembling the glands seen in colonic mucosa. The tumor cells are arranged in the form of glands and papillae. Tumor cells produce mucin.
2. **Diffuse:** In the diffuse type of gastric carcinoma, malignant cells are small in size, show a "signet ring" cell-appearance, the mucin pushing the nucleus to the periphery. Grossly, such tumors give the appearance of "linitis plastica" or leather bottle-like appearance.

Contd...

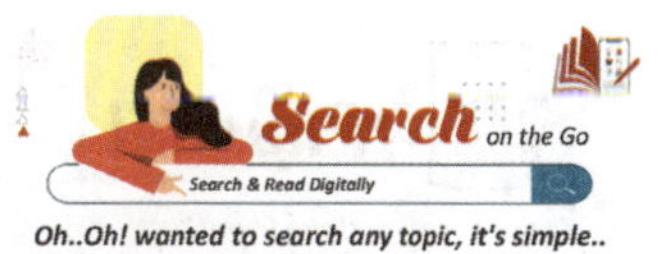

Differences between diffuse and intestinal gastric carcinoma are as follows:

Intestinal gastric carcinoma	Diffuse intestinal gastric carcinoma
Expansile growth pattern– Pushing margins	Diffuse infiltrative pattern
Frequently associated with intestinal metaplasia and dysplasia	Infrequent
Large cells with abundant cytoplasm and hyperchromatic nuclei, Forming glands, tubules Mucin is seen as apical vacuole/gland lumina	Individual dyscohesive cells No glands "signet ring" cells Strong mural desmoplasia causing rigidity of wall
M:F ratio is 2:1	M:F ratio is 1:1 more often in younger patients
More in high-risk area Good prognosis	Relatively constant Poor prognosis
APC/β-catenin mutation	E cadherin mutation
Frequently ulcerative, more commonly appear in the antrum and lesser curvature of the stomach	Develops throughout the stomach (including the cardia) infiltrate and thicken the stomach wall without forming a discrete mass

Sites of Predilection

- Antrum
- Pylorus
- Gastric cardia
- Remaining lesions occur in the body and fundus. Out of the two curvatures, lesser curvature is more frequently involved.

Spread of Gastric Carcinoma

- Direct: Spreading to the adjacent organs—esophagus, duodenum, spleen, pancreas, CBD, liver.
- Hematogenous: *Via* blood stream to the lungs, liver and bone.
- Transcoelomic: The tumor may spread through the abdominal cavity to involve the ovaries bilaterally, known as the Krukenberg tumor.
- Through the lymphatics: Involves the regional/distant lymph nodes.
- Left supraclavicular lymph node involvement is referred to as the Virchow's node (Virchow's sign).
- Left axillary lymph node—irish node.
- Involvement of the umbilicus—Sister Mary Joseph nodule.

MUST KNOW

Differences between benign and malignant gastric ulcers

Feature	Benign gastric carcinoma	Malignant gastric ulcer carcinoma
Age involvement	Younger age group	Elder age group
Size	Usually, small	Usually, large >4 cm
Appearance	Punched out	Irregular
Base	Clean, may show hemorrhagic foci	Shows necrotic slough
Margins	Flat	Heaped up
Mucosal folds	Radiating in a wheel-like manner from the ulcer	Discontinuous and interrupted by the malignant lesions

Linitis Plastica (Leather Bottle Stomach)

- Generalized/ localized, commonly involving the antrum. No exophytic growth identified grossly.
- Extensive wall thickening is noted giving the stomach a rugged appearance resembling a leather bottle.
- The stomach in later stages shows a decreased volume and reduced distensibility.
- On opening the stomach, mucosa appears diffusely thickened with a distortion/loss of folds.
- Extensive fibrosis of the submucosa and muscularis propria leads to wall thickening which on sectioning appears firm.
- Perigastric lymph nodes are usually present.
- Such cases show a poor prognosis.

COLORECTAL CANCER

Colorectal cancer represents the most common malignancy of gastrointestinal tract.

Clinical Presentation

- Altered bowel habits—diarrhea or constipation.
- Bleeding in the stools (hematochezia).
- Anemia due to loss of blood.
- Loss of appetite.
- Loss of weight (anorexia).

Risk Factors for the Development of Colorectal Cancer

Population affected: It is frequently seen in elder adults (peaking between 60–70 years of age). There is a predilection for upper socioeconomic strata.

Diet: Populations of wealthy countries especially consume diets low in fiber with a higher proportion of dietary fat and carbohydrates. The reduced fiber component in the diet leads to a decreased stool bulk. Diminished stool bulk increases the contact time between feces and the colonic epithelium as transit times are prolonged. In addition the gut flora is altered. As the stool remains in the colon for longer times, metabolic products toxic to the system are elaborated.

Intake of meat: Red/processed meat increases cholesterol. This in turn increases bile production. The metabolic products in turn are carcinogenic.

Reduced physical activity and obesity: This promotes accumulation of body fat which in turn promotes insulin resistance and higher concentrations of IGF-1 are seen. This stimulates proliferation of colonic mucosa.

History of prior intestinal disease: The presence of chronic inflammation in the bowel such as the presence of inflammatory bowel disease and diverticulitis (inflammation in a diverticular outpouching) is a risk factor for the development of colorectal cancer. Inflammatory bowel disease cases especially involving the entire colon (pancolitis) leads to a definite higher risk.

Genetic influences: Certain hereditary conditions, predispose to colorectal oncogenesis such as:

- **Familial adenomatous polyposis (FAP):** Autosomal disorder associated with APC gene defects and showing multiple adenomas (at least a 100 for diagnosis). Untreated cases have a very high risk of developing cancer ,even at a young age (<45 years).

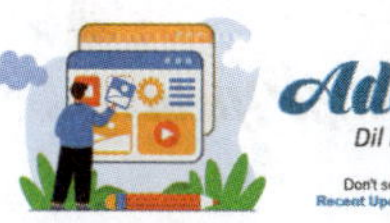
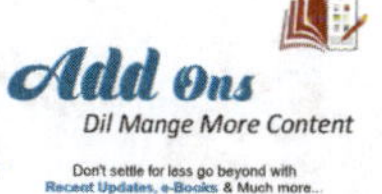

- **Hereditary non polyposis coli (Lynch's syndrome):** Autosomal dominant disease due to mutations in mismatch repair genes. Faster rate of tumor progression is seen. Amsterdam criteria for diagnosis is the presence of 3 or more relatives with colorectal cancer, one of whom is a first-degree relative of the other two ,one or more cases of colorectal cancer diagnosed before age 50 in the family, colorectal cancer involving at least two generations and exclusion of FAP.
- MUTYH gene mutation-associated polyposis.
- Peutz-Jegher's syndrome.

Pathogenesis

Pathogenesis of colorectal cancer (CRC) has been depicted in Figure 10.12.

Molecular pathways implicated in the diagnosis of colorectal carcinoma include:

- **Adenomacarcinoma sequence:** This involves a stepwise accumulation of mutations as well as epigenetic changes.
  The epithelial lining first becomes hyperplastic (*via* APC gene mutations) subsequently forming an adenoma,acquiring further mutations (K-RAS, BRAF, SMAD2, 4, CDC4) to show dysplastic change and in turn at later stages of the pathway, p53 mutations enable progression to in situ and invasive colorectal cancer.
- **Microsatellite instability pathway:** 10–15% of colorectal cancer is characterized by a unique pathogenetic mechanism- microsatellite instability. This shows a failure of the DNA mismatch repair system. It is defined as the presence of additional alleles at a microsatellite vs normal area. A microsatellite is a short repeating sequence occurring throughout the genome of one or two base pairs. When DNA replicates, if there are any errors in pairing up of bases, an entire system of genes (mismatch repair genes) gets into action to correct the error. Microsatellite areas are a bit prone to errors because of the repetitive nature of sequence causing errors when DNA strands realign after replication. When the mismatch repair genes (MLH1, MSH2, PMS2, MSH6) are lost or deficient, potential for colorectal carcinogenesis exists. Testing is important as MSI related cancers have a better prognosis and is done by immunohistochemistry and mutational analysis (PCR/NGS assays).

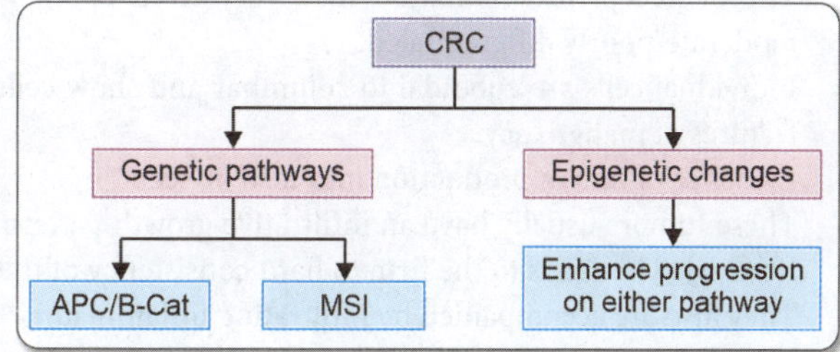

Figure 10.12: Pathogenesis of colorectal cancer

Abbreviations: APC, gene; B-cat, β-catenin gene; CRC, Colorectal cancer; MSI, microsatellite instability

EXTRA EDGE

Mismatch repair (MMR) deficient colorectal cancers have unique histopathological features:

1. Mucinous histology.
2. Tumor infiltrating lymphocytes.
3. Crohn's disease like peritumoral lymphocyte predominance.
4. Lack of differentiation.

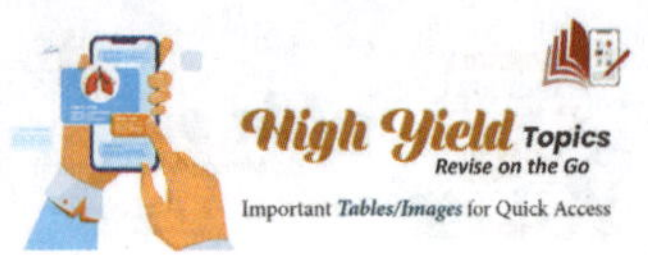

Pathological Changes

Gross

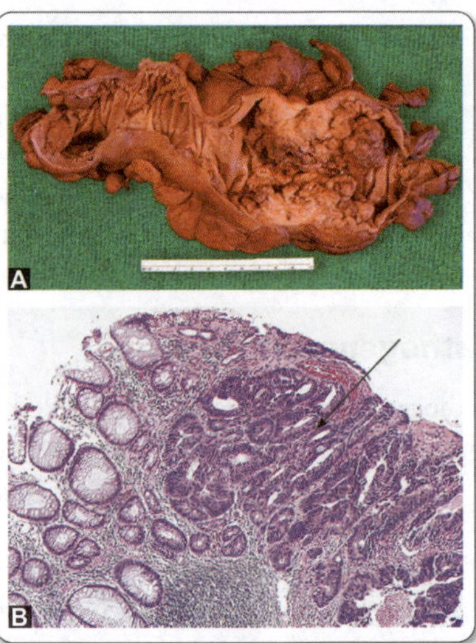

Figures 10.13A and B: **A.** Colon carcinoma (gross appearance); **B.** Colon adenocarcinoma (microscopic appearance)

Depending on the site of the tumor:

- Right colon-fungating ulceroproliferative masses.
- Left colon-Napkin ring annular constricting, infiltrating masses (Fig. 10.13A).
- Sometimes the lesion may present as a polypoidal mass projecting into the lumen.
- Cut surface: Firm, white, hard sometimes with areas of necrosis.

Microscopy

Most colorectal cancers are adenocarcinomas. As discussed previously, adenocarcinomas are tumors comprised of malignant glands showing back to back arrangement, complex branching and at times papillary formations (Fig. 10.13B).

- The degree of differentiation may vary from being well/ moderate/poorly differentiated.
- Individual cells are cuboidal to columnar and show cellular features of malignancy.
- Evidence of mucin production may also be seen.
- These tumors usually have an infiltrative growth pattern and are accompanied by desmoplasia (intense fibrosis). This leads to the firm to hard consistency of the tumor.
- They also are accompanied by infiltrating inflammatory cells, usually lymphocytes.
- Morphological variants include signet ring cell carcinoma, mucinous carcinoma. Other types of malignancies involving the colon and rectum include adenosquamous carcinoma and neuroendocrine carcinoma.

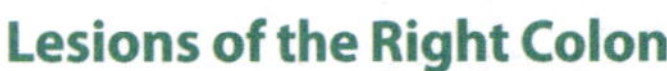

Lesions of the Right Colon

In the right colon, the stool is still in liquid state, lesions therefore have enough space to proliferate and expand to form large soft fungating cauliflower like masses accompanied by chronic, insidious blood loss leading to anemia. Obstruction is less frequent.

Lesions of Left Colon

Because stool becomes more formed as it passes into the transverse and descending colon, tumors arising there tend to impede the passage of stool, resulting in the development of abdominal cramping, tenesmus, occasional obstruction, and constricting lesions called as "napkin-ring" tumors.

The salient differences between right and left sided lesions have been discussed in Table 10.1.

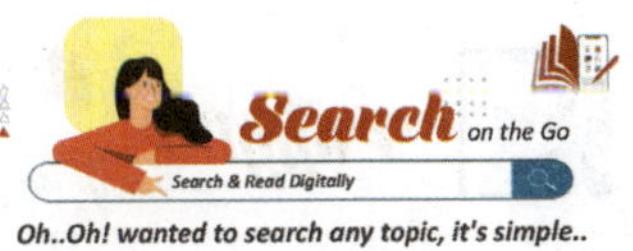

Table 10.1: Salient differences between right and left sided lesions

Feature	Right sided colorectal cancer	Left sided colorectal cancer
Gender predilection	Females	Males
Age	Elderly	Young
Clinical features	Anemia, passage of fresh blood per-rectum (hematochezia)	Obstruction, altered bowel habits
MSI	Associated with microsatellite instability and Lynch syndrome	Follow APC gene mutation pathway more, associated with FAP
Gross	Initially flat sessile lesions which escape notice Later: Fungating, friable, cauliflower-like	Napkin ring, circumferential
Microscopy	More infiltrating T-lymphocytes	Less
Prognosis	Slightly better	Worse

Spread

The tumor spreads to adjoining structures by direct extension.

Spread through lymphatics to the local mesenteric lymph nodes in the pericolic fat and then to non-regional lymph nodes.

Hematogenous spread to the liver, bones, brain, lungs.

Staging (Fig. 10.14)

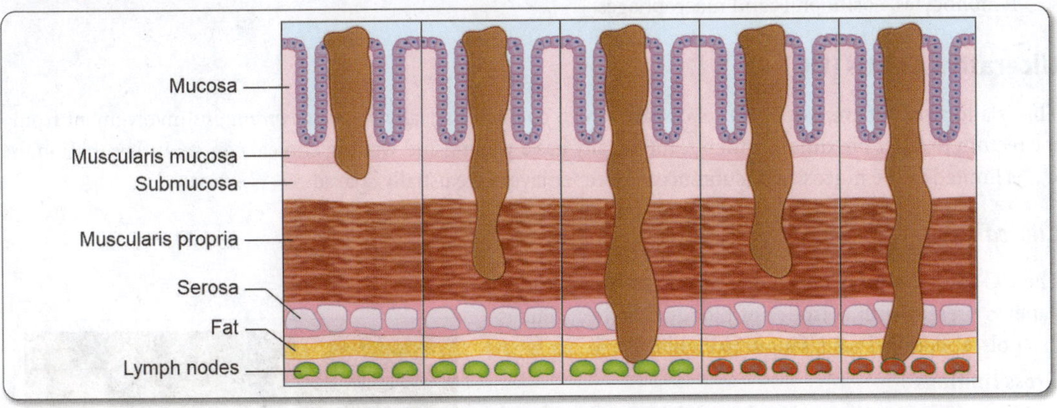

Figures 10.14: Staging of colorectal cancer

T1 - (till submucosa)
T2 - (till muscularis propria)
T3 - (till subserosa)
T4 - (other organs)
N1 - (1–3 LN)
N2 - (>4 LN involved)

Poor Prognostic Factors

- Tumor spread to regional lymph nodes and number of regional lymph nodes involved.
- Tumor penetration through the bowel wall (i.e., increased depth of invasion).
- Poorly differentiated histology.
- Presence of lymphovascular emboli.
- High levels of CEA (>5 ng/mL) before surgery.

INFLAMMATORY BOWEL DISEASE

This is a group of diseases which, as the name suggests, is characterized by inflammation of the intestine. This shows a waxing and waning course with frequent exacerbations and remissions. Though traditionally believed to be a disease affecting the Western population,its incidence is on the rise in the Indian population. The two main types of inflammatory bowel disease described include:

1. Ulcerative colitis
2. Crohn's disease

Pathogenesis of Inflammatory Bowel Disease (IBD)

The pathogenesis of IBD is multifactorial.

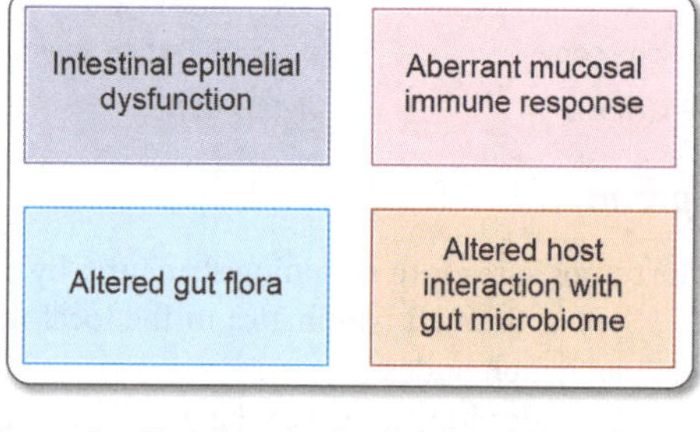

- A genetically susceptible host for IBD bears polymorphisms in molecules such as DLG5, NOD2 (Crohn's disease), CARD9, autophagy genes IRGM, ATG16L1, PTPN2.
- The host fails to recognize and respond to microbial pathogens.
- Exaggerated mucosal immune response to gut flora and microbial pathogens.
- Altered intestinal epithelial barrier leading to a leaky gut through which bacterial entry is easy.
- Liberation of cytokines -IL-1, IL-12, IL-21, IL-17, TNF-α, this leads to recruitment of neutrophils, lymphocytes, eosinophils and macrophages.

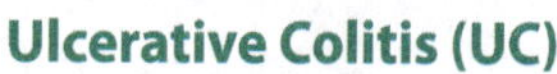

Ulcerative Colitis (UC)

This is a form of inflammatory bowel disease which characteristically shows a *continuous* involvement from the rectum to other proximal segments. It typically has a waxing and waning clinical course. Inflammation in UC is limited to the mucosa and submucosa. Deeper layers are usually spared.

Clinical Features

The UC commonly presents in the second to fifth decades. Patients present with episodes of bloody diarrhea, mucus in stools, abdominal pain, fatigue, weight loss.

Gross findings

- **In acute cases,** the mucosa is **reddish, congested** and granular and uneven.
- The intervening mucosa regenerates and forms **pseudopolyps**.
- Numerous **ulcers** may be seen on the mucosal aspect.
- Mucosal **edema** is generally seen.
- There is a sharp transition between the involved and uninvolved part of the colon.

Features of chronic ulcerative colitis:

- The mucosa appears atrophied (Fig. 10.15).
- Unlike Crohn's disease, there is no stricture formation.

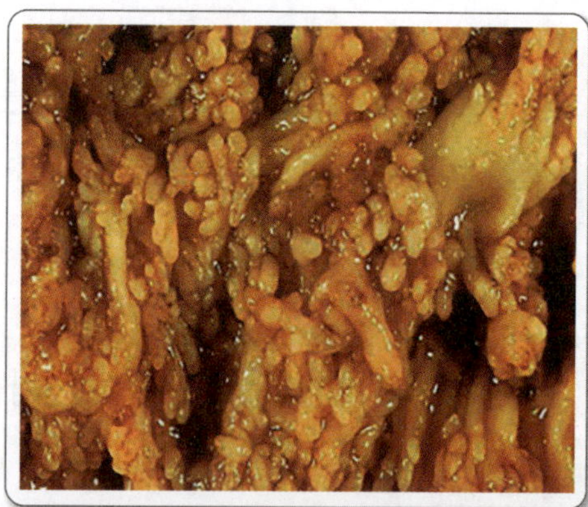

Figure 10.15: Ulcerative colitis

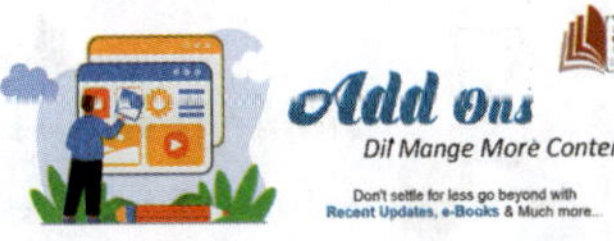

Microscopic features

- Disorganization of glandular architecture with crypt budding and branching and varying size.
- Mucosal eosinophilia.
- Cryptitis: Neutrophils in crypt epithelium.
- Crypt abscesses: Neutrophils in crypt lumen.
- Basal plasmacytosis and the presence of lymphoid cell collections.
- Basal lymphoid aggregates.

Chronic cases show

- Mucosal gap, i.e., due to crypt destruction, there is a widening between crypts and increased distance between crypt bases and muscularis mucosa.
- Mucin depletion, with loss of goblet cells.
- Paneth cell metaplasia.

Complications of Ulcerative Colitis

- Perforation
- Peritonitis
- Profuse bleeding
- Malignant transformation

Crohn's Disease

This form of IBD is characterized by segmental involvement of the bowel, i.e., involved areas alternate with uninvolved areas. It shows knife like piercing ulcers and preferentially involves the terminal ileum and caecum. Inflammation in Crohn's disease is frequently transmural ,ie involving all layers of the affected segment. Smoking is a well-established risk factor in the development of Crohn's disease.

Clinical Features

Episodes of diarrhea, fatigue, bloating, abdominal cramps, bloody stools, oral ulcers, reduced appetite and anorexia.

Pathological Changes

Gross features:

- The involved intestine shows a thickened wall.
- Lumen of the intestine is narrowed.
- Strictures and perforation are common.
- Perianal fistula formation is seen in cases where the anorectum is involved.

Mesenteric fibrosis leads to a characteristic gross finding—"creeping fat" (Fig. 10.16A).

Microscopic features:

- Deep, penetrating knife like ulcers of the mucosa.
- Mucosa can also be thrown into villiform folds.
- Crypt architecture is distorted-branching, loss and cryptitis is usually present.
- Full thickness inflammation, often mixed acute on chronic with lymphoid follicles.
- The presence of small noncaseating granulomas (Fig. 10.16B) usually in the mucosa, also called as microgranulomas.
- Submucosal fibrosis.
- Muscle layer hypertrophy.

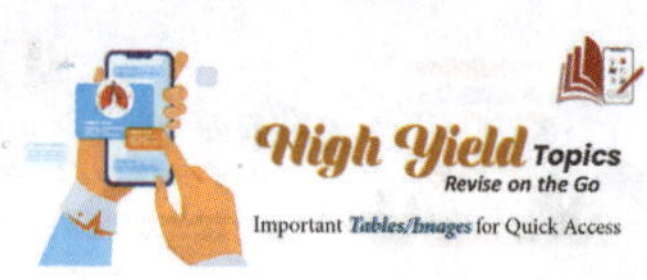

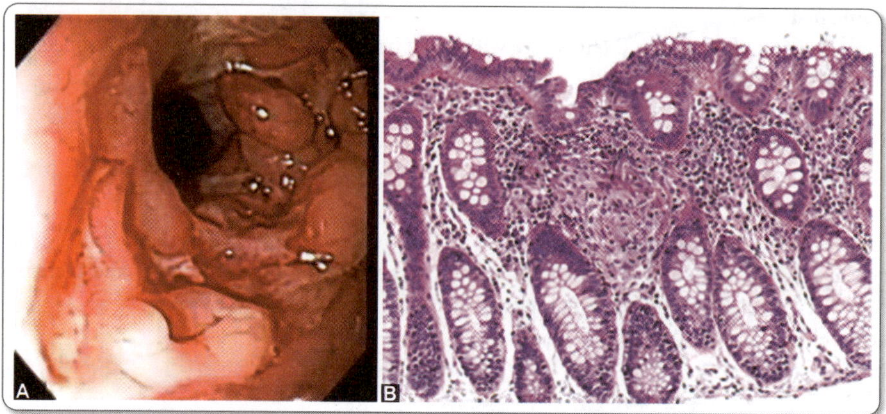

Figures 10.16A and B: Crohn's disease A. Gross appearance; B. Microscopic appearance (noncaseating granuloma)

MUST KNOW

All biopsies involved by inflammatory bowel disease must be examined for the presence or absence of dysplasia.

Laboratory Diagnosis of Inflammatory Bowel Disease

- **Elevated acute-phase reactants**—CRP, ESR
- **Serological tests:** Perinuclear antineutrophil cytoplasmic antibodies (pANCA): positivity is seen in 75% cases of ulcerative colitis.
  - Antibodies to saccharomyces cerevisae: Crohn's disease (Tables 10.2 and 10.3).
  - Fecal lactoferrin- is a sensitive and specific marker in the diagnosis of IBD.
  - Fecal calprotectin levels are elevated in cases with active inflammation and can predict relapses.
- **Hematological tests**: Anemia is frequent—which many be normocytic normochromic or microcytic hypochromic.

Total leukocyte count elevation is seen in phases of exacerbation.

Table 10.2: Gross features: Crohn's disease versus ulcerative colitis

Feature	CD	UC
Site	Ileum and colon Rectum usually spared	Colon only Rectum—100%
Distribution	Skip lesion	Continuous
Stricture	Common	Rare/late
Bowel wall	Thick	Thin
Mesentery	Creeping fat	N
Serosa	Serositis	Usually N
Mucosa	Linear serpiginous ulcer cobblestone	Superficial broad based ulcer, Red granular
Pseudo polyp	Uncommon	Common
Fistula and sinuses	Yes	Rare

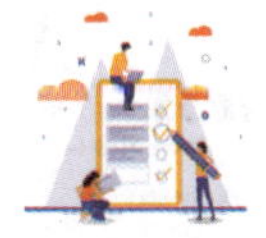

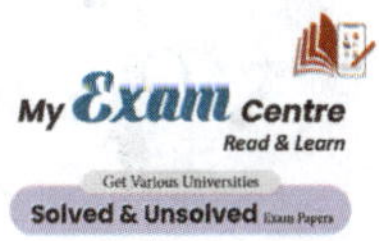

Table 10.3: Microscopic features: Crohn's disease versus ulcerative colitis

Feature	CD	UC
Inflammation	transmural	Superficial upto mucosa/submucosa
Ulcer	Deep linear	superficial
Granuloma	+ve	–ve
Lymphoid follicle	Common throughout wall	Limited to mucosa
Crypt abscess	+	More common
Fissures	+	–
Fibrosis	+	–
Pseudo polyp	Moderate	Marked

SUMMARY

- The peptic ulcer ultimately develops due to imbalance between gastroprotective mechanisms and aggressive factors.
- *H. pylori* is a common cause of chronic gastritis.
- Lesions due to typhoid are more frequent in the terminal ileum.
- Leucoplakia is a premalignant lesion of the oral cavity.
- The most common oropharyngeal site of involvement for squamous cell carcinoma is the base of tongue (posterior 1/3rd).
- Mutations in proteins such as CDKN2A, PIK3CA accumulate, accompanied with changes in gene expression and inactivation of tumor suppressor genes.
- The two main histological types of esophageal carcinoma are squamous cell carcinoma and adenocarcinoma.
- Esophageal SCC develops by a progressive accumulation of genetic alterations.
- Squamous cell carcinoma is the most frequent histological type of esophageal cancer in India.
- As per the WHO, squamous cell carcinomas are graded based on nuclear atypia, mitotic activity and keratin production.
- Esophageal adenocarcinomas are characterized by a specific cytokeratin pattern as CK7, CK 19, and CK 20.
- The most common histological type of gastric cancer is the adenocarcinoma.
- Early Gastric Carcinoma (EGC) is limited to mucosa and submucosa irrespective of lymph node status.
- Advanced Gastric Carcinoma (AGC) infiltrates muscularis propria and beyond.
- Two main histological types of gastric carcinoma include intestinal and diffuse.

ASSESS YOURSELF

Long Answer Questions

1. Explain pathology of gastric cancer.
2. Differentiate between intestinal and diffuse gastric carcinoma.
3. Distinguish between Benign gastric ulcer and malignant gastric ulcer.

Write Short Notes

1. Define typhoid fever.
2. What is buccal carcinoma?

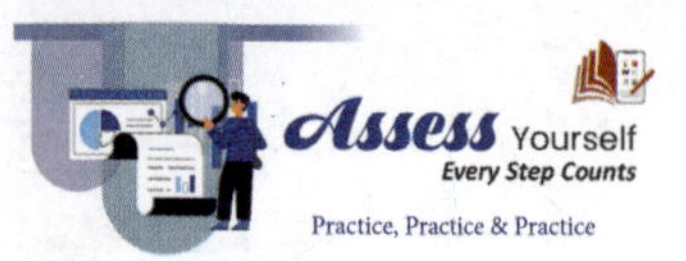

3. Write short notes on:
   i. Leukoplakia
   ii. Esophageal carcinoma

Multiple Choice Questions

1. **Select the option that completes the given analogy**
   Pneumonia: Streptococcus pneumoniae :: Typhoid:
   a. Plasmodium falciparum
   b. Hemophilus influenzae
   c. Salmonella typhi
   d. Wuchereria bancrofti
2. **The stage of cancer of the colon in which the tumor extends more deeply into or through the wall of the colon or rectum and may have invaded nearby tissue, but cancer cells have not spread to the lymph nodes is:**
   a. Stage I
   b. Stage II
   c. Stage III
   d. Stage IV
3. **An artificial opening made into the large bowel in order to divert feces (and flatus) to the exterior, where they may be collected in an adhesive bag is termed:**
   a. Colostomy
   b. Volvulus
   c. Diverticulum
   d. Veside abdominal fistula
4. **All the following statements about the influence of diet and lifestyle on lower esophageal sphincter (LES) function are true; Except:**
   a. Cigarette smoking produces no significant changes in LES pressures.
   b. High-protein diet increases LES pressure.
   c. A fat meal results in sustained decrease in LES pressure.
   d. Chocolate ingestion causes a decrease in LES pressure.
5. **First-line therapy for routine peptic duodenal ulcer disease includes:**
   a. Vagotomy and antrectomy
   b. Upper endoscopy and biopsy to rule out tumor
   c. Evaluation for *Helicobacter pylori*
   d. Serum gastrin determination
6. **Which of the following is NOT a causative agent for a peptic ulcer?**
   a. NSAIDs
   b. *Helicobactor pylori*
   c. Physiological stress
   d. Augmentin
7. **What are the complications of a peptic ulcer?**
   a. Barrett's
   b. GI bleed
   c. Perforation
   d. Dysphagia
   e. A & D
   f. B & C
8. **Both gastric ulcers and *H. pylori* infection are highly associated with _______________.**
   a. Closteidium difficile infection
   b. Gastric malignancy
   c. Uveitis
   d. Esophageal neoplasms

Answer Key

1. c	**2.** b	**3.** a	**4.** a	**5.** c	**6.** d
7. f	**8.** b				

Chapter 11

Liver, Gallbladder and Pancreas Diseases

LEARNING OBJECTIVES

After the completion of the chapter, the readers will be able to:

- Know about diseases of liver, such as jaundice, liver cirrhosis, liver abscess, hydatid cyst and tumors.
- Understand diseases of gallbladder such as cholecystitis and tumors.
- Discuss various diseases of pancreas, such as pancreatitis and pancreatic tumors.

CHAPTER OUTLINE

- Overview of Liver, Gallbladder and Pancreas

Diseases of Liver

- Hepatitis
- Jaundice
- Liver Cirrhosis
- Alcoholic Liver Disease and Cirrhosis
- Nonalcoholic Liver Cirrhosis/Disease
- Primary Sclerosing Cholangitis
- Liver Function Tests
- Autoimmune Diseases of Liver
- Liver Abscess
- Hydatid Cyst Disease
- Tumors of Liver

Diseases of Gallbladder

- Cholecystitis
- Tumors of Gallbladder
- Disease of Pancreas
- Tumors of Pancreas

KEY TERMS

Hepatotropic viruses: Viruses with a predilection of infecting the liver exclusively.

Intestinal metaplasia: A transformation of the cells in the lining of an organ, e.g., gallbladder.

Mucocele: A mucus-filled cyst that may appear in the gallbladder.

OVERVIEW OF LIVER, GALLBLADDER AND PANCREAS

The liver, gallbladder, and pancreas are vital organs located in the abdominal cavity, each playing a crucial role in the digestive and metabolic processes of the body (Fig. 11.1).

Liver

The liver is a large, reddish-brown organ situated on the right side of the abdomen, just below the diaphragm.

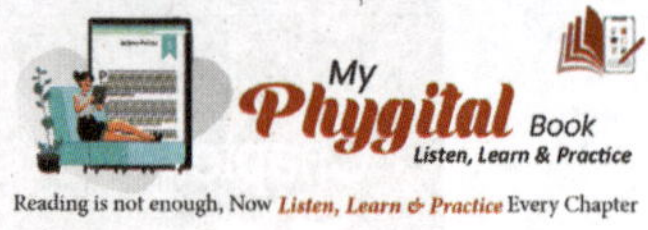

Functions of Liver

- **Metabolism:** The liver is a metabolic powerhouse responsible for processing nutrients, storing glycogen, and regulating blood sugar levels.
- **Detoxification:** It filters and detoxifies blood, removing harmful substances and metabolizing drugs.
- **Bile production:** The liver produces bile, a digestive fluid that emulsifies fats, aiding in their digestion and absorption in the small intestine.
- **Protein synthesis:** The liver synthesizes proteins, including clotting factors and albumin.

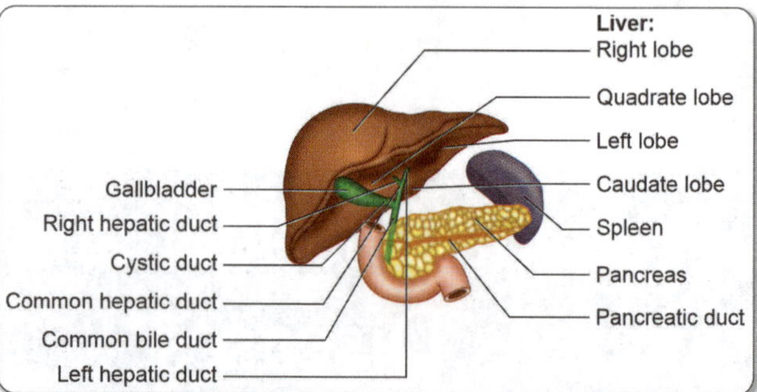

Figure 11.1: Accessory organs of digestive system—liver, gallbladder and pancreas

Gallbladder

The gallbladder is a small, pear-shaped organ located beneath the liver.

Functions of Gallbladder

- The gallbladder stores and concentrates bile produced by the liver.
- After upon the ingestion of fatty foods, the gallbladder contracts, releasing bile into the small intestine to aid in the digestion and absorption of fats.

Pancreas

The pancreas is a long, flat gland located behind the stomach.

Functions of Pancreas

- **Endocrine function:** The pancreas contains clusters of cells called the islets of Langerhans, which secrete hormones such as insulin and glucagon to regulate blood sugar levels.
- **Exocrine function:** The pancreas produces digestive enzymes, including lipases, proteases, and amylases, which are released into the small intestine to break down fats, proteins, and carbohydrates, respectively.

DISEASES OF LIVER

HEPATITIS

This is a disease accounting for substantial morbidity and is commonly caused by viral infections leading to inflammation and destruction of the hepatic parenchyma.

Various viruses may cause hepatitis. These include hepatotropic viruses:

- Hepatitis A
- Hepatitis B
- Hepatitis C
- Hepatitis D
- Hepatitis E
- Other viruses causing hepatitis include—cytomegalovirus (CMV), arbovirus, like dengue, Epstein-Barr virus, adenovirus, etc.

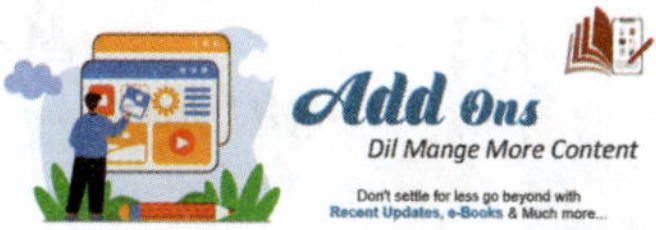

Clinical Features

- **Preicteric phase:** Fever, malaise, loss of appetite, myalgia, diarrhea.
- **Icteric phase:** The patient has visibly yellow sclera and passes yellow colored urine. Stool may be of lighter color in cases where inflammation also involves the biliary tract and some patients may complain of itchiness due to accumulation of bile salts.
- **Resolving phase:** As symptoms decline, transaminases (liver enzymes) may still be abnormally elevated and can take weeks to months to reach baseline normal values.

Complications of Acute Hepatitis B:
- Chronic hepatitis
- Fulminant hepatitis
- Cirrhosis

Hepatitis A Infection

- **Mode of transmission:** Orofecal route.
- **Risk factors:** Factors favoring transmission include poor hygienic conditions and lower socio-economic strata.
- **Incubation period:** 15–45 days.
- **Age:** Children and young adults, although elders may also be affected.
- **Pathogenesis:** Hepatitis A usually is self-limiting infection, with full recovery. Illness is usually mild with no chronicity or carrier state. In rare instances, fulminant hepatitis is seen or triggering of autoimmune infection may be noted.

Lab Diagnosis

- **In blood during incubation period:** Infection can be seen during incubation period by detecting virus in blood stream.
- **In feces:** Excretion in feces (2–3 weeks before jaundice appears and 1 week after development of jaundice).
- **In serum:** IgM antibody to HAV appears in the bloodstream and persists for 3–6 months, reliable marker to diagnose infection. IgG antibody to HAV, appears shortly after IgM antibodies appear in the bloodstream and gives lifelong protection.

Serological Tests

- HAV IgM in serum by ELISA in chronic phase.
- HAV IgG in serum by ELISA to detect a past infection.

Hepatitis B Virus (HBV) Infection

The HBV is a partly double stranded DNA virus.

Mode of transmission:
- Needlestick injury with contaminated needles.
- Blood transfusion with infected blood, intravenous drug abuse.
- Sexual contact with infected individuals.
- Transplacental spread to fetus by lactation to newborns.

Incubation period: 30–180 days.

Age: All age groups.

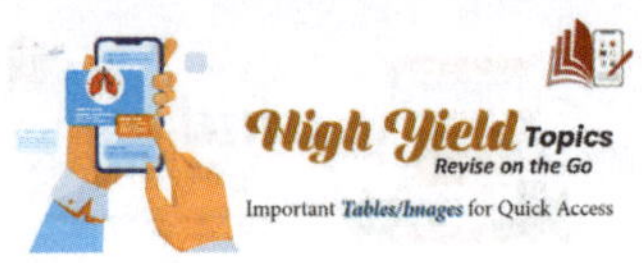

Lab Diagnosis

Hepatitis B, like other acute viral hepatitis infections, presents with elevated liver enzymes and serum bilirubin. Serological markers to diagnose infection include:

Serum Markers to Diagnose Hepatitis B

- **HBsAg:**
  - This is the first marker to appear in the course of disease. This marker indicates infection and peaks in the icteric phase.
  - Appears 4–28 weeks (1–7 months) after infection.
  - Appears before the elevation of liver enzymes and before the development of clinical symptoms.
  - Usually becomes undetectable 3–6 months after the clinical (symptomatic) phase. Persistence beyond this time frame indicates chronic hepatitis B infection.
- **Anti-HBs:**
  - This is the antibody to hepatitis B surface antigen (HBsAg) and is seen after HBsAg has cleared out. Anti-HBs indicates the beginning of the resolving phase or *recovery phase* and confers protection against infection.
  - The appearance of anti-HBs may not be immediately after infection and this time lag is referred to as window period.
- **HBeAg:**
  - This marker appears at the same time as HBsAg. It appears in the preicteric phase and is seen maximally in the acute phase.
  - HBeAg is a marker of active viral replication and signifies ongoing infection and liver injury. Its disappearance corresponds to an improvement in clinical course.
  - Reappearance corresponds to reactivation of infection.
- **Anti-HBe antibody:** Appears when HBeAg disappears and signifies the end of infective phase.
- **HBV DNA:** It is also a marker of viral replication and infectivity similar to HBeAg and is more sensitive, especially for mutant variants. It is often used as a tool to monitor response to therapy in cases of chronic hepatitis.
- **HBcAg:** Not detectable routinely in serum as it is a protein that is found in the nucleocapsid core and is hidden in the deeper virion core.
- **Anti-HBc:** This is of two types—IgG and IgM. This is an excellent marker for the window period. The IgM antibody is indicative of acute infection while the IgG antibody indicates chronic infection.

The summary of hepatitis B serological markers is given in Table 11.1.

Table 11.1: Summary of hepatitis B serological markers

	HBsAg	HBeAg	Anti-HBc	Anti-HBe	Anti-HBs	HBV DNA
Acute infection	+	+	IgM+	–	–	+
Chronic infection	+	–/+	IgG+	+/–	–	+/–
Healthy carrier	+	–	+	+	–	–
Vaccinated	–	–	–	–	+	–
Past infection	–	–	+	+/–	+	–

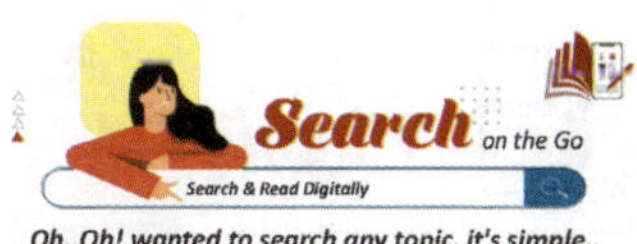

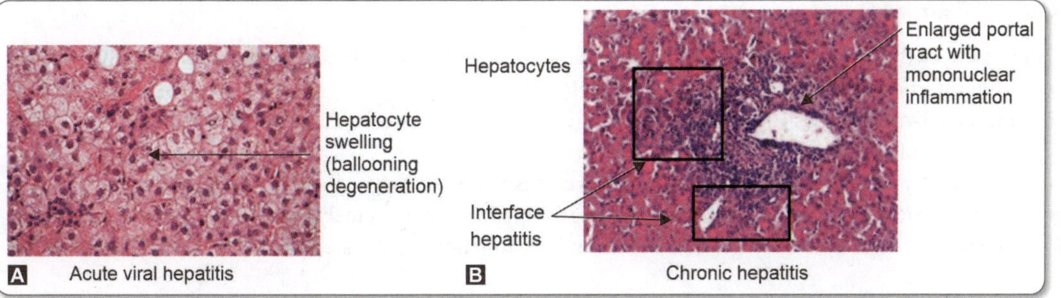

Figures 11.2A and B: Histological changes: **A.** Acute hepatitis; **B.** Chronic hepatitis

Pathological Changes

Gross appearance: There is a loss of normal lobular architecture.

- **Lobular inflammation:** Foci of lobular inflammation are seen throughout the hepatic parenchyma in varying degrees.
- **Changes in portal tract:** Expansion of the portal tract by a mixed inflammatory infiltrate comprising lymphocytes and neutrophils and macrophages. Interface activity is usually seen in varying degrees and refers to inflammation crossing over the portal tract boundary.

Histological changes: The changes in hepatocytes noted in hepatitis B infection include the following (Figs 11.2A and B).

- **Ballooning degeneration:** In acute case of viral hepatitis, hepatocytes undergo cloudy change or hydropic swelling resulting in the hepatocytes assuming a swollen or ballooned appearance.
- **Hepatocyte necrosis:** Hepatocyte necrosis may involve single hepatocyte (dropout necrosis), groups of hepatocytes in the limiting plate (piecemeal necrosis), hepatocyte necrosis in a band-like fashion (portoportal, portovenous/venovenal), and diffusely present (fulminant).
- **Apoptotic bodies:** Some hepatocytes may go through cell death *via* the pathway of apoptosis forming an eosinophilic globular body with a pyknotic nucleus giving a mummified appearance. This is also called the "councilman body".
- **Ground glass hepatocytes:** The cytoplasm of the hepatocytes has a coarse pinkish appearance which are nicely highlighted by HBSAg immunohistochemical markers.
- **Intrahepatocytic cholestasis:** In a hepatitic pathology, where inflammation usually involves the hepatic parenchyma, mild degrees of cholestasis may be seen.
- **Collapse of the reticulin framework:** It is seen in cases of severe hepatitis.

Hepatitis C Virus Infection

- **Etiology:** Hepatitis C virus is a single-stranded enveloped RNA virus.
- **Modes of transmission:** Parenteral route is the most common route of transmission. This includes usage of infected medical equipment:
    - IV drug abuse
    - Needle stick injury
    - Transfusion of contaminated blood and transmission during hemodialysis procedures
    - Sexual contact with an infected person also represents a mode of infection, though less frequent
- **Incubation period:** 2 weeks–6 months.

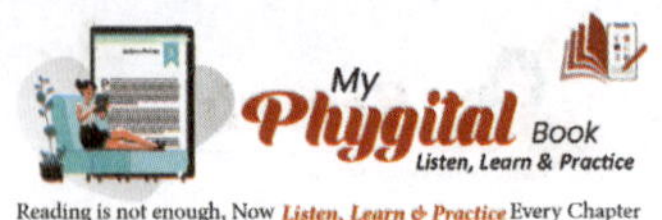

Clinical Features

Patients infected with hepatitis C virus can show an entire spectrum of clinical presentations ranging from:

- Mild infections in which the patient is asymptomatic.
- Elevated liver enzymes (transaminases) with complaints consistent with acute hepatitis such as nausea, fever, loss of appetite.
- Chronically infected cases may show features consistent with chronic liver disease and signs of cirrhosis.
- A small group of patients can progress to acute liver failure, are extremely sick, show progressive jaundice, persistently high liver enzymes and declining liver functions. They are referred to as having fulminant hepatitis.

Disease Course

Progression to chronicity and acquisition of carrier state is well known. It is also known to cause cirrhosis and is a predisposing factor for the development of hepatocellular carcinoma.

Pathological Features

In addition to the histopathological features seen in a case of chronic viral hepatitis which includes hepatocytic changes such as focal/diffuse necrosis, foci of lobular inflammation, ballooning degeneration, portal tract inflammation and varying degrees of inflammation, interface hepatitis and fibrosis, histopathological features unique to chronic hepatitis C infection are as follows:

- Steatosis/fatty change
- The presence of lymphoid aggregates with lymphoid follicle formation in the portal tracts. Lymphocytes are seen in the sinusoids.

Lab Diagnosis

- IgM and IgG anti-HCV antibodies in serum are used to detect acute and chronic infection respectively.
- HCV RNA is seen in the acute phase of illness.

Hepatitis D (Delta Virus) Infection

This is a single-stranded RNA virus which is seen along with Hepatitis B virus infection (co-infection). The reason behind this is that Hepatitis D virus is incapable of replication on its own. It requires a coat of HBSAg to replicate. It is also known as the "satellite virus". HDV antigen is present in association with the single-stranded RNA.

MUST KNOW

- Coinfection is when both infections occur simultaneously.
- Superinfection is when a person infected with HBV is subsequently infected with HDV.

- **Mode of transmission:** Occurs like HBV parenterally, i.e., through intravenous drug abuse, needle stick injuries, sexual contact, direct contact with infected blood/body fluids and rarely, transplacentally.
- **Incubation period:** 2–8 weeks.

Disease Course

1. Resolution of acute infection. The acute infection may progress to a fulminant hepatitis.
2. Carrier state or chronicity may be seen in which cirrhosis may develop and as a subsequent event fulminant hepatitis may occur.

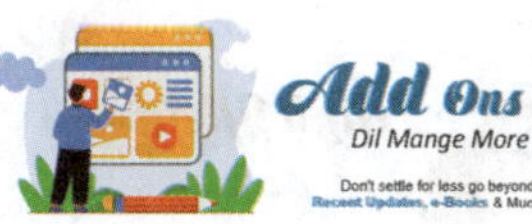

Lab Diagnosis

- IgM and IgG anti-HDV antibodies in serum are used to detect acute and chronic infection respectively.
- HDV RNA is seen in the acute phase of illness.

Hepatitis E Virus Infection

This is a single-stranded, non-enveloped RNA virus with the clinical picture and mode of transmission being similar to Hepatitis A. It spreads through consumption of water contaminated with infected fecal matter (enteric transmission) and its clinical course is usually self-limiting.

No progression to chronicity or acquiring of carrier state is known. In pregnant females, however it may show higher mortality (up to 20%).

- **Incubation period:** 2–6 weeks.
- **Lab diagnosis:** IgM, IgG anti-HEV antibodies in serum are used to detect acute and chronic infection respectively.

JAUNDICE

Jaundice is a condition in which the skin, white portion of eyes and mucous membranes become yellow.

Types of Jaundice

There are three main types of jaundice:

1. **Prehepatic jaundice:** Develops when unconjugated bilirubin is produced faster than the liver is able to conjugate it for excretion.
2. **Hepatocellular jaundice:** Arises when liver cells are damaged so severely that their ability to transport bilirubin diglucoronide into the biliary system is reduced, allowing some of the yellow pigment to regurgitate into the bloodstream.
3. **Posthepatic jaundice:** It occurs most often due to biliary obstruction by a stone in the common bile duct or by carcinoma of the pancreas.

Clinical Features

Yellow discoloration of the sclera, skin and mucous membranes (Fig. 11.3) indicate hyperbilirubinemia.

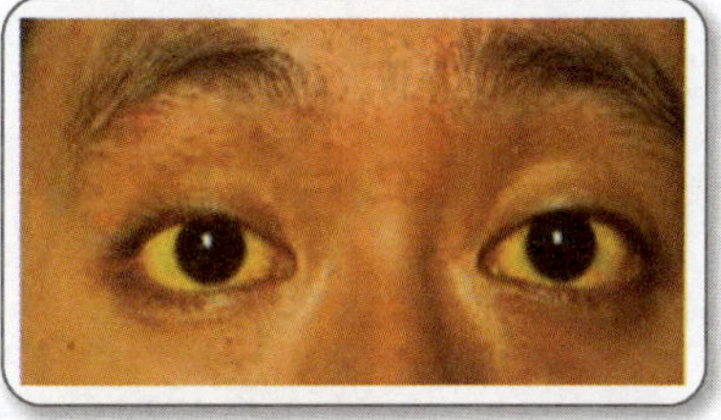

Figure 11.3: Yellow discoloration of the sclera, skin mucous membrane

Etiology

Jaundice appears may be due to the following causes:

- Viral infections (such as hepatitis A, B, C, D or E).
- Cirrhosis (scarring of the liver) or heavy consumption of alcohol.
- Autoimmune disease, such as primary biliary cholangitis.
- Hereditary conditions, such as Dubin-Johnson syndrome and Gilbert syndrome.
- Some medicines such as acetaminophen or certain heart medications.
- Pregnancy.

Risk Factors

- Obesity
- Diabetes
- Histology of recent travel
- Prior blood transfusion

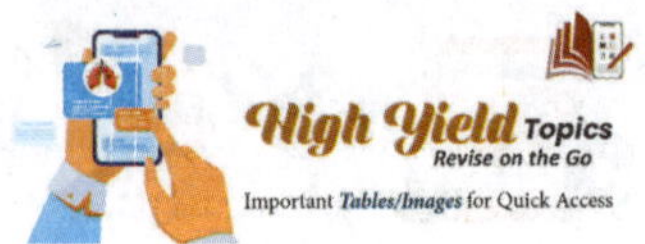

MUST KNOW

The liver can excrete six times the normal daily load before bilirubin concentrations in the plasma rise. Unconjugated bilirubin is insoluble and is not excreted in the urine.

Pathogenesis

The metabolism of bilirubin takes place through the hemolysis of red blood cells (RBCs), which leads to the release of hemoglobin. The heme oxygenase degrades heme into biliverdin and carbon monoxide within the reticuloendothelial system. Biliverdin is then converted to unconjugated bilirubin by biliverdin reductase. Unconjugated bilirubin binds to albumin in the blood to be transported to the liver. In the liver, it is taken up by hepatocytes and conjugated with glucuronic acid to make it water soluble (Fig. 11.4). Conjugated bilirubin is excreted in bile into the duodenum. The unconjugated bilirubin binds to albumin and is transported to the liver. The unbound unconjugated bilirubin is toxic to the central nervous system as it can cross the blood-brain barrier (BBB). In short, jaundice occurs when there is any one or more of the following:

- Bilirubin overproduction
- Hepatitis
- Obstruction to the flow of bile
- Destruction of red blood cells

Lab Diagnosis

The jaundice is tested from samples of blood, urine and feces as given in Table 11.2; and with the help of liver function tests.

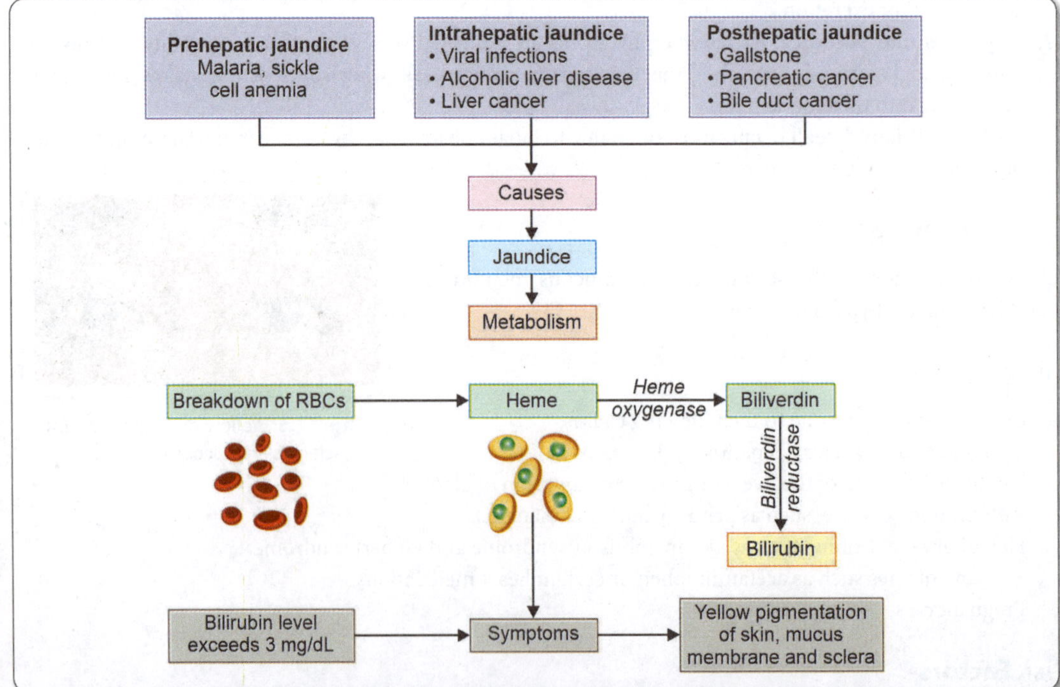

Figure 11.4: Pathogenesis of jaundice

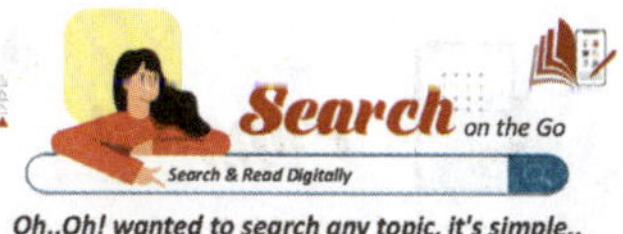

Table 11.2: Differential diagnosis of jaundice

	Hemolytic	Hepatocellular	Obstructive
Cause	Excessive RBC destruction	Parenchymal disease/ inflammation	Any obstruction in biliary tree
S. Bilirubin	↑ (unconjugated)	↑ (unconjugated + conjugated)	↑ (Conjugated)
Bilirubin in urine	–	+	+
Colour of urine	Normal	Dark	Dark
Urobilinogen in urine	↑	–/+	Reduced/–
Bile salts	–	+	+++
Pruritus (Itching)	–	+	+
Fecal stercobilinogen	↑↑	Reduced	Reduced/–
Color of feces	Dark	Pale	Clay
Transaminases	+/++	++++	Mild elevation upto 300 IU/L
Alkaline phosphatase	+/–	+	+++
Prothrombin time	↑/N	↑	↑, correction after inj vitamin K

LIVER CIRRHOSIS

CASE SCENARIO 1

A 60-year-old male presents to the OPD with yellowish discoloration of the eyes, loss of appetite, abdominal distension and a history of hematemesis (vomiting blood) the night before.

Liver cirrhosis is characterized by the loss of normal hepatic lobular architecture. It is a diffuse process wherein normal hepatic parenchyma is replaced by parenchymal nodules separated by fibrous bands also known as fibrous septa. This is also accompanied by remodeling of the hepatic vascular channels leading to elevated portal pressure (portal hypertension).

Types of Cirrhosis

On the basis of size of the nodules:

Micronodular: The size of the parenchymal nodules is small with individual nodule size being <3 mm.

Causes of micronodular cirrhosis:

- Budd-Chiari syndrome (BCS) and other hepatic vasculopathies.
- Biliary cirrhosis.
- Hemochromatosis (metabolic disease).
- Indian childhood cirrhosis.
- Jejunoileal bypass.

Macronodular cirrhosis: When the individual nodule size >3 mm and the nodules show variation in size and are separated from each other by broad fibrous bands.

Causes of macronodular cirrhosis:

- Alcoholic liver disease
- Viral hepatitis
- Wilson's disease

Mixed cirrhosis: When both sizes of nodules are seen in the liver.

On the basis of etiology, liver cirrhosis can be classified as:

- Alcoholic cirrhosis—as a sequelae to alcoholic steatohepatitis.
- Post-hepatitic (postnecrotic) cirrhosis—due to hepatitis virus/other viral infectious agents.
- Biliary cirrhosis (primary/secondary).
- Autoimmune cirrhosis-immune mediated damage.
- Reverse/venous cirrhosis (seen in Budd-Chiari syndrome and other vasculopathies).
- Metabolic cirrhosis (hemochromatosis, Indian childhood cirrhosis, alpha-1 antitrypsin deficiency, non-alcoholic steatohepatitis associated with metabolic syndrome).
- Idiopathic (cryptogenic) cirrhosis—when the cause is not known.

Based on the clinical scenario, the liver cirrhosis, can be:

- **Compensated cirrhosis:** Despite the scarring of the liver parenchyma, the liver is able to maintain basic functionality and the patient can remain in this phase for many years. Patients are asymptomatic or mildly symptomatic.
- **Decompensated cirrhosis:** The liver functions begin to evidently dip and the patient presents with complications such as ascites and upper gastrointestinal bleeding.

Clinical Features

A whole constellation of symptoms and signs characterize hepatic cirrhosis which must be recognized by the medical professionals dealing with such cases. Various clinical features are as follows:

Jaundice, which may or may not be present in cases of compensated cirrhosis; loss of appetite, anorexia, right upper quadrant pain; palmar erythema; spider nevi; caput medusae; ascites; endocrine abnormalities (testicular atrophy), feminization in men, gynecomastia, irregular menstrual cycles in women; portal hypertension-presenting as hematemesis, melaena; coagulopathy—petechiae, purpura; pruritus; nail changes—clubbing, white nails (leuconychia); flapping hand tremors (asterixis), seen in cases of hepatic encephalopathy.

Etiology

Multifold etiologies lead to hepatocyte injury and necrosis.

Alcohol represents an important cause of cirrhosis. (The salient features of alcoholic liver disease are hence discussed separately in this chapter).

Pathogenesis

In a normal healthy liver, type 4 collagen predominates. The process of fibrosis involves the laying down of type 1 and type 3 collagen fibers. This is done by the stellate cells which are perisinusoidal and which are activated by injurious insults to the liver.

Stellate cells normally act as storage cells of vitamin A. These cells change to myofibroblast cells on activation. A large number of cytokines are released including TGF beta and platelet-derived growth factor (PDGF) stimulate myofibroblasts to produce collagen leading to bridging fibrosis and the eventual formation of hepatic nodules.

The fibrosis also has vascular effects with blood being shunted from the portal tracts to the central vein (portovenous shunts) and there is a loss of fenestrations at the level of the sinusoids in due course of time leading to portal hypertension.

Pathological Changes

Gross appearance (Fig. 11.5A): The liver is nodular in appearance and initially may be normal/enlarged in size and then gradually decreases in size.

Cut surface: It is hard in consistency and shows the presence of varying sized nodules.

Histological changes (Fig. 11.5B): Parenchymal nodules of varying sizes:

- Nodules separated by septa.
- Infiltration by mononuclear cells which may be of varying degrees.
- The portal tracts show varying degrees of inflammation.

In cases where hepatitis is involved in etiological causation, features specific to that type of hepatitis may be seen, such as ground glass hepatocytes, sanded nuclei in cases of hepatitis B, lymphoid follicles in the case of hepatitis C, nuclear glycogenation in the cases of Wilson's disease.

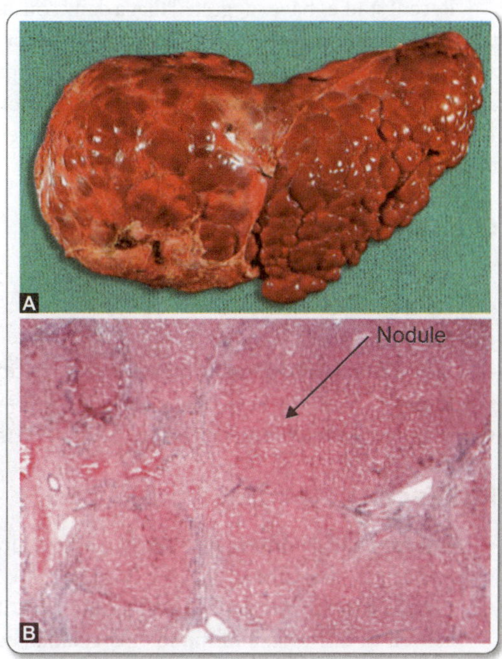

Figures 11.5A and B: Liver cirrhosis: **A.** Gross; **B.** Histology showing nodes

Lab Diagnosis

Radiological findings: Ultrasonography is frequently the first-line modality by which liver disease is assessed. It frequently shows a coarse echotexture in cases of cirrhosis and detects collateral vascular channels indicating portal hypertension.

After USG findings suggestive of cirrhosis and portal hypertension are noted, the next step is to evaluate the presence or absence of esophageal varices and their grading is done using upper GI endoscopy.

EXTRA EDGE

Fibroscan

- Fibroscan is now the most frequently used modality in the further imaging workup of cases of cirrhosis. This is a method (transient elastography) in which a probe is placed at various areas of the liver and the mean stiffness of hepatic parenchyma is calculated.
- Values of >14.0 kPa are consistent with cirrhosis.

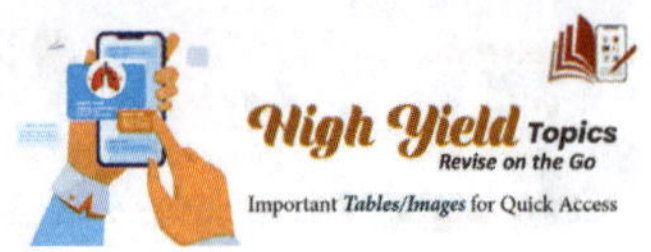

ALCOHOLIC LIVER DISEASE AND CIRRHOSIS

Alcoholic Liver Disease

Alcoholism is prevalent in our society and in recent times the incidence of alcohol-related liver disease is steadily increasing. There are three forms of alcoholic liver injury—steatosis, steatohepatitis and steatofibrosis (alcoholic cirrhosis).

Recent studies have suggested that a daily consumption of 30 g of neat/pure alcohol over 10 years increases the risk of alcohol-related liver illness. A daily consumption of about 80 g of pure alcohol per day ("heavy alcoholism") corresponds to a 100% risk of developing liver disease. The National Institute on Alcohol Abuse and Alcoholism has defined a standard drink as one glass of wine/12 oz of beer/one drink with 40% spirit. A standard drink has about 14 g of alcohol. Hence, as per recent data even two drinks a day pose a threat to liver health.

Clinical Features

Alcohol is a toxic agent and leads to the following effects:
- Lipid peroxidation.
- Fatty change.
- Impaired mitochondrial and microtubule structure and function.
- Impaired autophagy.
- Impaired endoplasmic reticulum function by inducing oxidative stress.

Risk Factors

- **Amount and duration:** As discussed above, alcohol-related liver injury is dependent on both the amount and duration of intake.
- **Coexistent chronic hepatitis:** Chronic hepatitis, especially secondary to Hepatitis B and C infections as well as due to autoimmune or metabolic etiologies weakens the liver. Superimposed alcohol intake increases the risk of severe liver disease.
- **Coexistent protein energy malnutrition:** Protein energy malnutrition is a known etiological factor for fatty change of the liver which is accentuated by alcohol-related injury.
- **Estrogen effect:** Females are more predisposed to alcoholic liver disease. Estrogen hormone increases the permeability of the intestine to endotoxins, increasing the expression of lipopolysaccharide receptor CD14 on the Kupffer cells. This, in turn, triggers the Kupffer cells to liberate proinflammatory cytokines.
- **Genetic variations:** Certain populations of Asians show genetic polymorphisms to ALDH2, a variant of alcohol dehydrogenase enzyme. Individuals with this polymorphism have a very low enzyme activity. Hence, acetaldehyde a metabolism product of alcohol is not processed adequately and the individual shows intolerancy to alcohol.

Pathogenesis

Pathogenesis of three major forms of alcoholic liver disease are as follows:
1. **Steatosis (fatty change):** Alcohol intake leads to cellular hypoxia, which in turn, leads to fatty change. In addition, increased free fatty acids enter the liver due to increased peripheral fat catabolism. With increasing intake of alcohol, the enzymes involved in its metabolism-alcohol dehydrogenase, acetaldehyde dehydrogenase produce more of NADH which promotes lipid synthesis. Lipoprotein assembly and transport is also affected by alcohol.

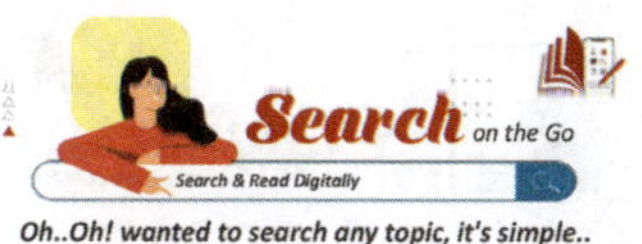

2. **Steatohepatitis:** When fatty change is accompanied by inflammation in the parenchyma, it is called *steatohepatitis*. The mechanisms behind this are:
   - Alcohol induces oxidative stress leading to lipid peroxidation and acetaldehyde adduct formation. This, in turn, damages cellular membranes.
   - Impaired autophagy contributes to increased risk of cell injury.
   - Ethanol increases the proliferation of the smooth endoplasmic reticulum, which in turn, induces the Cytochrome P450 enzyme system. This causes reactive oxygen species to bind with cell membranes damaging them and also promotes lipid peroxidation.
   - Cellular injury causes the release of proinflammatory cytokines such as IL-2, IL-6, TNF-α.
3. **Steatofibrosis/cirrhosis:** Chronic alcohol intake as discussed above leads to increased reactive oxygen species (ROS) and lipid peroxidation along with elevated gut derived endotoxin levels. All this leads to activation of the hepatic stellate cells and liberation of the fibrogenic cytokine TGF-beta promoting laying down of collagen leading to fibrosis and eventually cirrhosis.

Complications of Cirrhosis

Portal hypertension: Persistent elevation of the portal venous pressure >10 mm Hg. Any factor that causes resistance to portal blood flow causes portal hypertension.

A portal venous pressure >20 mm Hg leads to clinical manifestations.

In cirrhosis, there is resistance to blood flow both at the level of the sinusoids and the hepatic parenchyma which is arranged in the form of nodules, compressing the vasculature. The sinusoids also show fibrosis.

- **Gastrointestinal bleeding:** With the onset of portal hypertension, porto-systemic shunts (collaterals) are formed leading to arterial vasodilatation. With increasing pressure, these can rupture and lead to massive GI bleeding and if untreated, even death.
  - Portosystemic shunts are formed at the esophagus-varices—upper GI bleed.
  - Portosystemic shunts are formed at the rectum—hemorrhoids—lower GI bleed.
  - Vascular shunting in cirrhosis: Portosystemic shunts are formed at the retroperitoneum/involving periumbilical veins- caput medusae, dilated veins all over the abdomen.
    These shunts form as an adaptation to reduce the elevated portal venous pressure.
- **Ascites:** Accumulation of fluid in the peritoneal cavity. This is due to:
  - Decreased synthetic of the liver leading to decreased serum albumin leading to edema due to decreased plasma oncotic pressure.
  - Elevated sinusoidal pressure due to sinusoidal fibrosis and compression by altered parenchyma
  - Transudation into the peritoneal cavity due to leaky abdominal capillaries
  - Increased inflow of lymph into the liver: In cirrhosis, interstitial fluid is more and the lymphatic system is activated to resorb excess fluid. This, in turn, increases intravascular hydrostatic pressure. In cirrhosis, there is impaired lymphatic drainage.
  - With advancing disease, blood flow to the kidneys is decreased leading to activation of renin-angiotensin aldosterone axis. This leads to increased serum aldosterone and retention of salt and water.
- **Spontaneous bacterial peritonitis:** This is a dreaded complication as it increases the risk of mortality by 40–70%. It is defined as an infection of ascitic fluid without any other causative intra-abdominal focus and is diagnosed on seeing >250 cells/cumm on ascitic fluid analysis along with clinical features of fever and abdominal pain. The causes are:
  - Overgrowth of gut flora
  - Diminished host immunity in cirrhosis

    - Leaky gut, i.e., altered intestinal mucosal-vascular barrier leads to increased permeability and bacterial translocation to vasculature causing infection.
- **Hepatorenal syndrome:** This is a life-threatening complication of cirrhosis in which portal hypertension leads to splanchnic vasodilatation, which in turn, leads to a decreased circulating blood volume. This in turn causes activation of the renin-angiotensin-aldosterone axis and renal vasoconstriction ensues. The patient presents with a decreasing urinary output and features to suggest acute kidney injury.
    - **Hypersplenism:** Congestive changes lead to splenomegaly. Increased splenic sequestration of hematopoietic elements in turn leads to decreased blood counts and even pancytopenia.
- **Hepatic encephalopathy:** Failure of the liver to detoxify leads to accumulation of nitrogenous waste products, especially ammonia in the blood stream leading to a very challenging complication called encephalopathy. The patient has altered mental sensorium, displays flapping tremors and may even develop coma. The outlook is poor once encephalopathy sets in.

Pathological Changes

Histological changes: Histological changes originate at perivenular zone 3 extending toward zone 1 (the portal tracts) gradually with increasing severity of injury.

Hepatocytic ballooning and degeneration:

- **Fatty change:** Microvesicular steatosis and in advanced cases mixed macro and microvesicular steatosis
- Foci of lobular inflammation.
- The presence of Mallory's hyaline that is ropy eosinophilic material, noted within the cytoplasm of the hepatocytes. This is immunohistochemically positive for CK 8,18.
- Neutrophilic satellitosis, i.e., the damaged hepatocytes are surrounded peripherally by neutrophils.
- Varying degrees of fibrosis which is more in zone 3 (perivenular) and sinusoidal, in cases of cirrhosis, the fatty change may disappear, when it is referred to as the "burnt out" phase.

NONALCOHOLIC LIVER CIRRHOSIS/DISEASE

This is liver cirrhosis secondary to biliary disease. Prolonged cholestasis or accumulation of bile either within the liver (intrahepatic) or in biliary channels outside the liver (extrahepatic) predisposes to the development of cirrhosis. Biliary cirrhosis may further be primary or secondary.

- **Primary biliary cirrhosis:** Primary biliary cirrhosis is an autoimmune disease affecting middle aged to elderly females and is characterized by itching, jaundice and fatigue. Histopathological features include chronic inflammatory infiltrate in the portal tract destroying the bile ducts. Granulomas are seen in the portal tracts along with ductular proliferation. In advanced stages, cirrhosis develops. Nodules are separated by loose fibrosis.

  Lab diagnosis includes: Positivity of AMA-M2 antibody along with elevated alkaline phosphatase.
- **Secondary biliary cirrhosis:** This is in response to a chronic obstruction or blockage of the bile duct due to stricture or the presence of stones anywhere in the biliary tree including the gallbladder. The liver shows the presence of regenerative nodules separated by septa showing varying degrees of chronic inflammatory infiltrate. Additionally, the bile ductules in the portal tracts show proliferation/destruction and bile lakes are seen. Canalicular cholestasis is also noted.

PRIMARY SCLEROSING CHOLANGITIS

This is a disease of the biliary tract, believed to have an autoimmune etiology.

The diagnosis is based on the imaging findings of multiple strictures in the bile duct giving a **beaded string** appearance on MRCP (magnetic resonance cholangiopancreatography) along with biochemical/histological pointers of cholestasis, such as elevated serum alkaline phosphatase.

Liver biopsy shows characteristic onion skin fibrosis of medium-sized bile ducts along with chronic inflammatory infiltrate around the bile ductules and ductular proliferation along with ductular cholestasis.

LIVER FUNCTION TESTS

- **Serum bilirubin:** Variable, may be normal in compensated cases, while may be markedly elevated in decompensated cases.
- **Elevated liver enzymes:** ALT, AST elevation is variable in cases of cirrhosis. They may be completely normal or minimally elevated in cases of compensated cirrhosis. Even in decompensated cases, elevations are usually <500 IU/L. AST/ALT ratio >2 is strongly suggestive of alcoholic liver disease.
- **Alkaline phosphatase:** May be mildly elevated and is usually less than three times of baseline.
- **Gamma-glutamyl transferase (GGT):** This is a marker of cholestatic pathology and is elevated in alcoholic liver disease.

Refer to Table 11.3 to understand clinical and lab criteria of liver function test.

Parameters Deranged Reflecting Diminished Synthetic Capacity

- **Serum albumin, total serum protein:** As liver functions decline, serum albumin decreases leading to ascites/generalized anasarca.
- **Prothrombin time elevation:** Coagulation pathways are deranged because of the diminished synthesis of clotting factors.
- **Hematological abnormalities:**
    - **Anemia of chronic disease:** Normocytic normochromic blood picture with interspersed target cells is common in cases of chronic liver disease.

MUST KNOW

Child Pugh's score:
The Child Pugh's score is a clinical score based on laboratory parameters and clinical features to further prognosticate cases of cirrhosis.

Table 11.3: Child pugh criteria to assess the progression of advanced chronic liver disease

Clinical and lab criteria	Points		
	1	2	3
Encephalopathy	(Grade 0)	(Grade 1 or 2)	(Grade 3 or 4)
Ascites	None	Mild to moderate (diuretic responsive)	Severe (diuretic refractory)
Bilirubin (mg/dL)	<2	2–3	>3
Albumin (g/dL)	>3.5	2.8–3.5	<2.8
Prothrombin time Seconds prolonged International normalized ratio	 <4 <1.7	 4–6 1.7–2.3	 >6 >2
Grade	**Description**	**Points**	
A	Mild; well-compensated disease	5–6	
B	Moderate; significant functional compromise	7–9	
C	Severe; decompensated disease	10–15	

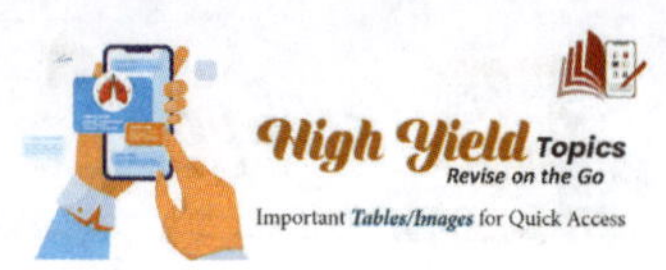

- **Macrocytic anemia:** Vitamin B_{12} deficiency is a frequent association due to inadequate nutrition leading to megaloblastic anemia.
- **Pancytopenia:** In advanced cases, all hematopoietic lineages may be suppressed leading to diminished blood counts.
- **Isolated thrombocytopenia:** Platelet counts are a prognostic factor in cirrhosis with low platelet counts seen in decompensated cirrhosis. Thrombocytopenia is due to reduced thrombopoietin levels and hypersplenism.

- **Ascitic fluid analysis:** This is frequently performed in cases of chronic liver disease in order to:
  - **Ascertain total leukocyte count (TLC):** Spontaneous bacterial peritonitis, a complication of cirrhosis is diagnosed when the number of cells is >250/cumm
  - **Calculate SAAG (Serum ascites-albumin gradient):** This is calculated by computing the difference between serum albumin and ascitic fluid albumin levels. SAAG>1.1 g/dL suggests alcoholic liver disease/cirrhosis.

AUTOIMMUNE DISEASES OF LIVER

Liver Cirrhosis Secondary to Autoimmune Hepatitis

Autoimmune hepatitis is an immune mediated injury of the liver that is diagnosed on the basis of laboratory investigations, such as elevated liver enzymes, elevated serum immunoglobulins (IgG) a positive autoimmune profile which could be either ANA/Anti-LKM-1/ASMA (Antismooth muscle antibody)/anti LC-1 positivity.

Clinical Features

- **Hepatic manifestations:** Mild elevation of liver enzymes to severe liver injury evidenced on liver biopsy as massive hepatic necrosis/steatosis (fatty change) or steatohepatitis with inflammation in the portal tract. Some cases show cirrhosis. Rhodanine stain for copper shows the presence of copper deposits around the portal tracts.
- **Neurological manifestations:** Degeneration of the basal ganglia occurs due to deposits of copper leading to tremors, seizures, loss of balance
- **Ocular manifestations:** Greenish-brown deposit of copper leads to the presence of Kayser-Fleischer rings on the iris as seen on slit lamp examination by an ophthalmologist.

Pathological Features

The histopathological features include interface hepatitis, plasma cells in the portal tract infiltrate, emperipolesis (lymphocytes infiltrating the hepatocytes) and hepatocytic rosetting.

Around one-third cases develop cirrhosis due to liver injury activating the stellate cells converting them into myofibroblasts leading to cirrhosis.

Nonalcoholic Fatty Liver Disease/Steatohepatitis (NAFLD/NASH)

This is a condition in association with metabolic syndrome, i.e. obesity, insulin resistance and diabetes. It is typified by fatty change (steatosis). It is difficult to distinguish from cases of alcoholic steatohepatitis but histological clues include zone1 fatty changes seen in at least >5% hepatocytes, ballooning degeneration, lobular inflammation and varying degrees of fibrosis. Perisinusoidal ("chicken-wire") type of fibrosis is characteristic for NASH. Severe cases progress to cirrhosis. Clinical history is important to exclude the intake of alcohol.

Wilson's Disease

This is a hereditary metabolic disease affecting copper metabolism and is autosomal recessive. It is seen in children and young adults and is usually diagnosed in patients aged between 5 and 40 years. Abnormal copper accumulation occurs in the liver and subsequently in organs apart from the liver. The patient may be completely asymptomatic or may present with hepatic dysfunction, neurological manifestations and ocular manifestations.

Laboratory Diagnosis

Laboratory investigations reveal a reduced serum ceruloplasmin (the protein that binds copper), increased hepatic copper content and increased urinary copper excretion.

Hemochromatosis

Hemochromatosis is a metabolic disorder characterized by abnormal deposition of iron in the liver. It can either be primary (hereditary) caused by mutation in HFE and related genes or secondary when it is usually secondary to multiple transfusions. Hereditary hemochromatosis is usually autosomal recessive. It is a multisystem disorder involving deposition of iron in the pancreas, thyroid, heart, skin and joints.

Clinical Features

Patients present commonly with fatigue. It is also called *"Bronze diabetes"* due to the diffuse hyperpigmentation of skin giving a bronze appearance. In addition, deposition in the pancreas reduces its function causing diabetes, while deposition in the heart causes cardiac dysfunction-arrhythmias and cardiomyopathy. Jaundice may or may not be present.

Laboratory Diagnosis

Liver enzyme derangement is frequent and up to 15% of cases show cirrhosis on liver biopsy. Serum iron and ferritin are both raised. In addition to parenchymal nodules, a Perl's stain is used to confirm the presence of iron deposition which is diffuse (and is in the hepatocytes in the hereditary form). In secondary hemochromatosis, the deposition would be in the Kupffer cells, i.e., cells of the reticuloendothelial cells.

Alpha-1 Antitrypsin Deficiency

This is a hereditary metabolic disease which is diagnosed in children and young adults. The patients may be asymptomatic or may present as severe liver disease with features of cirrhosis on imaging. Patients may also develop lung disease (emphysema). It is characterized by a deficiency of the enzyme alpha-1 antitrypsin (PiZZ) due to mutation in alpha-1 antitrypsin gene (AAT/SERPINA-1). The mutation causes abnormally folded proteins, which accumulate within the hepatocytes.

Histopathological Changes

Liver histology may reveal parenchymal nodules along with the presence of eosinophilic cytoplasmic globules within the hepatocytes. These globules are positive on PAS stain and resistant to diastase and are frequently seen around the portal tracts.

Mild fatty change and inflammation in the portal tracts may also be noted.

Indian Childhood Cirrhosis

An uncommon type of cirrhosis documented in the pediatric age group (6 months – 3 years) and with an unusual geographic predilection for the Indian subcontinent. Clinically, affected children show progressive liver failure. It is believed to occur due to abnormal copper metabolism. It is histologically characterized by parenchymal nodules with hepatocytes showing ballooning degeneration, abundant Mallory hyaline, marked fibrosis around the hepatocytes (pericellular fibrosis) and diffuse deposition of copper as seen on rhodanine stain.

LIVER ABSCESS

Clinical Features

The patient presents with fever, right upper quadrant pain, general malaise and sometimes jaundice. On examination, the liver is usually enlarged and painful on touch (tender hepatomegaly).

Etiology

- **Causative organism:** *Entamoeba histolytica* has a tendency to destroy or cause lysis of the tissue it infests.
- **Site predilection:** Right lobe of the liver, postero-superior portion.

Pathogenesis

Entamoeba histolytica is transmitted *via* food, and water, contaminated with human feces (oro-fecal route). It usually infects the colon where it causes amoebic colitis. However, infection may also be extraintestinal when amoebic trophozoites breach the gut mucosa and reach the portal vein to enter the liver.

Complications

- Abscess rupture can lead to peritonitis.
- Rupture into pericardium; can lead to fatal pericarditis.
- Superadded bacterial infection.

Lab Diagnosis

- Clinical assessment.
- **Radiological modalities (Ultrasound):** Usually solitary hypoechoic mass rimmed by a fibrous capsule.
- **Serological tests:** Antibodies to Entamoeba (especially IgG): Positive in most cases, may take a week to develop.
- **Stool test:** For cysts, though least reliable.
- **Pathological diagnosis:** Cytological analysis of drained content/tissue for histopathology may reveal amoebic trophozoites that are PAS positive.

Pathological Changes

Gross Appearance

- The abscess cavity is usually solitary, but can be of variable size (Fig. 11.6A).
- The necrotic cavity has brownish red pus-like content, classically described as the "anchovy sauce"/"anchovy paste" appearance.
- The abscess wall is comprised of connective tissue along with sloughed off, necrotic liver parenchyma.

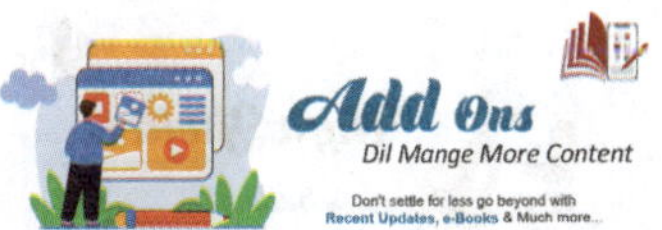

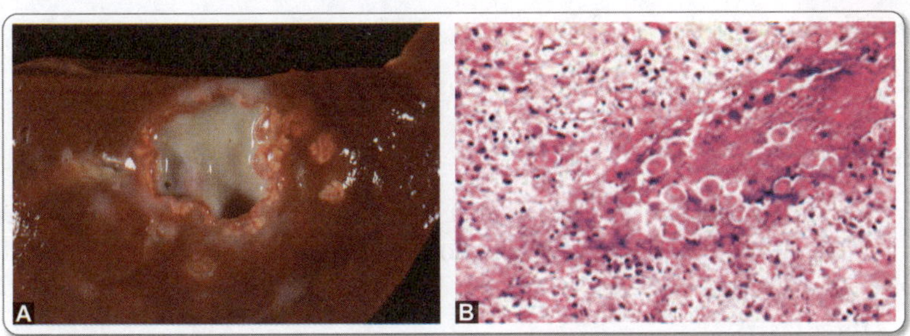

Figures 11.6A and B: Liver abscess: **A.** Gross; **B.** Histology

Histological Changes

- Within the necrotic cavity are degenerated leukocytes, hepatocytes, red blood cells and debris (Fig. 11.6B).
- Necrosis is usually liquefactive.
- Extensive inflammation is not a characteristic as the trophozoites also ingest the neutrophils.

EXTRA EDGE

Pyogenic liver abscess versus amoebic liver abscess

Another form of the liver abscess is the pyogenic liver abscess, caused by bacteria. The differences between pyogenic liver abscess and amoebic liver abscess are shown hereunder:

Pyogenic liver abscess	Amoebic liver abscess
Solitary/multiple	Usually, solitary
Older individuals (>50 years)	Younger age group, 20–40 years of age
Coexistent debilitating illness common	Uncommon
Cyst content—Frank yellowish pus	Anchovy sauce like pus
Bacterial colonies on aspirate/tissue	PAS positive amoebic trophozoites
Leucocytosis more, with left shift	Leucocytosis—lesser degree
Serology for Entamoeba—Negative	Usually, positive
Blood culture—positive for bacteria	Negative, unless superadded infection
Treatment—antibiotics, drainage	Antiprotozoal drugs

HYDATID CYST DISEASE

A unique parasitic disease that primarily affects the liver and is endemic in many parts of the world (Fig. 11.7).

Clinical Features

Abdominal pain, nausea and vomiting. When the lung is affected, clinical signs include chronic cough, chest pain and shortness of breath.

Etiology

A common parasitic disease produced by the larval stage of the Echinococcus tape-worm. *E. granulosus* is a more frequent cause of hydatid disease in humans than *E. multilocularis.*

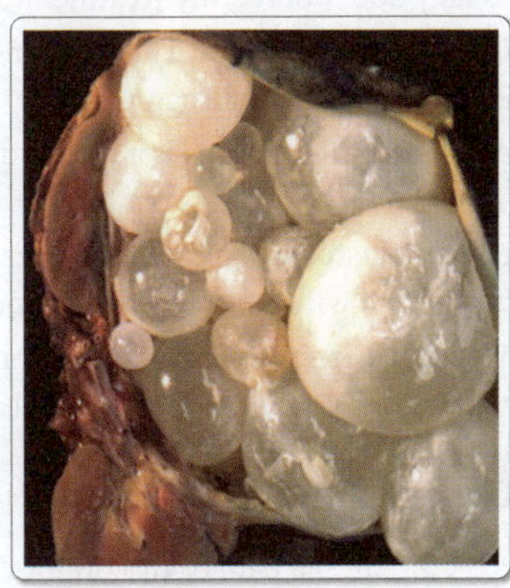

Figure. 11.7: Hydatid cyst in liver

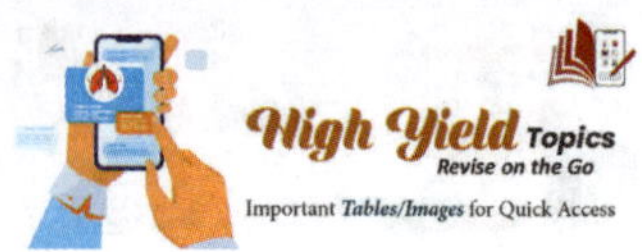

Mode of Infection

Eating contaminated food or through contact with dogs.

Pathogenesis

The hydatid cyst occurs by accidental infection of the human with the eggs of *Echinococcus granulosus*, followed by the development of the larvae, most commonly in the liver (50–70% of cases), and less commonly in the lungs, spleen, kidneys and brain.

Hydatid cyst has three layers:

1. **The outer pericyst** which forms a fibrous and protective zone.
2. **The middle, laminated, acellular membrane** for nutrient passage.
3. **Thin inner germinal layer** from which infectious embryos of tapeworms emerge.

Lab Diagnosis

- Blood tests to check elevated levels of antibodies to the Echinococcus (IgM, IgG-ELISA based test).
- X-ray, CT scan or ultrasound to examine the cysts.

TUMORS OF LIVER

Liver tumors can be either benign (noncancerous) or malignant (cancerous). The most common type of liver cancer is hepatocellular carcinoma (HCC), but there are other types as well.

Types

Hepatocellular carcinoma (HCC): This is the most common form of liver cancer and usually develops in people with chronic liver diseases, such as cirrhosis.

Hepatic angiomas (HA): This is a benign tumor composed of tangled blood vessels. Most hepatic hemangiomas do not cause symptoms and do not require treatment. They are often found incidentally during imaging studies for other reasons.

Hepatic adenoma: This is a benign tumor that is more common in women, especially those who use oral contraceptives. In some cases, hepatic adenomas can rupture and cause bleeding.

Focal nodular hyperplasia (FNH): This is another benign liver lesion. It is often discovered incidentally and usually does not require treatment. FNH is not considered to be precancerous.

Cholangiocarcinoma: This is a cancer that arises from the bile ducts within the liver. It is less common than HCC but can be quite aggressive.

Angiocarcinoma: This is a rare and aggressive form of liver cancer that originates in the blood vessels of the liver.

Hepatoblastoma: This is a rare liver cancer that usually affects children under the age of 3. It is more common in children with certain genetic conditions.

Metastatic liver cancer: Cancer from other parts of the body can spread (metastasize) to the liver. The liver is a common site for metastases because of its rich blood supply.

Clinical Features

- Abdominal pain or discomfort, especially in the upper right side.
- Jaundice (yellowing of the skin and eyes).

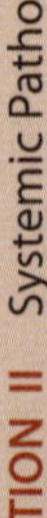

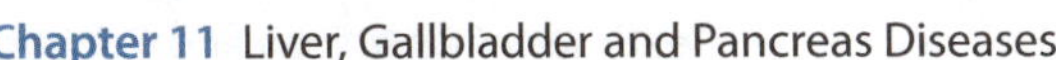

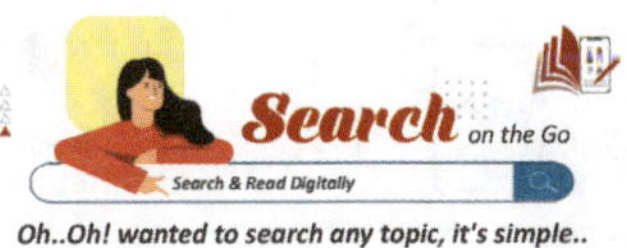

- Unexplained weight loss.
- Loss of appetite.
- Fatigue.
- Enlarged liver.

Etiology

- Exposure to certain chemicals, such as vinyl chloride or arsenic.
- Certain liver diseases, bile duct diseases, and chronic inflammation of the bile ducts.
- Chronic viral hepatitis (B or C), alcohol-related liver disease, nonalcoholic fatty liver disease (NAFLD).
- Certain genetic disorders.
- Hormonal factors and may grow in size during pregnancy.

Carcinogenic stimulus
↓
Genetic mutations
↓
Mutated gene inactivates the tumor suppresses genes
↓
Uncontrolled hepatocyte proliferation
↓
Leads to liver cancer

Figure 11.8: Pathogenesis of liver tumor

Pathogenesis

The carcinogenic stimulus leads to mutations in genes. The mutated genes inactivate the tumor suppressor genes. This prohibits the normal cell growth and leads to uncontrolled growth of tumor cells (Fig. 11.8).

Pathological Changes

Refer Figures 11.9A and B to understand the pathological changes of liver tumor.

- Multifocal, multiple scattered cells in the liver.
- Masses of various sizes and patterns.
- Central necrosis and hemorrhage.

Lab Diagnosis

- Biopsy
- Elevated serum enzymes and bilirubin
- Elevated level of alpha fetoprotein
- Radiographic studies

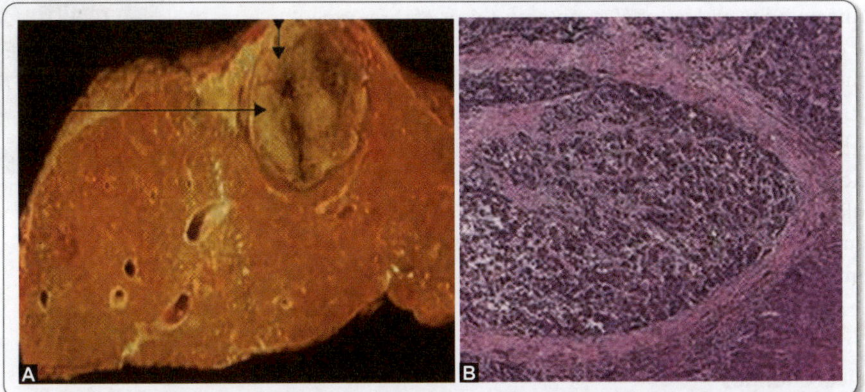

Figures 11.9A and B: HCC: **A.** Gross; **B.** Histology

DISEASES OF GALLBLADDER

CHOLECYSTITIS

CASE SCENARIO 2

A 35-year-old female presents to the casualty with severe pain in the right upper abdomen, nausea and vomiting. The patient never had any such complaint before and reported that the pain was worse after taking a heavy, fatty meal.

Cholecystitis is a term used for inflammation of the gallbladder.

Risk Factors

- Stones in the gallbladder (cholelithiasis)
- Burns
- Bacterial infections and sepsis
- Trauma
- In postpartum females
- Immunocompromised states, like diabetes mellitus

Pathogenesis

- Obstruction of the gallbladder by the presence of a stone leads to distension of the gallbladder (Fig. 11.10), and a reduced blood supply leading to reduction in blood supply (ischemia). The stone also leads to mechanical irritation and damage to the mucosal lining cells.
- Blockage at the level of the cystic duct by an impacted stone/biliary sludge is common causing pain.
- Fatty meals need more bile for optimal digestion, bile is stored in the gallbladder. If the gallbladder motility and emptying mechanism is slow or hampered, this also favors stone formation and subsequent pain.
- Direct infection by bacteria such as *E. coli*, Klebsiella, Salmonella.
- Irritated mucosal epithelial cells release phospholipase that hydrolyzes lecithin to lysolecithin which further damages the mucosa.

Figure 11.10: Cholelithiasis

Classification of Cholecystitis

Based on the duration and onset of symptoms, this is of three types:
- Acute cholecystitis
- Chronic cholecystitis
- Acute-on-chronic cholecystitis

Based on the presence of stones, cholecystitis may be classified on the basis of the presence or absence of gallbladder stones as:
- Calculous cholecystitis (representing the most common cause)
- Acalculous cholecystitis

Here, main types are discussed.

Acute Cholecystitis

Pathological Changes

Gross appearance: Gallbladder—normal/enlarged in size, tense.
- **Lumen:** May show the presence of stones.
- **Serosa:** Covered with fibrinopurulent exudate.

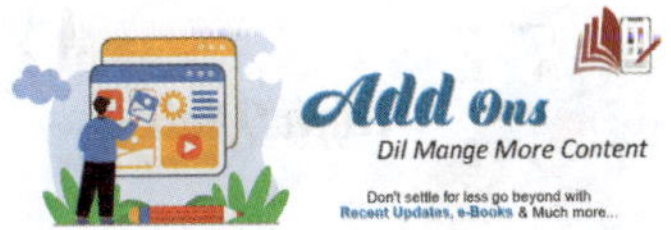

- **Wall of gallbladder:** Shows edema.
- **Mucosa:** Hyperemic.

In severe cases, perforation of the wall may also be noted.

Histological changes:

- Epithelial lining sloughed off (denuded/ulcerated).
- Varying degrees of neutrophilic infiltrate and edema in the lamina propria extending beneath the mucosa also.
- Dilated and congested vessels.

In severe cases—breach in the serosa.

Chronic Cholecystitis

This is the usual condition for which the patient is operated on. It is a consequence of numerous episodes of acute or acute on chronic cholecystitis.

Clinical Features

Upper abdominal pain, nausea, vomiting, fever–intermittent.

Complications of cholecystitis: Empyema (distension of the gallbladder with pus), hydrops, mucocele, gangrene, perforation, fistula, gallstone ileus.

Pathological Changes

- **Gross appearance:**
  - The gallbladder may be normal, shrunken or slightly increased in size
  - The outer serosa is dull and sometimes may show fibrous bands and adhesions
  - The gallbladder wall thickness is increased and the wall is firm
- **Histological changes:**
  - The lining epithelium may be normal or ulcerated or may show metaplastic change which includes intestinal metaplasia.
  - Mucosa may be partly preserved/completely atrophic
  - The lamina propria shows varying degrees of inflammation.
  - In cases with associated cholesterolosis, sheets of foamy macrophages are seen in the lamina propria.
  - In long standing cases, foci of calcification may also be seen in the wall; when this is diffuse, this is called porcelain gallbladder.

Acalculous Cholecystitis

It is a form of cholecystitis caused by dysfunction or hypokinesis of gallbladder emptying.

Clinical Features

- Acalculous cholecystitis should be considered in patient with right upper quadrant (RUQ) pain.
- Occurring 2–4 weeks after major surgery.
- Common in AIDS patients, due to weak immune system.

Etiology

- The more commonly encountered condition of cholecystitis is caused by a mechanical blockage of the gallbladder outlet at the cystic duct, usually by a gallstone. Causes when stones are absent include.
- Trauma, burns, diabetes, torsion.
- May be caused by infectious agents (cytomegalovirus, cryptosporidiosis, or microsporidiosis).

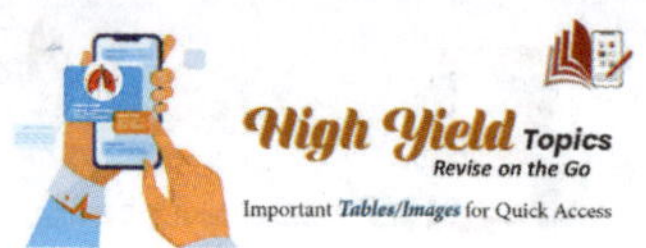

TUMORS OF GALLBLADDER

Gallbladder cancer is relatively rare, and its prognosis can be poor, especially if diagnosed at an advanced stage. Early detection and treatment can significantly improve outcomes.

Types

- **Gallbladder adenocarcinoma:** HIS is the most common type of gallbladder cancer. Adenocarcinomas arise from the glandular elements within the gallbladder.
- **Gallbladder polyps:** These are growths or lesions that develop on the inner surface of the gallbladder. Most gallbladder polyps are benign, but some may have the potential to become cancerous over time.
- **Papillary adenoma:** This is a rare, benign tumor that arises from the glandular cells of the gallbladder lining.

Clinical Features

It is important to note that symptoms of gallbladder cancer may not appear until the disease is advanced. Gallbladder polyps, may not cause any symptoms and are often discovered incidentally during imaging studies for unrelated issues. The symptoms seen are:

- Abdominal pain, particularly in the upper right side
- Jaundice (yellowing of the skin and eyes)
- Unexplained weight loss
- Loss of appetite
- Nausea and vomiting
- Abdominal bloating
- Fever

Risk Factors

Gallstones, chronic inflammation of the gallbladder (cholecystitis), and certain conditions, like porcelain gallbladder (calcification of the gallbladder wall).

Pathogenesis

The mechanism of tumarigenesis is associated with mutated genes which leads to suppressing of tumor suppressor cells (Fig. 11.11). It produces the following features of gallbladder tumor:

- Irregular areas of thickening and induration of gallbladder.
- Deep ulceration in the wall of gallbladder.
- Friable, papillary or cauliflower-like growths.

Cholecystitis
↓
Constant inflammation
↓
Cell turnover
↓
Accumulation of mutations
↓
Carcinogenesis (cancer formation)

Figure 11.11: Pathogenesis of gallbladder tumor

Lab Diagnosis

- Imaging studies such as ultrasound, CT scans, or MRI.
- In some cases, guided FNAC may be performed to confirm the presence of cancerous cells.

DISEASE OF PANCREAS

Pancreatitis

Inflammation of the pancreatic parenchyma. Pancreatitis is commonly described as autodigestion of the pancreas (Figs 11.12A and B). It is mainly of two types:

1. **Acute:** Emergency condition.
2. **Chronic:** Prolonged and frequently lifelong disorder resulting from the development of fibrosis within the pancreas.

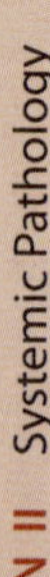

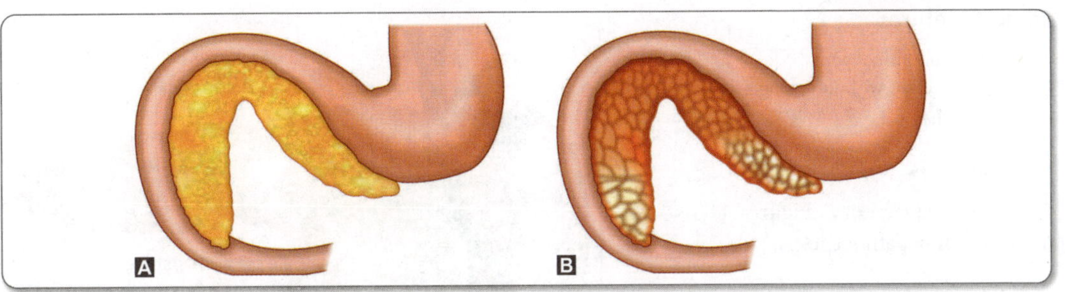

Figures 11.12A and B: **A.** Normal pancreas; **B.** Pancreatitis

Acute Pancreatitis

The degree of inflammation varies from mild edema to severe hemorrhagic necrosis (Fig. 11.13). Pancreatitis is most common in middle-aged men and women. It affects male and female, men and women, equally.

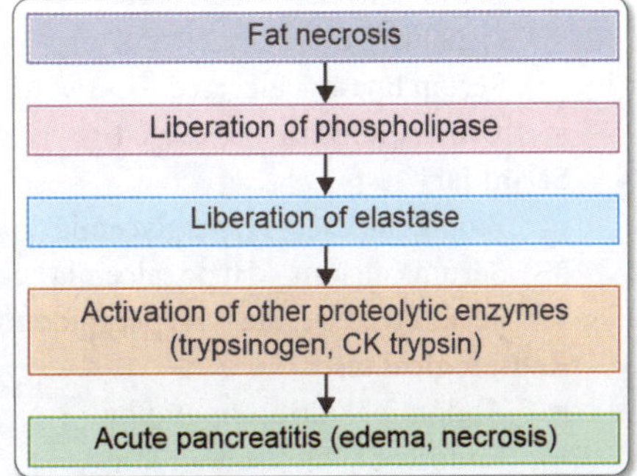

Figure 11.13: Pathogenesis of acute pancreatitis

Clinical Features

- Severe abdominal pain in upper quadrant and mid epigastrium.
- Severe, deep piercing and steady in nature.
- Hypotension, nausea, vomiting.
- Crackles present over the lungs.

Pathogenesis

Pathogenesis of acute pancreatitis have been depicted in Figure 11.13.

Pathological Changes

- Grey-Turner's spots (bluish flank discolouration) Cullen's sign (a bluish peri umbilical area).
- Tachycardia and jaundice.
- Bowel sounds may be decreased or absent.
- Shock may arise due to hemorrhage, toxemia from activated enzymes.
- Hypovolemia as a result of fluid shift.

Figure 11.14 shows the condition of acute pancreatitis.

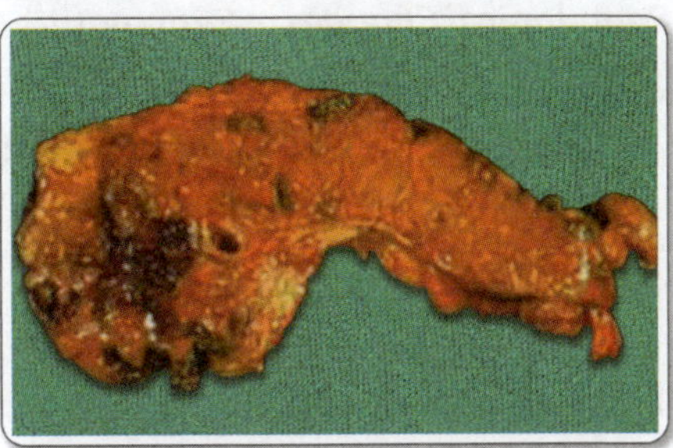

Figure 11.14 Acute pancreatitis

Chronic Pancreatitis

Chronic pancreatitis (Fig. 11.15) is a continuous, prolonged, inflammatory and fibrosing process of the pancreas. Progressively, the pancreas is destroyed and it is replaced with fibrotic tissue. Strictures and calcification may also occur in pancreas. It has two major types:

1. Chronic obstructive pancreatitis.
2. Chronic calcifying pancreatitis.

MUST KNOW

Hallmark of Pancreatitis

- Epigastric abdominal pain radiating to the back.
- Steatorrhea.
- Malnutrition.
- Diabetes mellitus.

Clinical Features

- Upper abdominal pain.
- Losing weight without trying.
- Steatorrhea.

Pathogenesis

Refer self-explanatory Figure 11.16, for understanding pathogenesis.

Figure 11.15: Chronic pancreatitis

Lab Diagnosis of Pancreatitis

- **Primary test**
  - Serum amylase – Increased (>200 U/L)
  - Serum lipase – Elevated
  - Urinary amylase – Elevated
- **Secondary tests**
  - Blood glucose – Hyperglycemia
  - Serum calcium – Hypocalcemia
  - Serum triglyceride – Hyperlipidemia
- **Radiological tests**
  - Abdominal ultrasonography
  - Endoscopic ultrasonography
  - Abdominal computed tomography scanning
  - Endoscopic retrograde cholangiopancreatography

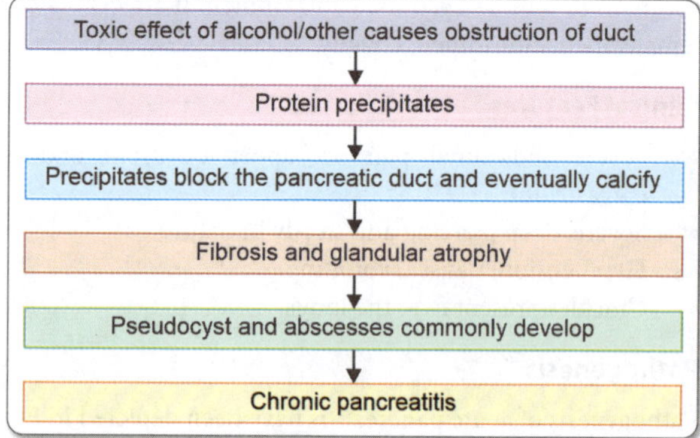

Figure 11.16: Pathogenesis of chronic pancreatitis

Pathological Changes in Pancreatitis

- **Gross appearance:** Necrosis is seen predominantly in peripancreatic fatty tissue while the parenchyma of the gland is usually less affected. There is loss of intracellular and extracellular compartmentation, by an obstruction of pancreatic secretory transport and by an activation of pancreatic enzymes.
- **Histological changes:** Necroinflammatory tissue reaction to functional and/or structural acinar cell damage and rarely duct cell necrosis.

TUMORS OF PANCREAS

Pancreatic tumors can be classified as either benign (non-cancerous) or malignant (cancerous). The vast majority of pancreatic tumors are malignant, and pancreatic cancer is a particularly aggressive form of cancer.

Clinical Features

Abdominal pain, malaise, obstructive jaundice, weight loss, weakness, anorexia. migrating thrombophlebitis (Trousseau's syndrome).

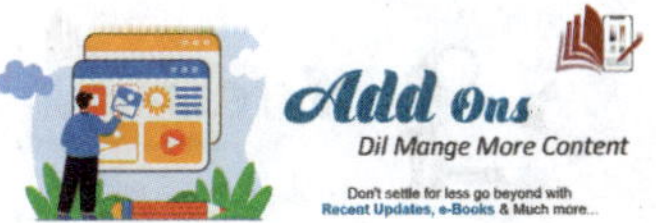

Types

- **Pancreatic adenocarcinoma:** This is the most common type of pancreatic cancer. It arises from the exocrine cells of the pancreas, which produce digestive enzymes. Pancreatic adenocarcinoma is often diagnosed at an advanced stage, making it challenging to treat.
- **Pancreatic neuroendocrine tumors:** These tumors arise from the endocrine cells of the pancreas, which produce hormones. PanNETs can be functional, meaning they produce hormones that cause symptoms, or non-functional. These tumors are generally less aggressive than pancreatic adenocarcinoma.
- **Serous cystic neoplasm:** These are typically benign cystic tumors that contain clear fluid. They are more common in women and are often discovered incidentally by imaging studies.
- **Mucinous cystic neoplasms:** These cystic tumors can be benign or malignant. They are more common in women and may be associated with mucin-producing cells.
- **Intraductal papillary mucinous neoplasms:** These are precancerous or potentially cancerous growths that occur in the pancreatic ducts. They can lead to the development of pancreatic adenocarcinoma if not treated.

Pathogenesis

Pancreatic cancer arises from two histological types of precursor lesions—PanINs and IPMNs. Through progressive stages of pathogenesis, molecular changes occur, leading to increasing degrees of nuclear and cytoskeletal abnormalities.

Pathological Changes

- **Gross appearance (Fig. 11.17A):** Usually hard stellate, gray white poorly defined masses.
- **Histology changes (Fig. 11.17B):** Cells arranged in glandular pattern.

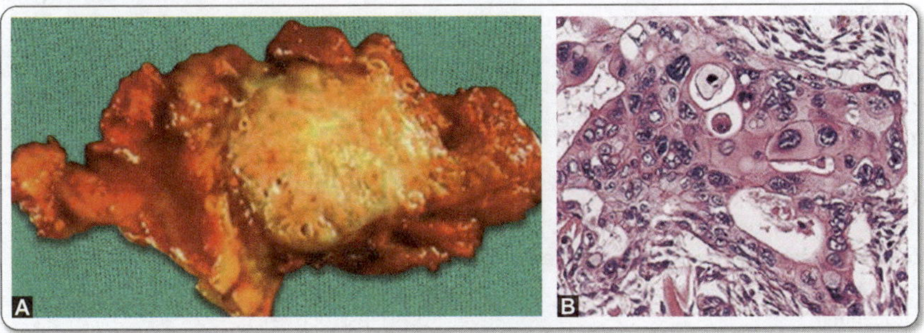

Figures 11.17A and B: Tumor of pancreas: **A.** Gross; **B.** Histology

SUMMARY

- Obstruction of the gallbladder by the presence of a stone leads to distension of the gallbladder and a reduced blood supply leading to reduction in blood supply (ischemia).
- The gallbladder motility and emptying mechanism is slow or hampered, this also favors stone formation and subsequent pain.
- The more commonly encountered condition of cholecystitis is caused by a mechanical blockage of the gallbladder outlet at the cystic duct, usually by a gallstone.

Contd...

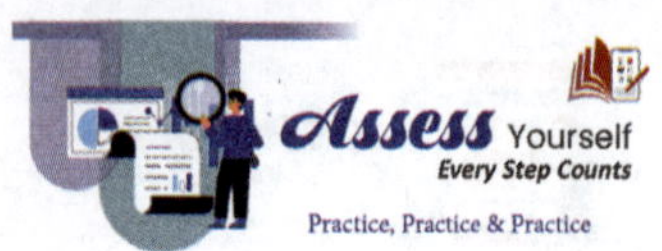

- Various hepatotropic viruses may cause hepatitis.
- Hepatitis B like other acute viral hepatitis infections presents with elevated liver enzymes and serum bilirubin.
- In acute, viral hepatitis, hepatocytes undergo cloudy change or hydropic swelling resulting in the hepatocytes assuming a swollen or ballooned appearance.
- Liver cirrhosis is a late stage of scarring (fibrosis) of the liver caused by many forms of liver diseases and conditions, such as hepatitis and chronic alcoholism.
- Various agents can injure the liver, including viral infections, toxins, hereditary conditions, or autoimmune processes.
- Portal hypertension is due to increased pressure in the portal vein; ascites, hepatic encephalopathy, esophageal varices.
- Histologically, cirrhosis is characterized by vascularized fibrotic septa that link portal tracts with each other and with central veins.
- The hydatic cyst occurs by accidental infection of the human with the eggs of *Echinococcus granulosus*, followed by the development of the larvae.
- Pancreatitis is commonly described as autodigestion of the pancreas.
- Chronic pancreatitis is a continuous, prolonged, inflammatory and fibrosing process of the pancreas.

ASSESS YOURSELF

Long Answer Questions

1. Describe etiopathogenesis of hepatitis B.
2. Discuss hepatocellular carcinoma.
3. Discuss hepatitis in detail.

Short Answer Questions

1. Define jaundice?
2. What is liver function tests?
3. Write short notes on:
   i. Hydatid disease
   ii. Liver cirrhosis

Multiple Choice Questions

1. **Jaundice in sickle cell anemia can be classified under:**
   a. Congenital hyperbilirubinaemia
   b. Hemolytic
   c. Hepatocellular
   d. Obstructive
2. **Jaundice in viral hepatitis can be classified under:**
   a. Congenital hyperbilirubinemia
   b. Hemolytic
   c. Hepatocellular
   d. Obstructive
3. **Jaundice in acute cholecystitis can be classified under:**
   a. Congenital hyperbilirubinemia
   b. Hemolytic
   c. Hepatocellular
   d. Obstructive
4. **A known case of cirrhosis suddenly developed severe jaundice and rapid deterioration of health. On examination liver was enlarged and tender. The most likely investigation is:**
   a. Alfa fetoprotein
   b. CT abdomen
   c. HBsAg
   d. Alkaline phosphatase
   e. LFT

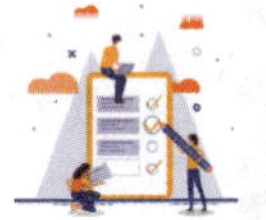
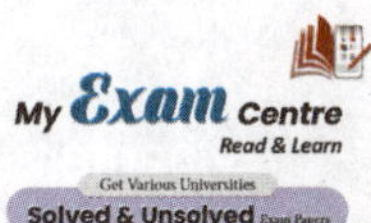

5. **Vertical transmission may be seen in**
   a. Hepatitis B virus
   b. Hepatitis C virus
   c. Hepatitis D virus
   d. All of these
6. **Hepatocellular carcinoma (Hepatoma) may be caused by**
   a. Hepatitis A virus
   b. Hepatitis C virus
   c. Both (a) and (b)
   d. None of these
7. **In a patient with liver cirrhosis, the recommended diet is?**
   a. Low protein
   b. High protein
   c. High fat
   d. Low fiber
8. **Which of the following is not an ultrasonic finding in acute cholecystitis?**
   a. Absence of gallstones
   b. Gallbladder wall thickness >6 mm
   c. Pericholecystic fluid
   d. Murphy's sign
9. **Signs and symptoms of acute cholecystitis usually include the following; except:**
   a. Jaundice
   b. RUQ pain
   c. Fever
   d. Elevated WBC count
   e. Nausea and vomiting
10. **Which of the following statements about chronic pancreatitis is/are correct?**
    a. Chronic pancreatitis is the inevitable result after repeated episodes of acute pancreatitis.
    b. Patients with chronic pancreatitis commonly present with jaundice, pruritus, and fever.
    c. Mesenteric angiography is useful in the evaluation of many patients with chronic pancreatitis.
    d. Total pancreatectomy usually offers the best outcome in patients with chronic pancreatitis.
    e. Pancreatic enzymes replacement and symptomatic therapy are useful.
11. **Which of the following statements about cancer of the pancreas is/are correct?**
    a. It is the most common cause of cancer death in the US
    b. Most cases occur in the body and tail of the pancreas
    c. Prognosis appears to be independent of the presence of metastasis, margin status or tumor diameter
    d. The most accurate screening test involves surveillance of α-fetoprotein
12. **Which of the following medical procedures has/have been associated with an increased risk of post-procedure acute pancreatitis?**
    a. Upper endoscopy
    b. Endoscopic retrograde cholangiopancreatography
    c. Paracentesis
    d. Colonoscopy

Answer Key

1. b	**2.** c	**3.** d	**4.** b	**5.** d	**6.** c
7. b	**8.** d	**9.** a	**10.** a and e	**11.** a	**12.** b

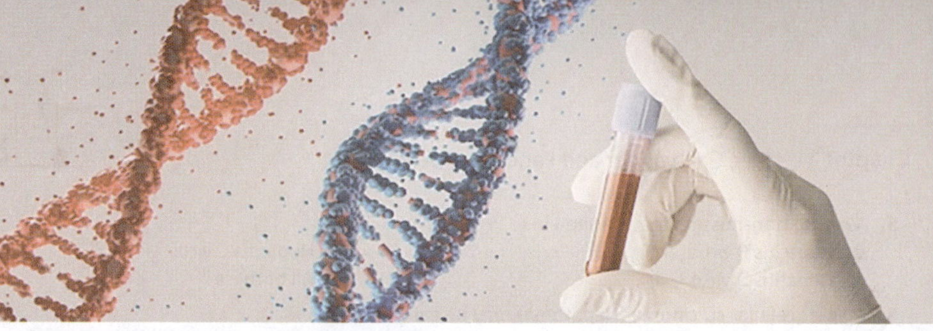

Chapter 12

Skeletal System Diseases

LEARNING OBJECTIVES

After the completion of the chapter, the readers will be able to:

- Learn about bone healing processes.
- Discuss disease conditions such as osteoporosis, arthritis and osteomyelitis.
- Explain bone tumors.

CHAPTER OUTLINE

- Overview of Skeletal System
- Structure of Bones
- Classification of Bones
- Bone Formation and Maintenance
- Bone Healing
- Osteoporosis
- Osteomyelitis
- Arthritis
- Bone Tumors
- Classification of Bone Tumors—WHO

KEY TERMS

Curettage: A surgical cleaning or scraping of a body part.

Denosumab therapy: Denosumab is a human monoclonal antibody for the treatment of osteoporosis, treatment-induced bone loss, metastases to bone, and giant cell tumor of bone.

Kyphosis: An exaggerated, forward rounding of the upper back.

Multipotent: Cells that can develop into more than one cell type, but are more limited than pluripotent cells. For example, adult stem cells and cord blood stem cells.

Osteoclast: Large multinucleated cell responsible for the dissolution and absorption of bone.

Osteophytes: Bony growths that form in joints or in the spine.

RANK-ligand: Receptor activator of nuclear factor kappa beta (NF κB ligand). It is also referred to as osteoprotegerin ligand (OPGL) or osteoclast differentiation factor (ODF) or tumor necrosis factor (TNF) related activation-induced cytokine (TRANCE).

Scoliosis: An abnormal lateral curvature of the spine.

OVERVIEW OF SKELETAL SYSTEM

The skeletal system is a complex structure in the human body that provides support, protection, and movement. It is composed of bones, cartilage, ligaments, and tendons.

The 206 bones in a human body are categorized into axial (skull, spine and ribcage) and appendicular (limbs, shoulder girdle and pelvic girdle) skeletons.

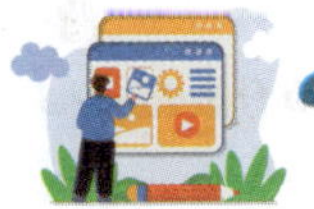

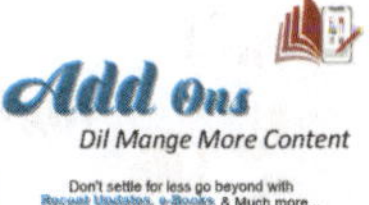

Functions of skeletons:

- Provide support, protection and mobility for organs and tissues.
- Store minerals, such as calcium and phosphorus, crucial for metabolic processes.
- Blood cells proliferate in the bone marrow.
- Joints enable movement and flexibility in mineral homeostasis.

STRUCTURE OF BONES

Bones are made up of a matrix of collagen fibers and minerals, primarily calcium and phosphorus. There are two main types of bone tissue: Compact bone (dense and strong) and spongy bone (porous and lighter). Zones of a normal bone are given in tabulated form (Table 12.1).

Table 12.1: Zones of a bone

Zone	Description
Epiphysis	• These are the ends of the bone which are partly covered with cartilage • In growing children, these are the most active areas of the bone • The epiphyseal plate shows endochondral ossification
Metaphysis	This is the junction of the end and the shaft where the bone shows a reduced diameter
Shaft (diaphysis)	This is the area between the two opposing metaphyses
The cells of a bone are:	• Osteoblasts bone producing mesenchymal cells • **Osteocytes:** Osteoblasts within the bone lacunae • Osteoid is unmineralized bone matrix • **Osteoclasts:** Multinucleated giant cells involved in bone resorption

CLASSIFICATION OF BONES

Bones:

The bones can be classified with different names based on different criteria which are as follows (Table 12.2).

Table 12.2: Classification of bones based on different criteria

Criteria	Types of bones
On the basis of gross sectioning	• **Cortical/compact bone:** Characteristically dense • **Cancellous/spongy bone:** Seen at the ends of long bones and shows a central spongy region
On the basis of types of bone tissue	• **Lamellar bone:** Mature developed bone which shows parallel arrangement of lamellae • **Woven bone:** Immature, undeveloped bone which shows disordered arrangement of bone. This is of low tensile strength.
On the basis of shape	• Long bones (e.g., femur) • Short bones (e.g., carpals) • Flat bones (e.g., skull bones) • Irregular bones (e.g., vertebrae)

- **Joints:** Two or more bones meet to form a joint. It allows movement of the bone. There are three main types of joints: Fibrous (immovable), cartilaginous (slightly movable), and synovial (freely movable).
- **Ligaments and tendons:** Ligaments connect bones to bones, providing stability to joints, while tendons connect muscles to bones, facilitating movement.

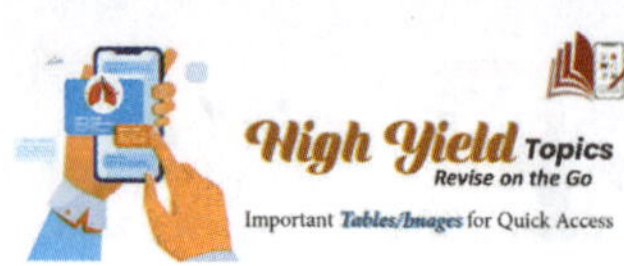

BONE FORMATION AND MAINTENANCE

- The skeletal system undergoes constant remodeling, with old bone tissue being replaced by new bone tissue. This process is crucial for maintaining bone strength and adapting to changing mechanical demands.
- Bones are formed through two processes—intramembranous ossification (for flat bones) and endochondral ossification (for long bones).
- Three main types of cells form the bones—osteoblasts (bone-forming cells), osteoclasts (bone-resorbing cells), and osteocytes (mature bone cells). These cells work together to maintain bone health and repair.
- Bones grow through a process called longitudinal growth, primarily occurring during childhood and adolescence at the epiphyseal plates (growth plates).

BONE HEALING

Bone healing is an intricate regenerative process which can be classified into primary (direct) and secondary (indirect) bone healing.

- **Primary healing:** There is no callus formation. The bony ends join and heal by osteoclast and osteoblast activity.
- **Secondary healing:** Involves both endochondral and intramembranous bone healing. This type of healing usually occurs with:
  - Nonoperative fracture treatment
  - Operative treatments where some motion occurs at the fracture site, such as external fixation, or intramedullary nailing.

Steps of Bone Healing

Just like cutaneous wound healing, fracture healing undergoes multiple steps (Fig. 12.1). The aim is to restore continuity of the damaged bone and ensure restoration of mechanical strength. The steps involved in this process include:

Step 1: Hematoma formation: (week 1): The fracture is accompanied by bleeding and this blood percolates into the gap between the bone and the surrounding soft tissue. The expanding blood may strip off the local soft tissue and periosteum leading to ischemic death of the osteocytes. This phase lasts for 1 week.

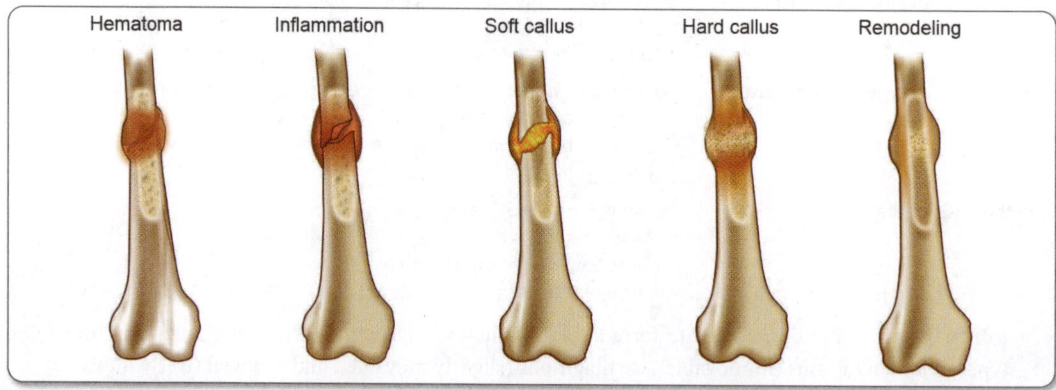

Figure 12.1: Steps of bone healing

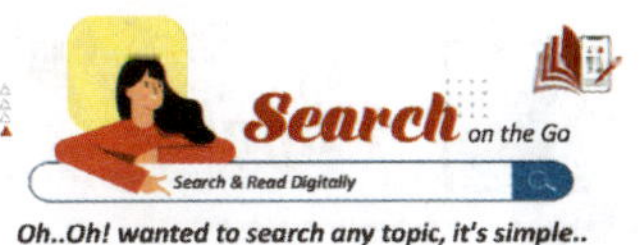

Step 2: Inflammatory cell recruitment and granulation tissue formation (week 2–3)

- Neutrophil recruitment at the site of fracture occurs in the next phase of healing. Eventually, proliferating blood vessels and fibroblasts lead to the formation of granulation tissue which bridges the gap between the fractured bone fragments as well as provides structural stability by stabilizing the area with the surrounding soft tissue.
- Platelets are also recruited to the injury site in this phase.

Step 3: Fracture callus formation: (from the end of the first month up to three months after injury): Granulation tissue is eventually replaced by mineralized bone. This process occurs when the granulation tissue itself after some time differentiates forming osteoblasts that lay down immature woven bone which undergoes calcification. This phase represents the completion process of bridging of the gap between the fractured bones.

Step 4: Resorption and remodeling (months to 2 years after the fracture): Immature woven bone is then replaced by lamellar bone. This is result of an increase in both osteoblastic activities laying down new bone and osteoclastic activity that helps in shaping the newly-formed bone in response to mechanical stress.

Step 5: Modeling of bone (many years): This is the final stage of bone strengthening. Modeling of the outer cortex and the periosteal surface occurs in response to mechanical loads and weight-bearing activities. The result is the bone that is indistinguishable from its previous unfractured state.

OSTEOPOROSIS

Osteoporosis or osteopenia is a metabolic bone disease, characterized by reduced bone mineral density. This is a consequence of increased bone resorption and increased porosity of bones. The bones are more prone to deformity and fracture. This disease has a predilection for women though both sexes may be affected. It is usually seen in patients above the fifth decade.

Common fracture sites include the spine (thoracolumbar), neck of femur and wrist.

Types of Osteoporosis

Osteoporosis may be:

- **Primary:** When it is not in association with any underlying disease.
- **Secondary:** When associated with other diseases.

Depending on the extent of involvement, osteoporosis can also be classified as localized or diffuse.

Clinical Features

Most patients of osteoporosis are usually asymptomatic. However, patients may present with joint pain and an increased tendency of bone fractures with even minor episodes of trauma.

Cases of spinal osteoporosis present with shortening of height due to compression of the vertebrae and kyphosis (forward bending)/scoliosis (side bending).

Etiology

- Age-related bone density reduction.
- Hormonal as in post-menopausal females, or in Cushing's disease.
- In bedridden patients, immobilization due to fracture/paralysis/other diseases.
- Dietary factors such as reduced intake of protein/malabsorption.
- Drug induced, as is seen in osteopenia which is a known complication of long-term intake of steroids.

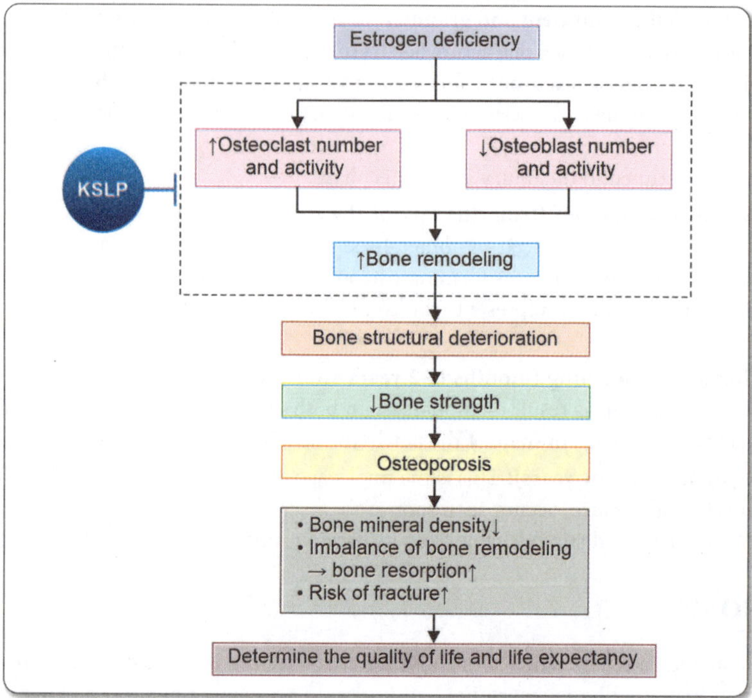

Figures 12.2: Pathogenesis of osteoporosis

Risk Factors

- Menopause
- Old age
- Steroids
- Endocrine disorders
- Nutrition disorders

Pathogenesis

Hormonal insufficiency, oversupply of osteoclasts and reduction in number of osteoblast enhances bone remodeling. The bone structure deteriorates with lessening of bone strength caused by osteoporosis (Fig. 12.2).

Pathological Changes

- **Gross (Fig. 12.3A):** The bony cortex is thinned out with expansion of the medulla.
    - **Appearance:** Standard X-rays may miss osteoporosis in the early stages. A minimum of 30% reduction in density must have occurred for changes to appear on X-ray. X-ray changes include:
        - Cod-fish appearance
        - Ground glass appearance due to reduced density
        - Reduced height of the vertebra
    - **Dexa densitometry:** This is an X-ray-based densitometric examination of bone density in which photons are emitted from absorption.
    - **Bone biopsy:** A pathological opinion is usually sought to exclude any malignant/other abnormal causes of reduced bone density. The following features may be seen:

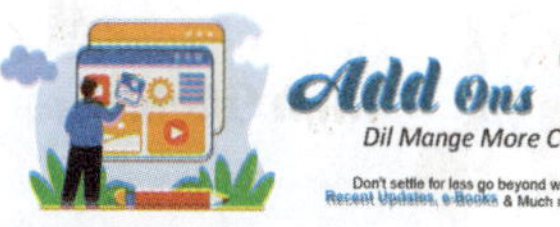

Histological changes (Fig. 12.3B):

- Bony trabeculae are thinned out or normal and comprise lamellar bone.
- Osteoblasts are diminished. In the active phase, osteoclasts or giant cells are increased.

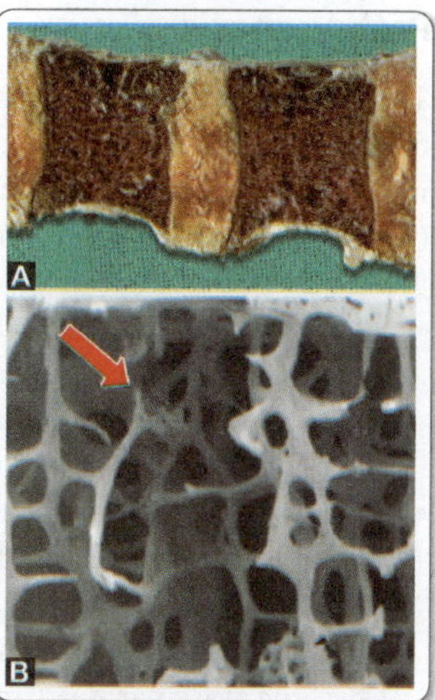

Figures 12.3A and B: Osteoporosis: **A.** Gross; **B.** Histology

OSTEOMYELITIS

Inflammation of bone and bone marrow, secondary to infection is osteomyelitis. It can result from an infection somewhere else in the body that has spread to the bone. It can start in the bone as a result of an injury. Although osteomyelitis is more common in younger children (five and under), it can happen at any age.

Relevant anatomy favoring vascular stasis and bacterial infection: The bony metaphysis is a highly vascular zone and shows a hair loop arrangement of blood vessels (Fig. 12.4). Such an arrangement favors vascular stasis and bacterial infection.

Types of Osteomyelitis

The types of osteomyelitis based on duration are tabulated here (Table 12.3). These are—acute, subacute and chronic.

Clinical Features

The patients are usually children or young adults who complain about pain and swelling toward the end of a bone. This is usually accompanied by fever, redness and swelling of the affected area. When the lesion spreads to the soft tissue, a well-defined abscess or sinus may be noted on clinical examination.

Epipysis
Metaphysis
Hair-pin arrangement
Medullary vein
Medullary artery

Figure 12.4: Bony metaphysis showing hair loop arrangement of blood vessels

Etiology

- **Bacteria:** *Staphylococcus aureus*, Streptococcus, Pneumococcus are common organisms causing osteomyelitis. In addition, *Mycobacterium tuberculosis* is an important causative organism in India.
- **Other infectious organisms:** Though osteomyelitis is of bacterial origin in the majority of cases, other infectious agents such as viruses, parasites and fungi may also be involved. This is especially the case in immunocompromised patients.

Table 12.3 Duration of osteomyelitis

Type	Duration
Acute	<2 weeks
Subacute	2–6 weeks
Chronic	>6 weeks

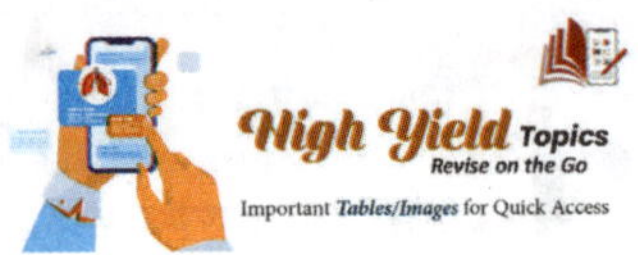

Pathogenesis

The causative organism reaches the bone *via* the bloodstream. Bacteria preferentially reside in the metaphysis. This causes an inflammatory response (Fig. 12.5). Inflammation is localized or may spread to the bones in multiple directions:

- **To the marrow, i.e., along the medullary cavity:** The blood vessels of the bony medulla is blocked by the pus and necrotic material leading to ischemia and necrosis of the bone.
- **To the cortex and beyond:** Inflammation spreads outward from the medulla to reach the cortex and involves the periosteum. The periosteum is lifted and the blood vessels beneath are disrupted thus causing the part of bone beneath to become avascular, dead and necrosed. This part of affected bone is called sequestrum.
  - A new layer of reactive bone is formed around the sequestrum called involucrum.
  - Pus is formed under the periosteum as a response to laying down of new bone, called the periosteal reaction.
  - Extension of inflammation to the adjoining soft tissue, sometimes leading to formation of an abscess. When an abscess does not respond to treatment or is untreated a sinus is formed wherein pus exudes out of an opening in the skin.

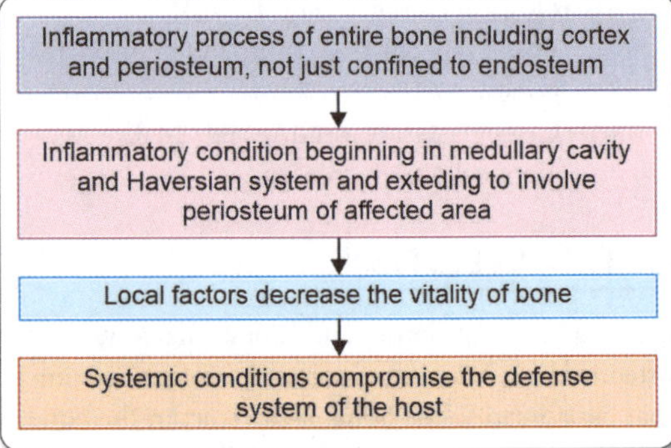

Figure 12.5: Pathogenesis of osteomyelitis

Complications of Osteomyelitis

- Acute osteomyelitis if persistent can lead to chronic osteomyelitis.
- **Pathologic fracture:** When the bone is weakened by the presence of pus, it becomes more susceptible to fractures.
- Secondary amyloidosis.
- **Growth abnormalities:** If the growth plate is involved, deformities can appear which include both shortening and lengthening of the bone.
- Endocarditis.
- Sepsis.
- Development of squamous cell carcinoma in the draining sinus tracts.
- Sarcoma in the infected bone.

Specific Forms of Osteomyelitis

Pyogenic Osteomyelitis

Clinical Features

The patient presents with pain in the affected limb, swelling associated with fever and an elevated total leukocyte count.

Etiology

This form of osteomyelitis is usually due to bacterial infections such as *Staphylococcus aureus*, *E. coli*, and *Streptococcus*.

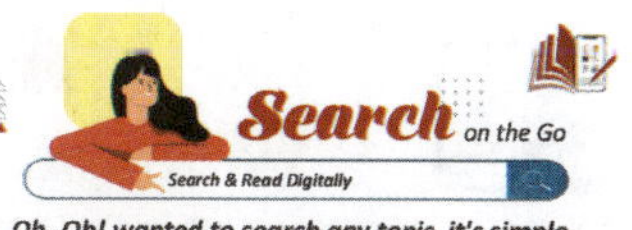

Pathogenesis

Organisms may reach the bone by hematogenous spread (*via* blood). Contiguous spread (*via* spread of infection from a neighboring site), or direct implantation (*via* infected foreign bodies). As described before, exudate formation lifts the periosteum. Reactive new bone is formed. This process is accompanied by necrosis (Fig. 12.6).

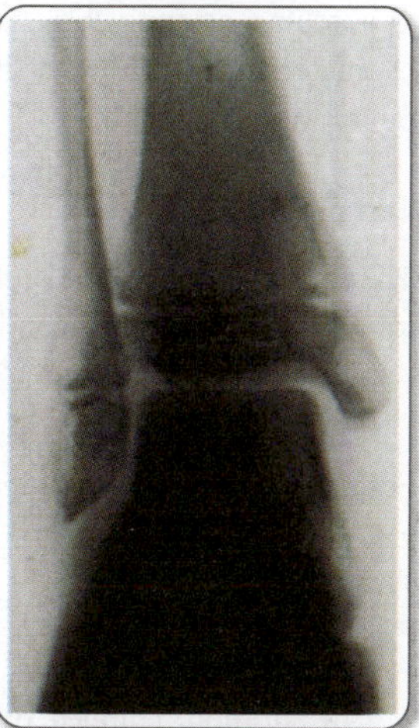

Figure 12.6: Pyogenic osteomyelitis

Site of Involvement

The common site involved is the metaphyseal area, especially in children.

Chronic Osteomyelitis

In 5%–25% of cases, acute osteomyelitis fails to resolve and persists as chronic infection (Fig. 12.7).

Pathogenesis

Chronic infections may develop when there is delay in diagnosis, extensive bone necrosis, inadequate antibiotic therapy or surgical debridement, or weakened host defenses. The course of chronic infections may be punctuated by acute flare-ups, usually spontaneous and may occur after years of dormancy.

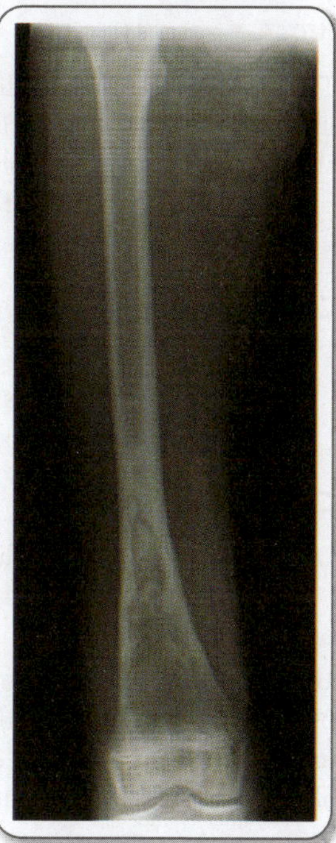

Figure 12.7: Chronic osteomyelitis

Diagnosis

Key diagnostic features to keep in mind are to note the presence of dead necrotic bone. This is avascular bone which is separated from the rest of the bone by chronic granulation tissue and is called sequestrum. The sequestrum serves as a nidus for reactive bone formation, known as involucrum.

Histological Changes

Dead necrotic pieces of chipped off bone are seen surrounded by a chronic inflammatory infiltrate.

Tubercular Osteomyelitis

This represents a common form of chronic osteomyelitis in developing countries. The causative organism is *Mycobacterium tuberculosis.*

Pathogenesis

Infection usually spreads from the lungs *via* hematogenous route and infrequently by direct extension of foci in the lungs or elsewhere. Tuberculous osteomyelitis (Fig. 12.8A) is usually a destructive process and is frequently seen in immunocompromised individuals. It involves the spine in roughly half of cases and is resistant to control vis-a-vis other forms of osteomyelitis. Involvement of the spine is called Pott's spine (Fig. 12.8B). The infection breaks through intervertebral discs to affect multiple vertebrae and extends into the soft tissues forming a paravertebral abscess.

Destruction of discs and vertebrae frequently results in permanent compression fractures. The result is scoliosis/kyphosis/neurologic deficits (secondary to spinal cord and nerve compression).

Tubercular osteomyelitis is frequently multifocal and characteristically shows a thin, watery discharge oozing out of the sinus tract.

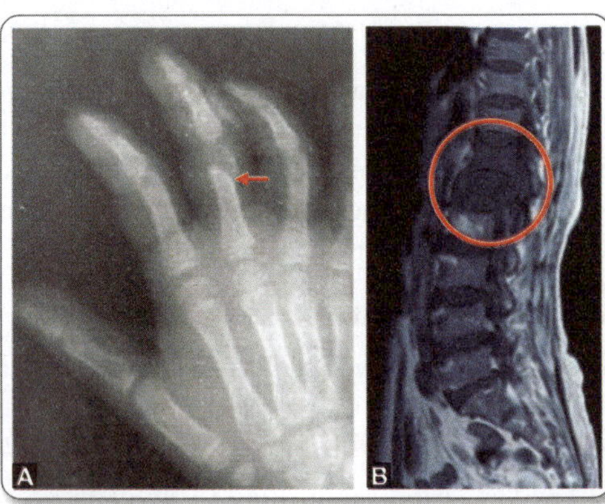

Figures 12.8A and B: A. Tubercular osteomyelitis; **B.** Pott's spine

Complications

The complications include tuberculous arthritis, sinus tract formation, psoas abscess, and amyloidosis.

Histological Changes

Features consistent with tubercular infection elsewhere are:

- Granulomas
- Epithelioid cells
- Langerhans giant cells
- Caseous necrosis (+/–)
- In addition, chipped off fragments of dead necrotic bone may be interspersed.
- Ziehl-Neelsen stain for acid fast bacilli may or may not be positive.

Brodie's abscess

This is a form of osteomyelitis which usually is subacute/chronic. It is frequently seen in young males after injury (Figs 12.9A and B). It is commonly caused by *Staphylococcus aureus* infection. It is basically a small abscess that frequently involves the cortex and is walled off by reactive thickened, sclerotic bone.

- **Site of involvement**: Femur, tibia.

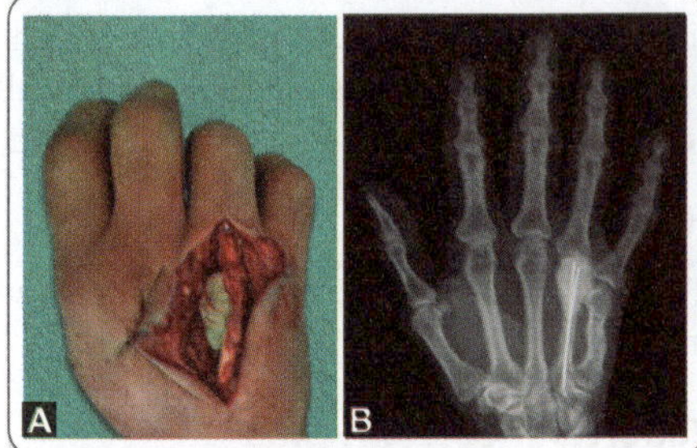

Figures 12.9A and B: Brodie's abscess: **A.** Gross; **B.** X-ray

Clinical Features

- The patient feels a deep, boring pain which increases at night time. Patients typically do not show systemic symptoms such as fever.

Gross Appearance

On examination, joint swelling may be noted.

X-rays reveal an oval radiolucent lesion which has a rim of sclerotic bone.

Histological changes: It may sometimes mimic malignancy and on biopsy, histopathological findings consistent with an abscess, i.e., a localized, walled off acute on chronic inflammatory infiltrate are seen along with granulation tissue.

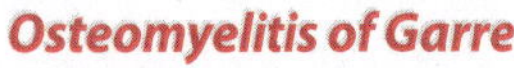

Osteomyelitis of Garre

Garre's osteomyelitis is a specific type of osteomyelitis which frequently involves the jaw and is seen in children and young adults (Fig. 12.10). It is precipitated by low grade periosteal infections or irritation to the oral cavity. It is a typically nonsuppurative osteomyelitis and patients do not present with discharging sinuses.

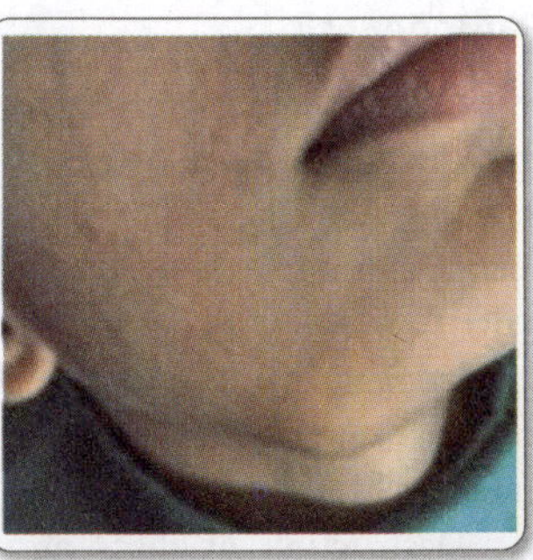
Figure 12.10: Garre's osteomyelitis

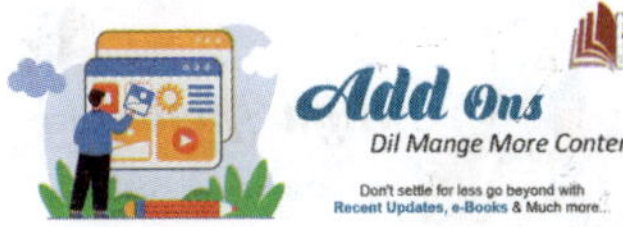

Site of involvement: It involves the mandible more than the maxilla and patients commonly present with jaw swelling. It can also involve the shafts of the femur and tibia.

Gross Appearance

- **X-ray finding:** It is characterized by an exaggerated periosteal reaction with "onion skin" multilayering which leads to swelling in the jaw area.
- **Bone biopsy:** This marked periosteal reaction can cause a diagnostic difficulty with malignant lesions such as Ewing's sarcoma and osteosarcoma. In such cases, a bone biopsy is commonly sent to the pathologist for analysis and hence awareness of this entity is important.

Treatment

Symptomatic relief.

ARTHRITIS

Arthritis is the swelling and tenderness of one or more joints. The main symptoms of arthritis are joint pain and stiffness, which typically worsen with age. The most common types of arthritis are rheumatoid arthritis and osteoarthritis.

Rheumatoid Arthritis

This is a chronic nonsuppurative inflammatory pathology and a multisystem disease affecting the joints bilaterally (symmetric pattern). Rheumatoid arthritis is a common disease which affects females, usually in the third to fourth decade. It usually afflicts smaller joints of the hand first, subsequently involving larger joints later in the course of disease.

Clinical Features

The patient presents with fatigue, stiffness of joints, joint pain, weakness along with myalgias (muscle pain). Multiple joints are usually affected. Morning stiffness is a characteristic feature.

Diagnosis

Clinical examination reveals swelling around the affected joint with limited range of mobility in established cases. With progression of disease, various joint deformities may also be seen. The recent ACR/EULAR diagnostic criteria of rheumatoid arthritis are outlined in Table 12.4.

Table 12.4: ACR/EULAR diagnostic criteria of rheumatoid arthritis

Joint involvement	Score
1 large joint	0
2–10 large joints	1
1–3 small joints, +/– large joint	3
>10 joints (at least 1 small joint)	5
Serology	
RF negative, negative anti CCP	0
anti CCP/RF low positive	2
anti CCP/RF strong positive	3
Symptom duration	
<6 weeks	0
≥6 weeks	1
Acute phase reactants	
Normal CRP, normal ESR	0
Abnormal CRP/ESR	1

Pathogenesis

The pathogenesis of rheumatoid arthritis involves an interaction of genetic factors and environmental exposure (Fig. 12.11). The histocompatibility markers associated with RA include HLA-DRW4/HLA-DR1. In genetically susceptible individuals, environmental triggers (an infectious/noninfectious agent) promote loss of tolerance to self-proteins that contain a citrulline residue.

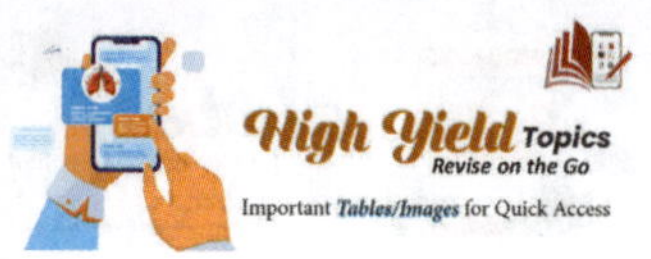

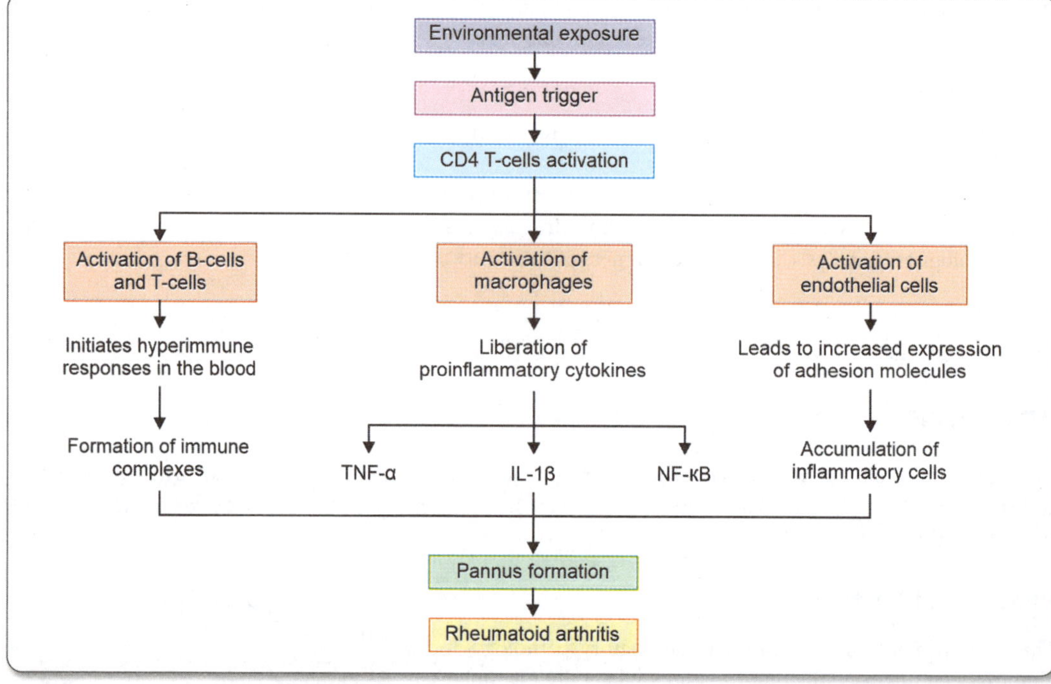

Figure 12.11: Pathogenesis of rheumatoid arthritis

- The antigen presented from the environment triggers CD 4 + T cell activation.
- Activation of T cells leads to cytokine production such as TNF-α, IL-1β, IL-6.
- This in turn causes endothelial cell activation further liberating more cytokines.
- The B cells also are activated leading to the production of antibodies against the Fc portion of native IgG molecule.
- Circulating antibodies cross react with the synovial lining of the joint causing damage and destruction extending to the joint itself leading to destruction and fibrosis.
- Anti-citrulline response is detected in both T-cells and B-cells.

Pathological Changes

Changes around the joints:

- The synovial surface shows the presence of fibrin with inflammatory cells comprising neutrophils and lymphocytes.
- Synovial hypertrophy is present which surrounds the cartilage forming a growth, like "pannus". Edema is also noted.
- The pannus erodes the surrounding articular cartilage.
- Chronic inflammation is noted in the underlying tissue comprising lymphocytes and plasma cells. Proliferating blood vessels are also seen.
- Hemosiderin deposition is noted.
- Articular cartilage becomes dull and gradually shows wear and tear.

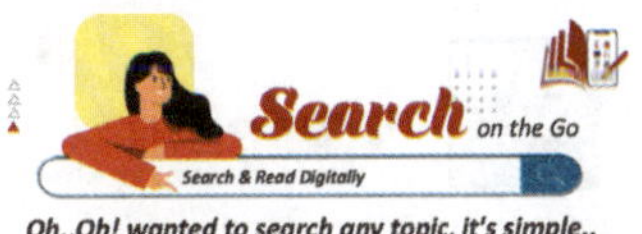

Changes outside the joints (extra-articular features):

- The cutaneous manifestations of rheumatoid arthritis include the presence of a rheumatoid nodule which comprises palisaded histiocytes, lymphocytes and plasma cells.
- Rheumatoid nodules are frequently seen over points on which pressure is applied such as the elbows and the sacrum.
  - They are usually present in the subcutaneous plane. However, in severe cases, rheumatoid nodules are also seen in internal organs.
- Inflammation may also be present in other organs, such as the heart, lungs, blood vessels (vasculitis), muscles and even the eyes.

Lab Diagnosis

- **Rheumatoid factor positivity** seen in 80% cases. These are IgM/IgG antibodies binding to Fc portion of IgG. However, this is nonspecific and may be seen in other autoimmune diseases.
- The presence of serum anticyclic citrullinated peptides (CCP) antibodies which is specific for rheumatoid arthritis.
- **Synovial fluid examination:** Sterile turbid fluid with decreased viscosity, poor mucin clot formation, inclusion bearing neutrophils.
- **Synovial biopsy:** Shows histopathological features as described before.
- **Hematological changes:** These include the presence of a normocytic normochromic anemia. The total leukocyte count may be elevated.
- **Elevated ESR:** A feature of all chronic inflammatory disease.

EXTRA EDGE

Deformities in Rheumatoid Arthritis

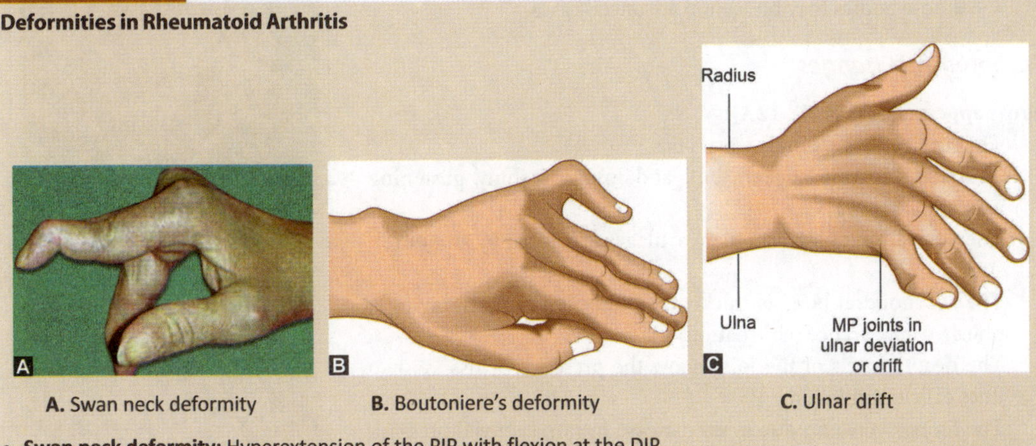

A. Swan neck deformity **B.** Boutoniere's deformity **C.** Ulnar drift

- **Swan neck deformity:** Hyperextension of the PIP with flexion at the DIP.
- **Boutoniere's deformity:** Flexion at PIP with hyperextension at DIP.
- **Ulnar drift:** Ulnar deviation of metacarpophalangeal joint.

Osteoarthritis

Osteoarthritis is a slowly progressing, noninflammatory degenerative joint disease which involves erosion of the articular cartilage and bone beneath (subchondral bone).

Classification of Osteoarthriritis

- **Primary osteoarthritis:** It is a common joint disease and frequently affects the middle-aged or elderly population. It has a multifactorial etiology and is seen due to senility (repeated wear and tear of the joint). This type is called primary osteoarthritis.
- **Secondary osteoarthritis:** It is seen secondary to other pathologies, such as fracture, sports injuries, chronic steroid intake, congenital deformities.

Clinical Features

Osteoarthritis primarily affects the large joints of the body, especially the lower limb, such as the knee joint and hip joint. It may also involve the spine and the hands.

The patient presents with pain which is worse on usage of the joint, inability to use the joint fully for instance in the lower limbs causes inability to walk, joint tenderness, swelling and stiffness. Some patients may feel a gritty sensation or instability while moving the joint.

Lab Diagnosis

- **Physical examination:** Reveals tenderness while examining, crepitus and limited movement. Bone deformities are also seen. In some cases of osteoarthritis, surrounding muscle appears atrophied.
- **X-ray:**
  - Joint space is reduced
  - The bone beneath is sclerosed
  - Projecting spurs of hypertrophied bone called "osteophytes" are seen.
  - Loose bodies may be seen in advanced cases.

Pathological Changes

Gross appearance (Fig. 12.12A):

- The surface of the joint is worn out.
- Articular cartilage appears dull and loses its shiny glistening appearance.
- The normally smooth articular cartilage is replaced by an uneven surface.
- The subchondral bone is thickened and becomes hard, giving a polished appearance (eburnation).
- The deeper levels of the joint show the presence of fissure, like lines called fibrillation.
- The lining synovium due to an increase in intrasynovial pressure shows the formation of subchondral cysts.
- Spur-like bony outgrowths are noted coming out from the margins of the joints. These are also called osteophytes.

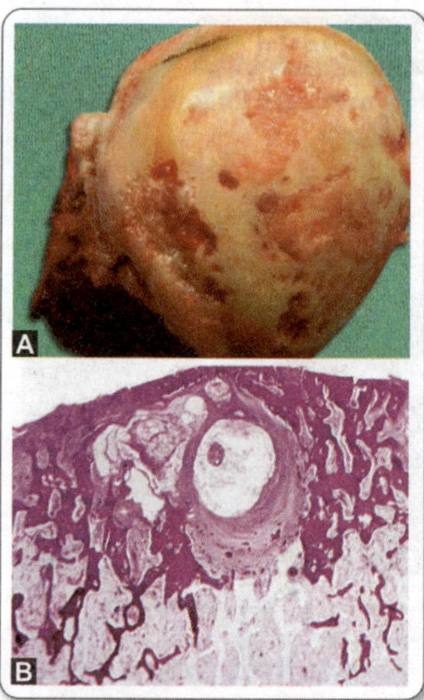

Figures 12.12A and B: Osteoarthritis: **A.** Gross; **B.** Histology

Histological changes (Fig. 12.12B):

- **Cartilage:** The cartilage shows cracks and vertical fissures. The number of chondrocytes is reduced in the cartilage. The cartilage matrix staining quality is altered.
  Tidal duplication is present, i.e., the tidal mark present at the junction of mineralized and nonmineralized bone is seen as two lines.

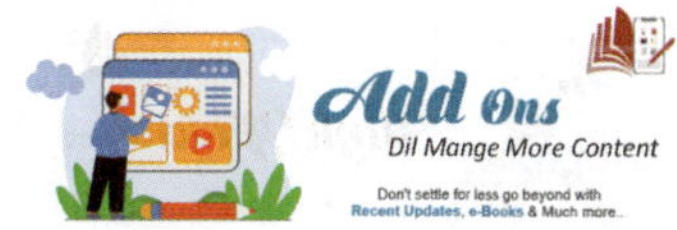

- **Synovial lining:** Hypertrophy, villous formations, edema and varying degrees of inflammation may be seen. Synoviocytes may also show giant cell change.
- **Bone beneath the cartilage (subchondral bone):** Shows thickening (reactive sclerosis).
- The bony trabeculae are widened. Bone cysts may be seen.
- **Loose bodies:** The synovial membrane may show embedded cartilaginous nodules which subsequently show endochondral ossification. This may fragment off to form loose bodies.

Differences between rheumatoid arthritis and osteoarthritis are given in Table 12.5.

Table 12.5: Differences between rheumatoid arthritis and osteoarthritis

Features	Rheumatoid arthritis	Osteoarthritis
Nature of disease	Autoimmune	Degenerative
Patient age	Common in 4–5th decade	Common in elderly age group
Distribution of involvement	Symmetric	Asymmetric
Type of joints	Smaller joints of hands and feet affected first	Larger joints affected
Stiffness	Characteristically in the morning	More in the evening/after exertion
Systemic symptoms	More frequently present	Absent
Deformity present	Swan, neck, ulnar drift, Boutonniere	• Heberden's nodes (DIP) • Bouchard's nodes (PIP)
Joint features	Swelling present, redness	Redness and swelling are often absent
Diagnostic serology	Anti-RF, anti-CCP positive	Anti-RF, anti-CCP negative

EXTRA EDGE

Deformities in Osteoarthritis

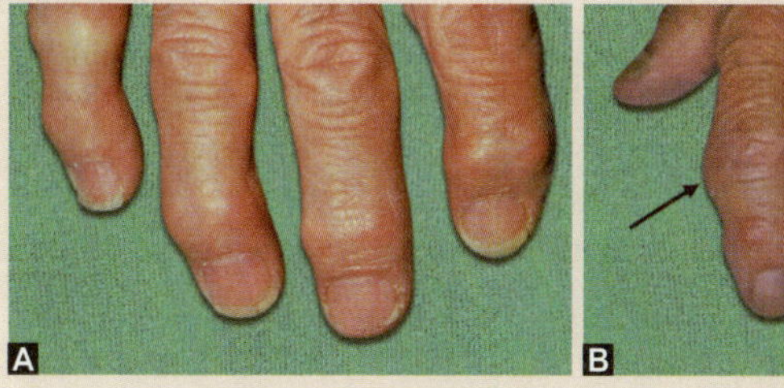

A. Heberden's nodes; **B.** Bouchard's nodes

- **Heberden's nodes:** Painless nodularity seen at the distal interphalangeal joint.
- **Bouchard's nodes:** Less common, seen at the proximal interphalangeal joint.

BONE TUMORS

Bone tumors develop when cells within a bone divide uncontrollably, forming a lump or mass of abnormal tissue. Most bone tumors are benign (not cancerous).

CLASSIFICATION OF BONE TUMORS—WHO

The histological classification of bone tumors is given in Table 12.6.

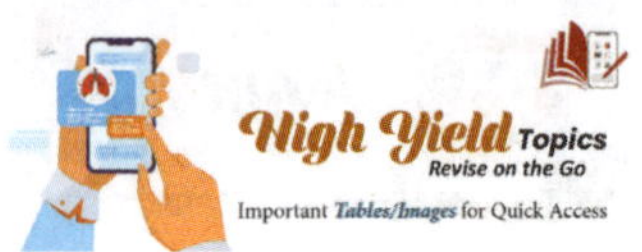

Table 12.6: Histological classification of bone tumors

Predominant tissue	Benign	Malignant
Bone forming	• Osteoma • Osteoid osteoma and • Osteoblastoma	Osteosarcoma • Central • Periosteal • Parosteal
Cartilage forming	• Chondroma • Osteochondroma • Chondroblastoma • Chondromyxoid fibroma	Chondrosarcoma • Juxtacortical chondrosarcoma • Mesenchymal chondrosarcoma • Dedifferentiated chondrosarcoma • Clear cell chondrosarcoma • Malignant chondroblastoma
Marrow tumors		• Ewing sarcoma • Primitive neuroectodermal tumor of bone (PNET) • Malignant lymphoma of bone • Myeloma

Bone Forming Tumors

Osteoma—Benign Tumor

An osteoma is a new piece of bone usually growing on another piece of bone, typically the skull (Figs 12.13A and B). It can be:

- **Homoplastic osteoma:** When the bone tumor grows on other bone
- **Heteroplastic osteoma:** When it grows on other tissue.

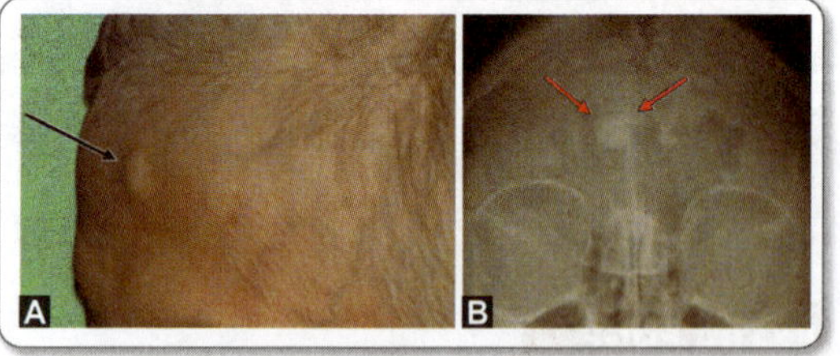

Figures 12.13A and B: Osteoma: **A.** Gross; **B.** Radiographic

Refer to Figures 12.13A and B to observe gross and radiographic images of osteoma.

Pathogenesis

Osteomas are the most common tumor involving the paranasal sinuses, arising from the normal bony walls of the sinus cavities.

Etiology

Supposed causes of osteoma development include congenital, inflammatory, or traumatic factors. In most cases, the cause of the osteoma is unknown.

Pathological Changes

Gross appearance: Lesion involves the surface of the bone and appears well marked, ovoid or the mushroom shaped with broad base of attachment to the cortex.

Osteoid Osteoma Benign Tumor

This is a benign bone producing tumor. This tumor has following predilections:

- **Age:** 10–30 years.
- **Site:** Metaphyseal, most lesions are seen in the bony cortex.
- **Bones involved:** Femur, tibia, humerus.

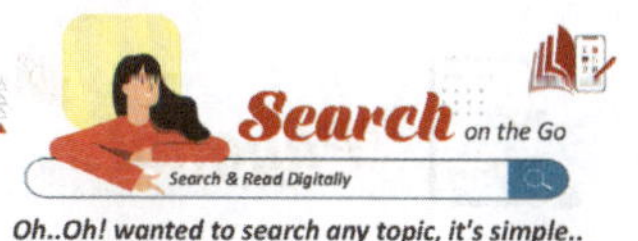

Clinical Features

The most striking feature is that the patient presents with intense pain relieved by medication, but which increases at night-time. An osteoid osteoma is a benign bone-forming tumor that has no potential to become malignant. It classically causes severe pain at night but it is relieved with nonsteroidal anti-inflammatory medications. Occasionally, it gets resolved without treatment.

X-ray findings represent osteoid osteomas as radiolucent central nidus surrounded by peripheral sclerosis.

Pathological Changes

- **Gross appearance (Fig. 12.14A):** A small well-circumscribed round to oval lesion
- **Cut surface (Fig. 12.14B):** Gritty, tan, focally hemorrhagic
- **Histological changes**: A central nidus is seen comprising of calcified osteoid (bony trabeculae) lined by plump osteoblasts. The stroma shows loose connective tissue with dilated, congested capillaries.

Osteoblastoma

Benign tumor

This is like osteoid osteoma—a bone-producing tumor.

Age: 10–30 years.

The key differences from an osteoid osteoma however, are:

- Larger nidus size.
- More frequently involves the spine.
- More frequently involves the bony medulla rather than the cortex.
- Clinically, the pain is less intense, being of a dull aching type rather than intense as seen in osteoid osteoma.
- Reactive bone formation is also less.

Histological features: Similar to the osteoid osteoma.

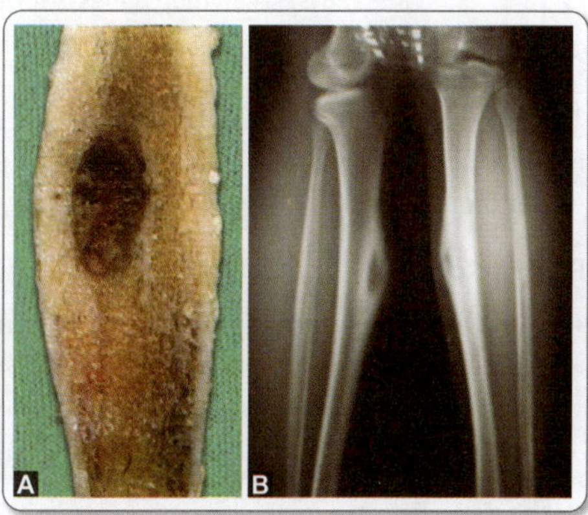

Figures 12.14A and B: Osteoid osteoma: **A.** Gross; **B.** X-ray

MUST KNOW

Histologically, osteoid osteoma and osteoblastoma are similar, containing osteoblasts that produce osteoid and woven bone. Osteoblastoma, is larger and tends to be more aggressive. It can undergo malignant transformation, whereas osteoid osteoma is small and benign.

Osteosarcoma

The most common primary malignant tumor of the bone, is characterized by formation of osteoid by malignant tumor cells.

Spread: Osteosarcoma spreads to the lungs and brain.

Classification of Osteosarcomas

Types of osteosarcomas according to site:

- Osteosarcomas may be classified as per their exact site in the bone or by the type of appearance they see on histological evaluation. Depending on the site within the bone, tumors may be:
  - **Parosteal:** On the cortical surface
  - **Periosteal:** On the surface of the bone, beneath the periosteum.

- **Central:** Within the medulla. This is either of high grade (classical) or low grade
- **Secondary osteosarcoma:** This refers to the development of osteosarcoma in those cases where there is a pre-existing risk factor.

Types of osteosarcomas according to histology:
Chondroblastic, fibroblastic, osteoblastic, small cell, giant cell, and telangiectatic.

Predilections

This tumor has the following predilections:

Age	It is seen in a bimodal distribution with 75% being seen in the younger age group (10–25 years) and a smaller group of elderly patients are also affected.
Sex	This tumor shows a male predilection
Site	Metaphyses, common bones involved include lower femur, upper tibia/fibula/proximal humerus.

Clinical Features

The patient presents with a painful mass. The pain is dull aching in nature with intermittent episodes of increased pain. There may be a restriction in joint mobility and the affected joint may show swelling and is tender on palpation.

Risk Factors

- Past history of receiving chemotherapy/radiation
- The presence of long-standing bone disease, such as osteomyelitis, paget's disease of the bone, presence of orthopaedic implants.

Pathogenesis

Pathological changes:

- **Gross appearance (Fig. 12.15A):** The osteosarcoma is typically a large grossly expansile mass lesion with infiltrative margins.
- **X-ray findings (Fig. 12.15B):** The osteosarcoma is an infiltrative mass which destroys the cortex, leading to an elevation of the periosteum. This forms a triangular area known as the Codman's triangle. On extension to the surrounding soft tissue, it displays a sunburst appearance on radiological imaging.
- **Cut surface:** Gray-white/brownish in color, hard and gritty to cut. Areas of necrosis and hemorrhage may be seen.
- **Histological changes (Fig. 12.15C):** The osteosarcoma comprises three major components:
  1. Pleomorphic spindle cells with features of malignancy, i.e., increased hyperchromasia and nucleocytoplasmic ratio.
  2. Lace-like irregularly mineralized osteoid matrix which in some areas shows a basophilic hue.
  3. The presence of giant cells in varying proportions. Additionally, frequent atypical mitoses are seen.

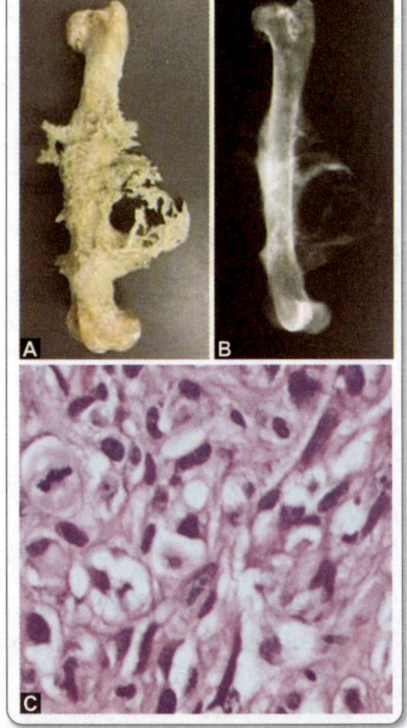

Figures 12.15A to C: Osteosarcoma: **A.** Gross; **B.** X-ray; **C.** Histology

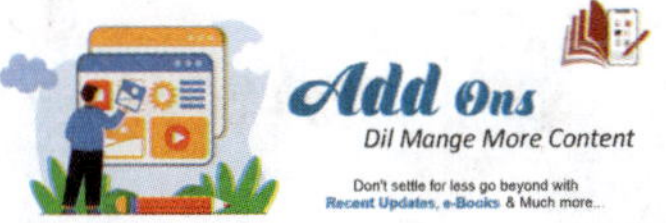

Cartilage Forming Tumors

Chondroma (Benign Tumor)

Chondromas are benign (not cancerous) tumors made of cartilage, which are found mostly in the small bones of the hand and feet. These tumors rarely produce symptoms but can cause the affected bone to easily fracture.

Pathogenesis

Chondromas are extremely rare, slow-growing tumors that arise from the cartilaginous portions of bones. They can occur in the humerus (upper arm), femur (thigh bone), and ribs. In the cranial region, this includes the bones of the skull base and paranasal sinuses. These benign (noncancerous) tumors are composed of mature cartilage.

Chordomas are thought to arise from primitive notochordal remnants along the axial skeleton.

Pathological Changes

- **Gross appearance (Fig. 12.16A):** Bulky often lobulated masses
- **Histological changes (Fig. 12.16B):** A lobulated architecture

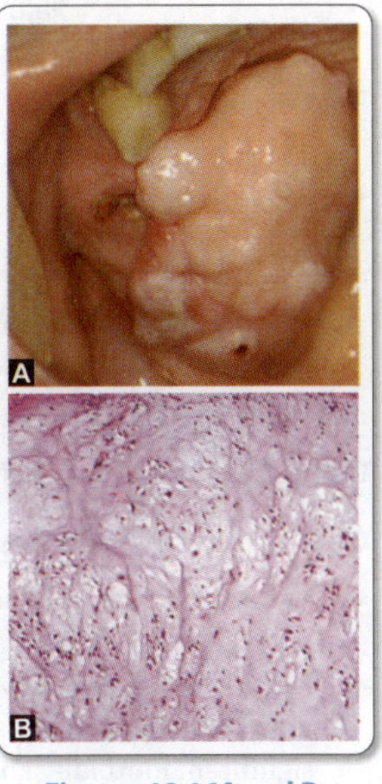

Figures 12.16A and B: Chondroma: **A.** Gross; **B.** Histology

Osteochondroma (Benign Tumor)

This is also called exostosis. Exostosis is the most common cartilage-producing tumor. The lesion protrudes out from the bone beneath and has a stalk. It is a benign tumor that is characteristically associated with presence of a cartilage cap—which is identified both grossly and microscopically.

Predilections

This tumor has the following predilections:

- **Age:** Affects young adults.
- **Sex:** Male predilection.
- **Site:** It is a metaphyseal lesion seen near the growth plate.

Clinical Features

The patient presents with a slow growing painful mass.

Pathological Changes

- **Gross appearance (Fig. 12.17A):** The lesion may be sessile/may show a stalk. A cartilaginous cap is present on the upper surface.
- **Histological changes (Fig. 12.17B):** Two distinct zones are seen:
  - The upper cartilaginous cap
  - The lower bony area showing trabeculae of lamellar bone enclosing marrow spaces.

Chondrosarcoma (Malignant Tumor)

This is a malignant bone tumor-producing cartilage. It is associated with IDH 1,2 mutations in half of the cases.

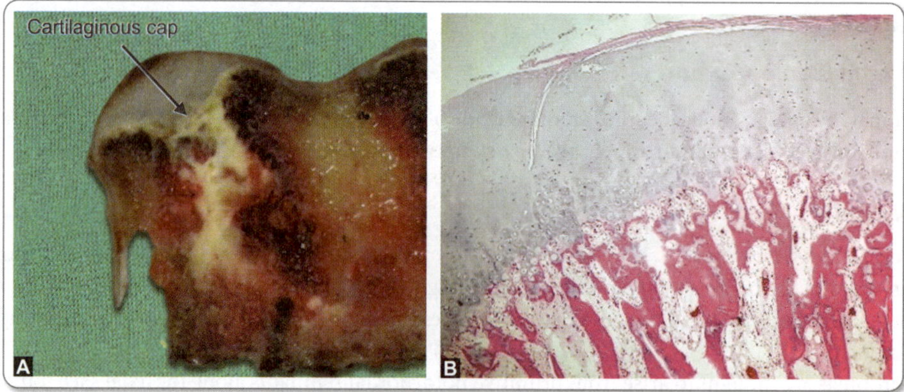

Figures 12.17A and B: Osteochondroma: **A.** Gross; **B.** Histological

Predilections

Chondrosarcoma has the following predilections:

Age	4–5th decade
Sex	Male predilection
Site	Frequently seen in pelvic bones and in sites such as the ribs and shoulders. It may also be seen in smaller bones of the hands/feet
Spread	The tumor can spread to the surrounding tissue. It may also spread to the lungs

Clinical features: The patient presents with a painful swelling/mass that shows an increase in size.

Classification of Chondrosarcoma

- **Juxtacortical chondrosarcoma or periosteal chondrosarcomas:** A rare malignant cartilaginous tumor arising from the external surface of bone.
- **Mesenchymal chondrosarcoma (MC):** A rare, aggressive small round blue cell malignancy that may arise in bone or soft tissue. It has high potential for hematogenous dissemination. It is associated with significant morbidity and mortality.
- **Dedifferentiated chondrosarcoma:** A rare, highly malignant tumor with a poor survival rate.
- **Clear cell chondrosarcomas:** Low-grade malignant cartilaginous bone neoplasms, found in the epiphyses and characterized by the presence of lobules of clear cells that contain an abundant clear or mildly eosinophilic cytoplasm with centrally-placed nuclei.

Pathological Changes

- **X-ray:** Shows a tumor with poorly-defined borders, often eroding the cortex. The tumor shows popcorn/spotty calcification.
- **Gross appearance (Fig. 12.18A):** Large-sized voluminous tumor mass which is largely solid but may also show cystic spaces.
- **Cut surface:** Firm to hard with a glistening myxoid appearance. The lesion is bluish-gray in color. Focal gritty areas correspond to areas of calcification. Focal necrosis may also be seen.
- **Histological changes (Fig. 12.18B):**
    - Chondrosarcoma is comprised of malignant chondrocytes showing varying degrees of atypia from very mild to marked pleomorphism.

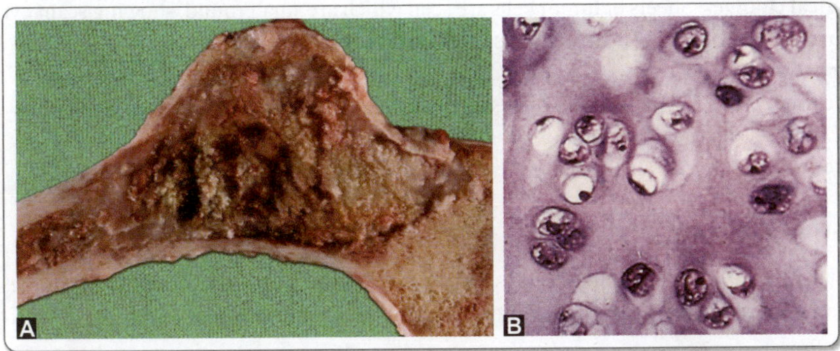

Figures 12.18A and B: Chondrosarcoma: **A.** Gross; **B.** Histology

- The cartilage shows a lobulated appearance. Within the cartilage, the chondrocytes may be two or more per lacuna.
- Areas of myxoid change and necrosis can be seen microscopically also.

Other important bone tumors:

Ewing's Sarcoma—Malignant

Ewing's sarcoma is a malignant tumor of the bone seen in young children and adolescents (Fig. 12.19A). On account of its typical histomorphology, it is one of the tumors coming under the nomenclature "small blue round cell tumors" of childhood (Fig. 12.19B).

Location and site:

It is typically a diaphyseal tumor (involving the shaft).

- **Long bones:** Humerus, tibia, femur, fibula are the common sites affected.
- **Origin:** Multipotent mesenchymal stem cell
- **X-ray:** Standard X-ray shows a lesion which is lytic, within the shaft and surrounded by layers of periosteal bone formation giving a characteristic "onion skin" pattern.

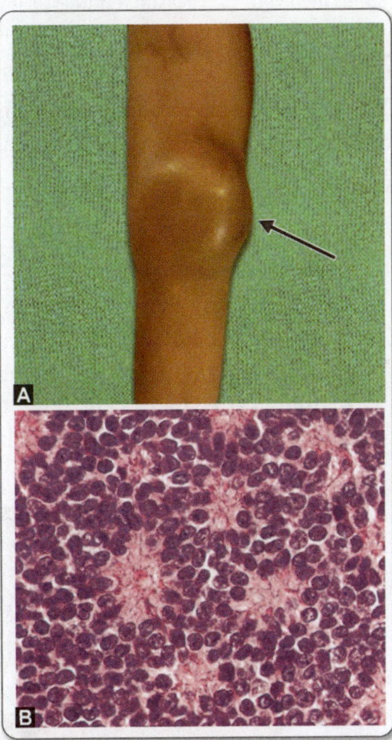

Figures 12.19A and B: **A.** Ewing sarcoma; **B.** Histological (small blue round cell)

Clinical Features

Patients are typically between 10 and 20 years of age, frequently males will a complain of pain and swelling around the affected joint. The patient may appreciate a definite mass around the affected area and sometimes may complain of fever. Overlying skin appears swollen. On examination the area is tender.

Pathological Changes

- **Gross appearance:** The tumor is grossly soft, gray-white, with foci of hemorrhage and necrosis. The bulk of the tumor is usually within the medulla of the bone and infiltrates surrounding areas.

- **Histological changes:** Sheets of tumor cells are seen which are small round, showing scant cytoplasm and hyperchromatic nuclei with inconspicuous nucleoli. Rosettes can also be seen.
- **Ancillary studies:**
  - **Cytochemistry:** Tumor cells are diffusely positive for PAS (cytoplasmic)
  - IHC -CD99 (diffuse membranous).
  - **Cytogenetics:** t(11,22) is the most common one seen in cases of Ewing's sarcoma.

Osteoclastoma

This is a bone tumor which is benign and is locally aggressive. However, it rarely undergoes malignant transformation. The neoplastic cell is the mononuclear stromal cell which expresses RANK-ligand and various cytokines.

Predilections

Giant cell tumour has predilections tabulated as follows:

Giant cell tumors

Age	Seen in young adults (20–40 years)
Site	It is typically an epiphyseal tumor and can extend to the metaphysis (epiphysiometaphyseal)
Cell of origin	Stromal mononuclear cells
Bones involved	Distal femur, proximal tibia, lower end of the radius, humerus

Clinical Features

The patient typically presents with pain, swelling around the affected joint, limited range of movement and sometimes joint deformity and effusion.

Pathological Changes

- **Gross appearance (Fig. 12.20A):** The giant cell tumor is a well-circumscribed tumor present at the epiphyseal end of the bone. The lesion has a brownish-red cut surface and shows foci of hemorrhage. Necrosis and cystic areas may or may not be seen.
- **X-ray (Fig. 12.20B):** Standard X-ray shows a lesion which is lytic, eccentrically placed within the shaft, expansile and multiloculated giving a characteristic "soap bubble" appearance.
- **Histological changes (Fig. 12.20C):** Sheets of numerous multinucleated osteoclasts type giant cells are uniformly distributed in a background of mononuclear cells (neoplastic) which are round to ovoid.

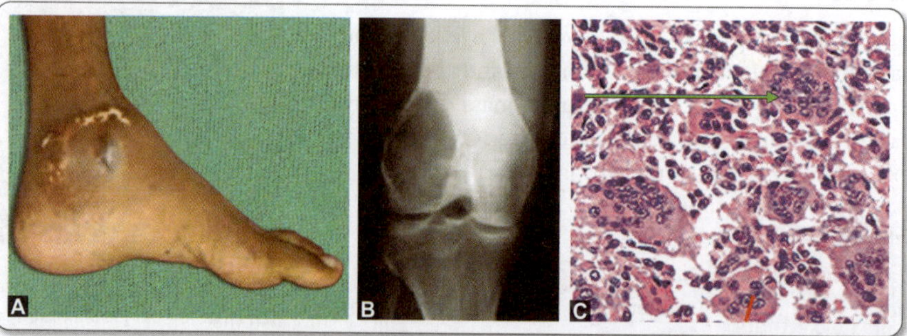

Figures 12.20A to C: Osteoclastoma: **A.** Gross; **B.** X-ray showing giant cell tumor; **C.** Histological changes

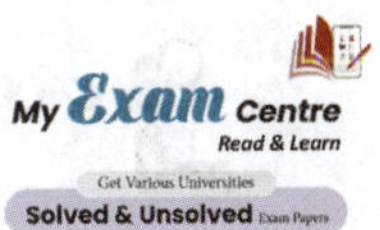

The nuclei of the giant cells resemble those of the mononuclear stromal cell and have indistinct nucleoli. Individual giant cells have up to 50–100 nuclei.

- **Ancillary studies:** Tumor cells are positive for p63, CD68.

Treatment

Curettage, Denosunab (rank-ligand inhibitor) therapy.

SUMMARY

- Bone healing is an intricate regenerative process.
- Osteoporosis or osteopenia is a metabolic bone disease, characterized by reduced bone mineral density.
- Depending on the extent of involvement, osteoporosis can also be classified as localized or diffuse.
- Cases of spinal osteoporosis present with shortening of height due to compression of the vertebrae and kyphosis or scoliosis.
- Inflammation of bone and bone marrow, secondary to infection is osteomyelitis.
- Pus under the periosteum as a response to laying down of newbon, fibroblasts is called the periosteal reaction.
- Tuberculous osteomyelitis is usually a destructive process and is frequently seen in immunocompromised individuals.
- Garre's osteomyelitis is a specific type of osteomyelitis which frequently involves the jaw and is seen in children and young adults.
- The most common types of arthritis are rheumatoid arthritis and osteoarthritis.
- Rheumatoid arthritis is a common disease which affects females, usually in the third to fourth decade.
- Pathogenesis of rheumatoid arthritis involves an interaction of genetic factors and environmental exposure.
- Circulating antibodies cross react with the synovial lining of the joint causing damage and destruction extending to the joint itself leading to destruction and fibrosis.
- Bone tumors develop when cells within a bone divide uncontrollably, forming a lump or mass of abnormal tissue.
- Ewing's sarcoma is a malignant tumor of the bone seen in young children and adolescents.
- The neoplastic cell is the mononuclear stromal cell which expresses RANK-ligand and various cytokines.
- Histologically, osteoid osteoma and osteoblastoma are similar, containing osteoblasts that produce osteoid and woven bone.
- The osteosarcoma is an infiltrative mass which destroys the cortex, leading to an elevation of the periosteum.
- Chondrosarcoma is comprised of malignant chondrocytes showing varying degrees of atypia from very mild to marked pleomorphism.

ASSESS YOURSELF

Long Answer Questions

1. Discuss bone healing in detail.
2. Describe osteomyelitis and its types.

Short Answer Questions

1. What is tubercular osteomyelitis?
2. Write about brodie's abscess.
3. What is garre's osteomyelitis?
4. Write short notes on:
   i. Rheumatoid arthritis
   ii. Ewing sarcoma
   iii. Osteoclastoma
   iv. Osteochondroma

Multiple Choice Questions

1. **True or false:**
   i. Acute osteomyelitis is most commonly caused by Staphylococcus aureus:
      a. True b. False
   ii. Rheumatoid arthritis is usually associated with a negative test for the rheumatoid factor during the active phase of the disease:
      a. True b. False
2. **Rheumatoid arthritis gives rise to ________________ deviation of the fingers.**
   a. Ulnar b. Radial
   c. Humeral d. None of these
3. **Infections in the bone can be secondary to:**
   a. Bacteremia b. Skin and soft tissue infections
   c. Trauma or surgical procedures d. All of these
4. **Synovial joints allow for:**
   a. Minimal movement b. A wide range of movement
   c. No movement at all d. Restricted movement
5. **Heberden's node usually affects:**
   a. Lumbar spine b. Proximal interphalangeal joints
   c. Symmetrical small joints d. Distal interphalangeal joints
6. **Which of the following benign bone tumors have a significant tendency to recur after excision?**
   a. Chondromyxofibromas b. Benign giant cell tumors of bone
   c. Osteochondromas d. Osteoid osteomas

Answer Key

1. (i) a (ii) b **2.** a **3.** d **4.** b **5.** d **6.** b

Chapter 13

Endocrine System Diseases

LEARNING OBJECTIVES

After the completion of the chapter, the readers will be able to:

- Know about various diseases of thyroid gland.
- Explain different types of goiter.
- Understand thyroid neoplasm.
- Describe diabetes mellitus.

CHAPTER OUTLINE

- Overview of Thyroid Gland
- Diseases of Thyroid Gland
- Overview of Pancreatic Gland
- Diabetes Mellitus

KEY TERMS

Cold nodule: A thyroid nodule that does not produce thyroid hormone.

Nuclear grooves: Longitudinal grooves along the length of the nucleus.

Nuclear pseudoinclusions: Cytopasmic invaginations inside the nucleus.

Orphan Annie-eyed nuclei: Optical clearing of nuclei due to fixation artefact resembling the cartoon character orphan Annie.

Psammoma bodies: Laminated deposits of calcium.

OVERVIEW OF THYROID GLAND

The thyroid is an endocrine gland, situated at the anterior aspect of the neck. It has a peculiar butterfly-like shape and is comprised of two lateral (left and right) lobes joined by an isthmus that overlies the 2nd to 4th rings of the trachea. Some individuals may show a small pyramidal lobe projecting from the left side of the isthmus. It is encased by a thin fibrous capsule. The thyroid is the largest endocrine gland with a weight of 15–25 g (Figs 13.1A and B).

Histology of the Thyroid Gland

The capsule invaginates inward to form septae that divide the thyroid parenchyma into various lobules comprised of follicles. The follicle represents the basic structural and functional unit of the thyroid and is filled with inspissated colloid. Colloid is a protein which contains thyroglobulin. The follicles are lined by

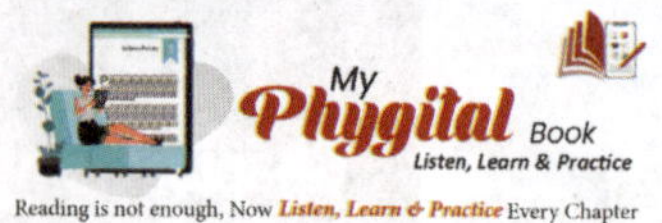

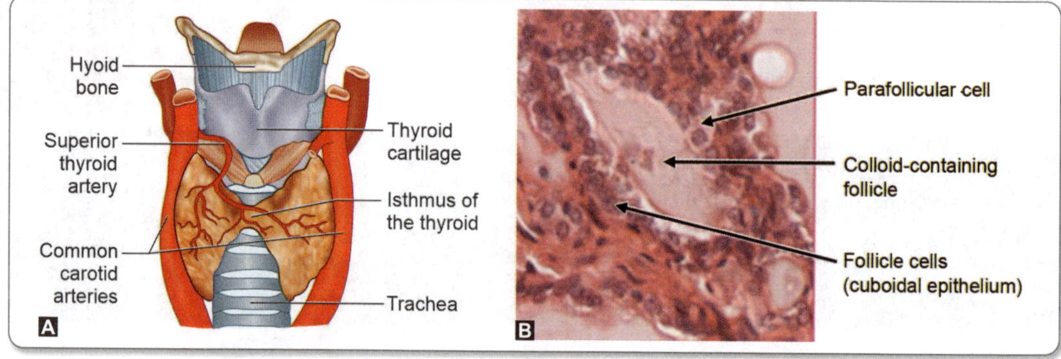

Figures 13.1A and B: Thyroid gland: **A.** Anterior view; **B.** Glandular tissue

low cuboidal to attenuated epithelium. In an active phase, these cells become plump cuboidal. Parafollicular C-cells are also present which are derivatives of the neural crest. These cells are ultrastructural and are not visible usually under standard microscopy and staining. The C-cells secrete the hormone calcitonin which lowers the calcium levels of the body.

Functions

- Thyroid gland is responsible for coordinating various functions important to achieving the body's homeostasis.
- Synthesis of thyroid hormones-T3 (more active form) and T4 (circulating form).
- Calcium metabolism.
- Regulation of the basal metabolic rate (BMR).
- Ensuring proper fetal growth and development.
- Brain development in children and functioning in adults as well as behavior.
- Regulation of body temperature.
- Regulating the function of other endocrine organs such as the pituitary and reproductive organs.
- Maintenance of normal heart rate and cardiac contractility.
- Maintenance of normal gut motility.

DISEASES OF THYROID GLAND

Goiter

Goiter is enlargement of the thyroid gland and is primarily of two types:

1. Simple goiter.
2. Multinodular goiter/nodular goiter.

Etiology

- Iodine deficiency—As iodine is required to produce thyroid hormone, its deficiency leads to goiter.
- Grave's disease—(autoimmune disease).
- Hashimoto's disease—(autoimmune disease).
- Pregnancy—hCG can induce goiter.

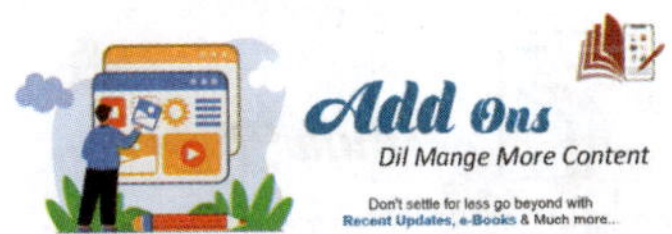

- Thyroiditis
- Thyroid cancer
- Secondary to pituitary carcinoma
- Eating goitrogens such as cauliflower, sarson, cabbage, turnips
- Taking drugs such as sulfonamides, phenylbutazone, para-aminosalicylic acid.

Risk Factors

- Obesity.
- Insulin resistance.
- Metabolic disorders.

Pathogenesis

The hormonal abnormality in goiter is reduced T3, T4 levels which in turn leads to an elevated TSH (Fig. 13.2).

Clinical features: Asymptomatic/neck swelling. If the swelling is large, it leads to pressure symptoms such as hoarseness and dysphagia.

Iodine lack → Goitrogens → Deficient thyroid hormone production → Excessive TSH stimulation → Cyclic hyperplasia-involution → Diffuse goiter → Repeated hyperplasia-involution → Fibrosis of involuted areas / Growth of hyperplastic areas → Nodular goiter

Figure 13.2. Pathogenesis of simple and nodular goiter

Simple Goiter

Simple goiter is also known as diffuse nontoxic goiter.

Age group involved: Young Adults

Simple goiter is characterized by the enlargement of thyroid gland; and the functional status of the thyroid may be euthyroid (normal functioning) or may show increased functioning (hyperthyroidism).

Types of Simple Goiter

1. **Endemic goiter:** This is characteristically associated with iodine deficiency which is normally seen in the Himalayan belt. It is also associated with the intake of goitrogens such as vegetables of the family Brassicaceae, sweet potato, etc.
2. **Sporadic goiter:** It has no geographical predilection. It is associated with:
   - State of altered demand in the body such as around puberty, lactation, or pregnancy
   - Drugs such as lithium, sulfonylurea
   - Metabolic defects

Pathological Changes

Gross appearance: The thyroid is grossly enlarged; weight of the gland increases.

Cut surface: Diffuse, brownish and homogenous.

Histological changes:

- Follicles are of varying size, many are distended by copious amounts of colloid.
- The lining epithelium is flattened/cuboidal.

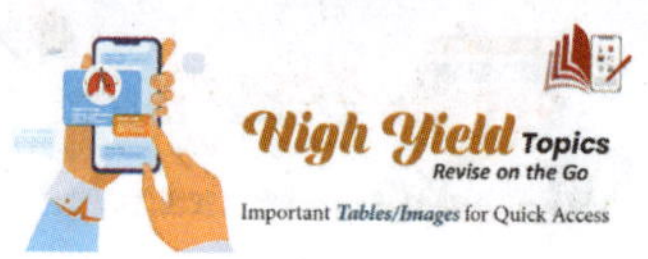

Multinodular Goiter

Multinodular goiter is characterized by enlargement of the thyroid with the presence of multiple nodules.

Pathogenesis

Reduced synthesis of T3 and T4 leads to an elevated TSH. This in turn leads to diffuse goiter. The thyroid follicular cells respond differently—some showing a higher proliferative rate which leads to the formation of nodules. Distension of the follicles with colloid leads to rupture of the follicles. This may also trigger accompanying inflammation.

Complications of Multinodular Goiter

- Pressure effects
- Hoarseness
- Dysphagia
- Foci of hemorrhage

Pathological Changes

Gross appearance: The thyroid gland enlarges.
- Weight of the thyroid gland increases.
- Nodules are of varying sizes and separated by thin strands of fibrous stroma.
- Foci of hemorrhage, calcification and necrosis may be present.

Histological changes: Various nodules of varying size are noted.
- The nodules are full of thick colloid.
- Follicular lining epithelium is flattened.
- Thin colloid is noted.
- Scalloping of colloid is noted.
- The follicular lining epithelium may also show papillary structures.

Lab Diagnosis

Checking levels of T3, T4, TSH; and correlation with USG, FNAC.

Thyroid Neoplasm

A neoplasm or tumor of the thyroid is called thyroid neoplasm. It can be a benign tumor such as thyroid adenoma, or it can be a malignant neoplasm (thyroid cancer), such as papillary, follicular, medullary or anaplastic thyroid cancer. The important tumors which will be elaborated upon and which form the bulk of neoplastic thyroid lesions are as follows:

Benign: Follicular adenoma

Malignant:
- Follicular carcinoma
- Papillary carcinoma
- Medullary carcinoma
- Anaplastic carcinoma

Etiology

Development of thyroid carcinomas is multifactorial and includes external influences, as well as constitutional predispositions and genetic factors. The environmental and constitutional factors affect genetic and epigenetic alterations resulting in cell proliferation and oncogenesis (Fig. 13.3).

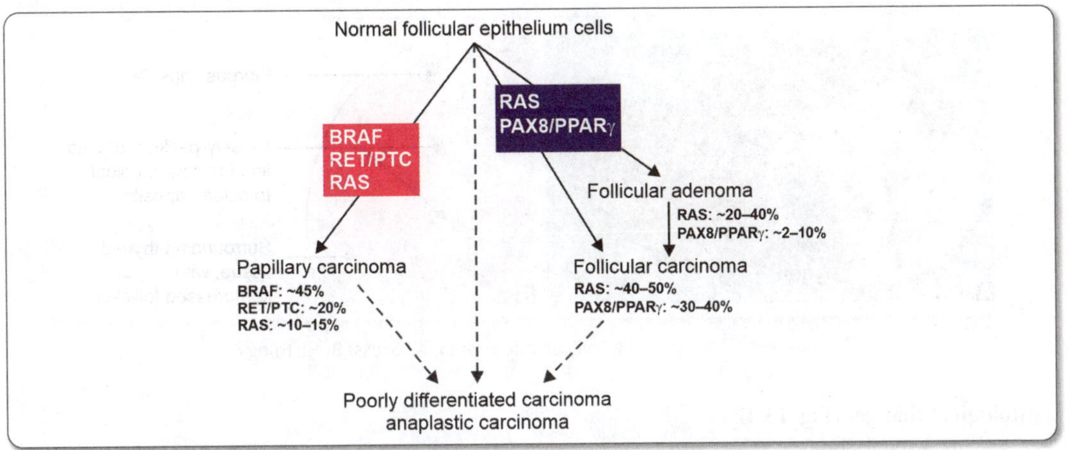

Figure 13.3: Development of thyroid carcinoma

Note: RAS are point mutations and PAX8-PPAR gamma rearrangement in thyroid tumors; RET is rearrangement of the RET gene, also known as RET/PTC; BRAF is a human gene that encodes a protein called B-Raf.

Follicular Adenoma of Thyroid

Follicular adenoma of thyroid represents the most common benign tumor of the thyroid which is encapsulated. It usually affects individuals in the fourth to fifth decade and is more common in females.

Risk Factors

- Exposure to radiation.
- Iodine deficiency or excess.
- History (personal or family) of thyroid conditions.

Pathogenesis

Monoclonal proliferation caused by mutations in the TSH receptor causes proliferation of follicular epithelial cells. K-RAS and N-RAS mutations may also be seen in cases with a predisposition to transform to the follicular carcinoma.

Clinical Features

Clinically the patient presents with a solitary nodule and is usually euthyroid, i.e., the thyroid shows normal function. Most cases are incidental and are detected during the diagnosis for some other condition. The patient may be completely asymptomatic.

Pathological Changes

The lesion is of follicular cell differentiation.

Gross appearance (Fig. 13.4A)

- Usually solitary and well-delineated.
- Firm, rubbery, gray-white in color. In cases when more colloid, a brownish color may be seen.
- Totally surrounded by a fibrous capsule (encapsulated).
- Cut surface: Homogenous, soft consistency.
- Usually, <3 cm in size.

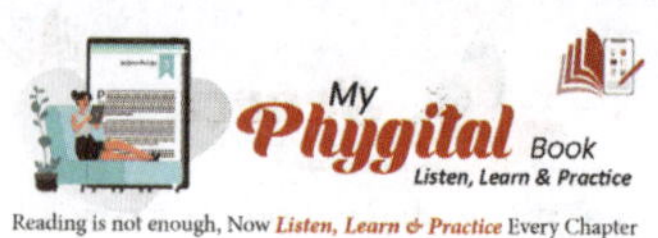

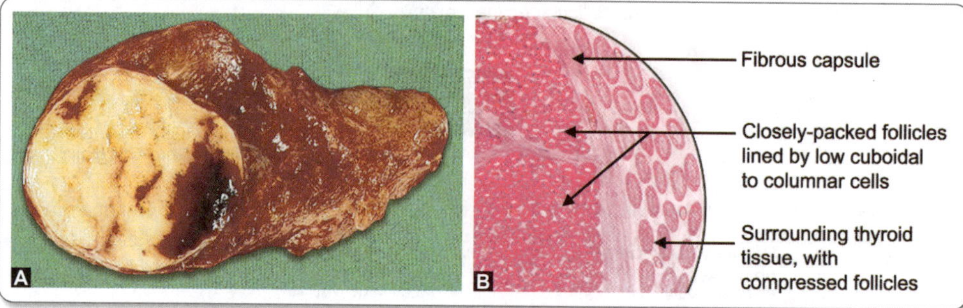

Figures 13.4A and B: Follicular adenoma: **A.** Gross; **B.** Histology

Histological changes (Fig. 13.4B)

- Encapsulated lesion.
- Closely-packed follicles.
- Of various types depending on the pattern of arrangement of cells—microfollicular (small follicle size), macrofollicular (large follicular size), and Hurthle cell type.
- Individual cells usually have regular chromatin with inconspicuous nucleoli and pleomorphism if present does not correlate with biological aggressiveness.
- Surrounding normal thyroid parenchyma (follicles) is compressed.
- Absence of capsular, vascular invasion and extrathyroidal extension differentiates this lesion from follicular carcinoma.

Follicular Carcinoma of Thyroid

Follicular carcinoma of thyroid is the second most common thyroid carcinoma (Fig. 13.4A) and usually occurs in the fourth to fifth decade. It is an aggressive tumor and the patient usually presents with a slowly enlarging neck mass, which is painless. Ultrasonographic examination reveals the presence of a solitary nodule. Metastasis through blood is seen frequently and this tumor spreads to the lungs, bones and liver.

Pathological Changes

Gross appearance (Fig. 13.5A): A solitary lesion which is encapsulated/partially encapsulated.
Cut surface: Soft to firm, pale gray-brown in color. Foci of necrosis and hemorrhage may be seen.
Histological changes (Fig. 13.5B): Tumor cells are arranged as follicles. In some areas, small sheets/trabecular arrangement may also be seen.

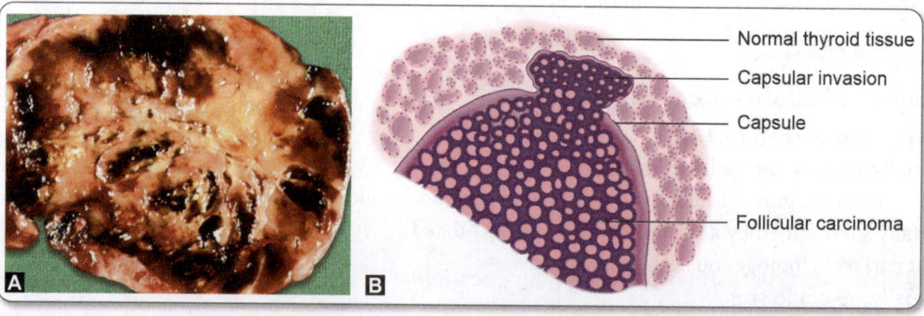

Figures 13.5A and B: Follicular carcinoma: **A.** Gross; **B.** Histology

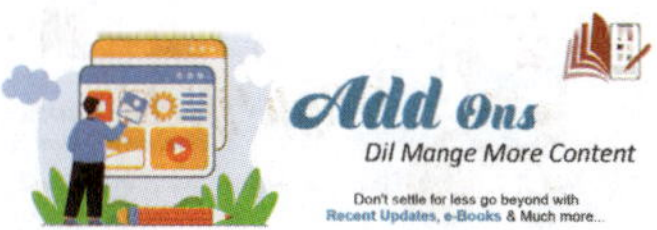

Individual tumor cells are cuboidal and have an increased nucleocytoplasmic ratio with nuclear hyperchromasia and clumped nuclear chromatin.

MUST KNOW

The key diagnostic feature is the presence of full thickness capsular invasion which distinguishes this from the follicular adenoma. Vascular invasion may also be seen.

A thorough sampling must be performed to rule out the presence of any papillary structures and any foci which show nuclear features similar to those seen in papillary carcinoma.

Papillary Carcinoma of Thyroid

Papillary carcinoma of thyroid is the most common malignancy of the thyroid. It is more common in women. The patients often present with a painless neck mass. Cancer spreads through lymph node metastases.

There may be a prior history of exposure to ionizing radiation or nuclear radiation. An association with Hashimoto's thyroiditis is also documented.

Types of Papillary Thyroid Carcinoma

Common variants of the papillary thyroid carcinoma include:

- Follicular variant
- Tall cell
- Columnar cell
- Hobnail

Pathological Changes

Gross appearance (Fig. 13.6A): The lesion is gray-white in color and may be solid or solid-cystic.

Cut surface is firm and may or may not show the presence of papillae grossly. Foci of calcification may also be seen.

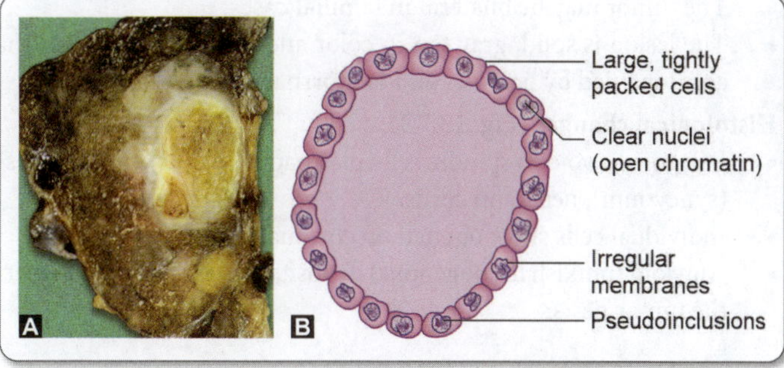

Figures 13.6A and B: Papillary thyroid carcinoma: **A.** Gross; **B.** Histology

Histological changes (Fig. 13.6B): Certain histological features are characteristic of a papillary carcinoma. These include:

- The presence of papillary structures with fibrovascular cores.
- Nuclear features include:
  - Nuclear pseudoinclusions
  - Nuclear grooves
  - Orphan Annie-eyed nuclei
  - Psammoma bodies
- The tumor shows an infiltrative growth pattern.

Immunohistochemistry: The morphological features of papillary thyroid carcinoma are usually sufficient for a diagnosis. However, in challenging cases, the IHC markers required to make a diagnosis include: CK7, PAX-8, Thyroglobulin.

In some cases when associated with BRAF mutation, IHC for BRAF may be positive.

Medullary Carcinoma of Thyroid

Medullary carcinoma of thyroid is a neuroendocrine tumor, the cell of origin being the parafollicular C cells. Medullary carcinoma is commonly seen in the 5th to 6th decade of life.

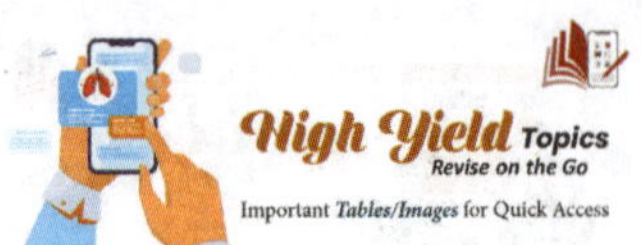

Etiology

Medullary carcinomas are rare in comparison to other tumors comprising <2% of all thyroid malignancies. RET gene mutations are important in the pathogenesis of familial medullary carcinoma.

Pathogenicity

In medullary carcinoma, calcitonin is produced, and elevated calcitonin level is an essential feature of this tumor. In some cases, other hormones such as somatostatin, ACTH and serotonin are produced. Most (70–80%) cases are sporadic (nonhereditary). The remaining cases are familial and are seen in association with MEN 2A/2B syndromes or neurofibromatosis.

Clinical Features

The patient presents with a neck mass with or without enlarged lymph nodes. In some cases, the tumor is detected incidentally on imaging. On thyroid scan, it is a "cold nodule".

Pathological Changes

Gross appearance (Fig 13.7A): Grossly, the tumor is either a single nodule (more common in the sporadic cases) or multiple (in familial cases).

- The tumor may be bilateral in familial cases.
- The lesion is solid, gray tan in color and larger sized lesions may be accompanied by necrosis and hemorrhage.

Histological changes (Fig. 13.7B):

- Polygonal/ovoid to spindle cells/plasmacytoid cells arranged as sheets (syncytium), nests and cords.
- Individual cells show opened up chromatin
- Amyloid (pinkish homogenous) deposits may also be seen in-between the tumor nests.

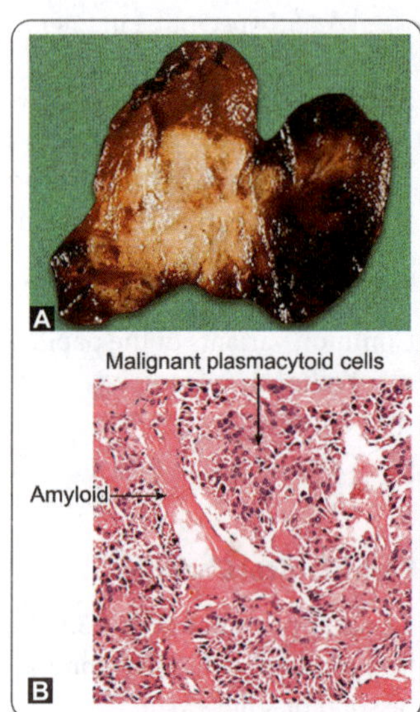

Figures 13.7A and B: Medullary carcinoma: A. Gross; B. Histology

Anaplastic Carcinoma of Thyroid

Anaplastic carcinoma of thyroid represents an infrequent type of thyroid malignancy with prevalence in most geographic areas being <5%.

Anaplastic carcinoma is a malignancy afflicting the elderly (patients in their 7–8th decade) and is biologically aggressive. The mortality rate is high reaching up to 90%.

Etiology

They are believed to arise due to dedifferentiation of previously existing more well-differentiated forms of thyroid carcinoma. p53 mutations are commonly seen in >50% cases.

Clinical Features

Patients usually present with shortness of breath (dyspnea), difficulty in swallowing (dysphagia) and voice hoarseness along with a neck mass that is unusually hard on palpation.

Imaging studies usually reveal a mass lesion displaying extensive invasion and destruction of surrounding structures such as the trachea, esophagus and regional soft tissue.

Pathological Changes

Gross appearance (Fig. 13.8A): Grossly, the tumor is large and irregular with a markedly hard consistency. The tumor commonly invades the surrounding structures.

Cut surface: Brownish/dirty-white in color, hard, having a variegated (variable) appearance with areas of necrosis and hemorrhage.

Histological changes (Fig. 13.8B): The tumor is poorly differentiated. Individual tumor cells may show varying shapes and sizes, i.e., they may be spindle shaped or be in the form of bizarre giant cells showing marked pleomorphism, hypercellularity and atypical mitotic figures. Some of the cells may appear squamoid/epithelioid. Foci of necrosis are usually seen with tumor cells displaying angiotropism (predilection to invade vessels).

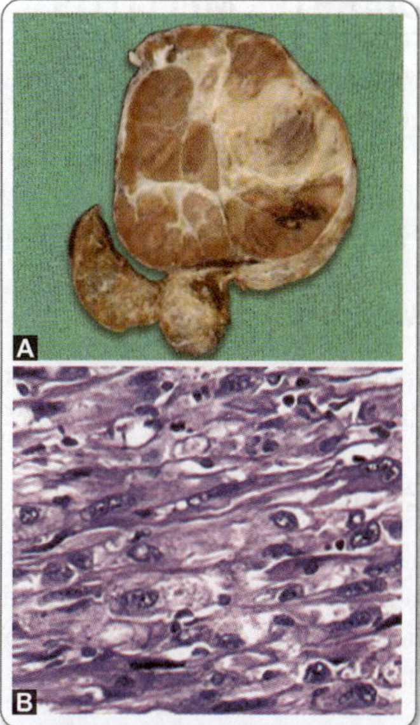

Figures 13.8A and B: Anaplastic carcinoma: **A.** Gross; **B.** Histology

OVERVIEW OF PANCREATIC GLAND

The pancreas (Fig. 13.9) lies transversely in the upper abdomen between the duodenum on the right and the spleen on the left. The pancreas is divided into four parts: Head, neck, body, and tail. The right side of the organ that is head lies on the inferior vena cava and the renal vein; and is surrounded by the C loop of the duodenum. The head is the widest part. The tapered left side extends slightly upward and is called the body of the pancreas, it ends near the spleen and is called the tail.

Functions

The pancreas has dual roles-it is an organ of the digestive system and of the endocrine system. The exocrine pancreas produces enzymes that help digest food, particularly protein. The endocrine pancreas makes the hormone insulin, which helps to control blood sugar levels.

Note that the pancreatitis and tumors of pancreas are given in chapter liver, gallbladder and pancreas. Here, in this chapter we are focusing on the disease caused due to dysfunction of pancreatic secretions and its impact on glucose metabolism.

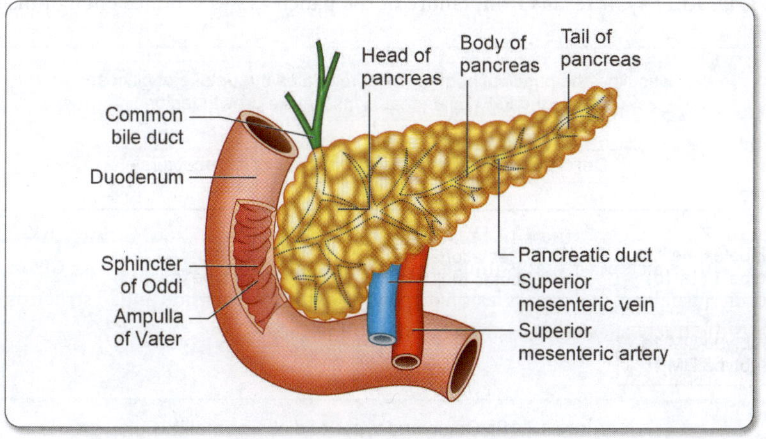

Figure 13.9: Anatomy of pancreas

DIABETES MELLITUS

Diabetes mellitus is a group of metabolic disease in which the blood levels of sugar are high over a prolonged period. The body obtains glucose from three main places:

1. The intestinal absorption of food.
2. The breakdown of glycogen, the storage form of glucose found in the liver.
3. Gluconeogenesis, the generation of glucose from noncarbohydrate substrates in the body.

Mechanism

Insulin is the principal hormone that regulates the glucose metabolism. Its dysregulation is associated with diabetes mellitus (DM) type I, DM type 2 and gestational DM (Fig. 13.10).

Etiology

The etiology of type 2 diabetes mellitus appears to involve complex interactions between environmental and genetic factors. Presumably, the disease develops when a diabetogenic lifestyle (i.e., excessive caloric intake, inadequate caloric expenditure, obesity) is superimposed on a susceptible genotype. Type 1 diabetes is mainly due to genetic factors.

Pathogenesis

Diabetes is due to either the pancreas not producing enough insulin or the cells of the body not responding properly to the insulin produced.

Insulin is released into the blood by beta cells (β-cells), found in the islets of Langerhans in the pancreas, in response to rising levels of blood glucose, typically after eating.

Lower glucose levels result in decreased insulin release from the beta cells; thereby resulting in the breakdown of glycogen to glucose.

This process is mainly controlled by the hormone glucagon, which acts in the opposite manner to insulin.

Classification of DM

There are three main types of diabetes mellitus:

Type 1: It is partly inherited, with multiple genes, including certain HLA genotypes, known to influence the risk of diabetes (Fig. 13.11A). It results from failure of the pancreas's to produce enough insulin. This form

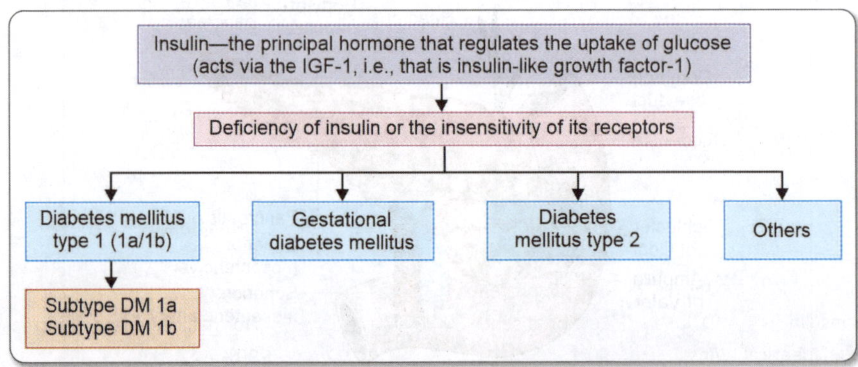

Figure 13.10: Origin and types of diabetes mellitus

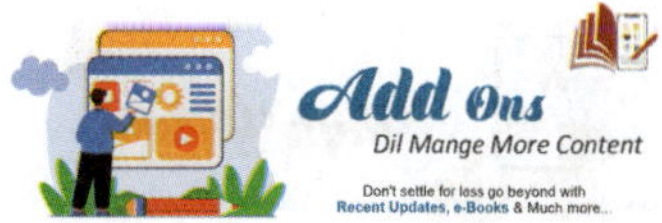

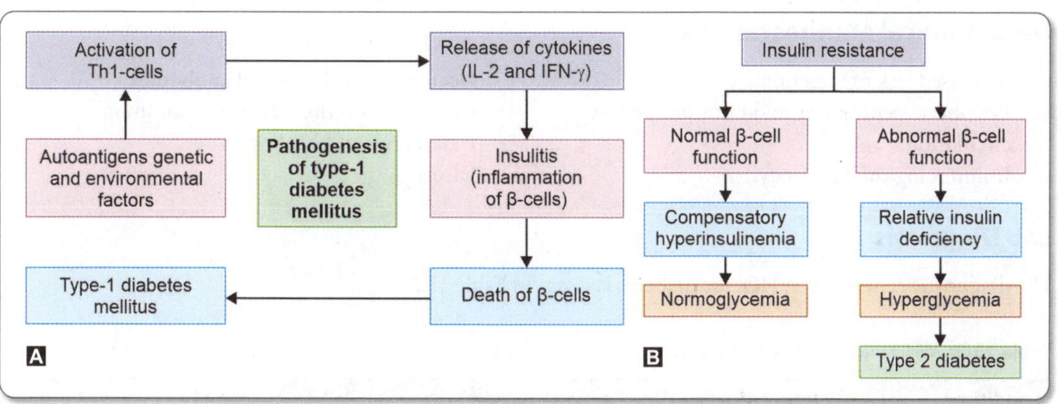

Figures 13.11A and B: Diabetes mellitus: **A.** Type 1; **B.** Type 2
Abbreviations: Th1, T helper cells; IL-2, Interleukin-2; IFN-γ, Interferon-gamma

was previously referred to as "insulin dependent diabetes mellitus" (IDDM) or "juvenile diabetes". The cause is unknown.

- In genetically susceptible people, the onset of diabetes can be triggered by one or more environmental factors, such as a viral infection or diet.
- Among dietary factors, gluten may lead to type 1 diabetes.

Type 2: Type 2 DM is characterized by insulin resistance. The defective responsiveness of body tissues to insulin is believed to involve the insulin receptor. Type 2 DM is primarily due to lifestyle factors and genetics (Fig. 13.11B). It begins with insulin resistance, a condition in which cells fail to respond to insulin properly. This form was previously referred to as "non-insulin-dependent diabetes mellitus" (NIDDM) or "adult-onset diabetes". The primary cause is excessive body weight and not enough exercise.

Gestational diabetes: It is the third main form and occurs in pregnant women without a previous history of diabetes.

Comparison between features of Type 1 and Type 2 diabetes mellitus is given in Table 13.1.

Clinical Symptoms

Frequent urination, increased thirst and increased hunger are some of the most common symptoms. It can cause many complications such as heart disease, stroke, chronic kidney failure, foot ulcers, damage to the eyes, diabetic ketoacidosis, nonketotic hyperosmolar coma, or death.

Table 13.1: Comparison between Type 1 and Type 2 diabetes mellitus

Features	Type 1 diabetes mellitus	Type 2 diabetes mellitus
Onset	Sudden	Gradual
Age at onset	Mostly in children	Mostly in adults
Body size	Thin or normal	Often obese
Ketoacidosis	Common	Rare
Autoantibodies	Usually present	Absent
Endogenous insulin	Low or absent	Normal, decreased or increased
Concordance in identical twins	50%	90%
Prevalence	~10%	~90%

Other Clinical Manifestations

- Increased risk of infection.
- Peripheral neuropathy and poor peripheral circulation.
- Immunological deficiency.
- Decreased production of antibodies.
- Candidal infections are more common.
- Delayed wound healing.
- Ulcers.

Lab Diagnosis

The diagnostic criteria by WHO, for diabetes is given in Table 13.2.

Table 13.2: WHO diabetes diagnostic criteria

Condition	2 hours glucose	Fasting glucose	HbA1c	
Unit	mmol/l (mg/dL)	mmol/L (mg/dL)	mmol/mol	DCCT %
Normal	<7.8 (<140)	<6.1 (<110)	<42	<6.0
Diabetes mellitus	≥11.1 (≥200)	≥7.0 (≥126)	≥48	≥6.5

MUST KNOW

GESTATIONAL DIABETES

Increased levels of insulin in a fetus's blood may inhibit fetal surfactant production and cause respiratory distress syndrome. In severe cases, perinatal death may occur, as a result of poor placental perfusion due to vascular impairment. Labor induction may be indicated with decreased placental function. A cesarean section may be performed if there is marked fetal distress or an increased risk of injury associated with macrosomia, such as shoulder dystocia.

Risks to the baby include:

- Macrosomia (high birth weight)
- Congenital heart defects
- Central nervous system abnormalities
- Skeletal muscle malformations
- Untreated gestational diabetes can damage the health of the fetus or mother.

Lab Diagnosis

It can be diagnosed by any method from the following:

- Fasting plasma glucose level ≥7.0 mmol/L (126 mg/dL)
- Plasma glucose ≥11.1 mmol/L (200 mg/dL) two hours after a 75 g oral glucose load as in a glucose tolerance test.
- Symptoms of high blood sugar and casual plasma glucose ≥11.1 mmol/L (200 mg/dL)
- Glycated hemoglobin (HbA1c) ≥48 mmol/mol (≥6.5 DCCT %)

SUMMARY

- The hallmark sign of goiter is reduced T3, T4 levels which in turn leads to an elevated TSH.
- Development of thyroid carcinomas is multifactorial and includes external influences, as well as constitutional predispositions and genetic factors.
- Follicular carcinoma of thyroid is an aggressive tumor and the patient usually presents with a slowly enlarging neck mass, which is painless.
- Papillary thyroid carcinoma is the most common malignancy of the thyroid. It is more common in women.
- Medullary carcinomas are rare in comparison to other tumors.
- In medullary carcinoma, calcitonin is produced, and elevated calcitonin level is an essential feature of this tumor.
- Anaplastic carcinoma is a malignancy afflicting the elderly (patients in their 7th-8th decade) and is biologically aggressive.

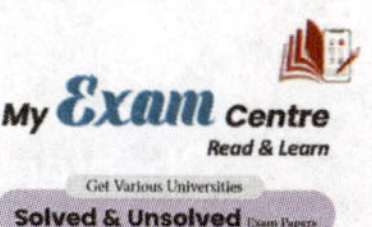

ASSESS YOURSELF

Long Answer Questions

1. Discuss carcinoma of thyroid in detail.
2. Explain diabetes mellitus in detail.

Short Answer Questions

1. Write in brief about papillary carcinoma.
2. What is anaplastic carcinoma?
3. Write short notes on:
   i. Type 1 and Type 2 diabetes
   ii. Types of goiter.

Multiple Choice Questions

1. **Iodine deficiency can cause:**
   a. Goiter
   b. Thyroid cancer
   c. Solitary thyroid nodules
   d. Thyroiditis
2. **Which of the following is correct about medullary thyroid carcinoma?**
   a. Arises from follicular cells
   b. May be associated with pheochromocytoma
   c. Low serum calcitonin is found
   d. Mutation of P53 is genetic marker
   e. Not hormone dependent
3. **Which of the following proteins is the precursor for the thyroid hormone, and also a marker of thyroidal cancer?**
   a. Thyroid albumin
   b. Thyroglobulin
   c. Thyroid binding globulin
   d. All of these
4. **Which of the following is the screening test for the diagnosis of thyroid disease?**
   a. Thyroid Stimulating hormone
   b. Total T3
   c. Total T4
   d. Free T3
5. **Which type of thyroid carcinoma comprises a large majority of all thyroid cancers? [Choose One]**
   a. Anaplastic
   b. Follicular
   c. Medullary
   d. Papillary
6. **Thyroglobulin secretion is preserved in __________ thyroid carcinoma. [Choose One]**
   a. Follicular
   b. Papillary
   c. A or B
   d. None of these
7. **Comparing follicular and papillary types of thyroid carcinoma, __________ carcinoma is more malignant and __________ carcinoma metastases are more responsive to radioiodine therapy. [Choose One]**
   a. Follicular; follicular
   b. Follicular; papillary
   c. Papillary; follicular
   d. Papillary; papillary
8. **Rapid thyroid enlargement that occurs alongside Hashimoto thyroiditis confirms a diagnosis of anaplastic thyroid carcinoma.**
   a. True
   b. False

Answer Key

1. a	**2.** b	**3.** b	**4.** a	**5.** d	**6.** c
7. a	**8.** b				

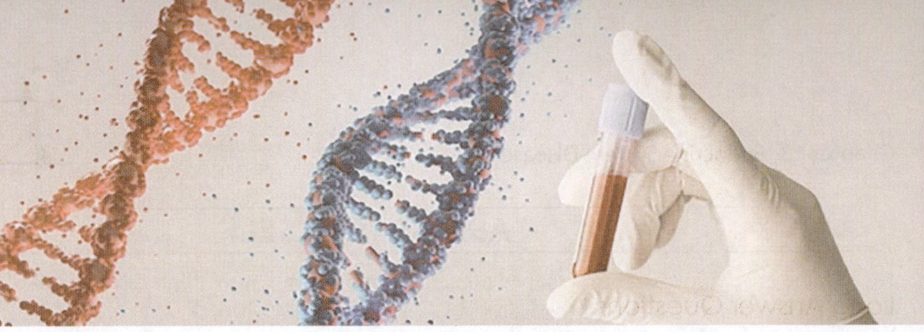

Chapter 14

Kidneys and Urinary Tract Diseases

LEARNING OBJECTIVES

After the completion of the chapter, the readers will be able to:

- Understand glomerulonephritis.
- Explain pathology of pyelonephritis.
- Know about renal calculi and cystitis.
- Understand renal cell carcinoma.
- Understand about renal failure.

CHAPTER OUTLINE

- Overview of Urinary System

Diseases of Kidney and Urinary Tract

- Glomerulonephritis
- Pyelonephritis
- Xanthogranulomatous Pyelonephritis
- Renal Calculi or Kidney Stones
- Cystitis
- Renal Cell Carcinoma
- Renal Failure

KEY TERMS

Anuria: No urine formation.

Azotemia: Increased blood urea nitrogen and creatinine, due to declining GFR.

Cystoscopy: Evaluating the urinary bladder with a fiber optic instrument.

Dialysis: A procedure for cleansing the blood of waste products in individuals with complete kidney failure or who have had kidneys removed by surgery.

Diffuse: Renal pathology involving all glomeruli.

Enuresis: Involuntary release of urine, most often in reference to bed-wetting.

Focal: Renal pathology involving some glomeruli.

Global: A process is global if the entire glomerulus tuft is involved.

Glomerulonephritis: Inflammation of the glomerular compartment of the kidney.

Hydronephrosis: Abnormal condition involving back up of urine into the kidney.

Lipiduria: Excretion of lipid into the urine.

Nephrosis: A noninflammatory disease of kidneys.

Nocturia: Frequently getting up and urinating during the night.

Oliguria: Reduced urine formation.

Polyuria: Frequent urination.

Proteinuria: Excretion of protein into the urine.

Segmental: Part of the glomerulus involved.

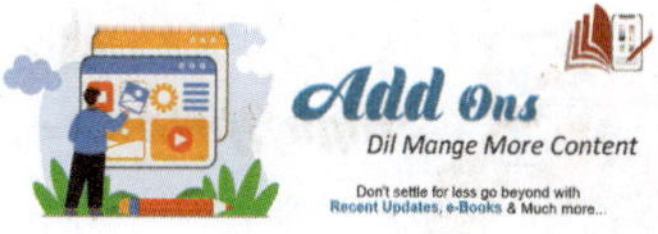

OVERVIEW OF URINARY SYSTEM

The kidneys are reniform or bean-shaped organs covered with an outer thin capsule. The kidney weighs 150 g in males and around 125–130 g in females.

Kidneys

Cut surface: On cut surface three major zones of the kidney are identified—outer cortex, inner medulla and renal pelvis.

1. **Cortex:** Shows the presence of nephrons represented by the glomeruli.
2. **Medulla:** Shows the presence of renal pyramids with the base toward the cortex and the apex of each pyramid representing the renal papilla.
3. **Renal pelvis with hilum:** Zone of the kidney where the urine collects briefly before being excreted out through the ureter. Minor calyces in this area act as conduits for urine in the renal papilla which further passes into the major calyces.

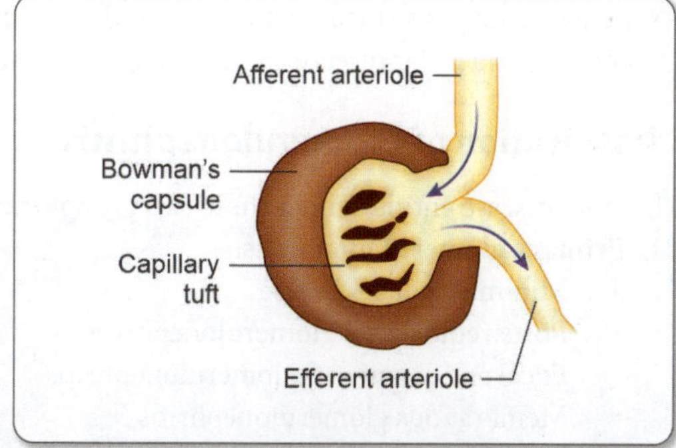

Figure 14.1: Glomerulus showing efferent and afferent arterioles

Histological compartments of urinary system kidneys:

All renal diseases can be categorized based on the four major histological compartments of the kidney—Glomeruli, tubules, interstitium and vessels.

1. **Glomerulus:** The glomerulus is a conglomerate of capillary tufts; the afferent arteriole enters the tuft and the efferent ("e"- exit) goes out of the tuft (Fig. 14.1).
2. **Tubular system:** The tubular system comprises proximal convoluted tubules, loop of Henle, distal convoluted tubules and collecting ducts (Fig. 14.2).
   - Proximal convoluted tubule is the longest part of the renal tubule lined by cuboidal epithelium with a brush border.
   - Loop of Henle has a thick descending portion (pars recta), a thin descending portion, a thin ascending portion, and a thick ascending portion. Its lumen is made up of simple squamous epithelium.
   - Distal convoluted tubules are less numerous than the proximal convoluted tubules and these are lined by cuboidal epithelial cells.
   - Collecting tubules are not part of the nephron. These are lined with cuboidal or columnar epithelium. Collecting tubules reasborb the water in response to the hormone vasopressin; and resorb sodium in response to the hormone aldosterone.

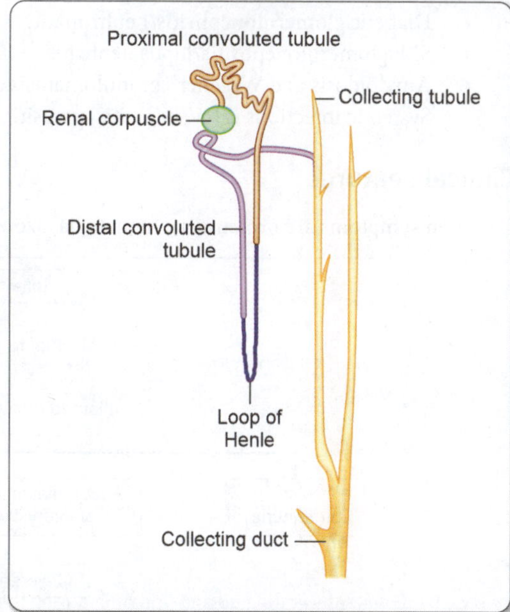

Figure 14.2: Tubular system

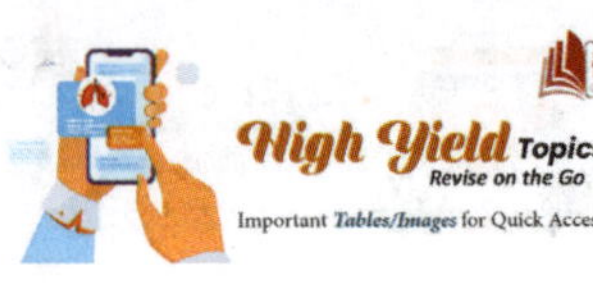

3. **Interstitium:** It is a supporting or connective tissue placed between the principal cellss of an organ or between structures in the body.
4. **Vessels:** Blood flows into kidney through renal artery. This large blood vessels are divided into smaller blood vessels until the blood reaches the nephrons.

DISEASES OF KIDNEY AND URINARY TRACT

GLOMERULONEPHRITIS

As the name suggests this refers to kidney disease in which there is inflammation/injury at the level of the glomeruli. Glomerular disease can be classified broadly as primary and secondary (systemic).

Classification of Glomerulonephritis

The main disease entities under these two groups include:

1. **Primary glomerulonephritis:**
   - Minimal change disease
   - Poststreptococcal glomerulonephritis
   - Focal and segmental glomerulonephritis
   - Membranous glomerulonephritis
   - Rapidly progressive glomerulonephritis (Crescentic glomerulonephritis)
   - Membranoproliferative glomerulonephritis
2. **Secondary (systemic) glomerulonephritis:**
   - Diabetic glomerulonephritis/nephropathy
   - SLE glomerulonephritis/lupus nephritis
   - Amyloidosis and Wegener's granulomatosis associated glomerulonephritis
   - Systemic infections (HIV, hepatitis, parasitic infections) causing glomerulonephritis

Clinical Features

Common symptoms are proteinuria, hematuria, azotemia, oliguria, anuria, edema, hypertension (Fig. 14.3)

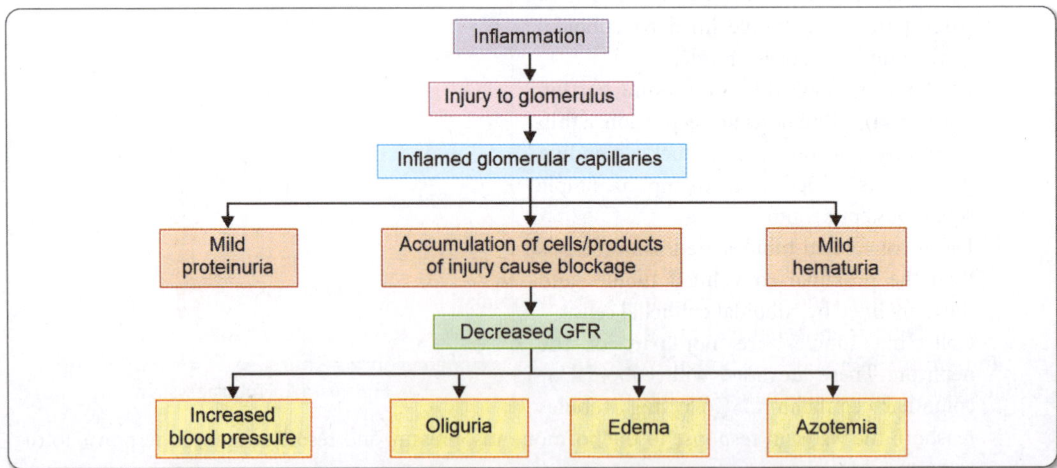

Figure 14.3: Clinical symptoms of glomerulonephritis

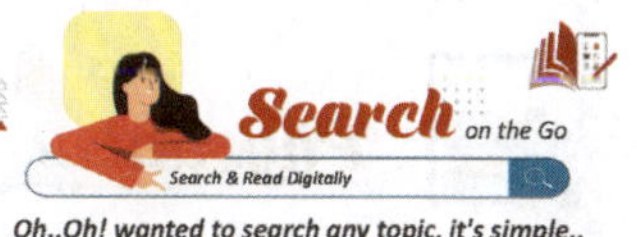

Etiology

Glomerulonephritis can be caused by various factors including:
- Viral infections, such as HIV, hepatitis B and C viruses.
- Toxins or drugs.
- IgA nephropathy.
- Lupus-related kidney inflammation.

Risk Factors

- Sore throat (due to streptococcal infection).
- Hereditary diseases.
- Diabetes.
- High blood pressure.
- Immune diseases such as SLE.
- Endocarditis.
- Vasculitis.
- Viral infections such as HIV, hepatitis B, hepatitis C.

Primary Glomerulonephritis

Minimal Change Disease

CASE SCENARIO 1

A 5-year-old child presents to the OPD with puffy eyes and retarded growth for the age.

Clinical Features

This disease affects young children (most cases between 2 and 5 years of age), presenting with massive proteinuria leading to renal edema (nephrotic range proteinuria). The glomerular basement membrane loses its integrity and spills protein, red blood cells and other substance into the urine (Fig. 14.4).

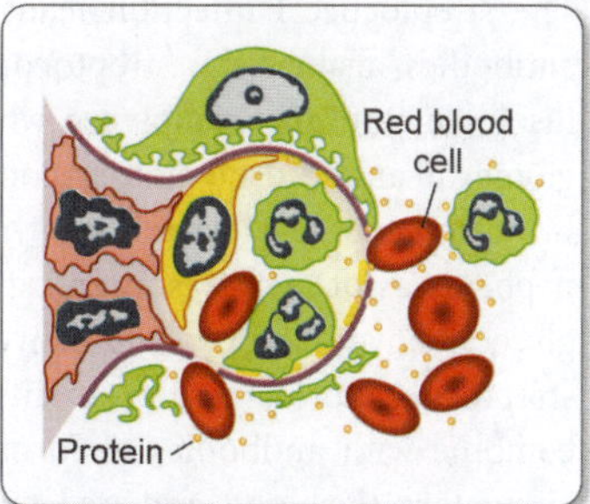

Figure 14.4: Minimal change disease

Pathogenesis

Minimal change disease is believed to be immune mediated despite the fact that immunofluorescence or electron microscopy does not reveal immune deposits per se.

Immune defects → Liberation of cytokines → Direct injury to the visceral epithelial cells → Reduced adhesion → Stripping off of the visceral epithelial cells → Proteinuria.

Pathological Features

Light microscopy: Reveals no significant change as the name suggests "Minimal change disease"

It is primarily a diagnosis by ultrastructural analysis, however, the observations under light microscope are as follows:
- **Glomeruli:** Normal size and cellularity.
- **Tubules:** Proximal and distal tubules may show accumulation of lipid, hence, the name is lipoid nephrosis. Proximal tubular epithelial cells can also show the presence of protein reabsorption droplets.
- **Interstitium:** May show the presence of foam cells, as evidence of proteinuria.
- **Vessels:** No significant changes seen.

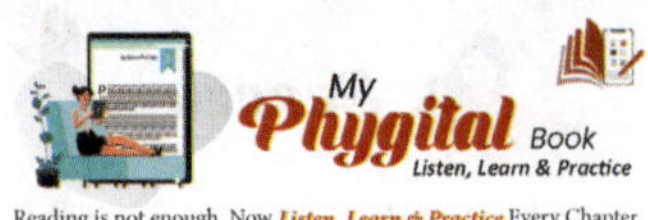

Electron microscopy: Reveals diffuse effacement of the foot processes.

- The glomerular basement membrane remains of normal thickness.
- There is a loss of slit diaphragm.

Immunofluorescence: No immunoglobulin highlighted/complement seen, i.e., no IgG/C3 deposits.
Prognosis: Usually responds to steroids, self-limiting

Poststreptococcal Glomerulonephritis

Poststreptococcal glomerulonephritis (PSGN) is a disease of children and the young, the most frequent age group is 5–15 years.

CASE SCENARIO 2

A 10-year-old child presents to the OPD with puffy eyes smoky urine and blood pressure of 170/100 mm Hg. There was a past episode of sore throat 2 weeks back.

Clinical Features

The patient presents with features of nephritic syndrome, i.e., smoky urine, puffy face, hypertension.

Risk Factors

A prior episode of pharyngitis; infection of skin or oral cavity (1–4 weeks earlier) is usual.

Pathogenesis

The streptococcal infection leads to formation of specific antibodies against the streptococcal antigen. These form insoluble immune complexes which get deposited in the glomeruli and leads to glomerulonephritis (Fig. 14.5).

Streptococcus bacterium has antigens which are nephritis-associated plasmin receptor (NAPLr), identified as glyceraldehyde-3-phosphate dehydrogenase (GAPDH); and streptococcal proteinase exotoxin B (SPEB). These antigens combine with antibodies to form immune complexes that circulate in the blood, and are later trapped in the glomeruli. Immune complex deposition in PSGN occurs either beneath the visceral epithelial cell (subepithelial), or beneath the endothelial cell (subendothelial), or within the mesangium. The trapped immune complexes also lead to inflammatory cell recruitment.

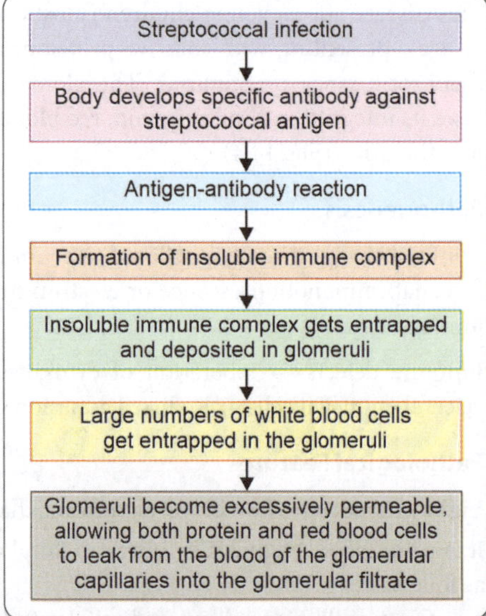

Figure 14.5: Pathogenesis of glomerulonephritis

Pathological Changes

Light microscopy: Reveals the following changes:

- **Glomeruli:** All show an increased cellularity and size (diffuse pathology). Hypercellularity is due to:
  - Mesangial expansion due to immune complexes.
  - The presence of polymorphonuclear cells/monocytes within the capillary lumina (>10 polymorphs/capillary lumina).
  - Swelling of endothelial cells and their proliferation, with presence of subendothelial deposits.
  - Thickening of the capillary wall due to subepithelial deposits resembling camel humps.

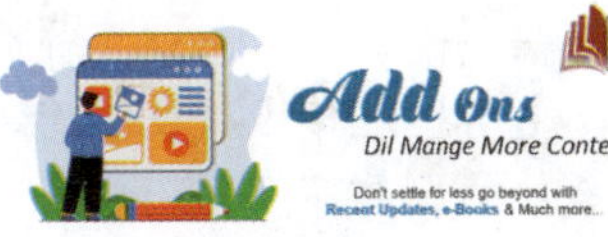

- **Tubules:** Mild inflammation may be seen.
- **Interstitium:** May show inflammation and edema.
- **Vessels:** No significant changes seen.

Electron microscopy: Reveals electron dense deposits in subepithelial or mesangial or subendothelial locations.

Immunofluorescence: 'Lumpy bumpy' or highly granular deposits of IgG, IgM and C3 in the mesangium, subendothelial or subepithelial location.

Other tests are as follows:

- Serum ASO—increased
- Serum C3 levels—decreased

Prognosis: Usually, a self-limiting illness with children recovering quickly and completely within a few weeks. Affected adults may develop chronic glomerulonephritis.

Focal and Segmental Glomerulonephritis

Focal and segmental glomerulosclerosis (FSGS) is a disease in which scar tissue develops on the glomeruli, the small parts of the kidneys that filter waste from the blood (Fig. 14.6). The patient presents with nephrotic range proteinuria. FSGS is not a specific disease per se but a manifestation of disease.

It is characterized by:

- Focal involvement, i.e., only a few glomeruli are involved.
- Segmental involvement, i.e., within a glomerulus, only a part of the glomerulus is affected. The key features are as follows:
  - Sclerosis, which is the obliteration of the capillary lumina by plasma proteins.
  - Foam cells.
  - Proliferating extracellular matrix material.

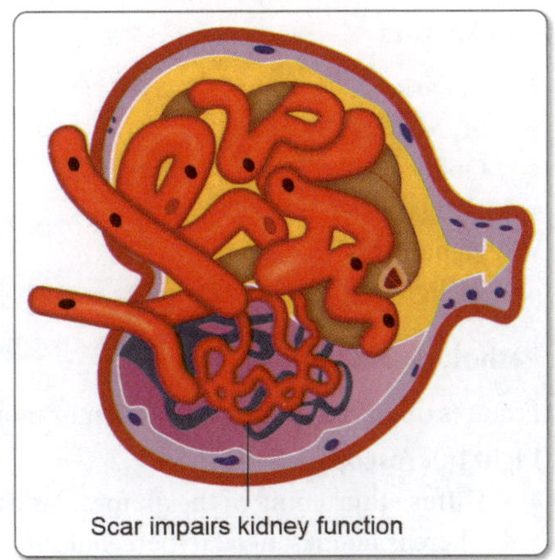

Figure 14.6: Focal and segmental glomerulonephritis

Pathological Features

- **Light microscopy:** Glomeruli present at the junction of the glomerular cortex and the medulla are involved, i.e., juxtamedullary involvement.
  - The visceral epithelial cell podocytes shows hypertrophy.
  - Fat cells accumulate in the capillary lumina.
  - Fat cells and endothelial lining degenerate.
  - Along with degenerated fat, plasma proteins precipitate forming an insudative lesion "hyalinosis".
  - Mesangial matrix is increased—sclerosis with or without hyalinosis.
  - Special stains reveal—accumulation of acellular PAS positive material.
  - Tubules—areas of tubular atrophy common.
- **Electron microscope:** Foot process obliterated, vacuolization of foot processes; no immune complexes.
- **Immunofluorescence:** Focal and segmental IgM, C3 deposits.
- **Prognosis:** Response to steroids is poor.

Special Variants of FSGS

- **Collapsing glomerulopathy:**
  - This is associated with HIV associated nephropathy

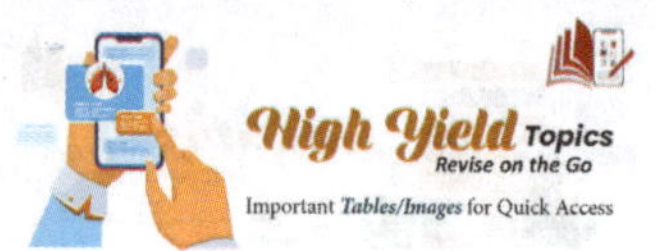

  - Precipitation of plasma proteins in the capillary lumina.
  - Marked alteration at the level of the visceral epithelial cells with evidence of enlargement and vacuolation.
- Glomerular tip lesion-segmental sclerosis, at the tip of capillary tufts.

Membranous Glomerulonephritis

Membranous glomerulonephritis is deposition of immune complexes on the glomerular basement membrane (GBM) with GBM thickening (Fig. 14.7). The patient presents with nephrotic range proteinuria.

Etiology

- Due to *in situ* immune complex deposition.
- Due to a planted antigen-antibody reaction.

Risk Factors

- Malaria
- SLE
- Gold
- Drugs
- Hepatitis B
- Malignancy

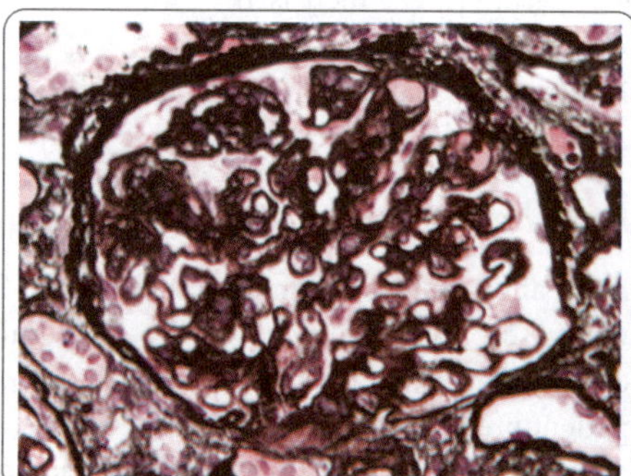

Figure 14.7: Membranous glomerulonephritis—histology

Pathological Changes

Features observed in the case of membranous glomerulonephritis are as follows:

Light microscopy:

- Diffuse thickening of the glomerular capillary walls.
- There is no mesangial hypercellularity.
- There are no inflammatory cells in the glomeruli.
- There are three further stages:
  1. Subepithelial deposits without spikes.
  2. Spikes between the subepithelial deposits. Deposits engulfed by thickened basement membrane.
  3. Spikes—positive on silver stain.

Immunofluorescence: Diffuse subepithelial or intramembranous deposits of IgG/C3; slow progression to renal failure.

Rapidly Progressive Glomerulonephritis

CASE SCENARIO 3

Previously healthy 55-year-old female came with complaints of macular hyperchromic lesions on the soles of her feet. After taking some medication, the patient developed oliguria, lower limb edema, and abdominal pain, mainly in the hypogastrium along with nausea and hyporexia.

Clinical Features

The patient presents with a rapid decline in kidney function with acute renal failure. The overall presentation is that of nephritic syndrome with affected patients presenting with a decline in urine output, hematuria, hypertension and nephritic range proteinuria.

Rapidly progressive glomerulonephritis (RPGN) is also known as crescentic glomerulonephritis in view of the histological presence of crescents in the glomeruli on analysis of renal biopsy tissue. Most authors have defined this as the presence of crescents in >50% glomeruli, though recent studies suggest even a cut off of 30% is appropriate for the diagnosis.

Etiopathogenetic Types

Type I: Antiglomerular basement membrane antibodies are found as linear deposits of IgG, C3 deposits in the glomerular basement membrane and along capillaries. In this type, antibodies to the GBM develop and deposit in the glomerular basement membrane and also potentially cross-react with the lung alveolar basement membrane, as seen in Goodpasture syndrome.

Type II: Granular IgG, C3 deposits in the glomerular basement membrane and capillary wall. This type is mediated by circulating immune complexes which are seen in postinfectious cases or autoimmune disease like SLE.

Type III (Pauci-immune): No deposits of IgG, C3 along the GBM/capillaries.

Histological Changes

Glomeruli: The key diagnostic hallmark is the presence of "crescents". This is nothing but an extracapillary proliferation of visceral epithelial cells and or fibrosis in the Bowman's capsule, i.e., crescents may be cellular or fibrous, the latter having a poor prognosis. In cases of cellular proliferation, the cells should be at least two layers thick partially or completely occluding the Bowman's space.

Tubules: Plasma proteins may precipitate forming hyaline droplets.

Interstitium: Varying degrees of chronic inflammation may be seen.

Vessels: Usually normal, however in cases with associated hypertension, splitting of the internal elastic lamina may be seen.

Prognosis

Crescentic glomerulonephritis represents a medical emergency and prompt institution of steroids is essential to improve outcomes which despite treatment are poor.

Membranoproliferative Glomerulonephritis

Membranoproliferative glomerulonephritis (MPGN) is a form of glomerulonephritis caused by an abnormal immune response. The patient presents with nephrotic range proteinuria in children and young adults. There is slow progression to renal failure.

Etiology

- Due to *in situ* immune complex deposition.
- Due to a planted antigen-antibody reaction.

Classification

These are of three types: (1) Type I, (2) Type II, (3) Type III depending on site of deposits.

Pathological Changes

Light microscopy:

- Lobular accentuation of the capillary tuft.
- Thick glomerular basement membrane.
- Increased cellularity of the glomeruli due to mesangial cell proliferation and endocapillary proliferation, hence, this condition is also called mesangiocapillary glomerulonephritis.

- Capillary loops show a "tram track appearance" or a "double contour" which is highlighted on Jones Methanamine Silver PAS stain.

  Immunofluorescence: Diffuse subepithelial/intramembranous deposits of IgG/C3.

Secondary Glomerulonephritis

Diabetic Glomerulonephritis Nephropathy

Diabetic nephropathy, also known as diabetic kidney disease is a complication of diabetes mellitus that affects the kidneys. It is a leading cause of end-stage renal disease (ESRD).

Etiology

Primarily associated with diabetes mellitus, both type 1 and type 2.

Risk Factors

- **Duration of diabetes:** The longer a person has diabetes, the higher the risk of developing diabetic nephropathy.
- **Poorly controlled blood sugar:** Inadequate management of blood glucose levels increases the risk of kidney complications.
- **Hypertension:** Hypertension is a common coexisting condition that accelerates the progression of diabetic nephropathy.

Pathogenesis

Prolonged hyperglycemia leads to the activation of various pathways, including the polyol pathway, protein kinase C (PKC) pathway, advanced glycation end products (AGEs) formation, and activation of the renin-angiotensin-aldosterone system (RAAS). These pathways contribute to oxidative stress, inflammation, and fibrosis in the kidneys, leading to structural and functional changes.

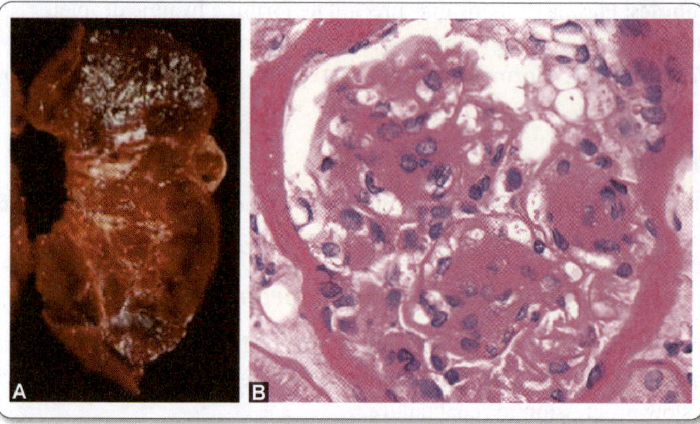

Figures 14.8A and B: Diabetic nephropathy: **A.** Gross; **B.** Histology

Pathological Changes

Gross appearance: Kidneys may appear normal or slightly enlarged in the early stages. In advanced stages, there may be evidence of renal hypertrophy (Fig. 14.8A)

Histological changes: The histopathological changes are depicted in Figure 14.9.

Early stage—Microalbuminuria mild proteinuria.

Management: Management of diabetic nephropathy involves tight glycemic control, blood pressure management, and the use of medications targeting the renin-angiotensin-aldosterone system (RAAS). Early detection and intervention are essential (Figs 14.8B and 14.9).

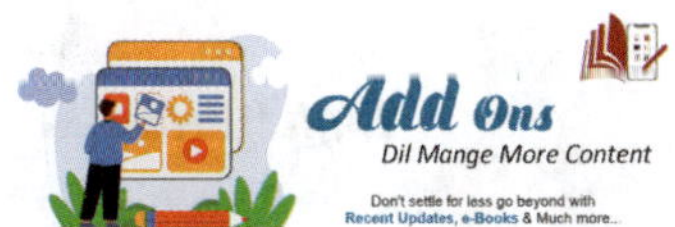

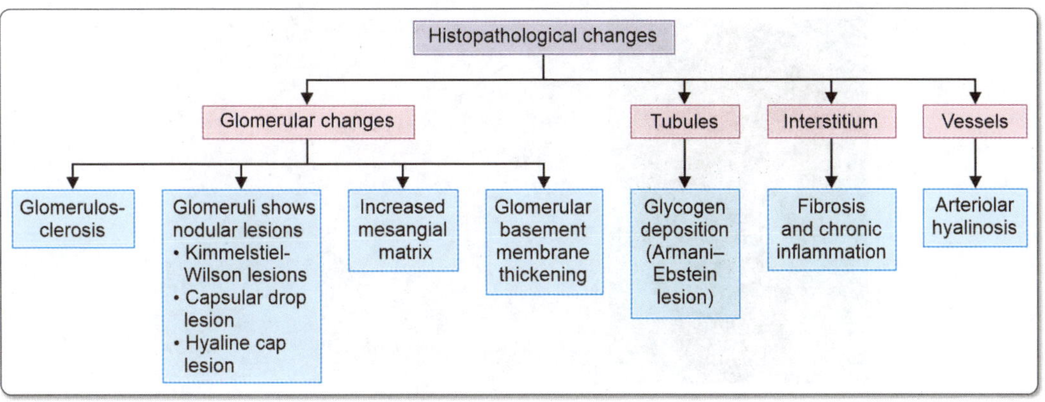

Figure 14.9: Histological changes in diabetic nephropathy

SLE Glomerulonephritis Lupus Nephritis

Lupus nephritis (LN) is a kidney disorder that arises as a complication of systemic lupus erythematosus (SLE), an autoimmune disease.

Etiology

- Associated with systemic lupus erythematosus (SLE), an autoimmune disease.
- The exact cause of SLE, consequently, lupus nephritis is not fully understood. Genetics, hormones, and environmental factors may contribute to its development.

Risk Factors

- **Gender:** Women are more commonly affected than men, with a female-to-male ratio of about 9:1.
- **Age:** Lupus nephritis typically develops in individuals between the ages of 15 and 45.
- **Ethnicity:** People of African, Asian, and Native American descent have a higher risk compared to individuals of European descent.
- **Genetics:** Family history of SLE may increase the risk.

Pathogenesis

Autoantibodies, particularly antidouble-stranded DNA antibodies, form immune complexes that deposit in the kidneys, triggering an inflammatory response. Further, activation of complement pathways and recruitment of immune cells contribute to tissue damage.

Pathological Changes

Gross appearance (Fig. 14.10A)

- Kidneys may appear enlarged and pale.
- Cortical scarring and atrophy can be presented in advanced stages.

Histological changes (Fig. 14.10B)

Class I: Minimal mesangial lupus: Mesangial immune deposits without evidence of structural abnormalities.

Class II: Mesangial proliferative: Mesangial hypercellularity and immune deposits with mild structural changes.

Class III: Focal lupus nephritis: Focal segmental glomerulonephritis with immune deposits and inflammation.

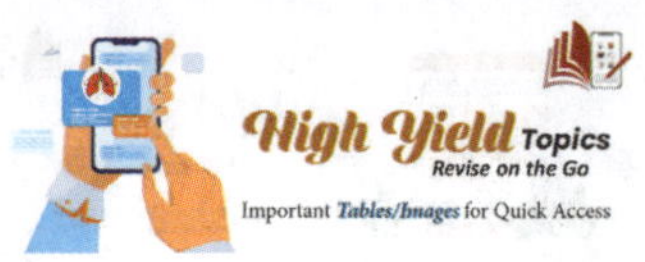

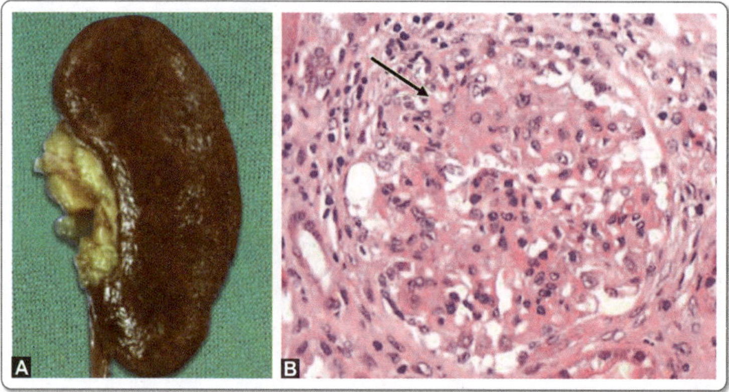

Figures 14.10A and B: Lupus nephritis: **A.** Gross; **B.** Histology

Class IV: Diffuse lupus nephritis: Diffuse global involvement with severe glomerulonephritis and immune deposits.

Class V: Membranous lupus nephritis: Global or segmental subepithelial immune deposits with or without mesangial alterations.

Class VI: Advanced sclerosing lupus nephritis: Advanced glomerulosclerosis and irreversible damage.

Hereditary Nephritis

Hereditary nephritis, also known as Alport syndrome, is a genetic disorder characterized by progressive kidney disease, hearing loss, and eye abnormalities.

Clinical Features

- Proteinuria
- Progressive hematuria
- Hearing loss
- Eye abnormalities

Etiology

Mutations in the COL4A3, COL4A4, and COL4A5 genes are responsible for the majority of cases. These genes are located on the X chromosome.

Risk Factors

The risk is increased in individuals with a family history of Alport syndrome (Fig. 14.11) since the disease is hereditary.

Pathogenesis

Mutations in the genes lead to abnormal synthesis and assembly of type IV collagen, resulting in structural defects in the basement membranes of kidneys, cochlea in the ear and the lens capsule in the eyes. Splitting and thinning of the glomerular basement membrane in the kidneys leads to progressive glomerular damage and kidney failure.

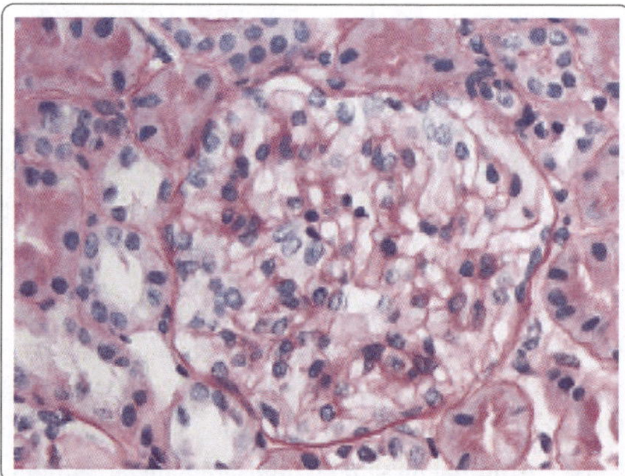

Figure 14.11: Alport syndrome: Histology

Pathological Changes

Gross appearance: Initially, the kidneys may appear normal or have subtle changes. In advanced stages, there may be evidence of renal atrophy and scarring.

Histological changes:

- **Glomerular basement membrane (GBM) abnormalities:**
  - Thinning and splitting of the GBM
  - Basket-weave appearance on electron microscopy
- **Tubulointerstitial changes:**
  - Interstitial fibrosis
  - Tubular atrophy

Vascular changes: Arteriolar changes.

Absence or abnormal staining of type IV collagen in the GBM under immunofluorescence test.

Management: Management involves supportive care, including monitoring and management of hypertension and proteinuria (Fig. 14.11).

PYELONEPHRITIS

Pyelonephritis belongs to the group of diseases known as tubulointerstitial nephritis. Tubulointerstitial nephritis means the infection is associated with inflammation of the tubules and interstitium. This group of diseases conspicuously spares the glomeruli, in contrast to glomerulonephritis where the main pathology is focused at the level of the glomeruli. Pyelonephritis is a type of tubulointerstitial nephritis in which the inflammation is prominent at the area of the renal pelvis and calyces (pelvicalyceal system) or the upper urinary tract.

Classification: It is primarily of two types; acute and chronic depending upon the duration of symptoms.

Acute Pyelonephritis

Acute pyelonephritis is an acute suppurative inflammation of the pelvicalyceal system.

CASE SCENARIO 4

The patient came to the casualty with a sudden onset of fever with chills and malaise; flank pain (unilateral/bilateral); an increased frequency of micturition; and pain during micturition. On examination, there was pain at the costovertebral angle.

Etiology

Ascending infection by Gram-negative bacilli such as *Klebsiella*, *E. coli* and Proteus, etc.

Risk Factors

- Usually, the patient has existing urinary tract infection with common pathogenic organisms such as *E. coli*, *Klebsiella*.
- In patients who are known diabetics, immunocompromised or in the case of pregnant females, the infection spreads from the lower urinary tract to the upper urinary tract. Spread of a systemic infection *via* blood stream (hematogenous) may also be seen in immunocompromised individuals/diabetics.

Pathological Changes

Gross appearance

- One/both kidneys may be affected.
- The kidney may be enlarged, swollen.
- Cortex is thinned out. In severe infection, corticomedullary differentiation is lost.
- Peripheral yellow-white colored abscesses beneath the renal capsule with foci of hemorrhage may be seen.

Microscopic changes

- **Tubules:** Tubular lumina studded with neutrophils (WBC casts in the urine). With time, the tubules are destroyed by the inflammation.
- **Interstitium:** Sheets of neutrophils are seen in the interstitium. This is the starting point of the disease process. With time, if not treated these extend to the tubules.
- **Glomeruli and vessels:** Spared in initial stages. If the infection is severe or persists, glomeruli and vessels involvement can also be seen.

MUST KNOW

Papillary necrosis: This is necrosis of the renal papillae as a result of acute pyelonephritis. It may also be seen in patients who are on NSAIDs for analgesic nephropathy/sickle cell disease.

Chronic Pyelonephritis

This is chronic inflammation of the tubulointerstitial compartment, with the pelvicalyceal system being predominantly affected as in the case of acute pyelonephritis. The end result is a kidney that progressively shrinks and scars, clinically manifesting as end-stage renal disease.

CASE SCENARIO 5

A patient presents to the OPD with complaints of headache, fatigue, reduced appetite, increased frequency of urination and intermittent flank pain.

Etiology

- **Vesicoureteral reflux:** A disease commonly is seen in children where the urine flows back in a reverse direction toward the renal pelvis and calyces.
- Obstruction anywhere in the urinary tract.

Pathological Changes

Gross appearance:

- Small contracted, shrunken kidney with the presence of irregular scars.
- Capsule is adherent.
- Loss of normal corticomedullary differentiation.
- Dilated pelvicalyceal system.

Histological changes

- Marked chronic inflammation in the tubulointerstitial compartment.
- Interstitial fibrosis—varying degrees.
- **Tubules:** Atrophy of tubular epithelial lining.

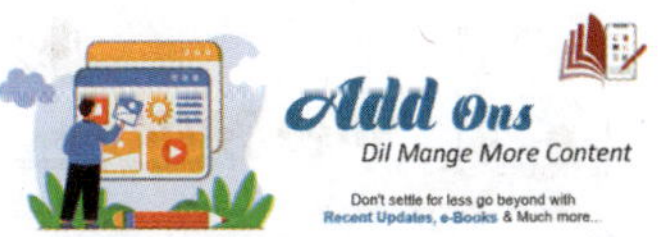

- **"Thyroidization" of the tubules:** Tubular lumina show eosinophilic cast material resembling the colloid seen in thyroid.
- **Glomeruli:** Heterogenous spectrum of glomerular involvement is seen. Glomeruli may be normal/show complete sclerosis.
  - Periglomerular fibrosis may be noted.
- **Vascular changes:** Hyaline change in the wall, also known as hyaline arteriosclerosis, occlusion of vessel lumina along with inflammation—obliterative endarteritis may also be seen (Fig. 14.12).

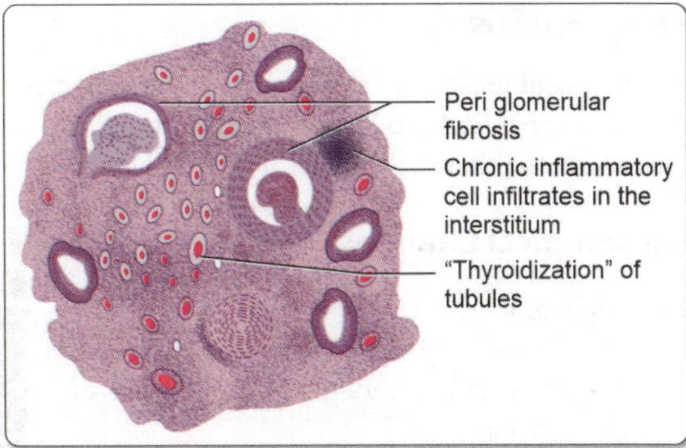

Figure 14.12: Chronic pyelonephritis: Histology

MUST KNOW

Difference between acute and chronic pyelonephritis

Acute pyelonephritis	Chronic pyelonephritis
Characterized by fever, flank pain, dysuria	Characterized by renal inflammation and fibrosis or persistent renal infection, vesicoureteral reflux or other causes of urinary obstruction
In case of potential life-threatening infection renal scarring occurs. Timely treatment leads to resolution.	Often associated with renal scarring that may lead to end-stage renal disease (ESRD)
Diagnosis—Outpatient setting history and urinalysis	Diagnosis—imaging studies such as ultrasound, CT scan

XANTHOGRANULOMATOUS PYELONEPHRITIS

Xanthogranulomatous pyelonephritis (XGP) is a rare and poorly understood form of pyelonephritis which is a type of kidney inflammation. This is characterized by the effacement of renal parenchyma by foamy lipid rich histiocytes ("xanthomatous" cells) rendering the kidney to become firm and even mimicking malignancy. Patients are usually women in the age group of 40–60, frequently present with fever and flank pain.

Etiology

Xanthogranulomatous glomerulonephritis (XGP) is caused by a chronic obstruction to the urinary flow, commonly due to a large staghorn calculus or due to recurrent infections with Gram-negative bacteria such as *E. coli*, *Proteus* and *Klebsiella*. It is believed the macrophage system is unable to effectively destroy the bacteria in this condition.

It is believed to be associated with chronic inflammation and is often considered a secondary phenomenon rather than a primary disease. XG can be seen in the context of chronic infections, obstructive uropathy, and other inflammatory conditions.

Risk Factors

- Chronic infections such as bacterial or fungal infections in the kidney.
- Conditions leading to urinary tract obstruction may predispose individuals to the development of obstructive uropathy.
- Chronic inflammatory conditions affecting the kidneys.

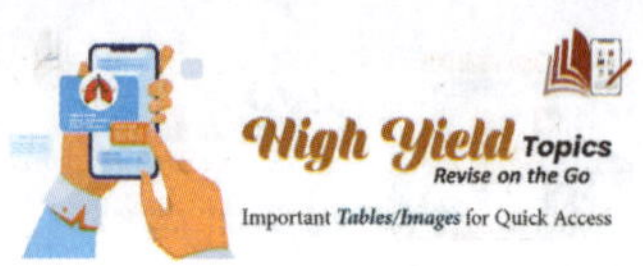

Pathogenesis

Xanthogranulomatous glomerulonephritis is characterized by the presence of lipid-laden macrophages, foam cells, and granulomatous inflammation within the renal parenchyma. The inflammation is often diffuse and can involve the glomeruli, interstitium, and blood vessels and can often mimic malignancy.

Pathological Changes

Gross appearance:

- The affected kidneys may appear enlarged due to chronic inflammation and infiltration of inflammatory cells.
- There may be yellowish nodules or areas within the renal parenchyma, representing accumulations of lipid-laden macrophages (Fig. 14.13A).

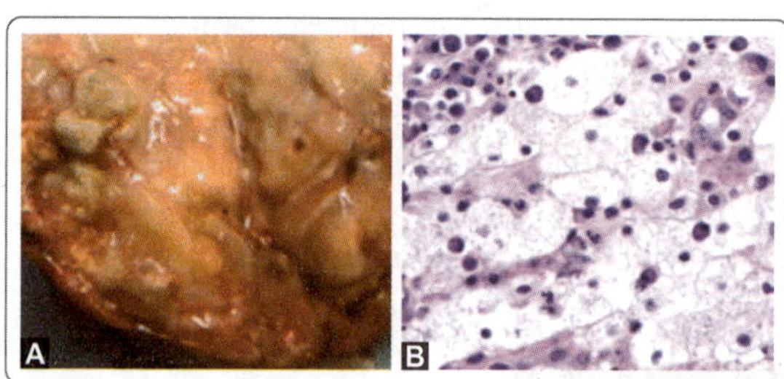

Figures 14.13A and B: Xanthogranulomatous glomerulonephritis: **A.** Gross; **B.** Histology

Histological changes

- Foamy macrophages loaded with lipid droplets is a hallmark of XG.
- Granulomas may be present in the interstitium.
- Glomeruli may show inflammatory changes, and sclerosis may occur.
- Inflammatory cells rimmed by granulation tissue and sheets of xanthomatous cells and giant cells including Touton giant cells (Fig. 14.13B).

NOTE

It is important to recognize this pathology correctly, as it may mimic clear cell variant of renal cell carcinoma. In addition, the treatment of the most cases is antibiotics and percutaneous drainage. Diagnosis should be timely done to prevent advancement of disease or till the requiremnet of nephrectomy.

Lab Diagnosis

- Requires a combination of clinical, radiological, and histopathological findings.
- On a CT scan, in some patients, the characteristic "bear paw" sign is seen in which the pelvis and calyces are dilated, hypoechoic and show peripheral enhancement.

RENAL CALCULI OR KIDNEY STONES

CASE SCENARIO 6

A 25-year-old male comes to the emergency with complaint of sharp, shooting, colicky flank pain. He also had experienced hematuria along with nausea, vomiting and fever.

When the urine becomes too concentrated with calcium, uric acid salts, and other chemicals dissolved in the urine, it can crystallize, forming a kidney stone, or renal calculus. This may also manifest as recurrent urinary tract infections.

Age group: 20–40 years.

Preferred site: Predilection to lodge at the renal pelvis and calyces, but may also occur in any other part of the urinary tract.

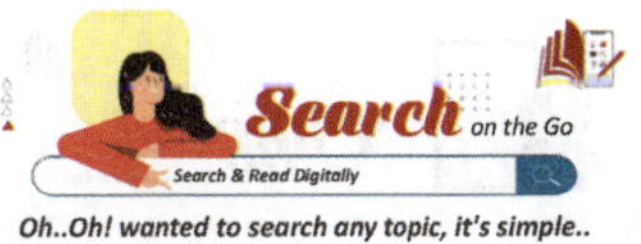

MUST KNOW

Stone/urinary calculus: Amorphous urinary crystalloids enmeshed in a mucoprotein matrix form a calculus or in common terms, a stone.
Urolithiasis: The presence of stones anywhere in the urinary tract.
Nephrolithiasis: The presence of stones, specifically in the kidney/renal parenchyma.

Types of Renal Stones

Main types of kidney stones are as follows:

- **Cystine stones:** Rare.
- **Calcium stones include calcium oxalates and calcium phosphates:** These represent the most frequent stones (75–80%) and comprise the major proportion of all calculi. Since when the urine pH is low or acidic.
- **Uric acid stones:** Associated with increased serum levels of uric acid.
- **Struvite stones:** These are also referred to as the triple phosphate stones/magnesium ammonium phosphate stones. These types of stones have a propensity to occupy the renal pelvis and calyces giving the appearance of a staghorn, hence the name staghorn calculi. This is associated with infection by urea splitting bacteria such as Klebsiella, Proteus and Pseudomonas. Urea production elevates urinary pH promoting the precipitation by phosphates.
- **Stones associated with intake of drugs:** Certain drugs are also associated with the formation of stones including sulpha drugs, drugs used to treat HIV like protease inhibitors such as indinavir (Fig. 14.14).

Clinical Features

- Obstruction leads to pain and in the long term it causes hydronephrosis.
- Propensity for infections is increased, both in the already dilated pelvicalyceal system—pyonephrosis or as recurring infections (urinary tract infections).
- Long standing calculi can also trigger metaplastic change from the normal urothelial lining to squamous lining epithelium. This squamous metaplasia may further serve as favorable environment for dysplastic change.

Etiology

Stones are formed due to:

- Increased crystalloid concentration in the urine.
- Reduced urinary volume due to dehydration.
- Naturally, increased excretion of crystalloids.

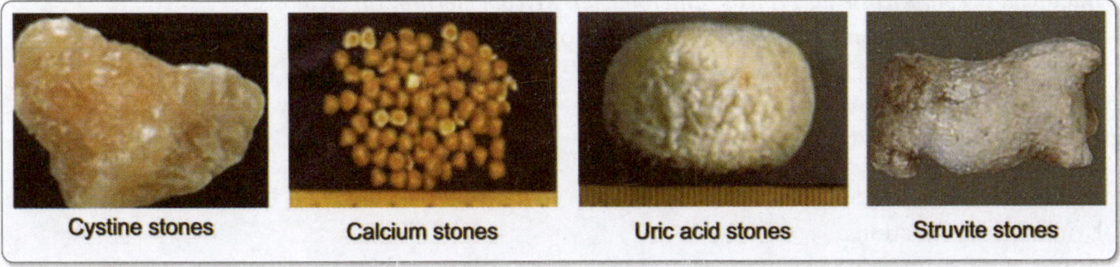

Figure 14.14: Types of Kidney stones

- Alteration in pH of the urine due to diet/infection, e.g., an acidic urine promotes the formation of calcium stones and an alkaline urine is favorable for formation of staghorn calculi.

Pathogenesis

Alteration in pH leads to supersaturation of urine. A nidus is formed with further deposition of crystalline material (Fig. 14.15).

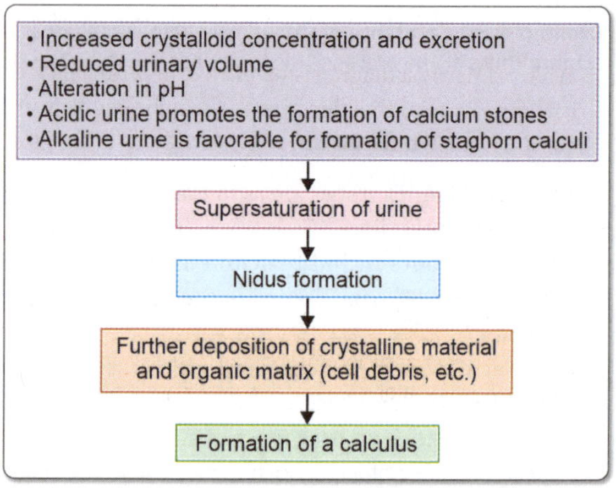

- Increased crystalloid concentration and excretion
- Reduced urinary volume
- Alteration in pH
- Acidic urine promotes the formation of calcium stones
- Alkaline urine is favorable for formation of staghorn calculi

↓

Supersaturation of urine

↓

Nidus formation

↓

Further deposition of crystalline material and organic matrix (cell debris, etc.)

↓

Formation of a calculus

Figure 14.15: Pathogenesis of renal calculi or kidney stones

CYSTITIS

Cystitis is a disease state charcterized by inflammation of the urinary bladder. The disease condition like other inflammatory diseases may be acute or chronic.

Types of Cystitis

- **Cystitis follicularis:** A type of cystitis in which the bladder mucosa shows the presence of lymphoid follicles.
- **Interstitial cystitis (Hunner's ulcer):** The presence of a deep ulcer extending from the mucosa into the submucosa accompanying by chronic inflammatory infiltrate, generally seen in middle-aged women.

Clinical Features

Clinically, the patient will present with lower abdominal pain, increased frequency of urination and pain during micturition (dysuria).

In chronic cystitis:

- Mucosa gets ulcerated, may assume a polypoid appearance with the presence of granulation tissue.
- Chronic inflammatory infiltrate comprised of lymphocytes, macrophages and histiocytes dispersing the muscle cells (myocytes) in the muscle layer.
- The mucosa, submucosa and muscle layer in chronic cases can show the presence of fibrosis.
- In the case of tubercular cystitis, there would be the additional presence of epithelioid cell granulomas, caseous necrosis may or may not be present.

Etiology

The common causative organisms include:

- **Bacteria:** *E. coli, Klebsiella, Proteus, Enterobacter, Mycobacterium tuberculosis.*
- **Fungi:** *Candida albicans*, especially in immunocompromised patients.
- **Parasites:** *Schistosoma hematobium.*

Risk Factors

Predisposing factors include:

- Urinary tract infections.
- Stones in the urinary bladder.

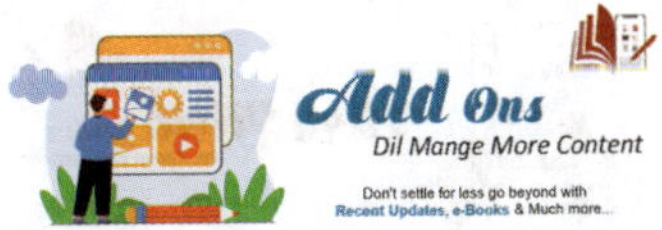

- Surgical instrumentation involves the urethra, urinary bladder.
- Immunocompromised state.

Pathological Changes

To have primarily a diagnosis by ultrastructural analysis, the specimen is observed as follows:

Gross appearance: Bladder mucosa may be reddish in color in acute cases. This is often accompanied by a fibrinopurulent exudate.

- **In acute cystitis:** The bladder mucosa may be ulcerated. Sheets of neutrophils in the mucosa are seen infiltrating the submucosa and muscle layer in cases of increased severity.
- **Submucosa:** Edematous

EXTRA EDGE

Ingestion of the drug cyclophosphamide causes a specific type of cystitis that is hemorrhagic cystitis, in which extensive mucosal sloughing along with areas of mucosal and submucosal hemorrhage are noted.

RENAL CELL CARCINOMA

This is also known by the name of hypernephroma/Grawitz tumor. Renal cell carcinoma (RCC) occurs in the elderly, predominantly in the 6th–7th decade and with a male predilection. It is the most frequent malignancy of the kidneys in adults and is associated with the highest rates of mortality amongst genitourinary cancers.

Cell of origin: Proximal renal tubular epithelial cell.

Clinical Features

The classical triad of presentation includes hematuria, abdominal mass and flank pain. Many cases are detected incidentally, while being evaluated for other conditions.

Risk Factors

- Consumption of tobacco.
- Obesity.
- Exposure to asbestos and industrial chemicals including heavy metals.
- Women on hormone replacement therapy, especially estrogen.
- Patients on long term dialysis.
- **Genetic factors:** Most cases are sporadic. The few cases (about 5%) that are inherited and associated with important syndromes include:
    - Von-Hippel-Landau Syndrome.
    - Tuberous sclerosis.
    - Polycystic kidney disease.

Pathological Changes

Gross appearance:

- It frequently involves one pole of the kidney with the upper pole being more frequently affected.
- Usually, unilateral or involving one of the kidneys.
- **Size:** Variable.

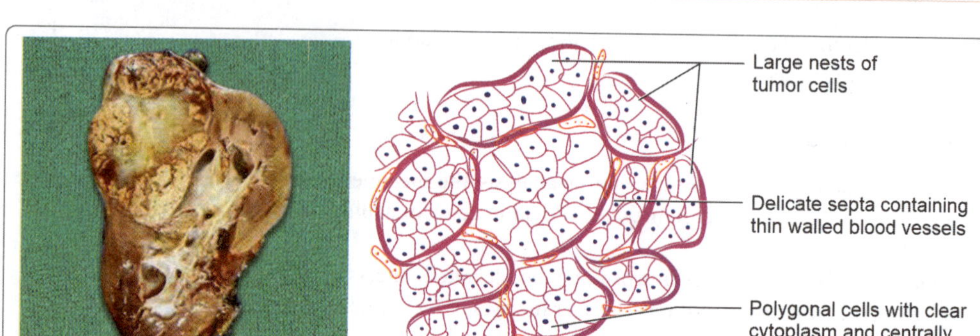

Figures 14.16A and B: Renal cell carcinoma: **A.** Gross; **B.** Histology

- **Color:** Brownish-yellow.
- **Cut surface:** The tumor is usually solid but may show areas of cystic change. RCC has a soft to firm consistency, is generally well-demarcated with a characteristic variegated appearance with areas of necrosis and hemorrhage. When the tumor increases in size, it can take the appearance of a fungating mass (Fig. 14.16A).

Histological changes:

- Tumor cells are arranged in nests.
- Fibrovascular septa are seen separating the tumor nests. The common histological types include clear cell, chromophobe, papillary, collecting duct and medullary.
- **Clear cell:** This is the most common type with individual cells have well-defined cellular outlines, clear cytoplasm (due to glycogen) and nuclei with nucleoli of varying conspicuousness (Fig. 14.16B).
- **Papillary:** Shows a papillary growth pattern.
- **Chromophobe:** Halo around nucleus, pale eosinophilic cytoplasm.
- **Collecting duct:** Glands in a fibrotic stroma.

Immunohistochemistry: When the diagnosis is difficult by morphology alone, immunohistochemical analysis aids in the diagnosis.

Tumor markers: Dual expression of CK and vimentin proteins is characteristic feature of RCC. This is accompanied by expression of CD10 and PAX8.

MUST KNOW

Paraneoplastic syndromes: RCC is notoriously associated with various paraneoplastic conditions which sometimes may even be the presenting feature of the case. This includes hypertension, hypercalcemia, cushing syndrome, polycythemia, eosinophilia.

RENAL FAILURE

Renal failure means inability of the kidneys to perform excretory function leading to retention of nitrogenous waste products from the blood. Renal failure is of two types: **acute and chronic**. Although with time, the conventional terminology of acute renal failure has been replaced by the term acute kidney injury, while

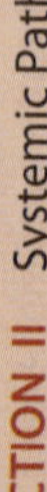

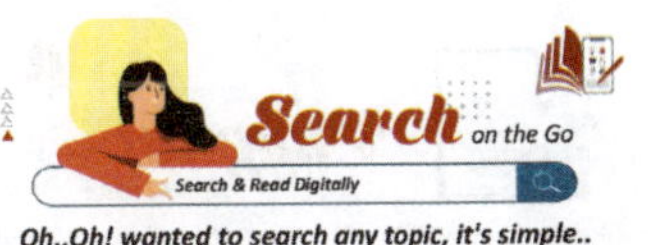

chronic renal failure is now commonly addressed as a stage V chronic kidney disease and is treated as per the clinical stage.

Acute Renal Failure (ARF) or Acute Kidney Injury (AKI)

Acute renal failure is a rapid and progressively declining glomerular filtration rate (within hours to days) and is manifested by a deranged renal function evidenced as increase in serum creatinine due to accumulation of nitrogenous waste products. About 50% of patients admitted in intensive care units for management develop AKI.

Etiology

Acute renal failure can be divided into three types—prerenal, intrarenal and postrenal.

Leading Causes of Acute Kidney Injury (AKI)

Prerenal:
- Dehydration
- Liver failure
- Heart failure
- Drugs such as NSAIDs, ACE inhibitors

Intrarenal:
- As a complication of severe glomerular disease (especially, rapidly progressive glomerulonephritis)
- Severe tubulointerstitial nephritis/pyelonephritis
- Vasculitis
- Acute tubular necrosis

Postrenal:
- Obstructive uropathy—enlarged prostate, stones, tumor.

Risk Factors

The risk factors for developing a new-onset AKI include:
- Advanced age.
- Diabetes mellitus.
- Coronary artery disease.
- Hypertension.
- Sepsis.
- Chronic liver disease.
- Use of vasopressor drugs during treatment.
- Post-traumatic injury.
- Burns.
- Usage of certain medications such as NSAIDs/ Diuretics/ACE-inhibitors/antibiotics such as aminoglycosides may predispose to AKI.

Clinical Features

The patient presents with decreased urinary output (oliguria/anuria), edema, nausea, confusion, tiredness, hypertension, discoloration of urine, acid base abnormalities, especially hyperkalemia and in some cases systemic manifestations depending on etiology such as fever, flank pain.

Pathogenesis

Acute renal failure is due to accumulation of nitrogenous waste products. This is also evidenced by an altered electrolyte balance leads to a deranged acid-base balance.

Lab Diagnosis

Kidney Disease Improving Global Outcomes (KDIGO) criteria are—frequently used for making the diagnosis of AKI. These include:

- Increase in serum creatinine by 0.3 mg/dL or more within 48 hours.
- Increase in serum creatinine to 1.5 times or more than baseline of the prior 7 days.
- Urine volume <0.5 mL/kg/hr for at least 6 hours.

MUST KNOW

Difference between acute and chronic kidney failure

Acute kidney failure	Chronic kidney failure
• Reduced urine output • Swollen legs, ankles, and feet • Weakness and fatigue • Confusion	• Abnormal blood and urine tests • Swelling on the face, hands, and feet • Headaches • High blood pressure

Chronic Renal Failure (CRF) or Chronic Kidney Disease (CKD)

The presence of kidney damage or a decline of estimated glomerular filtration rate to <60 mL/min/1.73 m^2 which is due to any cause, for a minimum duration of three months.

Evidence of kidney damage may be:

- Pathological changes seen on a renal biopsy.
- Persisting proteinuria.
- Abnormalities seen on imaging.
- Other derangements seen on urine analysis, e.g., hematuria.

Clinical Features

The important clinical features of CKD include:

- Fatigue.
- Lethargy/drowsiness.
- Nausea/vomiting.
- Reduced urine output.
- Skin itching.
- Hypertension.
- Edema.
- Shortness of breath due to anemia.
- Dullness of the mind.

Etiology

- Chronic renal disease such as chronic glomerulonephritis, chronic tubulointerstitial nephritis including pyelonephritis.
- Chronic systemic disease with renal manifestations such as diabetes, amyloidosis.
- As a sequel to chronic obstructive uropathy, vascular diseases, especially malignant nephrosclerosis.

Risk Factors for Progression of Chronic Kidney Disease

- Advanced age.
- Long standing diabetes mellitus.

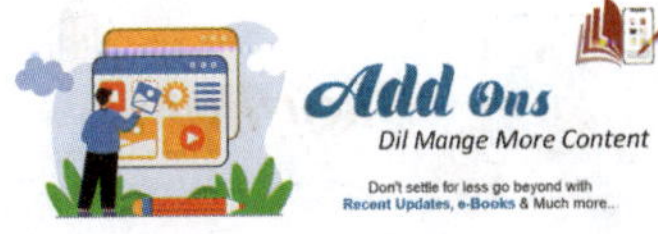

- Lifestyle diseases-hypertension, obesity
- Persistent albuminuria (Category A3)
- Chronic smoking
- Prior history of episodes of AKI
- Family history of kidney disease
- African-American descent
- Chronic usage of NSAID
- Hyperlipidemia
- Single nucleotide polymorphisms in genes TCF7L2 and MTHFS.

Pathogenesis

There is decrease in effective functioning of glomeruli which are evidenced histologically as sclerosed glomeruli, interstitial fibrosis with tubular atrophy. There is also a loss of concentrating ability of the kidneys with the change in specific gravity of excreted urine (having specific gravity equivalent to protein free plasma as 1.010). Other biochemical abnormalities include azotemia, metabolic acidosis (due to reduction in serum bicarbonate) and hyperphosphatemia.

In later stages the patient also develops clinical features of anemia and hypertension.

Staging of CKD (Table 14.1): Chronic kidney disease is clinically subdivided into various stages 1–5. The recent KDIGO staging system also stages CKD based on urine albumin-creatinine ratio on the early morning spot urine sample (Table 14.2).

Table 14.1: Chronic kidney disease stage and estimated glomerular filtration rate

CKD Stage	Estimated GFR (eGFR)
1	>90
2	60–89
3a	45–59
3b	30–44
4	15–29
5	<15

Table 14.2: Albumin creatinine ratio

Albumin	Albumin creatinine ratio
A1	<30 mg/g
A2	30–299 mg/g
A3	>300 mg/g

eGFR calculation formula:

GFR = 175 × $(Scr)^{-1.154}$ × $(age)^{-0.203}$ × (C)0.742 (if female) × 1.212 (if Black)

Scr = serum creatinine in mg/dL

Stage 5 represents end-stage renal disease or chronic renal failure, leading to the destruction of nephrons and consequent accumulation of nitrogenous wastes leading to uremia.

Stage five is subdivided as:

- 5D: Patients on dialysis, and
- 5T: Patients with kidney transplant

Pathological Changes

- Tubular necrosis with disrupted, necrotic or regenerating tubular epithelium.
- Uniform diffuse necrosis of proximal convoluted tubules.
- Crescents inside the Bowman's capsule.

Histopathological Features

The key histopathological features seen on renal biopsies are:

- Numerous sclerosed glomeruli.
- Interstitial fibrosis.

- Tubular atrophy
- Varying degrees of chronic tubulointerstitial inflammation
- Sclerosed vessels
- There is also a loss of concentrating ability of the kidneys with the excreted urine having a specific gravity equivalent to protein free plasma (1.010).
- Other biochemical abnormalities include azotemia, metabolic acidosis (due to reduction in serum bicarbonate) and hyperphosphatemia.

NURSING CONSIDERATIONS

The care of CKD patients is multidisciplinary and involves some key points:
More than 80% symptomatic cases suffer from an elevated blood pressure (BP). BP monitoring twice a day is important to ensure that it remains in controlled.

Diet:

- CRF patients suffer from uremia and accumulation of nitrogenous wastes. This would be worsened by taking more proteins, hence a low protein diet must always be given.
- The key electrolyte abnormality is seen hyperkalemia. Hence, potassium rich foods are to be avoided at all costs that include black eyed beans, avocadoes, potatoes, sweet potatoes, oranges.
- Sodium restriction is also a part of management to prevent worsening of edema.

SUMMARY

- All renal disease can be categorized based on the four major histological compartments of the kidney—Glomeruli, tubules, interstitium and vessels.
- Glomerulonephritis refers to kidney disease in which there is inflammation/injury at the level of the glomeruli.
- Minimal change disease affects young children (most cases between 2 and 5 years of age), presenting with massive proteinuria leading to renal edema.
- PSGN is a disease of children and the young, the most frequent age group is 5–15 years.
- Immune complex deposition in PSGN occurs either beneath the visceral epithelial cell (subepithelial), or beneath the endothelial cell (subendothelial), or within the mesangium.
- Focal segmental glomerulosclerosis (FSGS) is a disease in which scar tissue develops on the glomeruli, the small parts of the kidneys that filter waste from the blood.
- Membranous glomerulonephritis has deposition of immune complexes on the glomerular basement membrane (GBM) with GBM thickening.
- Pyelonephritis belongs to the group of diseases known as tubulointerstitial nephritis.
- Pyelonephritis is a type of tubulointerstitial nephritis in which the inflammation is prominent at the area of the renal pelvis and calyces.
- Renal calculi are formed when it becomes too concentrated, to cause crystallization of calcium, uric acid salts, and other chemicals dissolved in the urine.
- Cystitis is inflammation of the urinary bladder.
- Renal cell carcinoma (RCC) is also known by the name of hypernephroma/Grawitz tumor.
- The classical triad of RCC includes hematuria, abdominal mass and flank pain.
- Renal failure means inability of the kidneys to perform excretory function leading to retention of nitrogenous waste products from the blood.

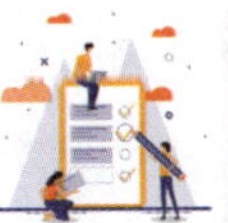
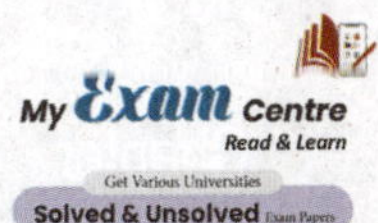

ASSESS YOURSELF

Long Answer Question

1. Discuss the etiology and pathogenesis of pyelonephritis.

Short Answer Questions

1. Write about pyelonephritis.
2. Write about the term renal cell carcinoma.
3. Write short notes on:
   i. ARF
   ii. Renal failure

Multiple Choice Questions

1. **Common nonspecific symptoms of chronic kidney disease include:**
   a. Increased urination at night b. Loss of appetite
   c. Swelling of hands and feet d. All of these
2. **A person can have chronic kidney disease without symptoms:**
   a. True b. False
3. **Which kidney disease is known to be inherited?**
   a. End-stage renal disease b. Protein disease
   c. Autoimmune kidney disease d. Polycystic kidney disease
4. **There are _____ stages of chronic kidney disease.**
   a. 3 b. 5
   c. 6 d. 7
5. **In distinguishing acute from chronic renal failure, which of the following is the most reliable evidence of CKD?**
   a. History of increased serum creatinine b. History of increased BUN
   c. Above normal plasma sodium d. Above normal serum calcium

Answer Key

1. d 2. a 3. d 4. b 5. a

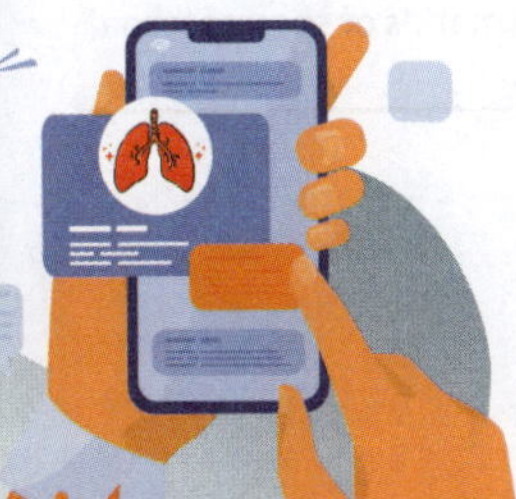
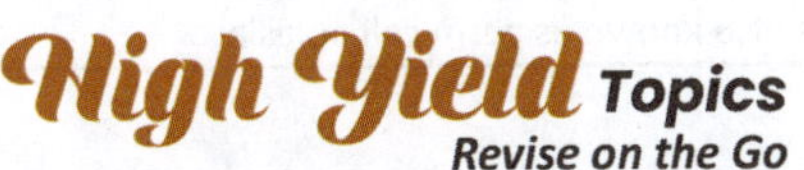

Get Topic-wise Selective **Images & Tables** with their description for LMR and Quick reference, based on the topics of University examination

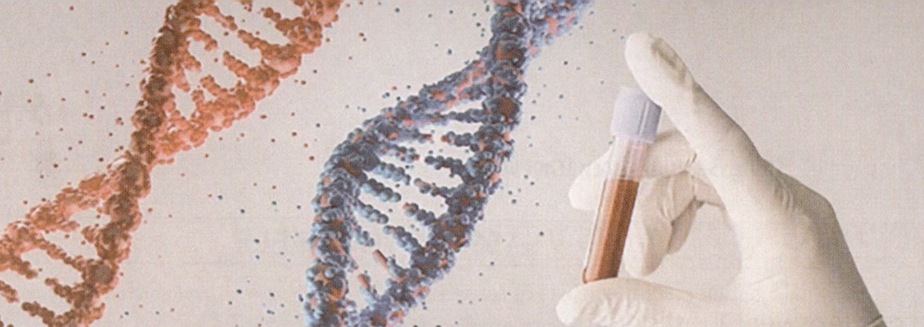

Chapter 15

Male Genital System Diseases

LEARNING OBJECTIVES

After the completion of the chapter, the readers will be able to:

- Describe the normal structure and function of the male genital system components.
- Pathological changes in various disease conditions of male genital system.

CHAPTER OUTLINE

- Overview of the Male Genital System
- Cryptorchidism
- Testicular Atrophy
- Benign Prostatic Hyperplasia
- Prostatic Carcinoma
- Carcinoma Penis

KEY TERMS

Aplasia: Testicular tissue is completely absent altogether.

Aspermia: Lack of semen on ejaculation.

Azoospermia: Lack of sperms on semen analysis.

Discordant pattern: Where the biopsy changes in the right and left testis are discrepant or dissimilar.

Hypospermatogenesis: Though maturation is seen from germ cells to spermatozoa in all tubules, the number of spermatozoa is less.

Incomplete spermatocytic arrest: Some tubules show a normal number of cells with adequate maturation, while others display a maturation arrest.

Late spermatocytic arrest: All cells, except mature spermatozoa are seen on the biopsy.

Maturation arrest: The germ cells that fail to complete maturation, i.e., spermatids and spermatozoa are absent.

Mixed pattern: When tubules showing germ cell aplasia coexist with tubules, showing only Sertoli cells.

Normal spermatogenesis: An orderly progression from germ cells to spermatocytes, spermatids and spermatozoa is seen in all tubules and the number of each cell type is adequate.

Oligospermia: A low sperm count on semen analysis, defined by <15 million sperms/1 mL of semen.

Sertoli cell-only (SCO) syndrome: When only sertoli cells are visualized and no germ cells, spermatids or spermatozoa are visualized, this is also known as germ cell aplasia.

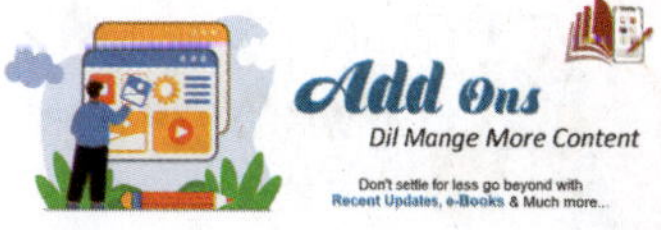

OVERVIEW OF THE MALE GENITAL SYSTEM

- The male genital system consists of several structures. The testes, situated in the scrotum are responsible for sperm production and testosterone secretion.
- The testes are paired organs present within the scrotal sac weighing approximately 20 g in human.
- Individual testis is covered by an outer fibrous capsule called tunica albuginea that is further covered by the serous covering called tunica vaginalis.
- The testis produces sperms and comprises coiled seminiferous tubules which represent the exact site where this process occurs.
- The seminiferous tubules are lined by germinal epithelium, i.e., spermatogonia. Primary spermatocytes change to secondary spermatocytes. These cells spermatids, finally lead to the formation of spermatozoa. Sertoli cells are interspersed in between.
- The tubules are interspersed in stroma which shows the presence of Leydig cells.
- Leydig cells have an endocrine function and it secretes testosterone. The functions of Sertoli and Leydig cells are given in Table 15.1.
- Connected to the testes is the epididymis, a coiled tube facilitating sperm storage and transport.
- The epididymis is present at the posterolateral aspect of the testis and is a coiled duct having a head, body and tail and leading up to the vas deferens which carries sperm from the epididymis to the urethra.
- The prostate gland, positioned below the bladder, produces prostatic fluid. Additionally, the bulbourethral glands release lubricating fluid before ejaculation.

Table 15.1: Functions of sertoli and leydig cells

Sertoli cells	Leydig cells
Sertoli cells are elongated and pyramidal cells.	Embedded in soft connective tissue surrounding the seminiferous tubule.
They provide nourishment to the sperms till maturation.	They are endocrine in nature.

MUST KNOW

Sertoli cells are also known as "nurse cells" and play role in nurturing and providing structural support for the sperm cells during their development.

CLINICAL CORRELATION

- There are two major zones of the prostate—inner periurethral zone and the peripheral zone
- The peripheral zone gives rise to carcinoma and the inner periurethral estrogen sensitive zone is the site for development of benign prostatic hyperplasia.
- Scrotum is located outside of the body as it helps in the thermoregulation of the testicles.

CRYPTORCHIDISM

This is a congenital anomaly in which there is failure of testicular descent, i.e., the process occurring during fetal development in which the intra-abdominal testes normally descend into the scrotal sac. The testes may be arrested at the level of the abdomen, the inguinal canal (most common) or other sites (Fig. 15.1).

- There is a complete or partial failure of the intra-abdominal testes to descend into the scrotal sac.
- Associated with testicular dysfunction and an increased risk of testicular cancer.
- Grossly, the testis is small, brown and atrophic.
- **Microscopically:** Atrophic tubules with thickened basement membrane, Leydig cells are spared and appear predominant.
- **Retractile or pseudocryptorchidism:** A retractile testicle descends into the scrotum but pulls back into the inguinal canal because of a hyperactive cremasteric reflex.

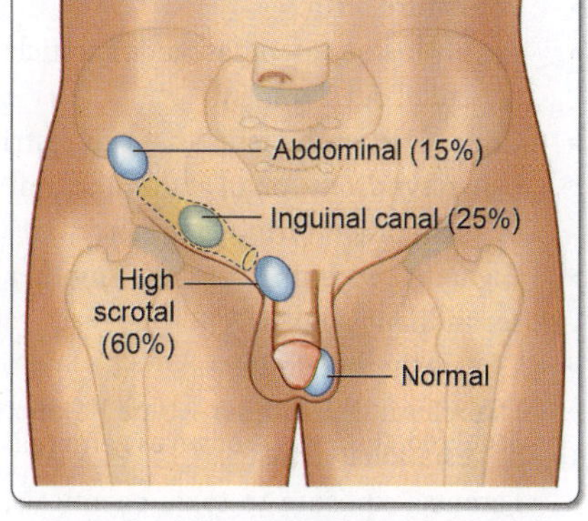

Figure 15.1: Cryptorchidism—most common site

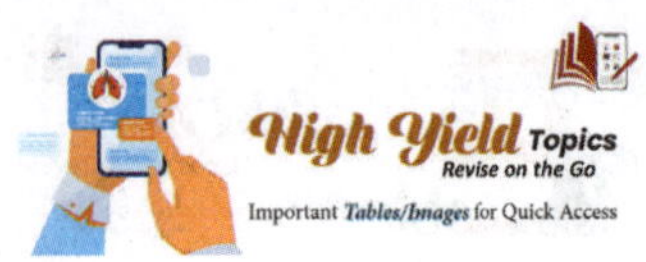

- **Palpable:** Also called prepubic or inguinal, the testicle is located anywhere from just above the scrotum to high in the groin.
- **Nonpalpable:** Testicle is in the boy's abdomen or is absent and not felt in the scrotum or inguinal canal.
- **Ectopic:** The testicle has taken the wrong path and ended in an unusual location in the groin area.

Clinical Features

The patient usually has no complaints (asymptomatic). The condition is often detected incidentally. Though the patient at presentation appears normal, this condition has longstanding clinical implications which include:

- **Male infertility:** An undescended testicle stays up in the body, and bears a higher temperature. This reduces sperm count and quality, hence, affects fertility of a male.
- An increased association with inguinal hernia/torsion of testis.
- Higher risk of testicular malignancy. This is usually unilateral (70–80% cases) and may be accompanied by other genitourinary/other congenital anomalies. Hence, a thorough physical examination is necessary to evaluate such patients.

Etiology

Exact cause is unknown as follows:

- A combination of genetical factors, maternal health, environmental factors might disrupt the hormones.
- Physical changes and nerve activity may also influence the development of the testicles.
- Blockage of the hypothalamic pituitary gonadal axis.
- Anatomical obstruction.
- Heredity or chromosomal anomalies.
- Short spermatic cord and artery mechanically prevent the descent.
- Ectopic attachment of the testes.

Risk Factors

- Low birth weight.
- Premature birth.
- Family history of undescended testicle or other problems of genital development.
- Conditions of the fetus that can restrict growth, such as Down syndrome or an abdominal wall defect alcohol use by the mother during pregnancy.
- Cigarette smoking by the mother or exposure to secondhand smoke.
- Obesity in the mother.
- Diabetes in the mother—type I diabetes, type II diabetes or gestational diabetes.
- Parents' exposure to toxic chemicals, e.g., pestisides or radiations.

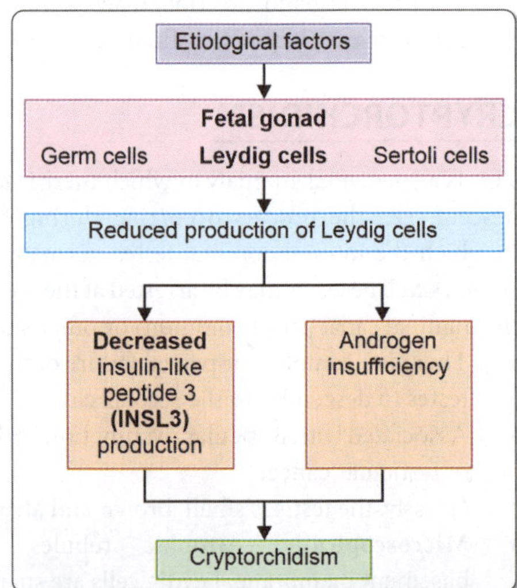

Figure 15.2: Pathogenesis of cryptorchidism

Pathogenesis

(Refer to Figure 15.2)

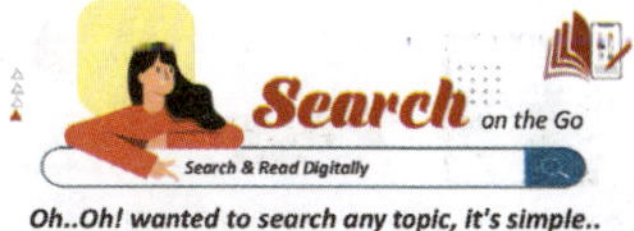

Pathological Changes

Gross Appearance

- **Size:** The testis may be normal or smaller in size due to changes of atrophy.
- **Consistency:** The testis may be firm due to fibrotic changes.

Histological Changes

- **Seminiferous tubules:** Show a thickened basement membrane along with hyalinization. There may be a complete absence/reduction in the number of germ cells with a relative increase in the number of Sertoli cells (Fig. 15.3).
- **Interstitium:** Leydig cell prominence with increased stroma.

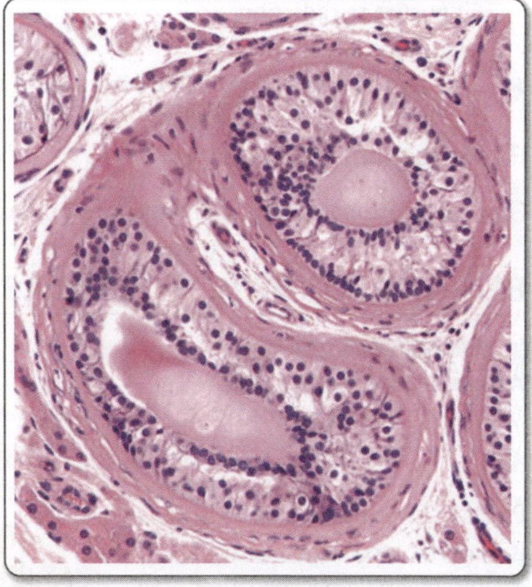

Figure 15.3: Histological changes in cryptorchidism

Diagnosis

- Physical examination.
- Gonadotropin-releasing hormone (GnRH) stimulation tests.

MUST KNOW

A surgical procedure called orchiopexy is used to bring the testis down into the scrotum.

TESTICULAR ATROPHY

This condition is characterized by a reduction in the size of the testis due to a reduction in the structural and/or functional elements of the organ (Fig. 15.4).

Clinical Features

The patient presents with the features:

- Sagging/soft testes.
- Diminished size of testes.
- Infertility.
- Reduced libido.
- Reduced muscle mass.

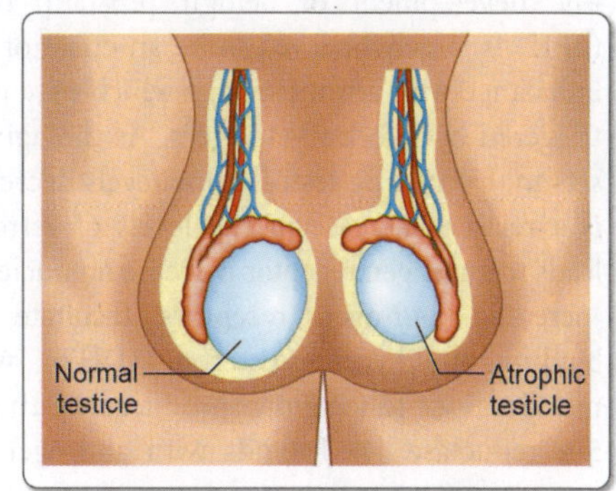

Figure 15.4: Testicular atrophy

Etiology

Cryptorchidism, as described above is one of the conditions leading to testicular atrophy. Other diseases causing testicular atrophy include:

- Senility.
- Malnutrition.
- Hypoxic ischemic injury due to atherosclerosis of testicular arterial vessels.
- Infectious disease, e.g., mumps, orchitis.

- Exposure to radiation.
- Hypopituitarism.
- Estrogen therapy administered in cases of carcinoma prostate.

Pathological Changes

Gross and histopathological changes are similar to those described for cryptorchidism.

BENIGN PROSTATIC HYPERPLASIA

CASE SCENARIO 1

60-year-old male presented to the surgical OPD with complaints of increased frequency of urination, pain during urination and urinary retention.

Prostatic hyperplasia (Fig. 15.5) is a common condition seen in elderly males, especially after 50 years of age. It is characterized by a nodular enlargement of the prostate, hence the name nodular hyperplasia. As, benign prostatic hyperplasia (BPH) is very frequently seen after 60 years of age, hence it is believed to be a part of the normal ageing process.

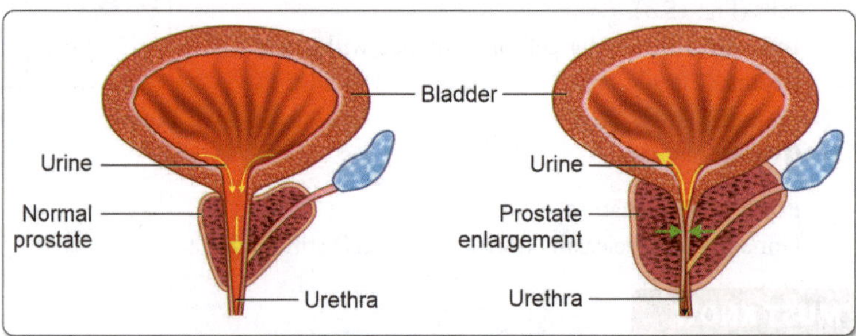

Figure 15.5: Prostate hyperplasia

Pathogenesis

The development of benign prostatic hyperplasia (BPH) is largely believed to be an effect of hormonal imbalance with advancing age which may possibly be triggered by infectious triggers. As the aging process sets in, circulating testosterone levels decrease. There is a relative increase in the levels of estrogen. This leads to androgen receptor increase on nuclear surface. Increased androgen receptors facilitate increased binding of dihydrotestosterone (DHT), which is a metabolite of testosterone produced by the action of 5-α reductase. DHT binds with androgen receptors present on the prostatic glands as well as in the prostatic stroma, promoting both epithelial and stromal proliferation (Refer to Figure 15.6).

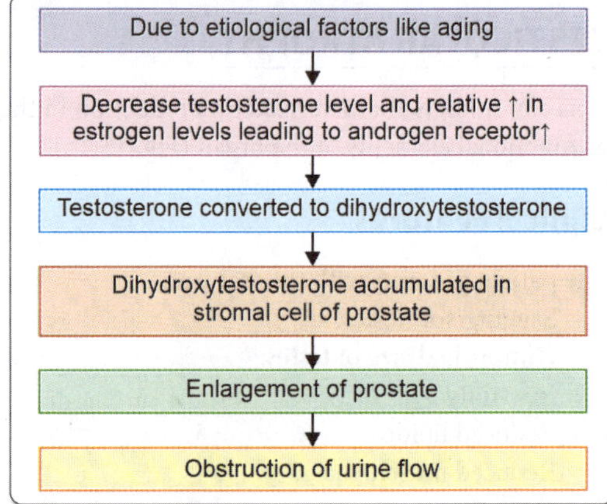

Figure 15.6: Pathogenesis of prostatic hyperplasia

Pathological Changes

Gross Appearance

The prostate gland gets enlarged in size and increased in weight. External surface usually is nodular with the presence of a capsule. With time the gland may become firm and fibrotic (Fig. 15.7A).

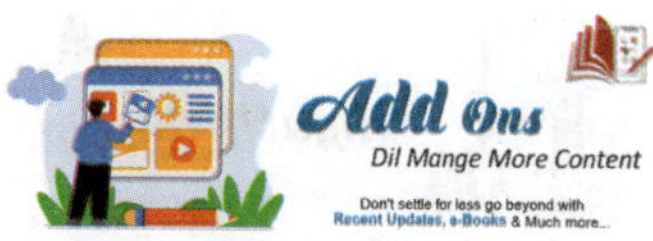

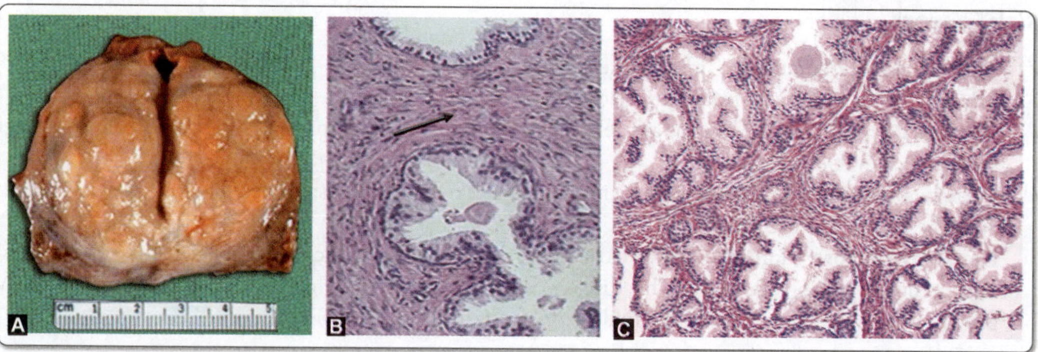

Figures 15.7A to C: Histological changes in benign prostatic hyperplasia: **A.** Gross showing nodular hyperplasia; **B.** Microscopy showing normal gland stroma; **C.** Microscopy showing glands (all are lined by two layers of cells) and stroma suggestive of benign prostatic hyperplasia

Cut surface: Largely solid and nodular, gray-white in color. Nodularity is more pronounced around the urethra (periurethral) and the nodules are of varying sizes.

- As per the component that predominates, if the nodules are predominantly stromal, the cut surface is solid/fibrotic.
- If nodules show more of glandular proliferation, nodules may be soft, gray-pink and show oozing of clear prostatic fluid.

Histopathological Changes

The prostate gland histologically comprises glands and stroma. In BPH both glands and stroma proliferate in varying degrees. Glands are of variable size and cystically dilated. Some may be filled with pink proteinaceous substance within the lumina called corpora amylacea. This is accompanied by fibromuscular hyperplasia (Figs 15.7B and C).

Clinical Testing

Prostate specific antigen (PSA) levels, ultrasonography, prostatic biopsy and histopathological evaluation.

PROSTATIC CARCINOMA

This is a common tumor afflicting men between 45 and 60 years of age and represents a leading cause of mortality in males.15–20% of prostatic carcinoma is incidentally detected during the course of evaluation of benign prostatic hyperplasia or other benign pathological conditions.

Clinical Features

The patient presents with symptoms of urinary outflow obstruction such as:

- Pain during micturition (dysuria).
- Increased frequency of urination (polyuria) and during night (nocturia).
- Urinary retention.
- Recurring urinary tract infection.
- In addition, patients may also present with hematuria and in cases of advanced disease general debility, anorexia and if the disease metastasizes to the bone, it causes bone pain.

Risk Factors

- **Age:** Prostatic carcinoma is commonly seen in elder males in the 5th—6th decades.
- **Ethnicity:** This is more common in African-Americans.
- **Hormonal influences:** Androgens are believed to promote the development of this tumor while estrogen therapy aids in its regression.
- **Dietary/environmental influences:** An intake of a diet rich in polyunsaturated fats, low fiber and obesity promotes prostatic oncogenesis.
- **Hereditary factors:** Families in which close relatives have had prostatic cancer are at a 50% increased risk of subsequently being affected by this disease. Similarly, families having BRCA 1 and 2 gene and ATM gene mutations are more susceptible to develop prostatic cancer.

Pathogenesis

The peripheral zone of the prostate is the area richer in glandular elements. Hence, the propensity to develop carcinoma is more in this zone. The transformation of a normal benign luminal epithelial cell of glands into a malignant cell is triggered by androgen receptor activation. This activation is mediated by testosterone, and a more potent form of testosterone called DHT. Once the androgen receptors (ARs) are activated they shift to the cell nucleus binding to androgen response elements (AREs). This in turn promotes transcription of genes promoting increased cellular proliferation and differentiation.

Additional factors such as coexisting chronic inflammation and genetic factors promote increase cell multiplication and eventual cancer (Refer Figure 15.8).

Diagnosis of Prostatic Carcinoma

Prostatic carcinoma may be completely asymptomatic and may be detected incidentally. In symptomatic cases, features may overlap with benign prostatic hyperplasia, initially. The three-method strategy is usually used to arrive at a diagnosis.

1. **Digital palpation (digital rectal examination):** The surgeon performs a per-rectal examination and feels the prostatic gland is nodular, hard and may be fixed to the surrounding structures. The peripheral part of the gland is easily palpated by this method and this is the common area where prostatic cancer develops.

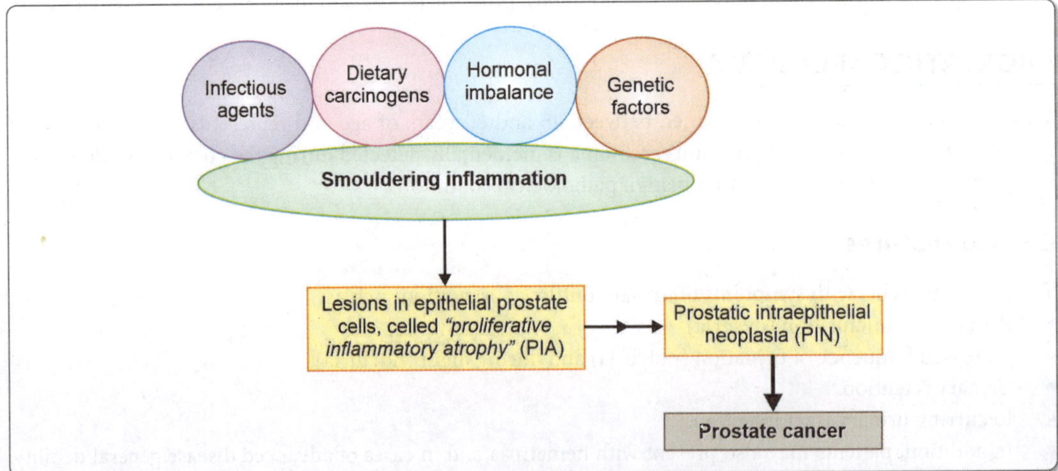

Figure 15.8: Pathogenesis of prostate cancer

However, in many cases of eventually biopsy proven prostatic carcinoma, no abnormality may be felt by this method. Hence, other tests are also necessary to arrive at the diagnosis.

2. **Serum tumor marker studies:** Sometimes, when clinical suspicion persists serial assessments of tumor markers are done.
   Prostate specific antigen (PSA): Normal value of total PSA is <4 ng/mL.
   Elevated values are associated with prostatic cancer. However, overlapping values may be seen in cases of benign prostatic hyperplasia and carcinoma. Hence, the surgeon uses a combination of techniques, including biopsy, to diagnose this cancer.
   Prostatic acid phosphatase (PAP): This was earlier used before the discovery of PSA. It is still relevant in cases where PSA levels are elevated, metastasis is present but the bone scan is negative for metastatic disease. PAP elevations in such cases favor extraprostatic extension of disease.
3. **Transrectal ultrasound (TRUS) guided needle biopsy:** The TRUS directed biopsy of the prostate forms the mainstay of diagnosis. In order to improve the diagnostic yield, recently MRI directed biopsies are also being performed.

MUST KNOW

Sometimes prostatic carcinoma is detected incidentally in tissue chips obtained during transurethral resection of prostate (TURP) which is a procedure performed in cases of BPH to relieve urinary obstruction.

Histological Changes

Biopsy/microscopic examination reveals (Fig. 15.9):

- An increased proliferation of glands infiltrating the surrounding tissue.
- Round generally monomorphic nuclei.
- Prostatic glands in prostatic carcinoma are typically small in size and are lined by atypical cells displaying an increased nucleocytoplasmic ratio.
- Nuclear enlargement, nucleolar prominence.

Figure 15.9: Histology of prostatic cancer

Histological grading of prostatic carcinoma:

Prostatic carcinoma is graded as per Gleason scoring system. The Gleason's scoring (Table 15.2) is the sum of the two most prevalent histological patterns is seen in the examined tissue.

Histological patterns associated with the Gleason grade groups:

- **Grade 1:** Only discrete well-formed glands.
- **Grade 2:** Predominately well-formed glands with a lesser component of poorly defined fused glands.
- **Grade 3:** Separate discrete malignant glands infiltrating into the tissue. Glandular lumen is appreciated.
- **Grade 4:** Glands which are fused/poorly formed/cribriform, i.e., their discrete borders are not appreciated and intervening stroma is sparse or absent.
- **Grade 5:** Malignant cells are seen as singly infiltrating cells arranged as cords or maybe seen as sheets/small nests. In other cases, comedo type necrosis is seen. Glandular lumina are not visualized in grade 5.

CARCINOMA PENIS

The most common histological type of carcinoma of penis (Fig. 15.10) is squamous cell carcinoma.

Age: This carcinoma is usually seen in the age group of 50–70 years.

Site involved: Glans/inner part of prepuce.

Table 15.2: Gleason scoring

Traditional gleason score	New grade group system
Gleason 3 + 3 = 6 Only individual discrete well-formed glands	Grade 1 – Gleason score 6 or less
Gleason 3 + 4 = 7 Predominantly well-formed glands with a lesser component of poorly-formed/fused/cribriform glands	Grade 2 – Gleason score 7 pattern 3 + 4
Gleason 4 + 3 = 7 Predominantly poorly-formed/fused/cribriform glands with a lesser component of well-formed glands	Grade 3 – Gleason score 7 pattern 4 + 3
Gleason 4 + 4 = 8 Only poorly-formed fused and cribiform glands or • Predominantly well-formed glands with and lesser component lacking gland formation or • Predominantly lacking glands with a lesser component of well-formed glands	Grade 4 – Gleason score 8 pattern 4 + 4/3 + 5/5 + 3
Gleason 9–10 Lacks gland formation (or with necrosis) with or without poorly-formed/fused/cribriform gland.	Grade 5 – Gleason score 9/10 pattern 4 + 5/5 + 4/5 + 5

Etiology

- Poor hygiene conditions.
- **Lack of circumcision:** Circumcision has a protective role by lessening the exposure to potential carcinogens in the smegma.
- Chronic inflammatory conditions/lichen sclerosis.
- Human papilloma virus (HPV) infection—high risk genotypes.
- Tobacco consumption.
- Premalignant lesions.

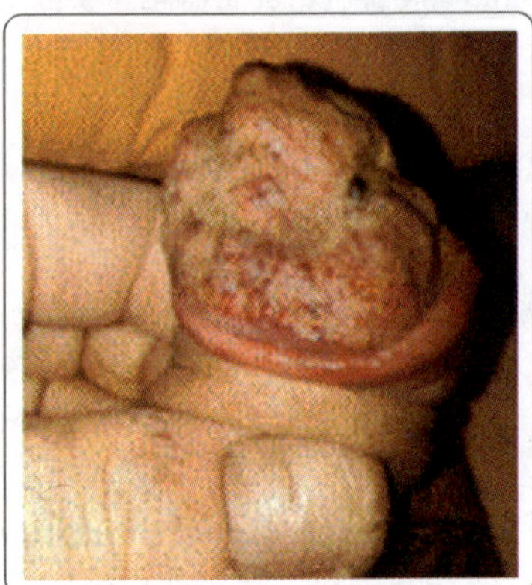

Figure 15.10: Carcinoma penis

Pathological Changes

Gross Appearance

Penile carcinomas can present in two forms:

1. Ulceroinfiltrative (endophytic)
2. Fungating (exophytic/cauliflower like)

Histological Changes

The tumor is usually a squamous cell carcinoma, displaying varying degrees of differentiation (Fig. 15.11). Spreads through lymphatics

- **Prognosis:** Related to tumor stage.
- **Other histological types:** Include verrucous, papillary and basaloid.

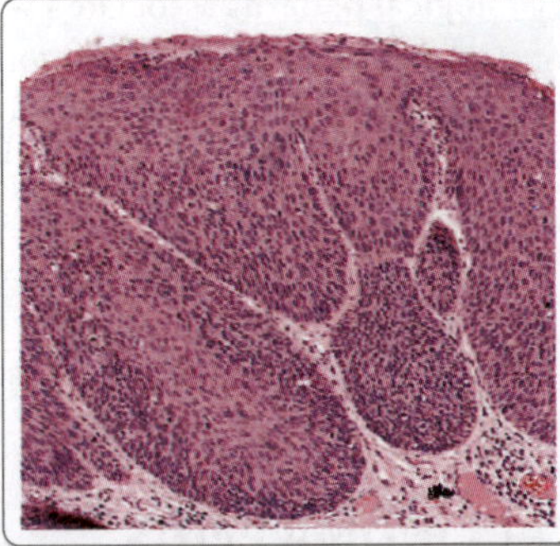

Figure 15.11: Histology of penile carcinoma

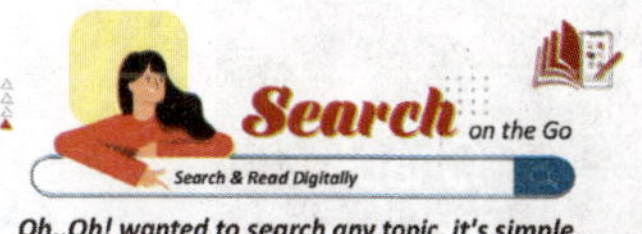

SUMMARY

- Cryptorchidism is a congenital anomaly in which there is failure of testicular descent.
- Cryptorchidism, is one of the conditions leading to testicular atrophy.
- Prostatic hyperplasia is a common condition seen in elderly males, especially after 50 years of age.
- BPH is very frequently seen after 60 years of age, hence it is believed to be a part of the normal ageing process.
- In BPH both glands and stroma proliferate in varying degrees.
- Prostatic carcinoma may be completely asymptomatic and may be detected incidentally.
- Prostatic carcinoma is graded as per Gleason scoring system.
- The most common histological type of carcinoma of penis is squamous cell carcinoma.

ASSESS YOURSELF

Long Answer Questions

1. What is etiopathogenesis of cryptorchidism?
2. Mention the pathogenesis and diagnostic approach to a case of prostatic carcinoma.

Short Answer Questions

1. Write about cryptorchidism.
2. Write about penile carcinoma.
3. Write short notes on:
   i. Benign prostate hyperplasia
   ii. Testicular atrophy

Multiple Choice Questions

1. **What do we call the failure of one or both testicles to descend into the scrotum?**
   a. Orchiopexy
   b. Testicular cancer
   c. Gynecomastia
   d. Cryptorchidism
2. **The prostate is about the size of a _____________.**
   a. Pea
   b. Dime
   c. Walnut
   d. Grape
3. **Prostate problems are common in men in their 30s.**
   a. True
   b. False
4. **Symptoms of an enlarged prostate may include:**
   a. Urinary tract infections
   b. Obstruction of urine flow
   c. Urinary retention
   d. All of these
5. **Which of the following is found in patients with prostate carcinoma, but not in patients that only have benign prostatic hyperplasia?**
   a. Prostate specific antigen (PSA)
   b. Prostatic acid phosphatase (PAP)
   c. CA19-9
   d. CCA

Answer Key

1. d **2.** c **3.** b **4.** d **5.** b

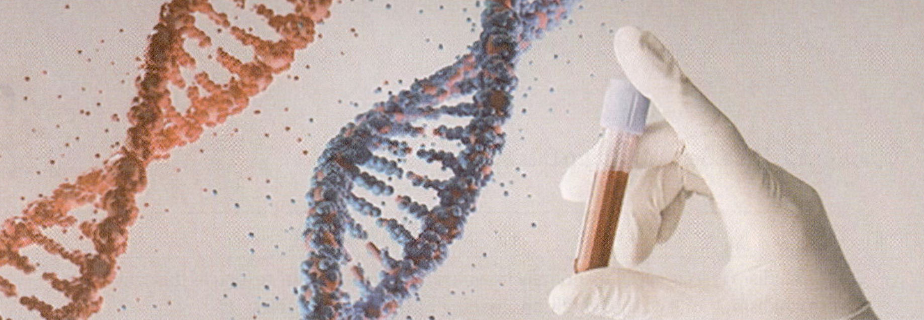

Chapter 16

Female Genital System Diseases

LEARNING OBJECTIVES

After the completion of the chapter, the readers will be able to:

- Describe cervicitis, leiomyoma, ovarian and endometriotic cyst.
- Explain carcinoma of cervix and endometrium.
- Discuss ovarian tumors, germ cell tumors of ovary, sex cord-stromal tumor and yolk sac tumor.
- Describe choriocarcinoma.

CHAPTER OUTLINE

- Overview of Female Reproductive/Genital System
- Cervicitis
- Ovarian Cysts
- Carcinoma Cervix
- Carcinoma of Endometrium
- Vesicular Mole and Choriocarcinoma
- Uterine Fibroid or Leiomyoma
- Ovarian Tumors

KEY TERMS

Cervical carcinoma: The growth of abnormal cells in the lining of the cervix.

Cervicitis: Inflammation of the cervix.

Endometrial carcinoma: A disease in which malignant (cancer) cells form in the tissues of the endometrium.

Hormone Replacement Therapy (HRT): A treatment used to relieve symptoms of the menopause.

Immunohistochemical markers: Proteins that help doctors tell the difference between different types of cancer.

Menarche: The first menstrual cycle.

OVERVIEW OF FEMALE REPRODUCTIVE/GENITAL SYSTEM

Internal reproductive organs in a female include the vagina, uterus, fallopian tubes, and ovaries.

- **Vagina:** It is a muscular, hollow tube extending from the vaginal opening to the uterus. The vagina is lined with mucous membranes to keep it protected and moist. The wall of vagina has four layers:
  i. Nonkeratinized stratified squamous epithelium
  ii. Lamina propria of connective tissue
  iii. Smooth muscle with bundles of circular and longitudinal fibers
  iv. Adventitia which has blood vessels, lymphatic ducts, and nerves.

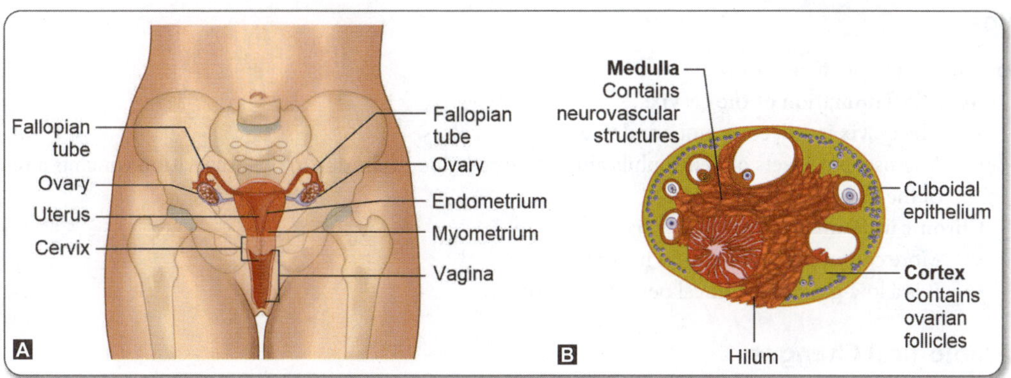

Figures 16.1A and B: Female reproductive system: **A.** Gross; **B.** Cut surface

- **Uterus:** The vagina connects with the uterus, at the cervix (lowest portion of uterus) which has strong, thick walls. Uterus has the strongest muscles composed of myometrium and endometrium, superficially lined by stratum functional (sloughs off during menstruation) and stratum basalis (rebuilds stratum functional).
- **Fallopian tubes:** Two **fallopian tubes** at the upper corners of the uterus connect the uterus to the ovaries.
- **Ovary:** The ovaries are important endocrine organs, which are central to the process of reproduction (Fig. 16.1A).

The ovaries are situated bilaterally on both sides of the uterus and represent the site for oogenesis or development of the ovum. Ovaries vary in size as per the age and hormonal status, however, normally they range in size from 3 cm to 5 cm and weigh 5–8 g.

The outer surface of the ovary is gray pink in color and smooth. The surface epithelial covering, called coelomic epithelium, is derived from the mesothelium.

Histology: On cut surface (Fig. 16.1B), two main zones exist:

i. **Outer cortex:** Cortical stroma has serpentine small spindle cells, fibroblasts and collagen.
ii. **Inner medulla:** Has smooth muscle cells.
   - The ovary shows numerous follicles existing in various stages of development. Follicles have an inner granulosa cell layer and an outer theca cell layer. The corpus luteum is a remnant of the ruptured ovarian follicles and secretes progesterone.
   - A third zone called the hilum also exists which harbors nerves, vessels and smooth muscle.
   - In the elderly, numerous acellular corpora albicans may also be seen.

CERVICITIS

Cervicitis refers to inflammation of the cervix.

Etiology

Sexually-transmitted infections (STIs), including gonorrhea, chlamydia, trichomoniasis and genital herpes and human papillomavirus (HPV). Other common infections include candidiasis/infection with anaerobic bacterium gardnerella.

Types

Cervicitis can be acute or chronic.

- **Acute inflammation of the cervix:**
  - The cervix is red, edematous and may show abscesses.
  - Microscopy: Sheets of neutrophils along with red blood cells due to the excoriation which is a result of the intense inflammation.
- **Chronic inflammation of the cervix:**
  - More common manifestation in India.
  - It is a low-grade subclinical persisting infection.

Pathological Changes

- **Gross appearance:** Inflamed indurated cervix, and may have a reddish appearance along with erosions.
- **Histological changes:** Sheets of lymphocytes with plasma cells, few histiocytes.
  - Epidermalization of endocervical glands.

OVARIAN CYSTS

The ovary may develop cysts at various ages either during the reproductive age group or later.

The cysts are commonly seen in the reproductive age group. They are derived from the normal follicles.

- **Cystic follicles:** When <3 cm in size, they are referred to as cystic follicles.
- **Follicular cysts:** When >3 cm, they are called follicular cysts. Histologically, they also have an inner granulosa layer and outer theca layer similar to normal follicles. These cysts are filled with clear fluid and when small they may spontaneously regress.

Polycystic Ovarian Disease (Stein-Leventhal Syndrome)

Polycystic ovarian disease is a common form of ovarian cyst afflicting the young, also called Stein-Leventhal syndrome (Figs 16.2A and B).

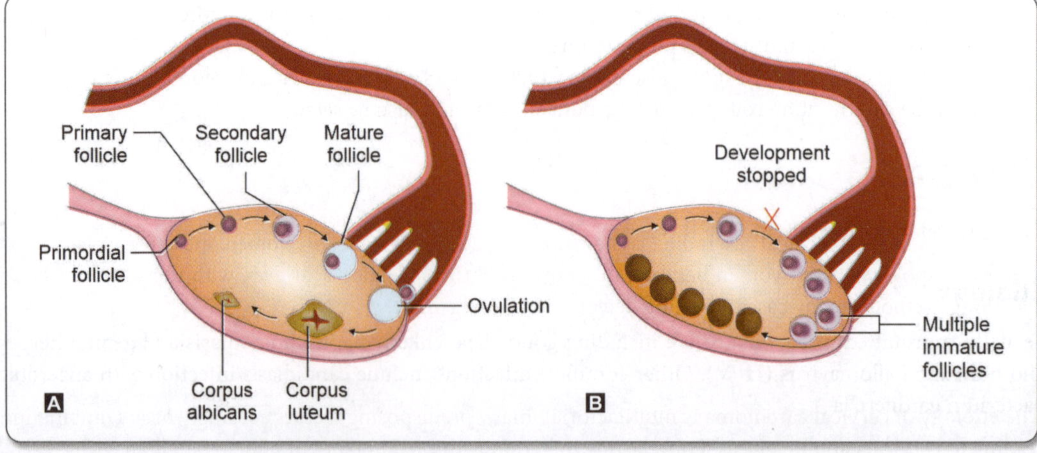

Figures 16.2A and B: Polycystic ovary syndrome: **A.** Normal ovary; **B.** Polysystic ovary

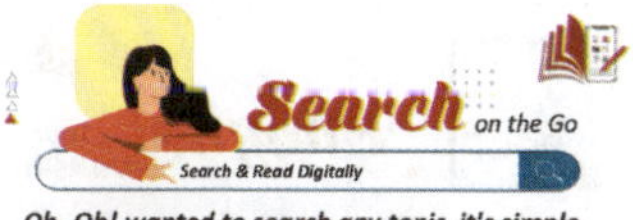

Clinical Features

Oligomenorrhea, hirsutism, obesity, anovulation, infertility with raised level of androgens (serum testosterone, androstenedione).

Pathological Changes

Gross appearance (Fig. 16.3A): Usually both ovaries are involved and enlarged, numerous cysts are seen in a "string of pearl" like appearance.

- **Cortex:** Thickened and collagenized
- Numerous cysts are seen,

Histological changes (Fig. 16.3B):

- Lined by luteinized theca cells and in similar phase of development.
- Corpus luteum is absent.

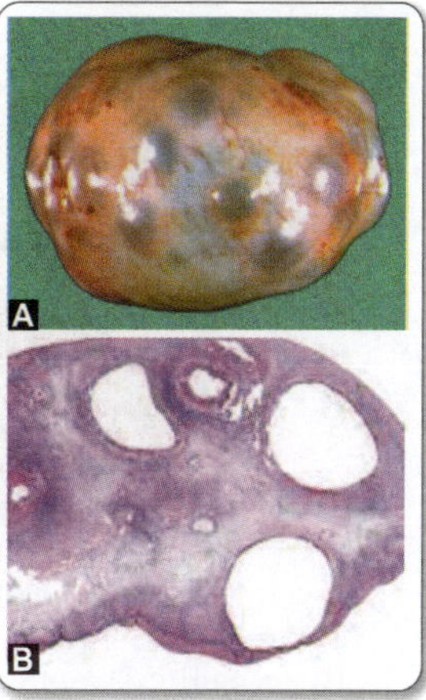

Figures 16.3A and B: PCOs: **A.** Gross; **B.** Histology

Corpus Luteal Cysts

Corpus luteal cysts are seen commonly in women of the reproductive age group. Corpus luteal cysts are usually >3 cm in size and microscopically have a characteristic undulating lining comprised of luteinized granulosa cells rimmed at the periphery by theca cells.

Pathological Changes

Refer to Figures 16.4A and B.

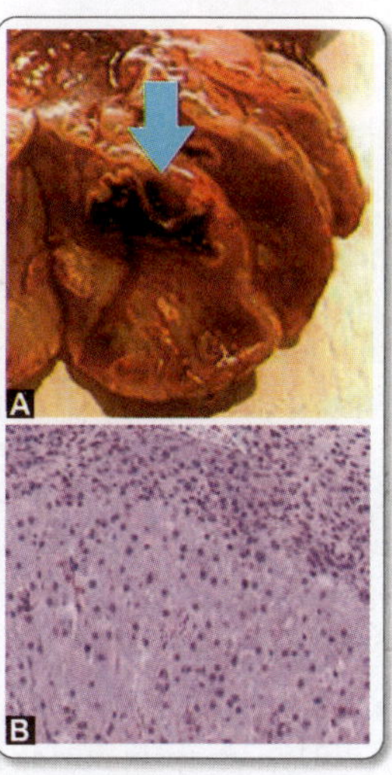

Figures 16.4A and B: Corpus luteal cyst: **A.** Gross; **B.** Histology

Endometriotic Cyst

Endometriotic cyst is also seen in the reproductive age group. The patient presents either with infertility or pain during menstruation.

Gross appearance (Fig. 16.5A): The ovary in such cases shows multiple cysts of varying sizes displaying thick chocolate-like material as the content giving the name of these cysts as "chocolate cysts".

Histological changes (Fig. 16.5B): Chocolate cysts are characterized by the presence of endometrial stroma and glands outside the uterus, i.e., inside the ovaries. Extensive hemorrhage is also seen along with the presence of numerous hemosiderin laden macrophages.

CARCINOMA CERVIX

Carcinoma cervix or cervical carcinoma is the most common malignancy in women after breast malignancy and is commonly seen in women between the fourth and fifth decades. However, with the advent of better screening methods, many cases are being detected at a younger age.

Etiology

The etiology of cervical carcinoma is multifactorial, many predisposing factors act singly or in combination, leading to cervical carcinogenesis. Long-lasting infection with certain types of human papillomavirus (HPV) is one of the major causes of cervical cancer.

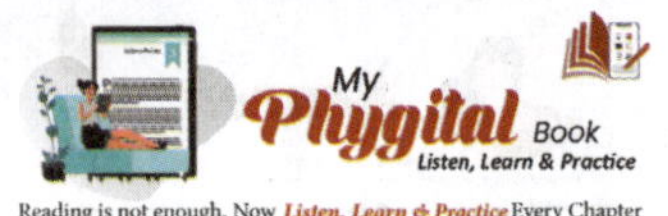

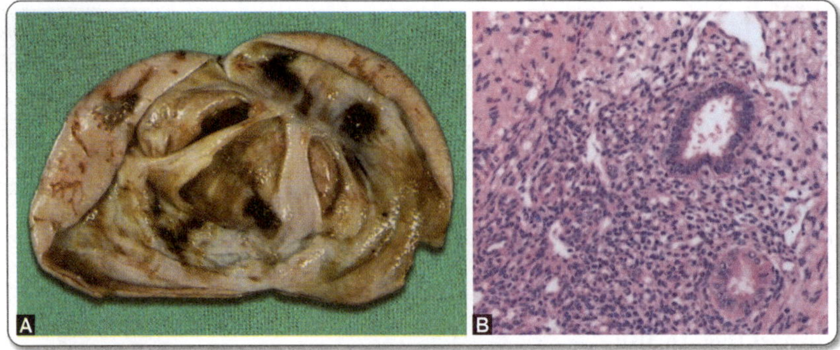

Figures 16.5A and B: Endometriotic Cyst: **A.** Gross; **B.** Histology

Risk Factors

- Having multiple sexual partners.
- Smoking.
- Infection with human papillomavirus.
- Early age at first intercourse.
- Multiparity.
- Poor personal hygiene.

Pathogenesis

The squamocolumnar junction represents an area of heightened activity with changing hormonal stimuli. The transformation zone refers to the zone where this junction keeps shifting at different ages and stages. This area is vulnerable to malignant transformation. It is believed that the human papilloma virus has a special role in the pathogenesis of cervical carcinoma. High-risk HPV genotypes include HPV 16, 18, 31, 33. HPV infection often occurs with sexual activity (Refer to Fig. 16.6).

MUST KNOW

- **High-risk HPV genotypes are HPV 16, 18, 31, 23, 52, 58**
- **Low-risk HPV genotypes are HPV 6, 11**

Clinical Features

- Vaginal bleeding, commonly after coitus.
- Dysuria (pain during micturition).
- Dyspareunia (pain on coitus).
- Foul smelling discharge.
- Per speculum examination—unhealthy cervix which may be red and/or inflamed.
- Vaginal discharge.
- Urinary obstruction in advanced cases.

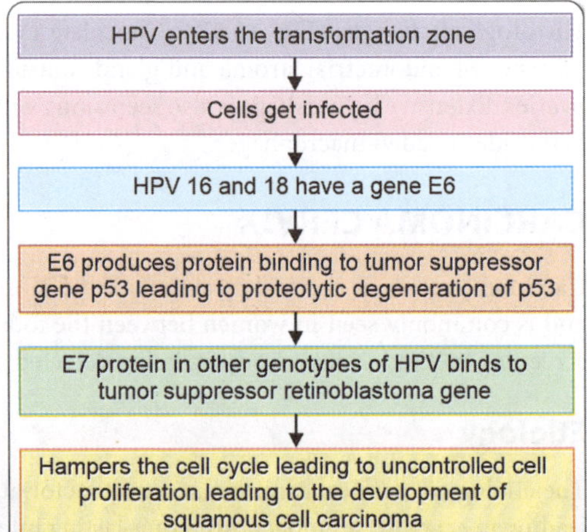

Figure 16.6: Pathogenesis of cervical cancer

Pathological Changes

Gross appearance: The tumor may have a fungating cauliflower-like growth (proliferative) which is friable and shows areas of hemorrhage and necrosis/an ulceroinfiltrative lesion which appears indurated and firm/may present as a polypoidal mass (Fig. 16.7).

Histological changes: The most common histological type of cervical carcinoma is squamous cell carcinoma (SCC). Other histological types include endocervical adenocarcinomas/ adenosquamous carcinomas. Squamous cell carcinoma may be keratinizing or nonkeratinizing. The salient histological features of SCC are:

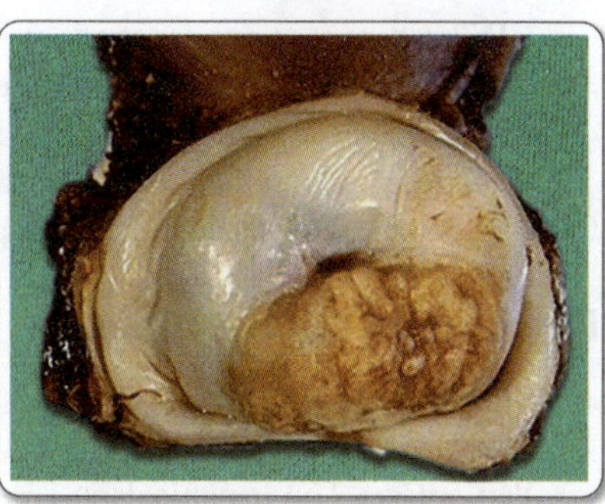

Figure 16.7: Carcinoma of cervix—Gross

- Sheets of cells displaying evidence of intracellular keratinization giving a pink color to the cytoplasm.
- Cells show intercellular bridges.
- Keratin pearls are seen in well-differentiated cases, keratinized cells are arranged as whorls.
- Features of malignancy, i.e., nuclear pleomorphism, nuclear hyperchromasia, increased nucleocytoplasmic ratio, clumped nuclear chromatin, infiltration of the underlying stoma by malignant cells, abnormal mitotic figures are noted.

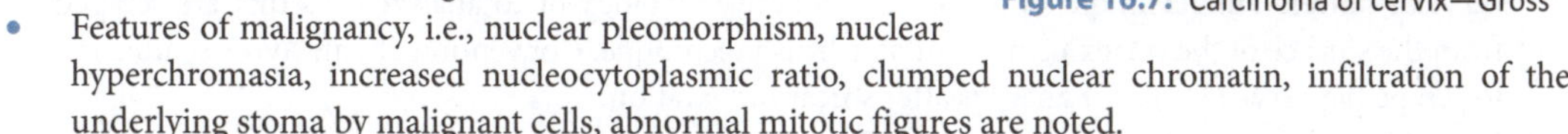

- Nonkeratinizing SCCs show the aforementioned features but without the presence of keratin pearls/ intracellular keratin.

Preneoplastic Lesions (Cervical Intraepithelial Neoplasia)

The sequence of precursor lesions for squamous cell carcinoma may be hyperplasia-metaplasia-dysplasia-CIS. Though all carcinomas do not develop through this sequence (Fig. 16.8) but many do which emphasizes the need for a timely diagnosis.

- **CIN1:** Changes of nuclear atypia are confined to the lower third of the lining squamous epithelium. HPV cytopathic change (presence of koilocytes) may be seen. CIN1 is also known as low grade squamous intraepithelial lesion (LSIL).

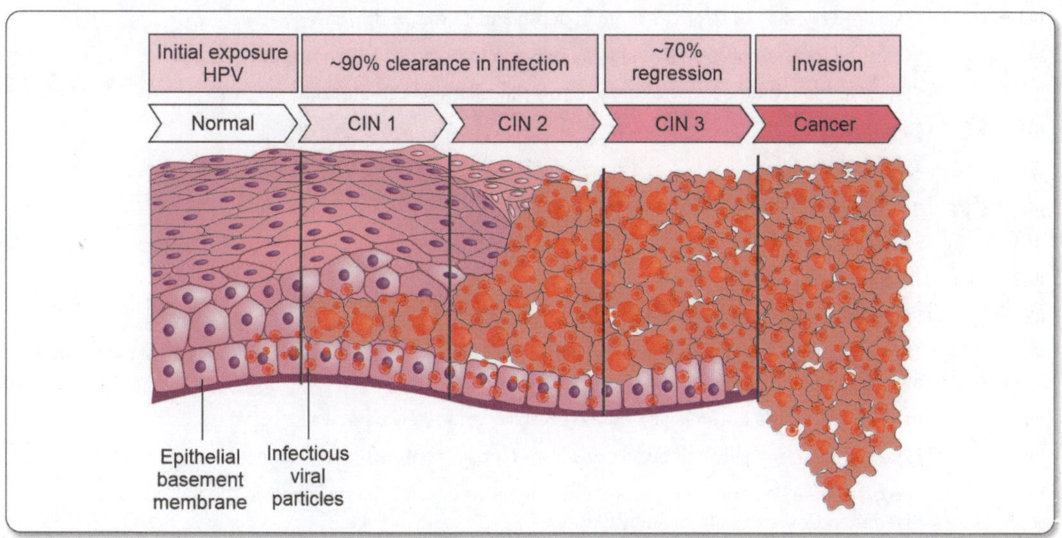

Figure 16.8: Preneoplastic lesions—cervical intraepithelial neoplasia

- **CIN2:** Changes of nuclear atypia are confined to the middle two-third of the lining squamous epithelium.
- **CIN3:** Changes of nuclear atypia are seen in the full thickness of the lining squamous epithelium. There is loss of nuclear polarity and loss of stratification. The basement membrane, however, remains intact, i.e., is no invasion into the underlying stroma is seen.

CIN 2,3 is also known as high grade squamous intraepithelial lesion (HSIL).

Detection of Cervical Cancer

- **Schiller test:** Application of Lugol's iodine solution to the cervix. Cancerous areas do not take up this stain.
- **Pap smear:** The Papanicolaou smear, also known as pap smear, has revolutionized the detection of cervical cancer. The technique is based on exfoliative cytology or to analyze cells that are scraped off from the surface of the cervix using a suitable brush technique. Conventionally, an Ayre's spatula is used to scrape the cervical cells for analysis after smear preparation.
- **Liquid-based cytology:** The two most important methods used to sample the cervix include the Sure Path and the ThinPrep techniques.
- Recent guidelines have suggested the concurrent testing of human papillomavirus by hybrid capture assay.

International Federation of Gynecology and Obstetrics (FIGO) criteria for staging of cervical cancer (Table 16.1)

Table 16.1: FIGO staging of cervical cancer

Stage	Description
IA	Invasive cancer identified only microscopically. Invasion is limited to measured stromal invasion with a maximum depth of 5 mm and no wider than 7 mm
IA1	Measured invasion of stroma ≤3 mm in depth and ≤7 mm width
IA2	Measured invasion of stroma >3 mm and ≤5 mm in depth and ≤7 mm width
IB	Clinical lesions confined to the cervix, or preclinical lesions greater than stage IA
IB1	Tumor ≤4 cm
IB2	Tumor >4 cm
IIA	Involvement till the upper 2/3 of the vagina
IIA1	Tumor ≤4 cm
IIA2	Tumor >4 cm
II8	Parametrial tumor involvement
III	The carcinoma has extended onto the pelvic sidewall and involves the lower third of the vagina and/or hydronephrosis and/or nonfunctioning kidney
IIIA	Involvement of the lower vagina but no extension onto pelvic sidewall
IIIB	Extension onto the pelvic sidewall or hydronephrosis/nonfunctioning kidney
IV	The carcinoma has extended beyond the true pelvis or has clinically involved the mucosa of the bladder and/or rectum (proven by biopsy).
IVA	Spread to bladder and/or rectum
IVB	Spread to distant organs

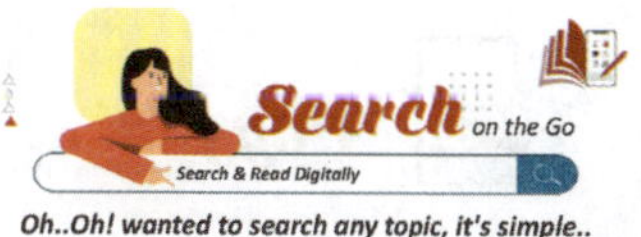

CARCINOMA OF ENDOMETRIUM

Carcinoma of endometrium arises from the lining of the uterus. Though common in Western females, it is still an important malignancy in Indian women. Generally, it is seen in peri/postmenopausal females.

Types of Endometrial Carcinoma/Carcinoma of Endometrium

Endometrial carcinoma has traditionally been classified into two types by Bokhman.

1. **Type 1 endometrial carcinomas:** Occurrs in a younger age group. These are related to hyperestrinism (unopposed estrogen), have a better prognosis being low grade and are associated with obesity/diabetes/HRT/early menarche and late menopause.
2. **Type 2 endometrial carcinomas:** On the other hand, type 2 endometrial carcinomas occurrs in post-menopausal females. These are independent of estrogen effects and have a poor prognosis. However, recently it has been observed that this classification is not representative of clinical behavior as overlapping features exist between these two types of carcinomas.

Subtypes of Carcinomas of Endometrium

The Cancer Genome Atlas (TCGA) has proposed four subtypes of endometrial cancer based on the tumor molecular profile (Table 16.2). Molecular profiling of endometrial cancer is based on three main parameters:

1. POLE molecule status.
2. Microsatellite instability status.
3. p53 mutation status.

Etiology

To remember etiology of endometrial cancer, use the mnemonic "COLD NUT".

MNEMONIC

"COLD NUT"

- **C**ancer – family history of hereditary nonpolyposis colorectal cancer—HNPCC syndrome
- **O**besity
- **L**ate menopause and early menarche
- **D**iabetes mellitus
- **N**ulliparity
- **U**nopposed estrogen as in PCOS and HRT
- **T**amoxifen which is used in breast cancer therapy

Table 16.2: Subtypes of endometrial cancer

Molecular subtype	Prognosis
POLE mutated	Good
Microsatellite instability	Intermediate
Low copy number mutations (No specific mutation)	Intermediate
High copy number mutations + p53 mutations (p53 mutated)	Poor

Risk Factors

- Women on hormone replacement therapy (HRT).
- Cases previously administered tamoxifen for breast carcinoma.
- Already diagnosed cases of endometrial hyperplasia.
- Obesity/hypertension.
- Early menarche/late menopause.

Pathogenesis

Refer to Figure 16.9.

Hormones stimulated by endogenous or exogenous estrogen
↓
Uninterrupted endometrial proliferation
↓
Unopposed by progesterone or progestins
↓
Leads from simple to complex forms of endometrial hyperplasia (EH)

Figure 16.9: Pathogenesis of endometrial carcinoma

Clinical Features

- The patient presents with abnormal uterine bleeding or postmenopausal bleeding.
- In advanced cases, the patient may present with an abdominopelvic mass.

Pathological Changes

Gross appearance (Fig. 16.10A):

- Necrotic mass/nodule obliterating the endometrial cavity which is usually friable, ulceroproliferative and extends to the adjoining myometrium.
- The lesion may sometimes be polypoidal and shows areas of hemorrhage and necrosis.
- In some cases, the endometrial cancer is infiltrative.

Histological changes (Fig. 16.10B):

- The tumor is comprised of malignant glands which are closely packed and admixed with individually dispersed atypical cells.
- The glandular lining epithelium is tall, columnar and shows pseudostratification with mild to moderate nuclear atypia. This may also be accompanied by a desmoplastic response comprised of fibroblasts and lymphocytes.
- Areas of squamous differentiation may also be seen in the form of small nests or morules, especially in low-grade endometrial carcinoma.

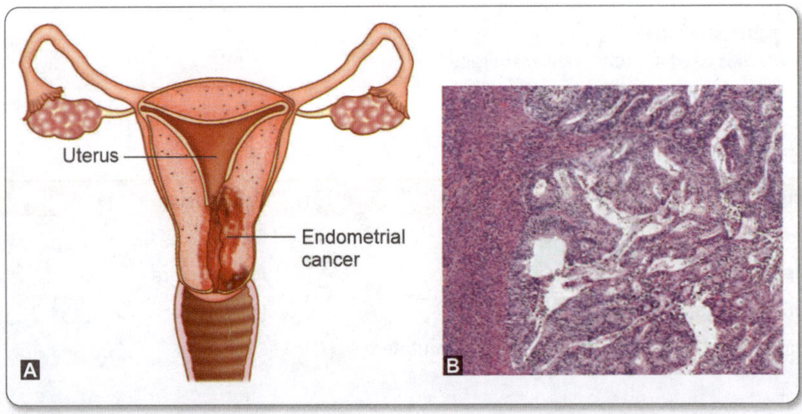

Figures 16.10A and B: Endometrial cancer: **A.** Gross; **B.** Histological changes

FIGO Criteria

Grading of endometrial cancer is done by FIGO criteria which is based on the percentage of solid, nonglandular areas (Table 16.3).

Table 16.3: FIGO criteria of grading endometrial cancer

Grade 1	<5% of solid area—Low grade
Grade 2	6–50% of solid area—Low grade
Grade 3	>50% of solid area—High grade

VESICULAR MOLE AND CHORIOCARCINOMA

CASE SCENARIO 1

A 40-year-old female presents to the gynecology OPD with complaints of amenorrhea of 12 weeks duration, accompanied by lower abdominal pain and heavy vaginal bleeding.

Vesicular moles and choriocarcinoma are part of an important group of disorders called gestational trophoblastic disease (GTD), i.e., tumors/tumor-like disease arising during gestation from the trophoblastic cells. Unlike hydatidiform mole, choriocarcinoma is a malignant and more aggressive form of GTD that spreads into the muscle wall of the uterus.

Vesicular Mole or Hydatidiform Mole

Age predilection: Females in the very young age group and those above 40 years.

Types of Hydatidiform Mole

1. Partial mole
2. Complete mole

Pathogenesis

In normal conception: One sperm(23X/23Y) fertilizes an ovum (23X) to form an embryo (46XX/46XY)

- **In partial Hydatidiform mole (Fig. 16.11A):** Two sperms (23X/23Y) (23X/23Y) fertilize an ovum (23X) to form a triploid conceptus (69XXX/69XXY/69XYY)
- **In complete Hydatidiform mole (Fig. 16.11B):** Two sperms (23X/23Y) fertilize an empty ovum to form a diploid (23X/23Y) conceptus (46 XX/XY) without any contribution from the ovum (androgenesis)

Pathological Changes

Gross Appearance

Complete mole: Swollen edematous grape-like translucent vesicular structures, filling and distending the entire uterine cavity.

- Hydropic change in all the villi causes them to swell up.

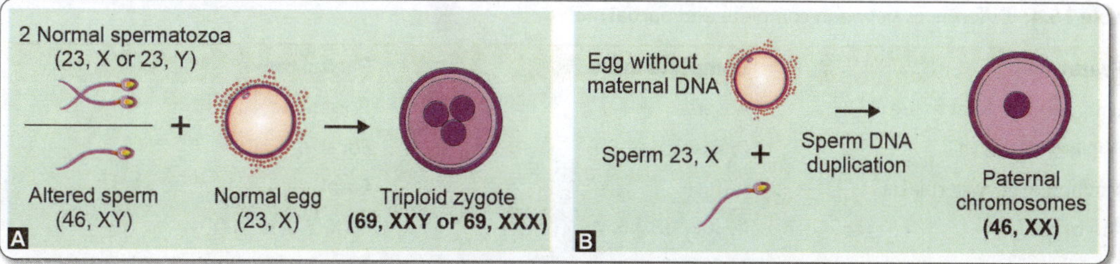

Figures 16.11A and B: Hydatidiform mole: **A.** Partial; **B.** Complete

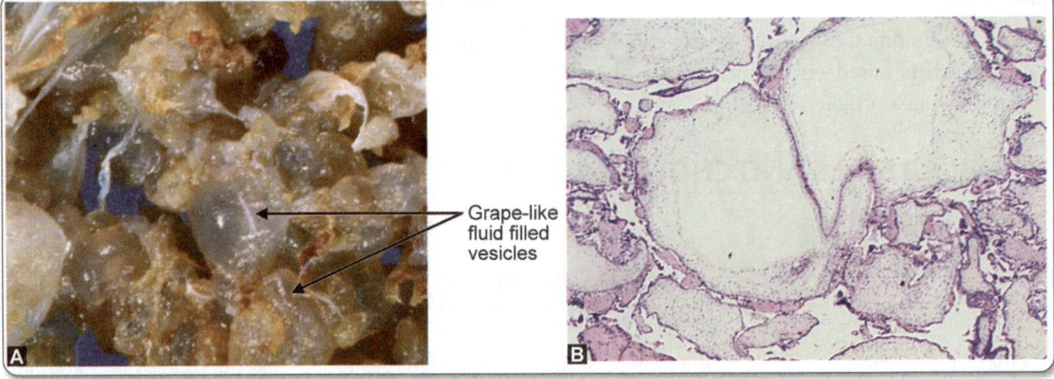

Figures 16.12A and B: Hydatidiform mole: **A.** Gross; **B.** Histology

- These vesicles are of variable sizes.
- On cutting open the vesicles, clear fluid is seen (Fig. 16.12A).
- No fetal parts/placenta are identified grossly.

Partial mole: Both enlarged swollen (hydropic) villi as well as normal sized villi are present.

- The number of vesicles and in turn the volume of conceptus is less than in the case of the complete mole.
- Fetal parts and gestational sac may also be seen.

Histological Changes

Complete mole:

- All villi show hydropic change.
- Some villi show swollen central portions that are fluid filled, called as "cisterns".
- Atypia and hyperplasia of both cytotrophoblasts and syncytiotrophoblasts is seen, i.e., diffuse and circumferential (Fig. 16.12B).
- Flow cytometric diagnosis: Diploid conceptus.
- IHC: p57 kip2 protein loss in trophoblasts.

Partial mole: Both hydropic villi and normal villi are seen.

- Mild trophoblastic atypia seen (less than the complete mole).
- Circumferential trophoblastic hyperplasia which is focal.
- Fetal parts may be identified microscopically.
- Flow cytometric diagnosis: Triploid conceptus.
- IHC: p57 kip2 protein presence in the trophoblastic tissue (nuclear positivity is seen).

The differences between the partial and complete mole are enumerated in Table 16.4.

Table 16.4: Differences between complete and partial mole

Feature	Complete mole	Partial mole
Embryonic or fetal tissue	Absent	Present
Swelling of the villi	Diffuse	Focal
Trophoblastic hyperplasia	Diffuse	Focal
Karyotype	46 XX (96%) or 46 XY (4%)	69 XXY or 69 XYY
Malignant changes	5–10%	Rare

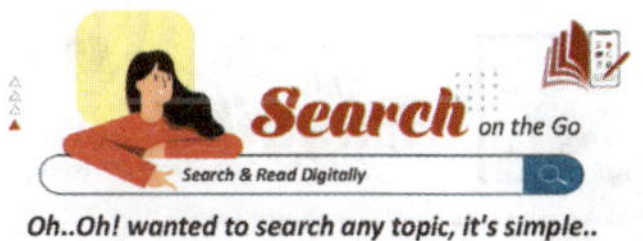

MUST KNOW

Invasive mole: This refers to the condition in which a complete hydatidiform mole demonstrates myometrial and/or vascular invasion.

Choriocarcinoma

CASE SCENARIO 2

A 42-year-old female presented to the OPD with complaints of persistent vaginal bleeding postabortion which is heavy. The patient also presented with shortness of breath.

Choriocarcinoma is a tumor which is known by the eponym gestational choriocarcinoma. The choriocarcinoma may also occur in the ovaries/testis at which time it is called nongestational choriocarcinoma. Treatment includes curettage and chemotherapy (methotrexate, etoposide).

Etiology

Choriocarcinoma usually has an aggressive biological course. It may arise:

- During the course of pregnancy.
- After a molar pregnancy.
- After a full-term pregnancy, miscarriage, ectopic pregnancy or abortion.

Risk Factors

- Previous history of hydatidiform mole especially complete hydatidiform mole.
- Previous abortion.
- Previous ectopic pregnancy.

Clinical Features

- **Persistent or irregular vaginal bleeding:** It is the most common symptom occurring after labor, abortion or evacuation of a vesicular mole. Bleeding can occur within days or months but rarely after 2 years.
- **Vaginal discharge:** Blood stained and offensive due to ulceration and infection.
- **Amenorrhea:** Due to continuous hCG production, pelvic pain or pressure, if an enlarged uterus or ovarian cysts are present, the patient may report pelvic pain or pressure.
- **Metastases:** The tumor commonly spreads to the lungs, liver, brain *via* the hematogenous route. Clinical features due to metastasis:
  - Dyspnea, cough, chest pain and hemoptysis are noticed with lungs metastasis.
  - Irregular and at times brisk hemorrhage in vaginal metastasis.
  - The appearance of neurological symptoms like hemiplegia, seizures, headache, dizziness and visual disturbances suggests brain metastasis.
  - Epigastric pain and jaundice in liver metastasis.
- Rapid growth, widespread dissemination, and a high propensity for hemorrhage make this tumor a medical emergency.

Pathological Changes

Gross appearance (Fig. 16.13A): Choriocarcinoma is highly hemorrhagic and necrotic tumor mass which is red, soft and friable. The tumor is frequently seen first in the uterine cavity and then extends through the cavity with time.

Histological Changes (Fig. 16.13B): A characteristic biphasic appearance is seen in which cytotrophoblasts alternate with sheets of syncytiotrophoblasts.

- An important diagnostic feature is the absence of villi.
- Trophoblast atypia is marked.
- Malignant trophoblasts infiltrate the myometrium, destroying the myocytes.
- Hemorrhage and necrosis are common
- Mitotic activity is high.

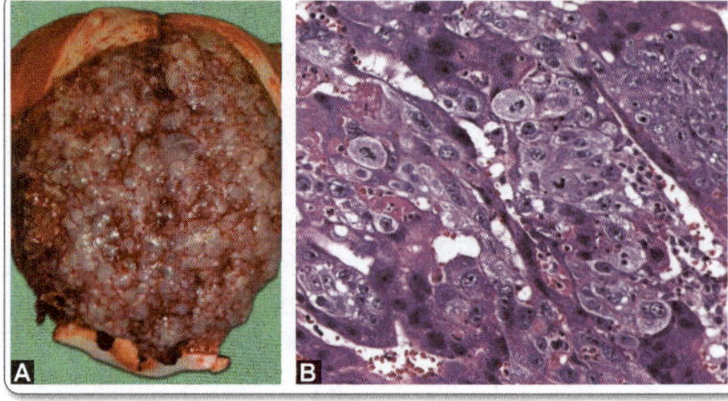

Figures 16.13A and B: Choriocarcinoma: **A.** Gross; **B.** Histology

Immunohistochemistry:

- Choriocarcinomas are positive for hCG, hPL and placental alkaline phosphatase.
- Tumor markers: Serum beta hCG levels are markedly elevated.

UTERINE FIBROID OR LEIOMYOMA

CASE SCENARIO 3

A 45-year-old female presented to the gynecology OPD with the complaints of heavy bleeding during menstruation and increased frequency of urination. Ultrasound showed a well-defined hypoechoic mass in the uterus.

The most common benign tumor of the uterus is uterine fibroid or leiomyoma. The tumor is of smooth muscle origin and is frequently seen in the third to the fifth decade.

Types of Leiomyoma

Depending on the site of occurrence of the leiomyoma:

- **Subserosal:** Just beneath the uterine serosa.
- **Intramural:** Within the wall of the uterus.
- **Submucosal**: Beneath the mucosa (endometrial lining).

Clinical Features

- Altered menstrual bleeding pattern- menorrhagia (heavy bleeding), polymenorrhea (more frequent cycles), metrorrhagia (bleeding in between cycles).
- Lower abdominal pain.
- Inability to conceive.
- Pressure symptoms: increased frequency of urination, retention of urine.

Pathogenesis

Leiomyomas are known to be dependent on the presence of estrogen. Certain molecular alterations are associated with the development of leiomyomas. The important ones include MED 12 mutations, HMGA1, HMGA2 rearrangements. Myometrial stem cells get transformed. Oxygen deprivation, growth factors influence and presence of steroids lead to uncontrolled growth of tumor cells (Fig. 16.14).

Some variations of the leiomyoma include:

- **Mitotically active leiomyoma:** A leiomyoma with more frequent mitoses than usual (6–14 mitoses/10 HPF).

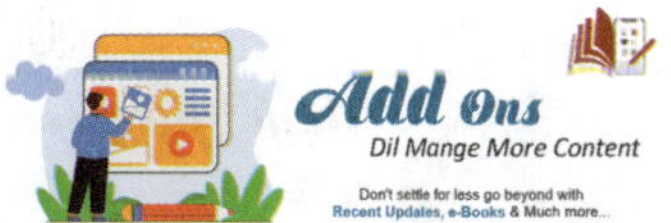

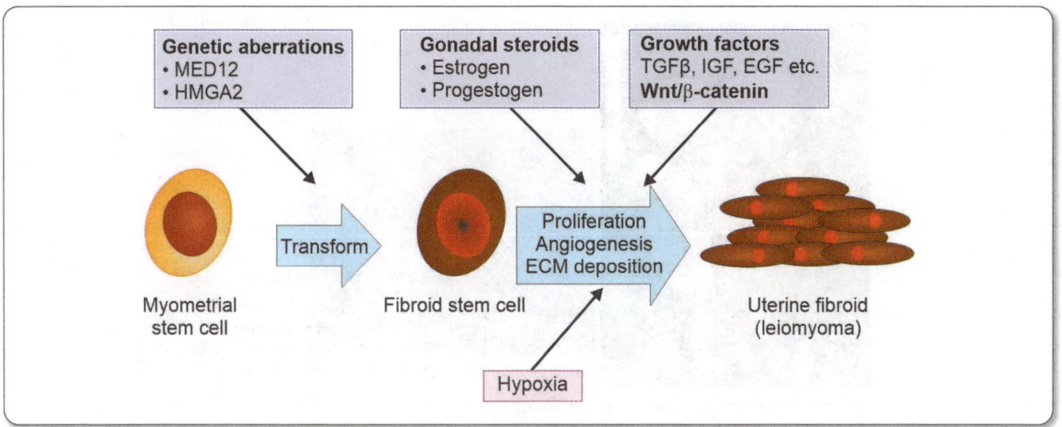

Figure 16.14: Pathogenesis of uterine fibroid

Note: MED12, HMGA2, TGFβ, IGF, EGF are mutations

- **Cellular leiomyoma:** A leiomyoma with more cellularity than the surrounding myometrium.
- **Hydropic leiomyoma:** A leiomyoma with edematous stroma.
- **Myxoid leiomyoma:** A leiomyoma with myxoid stroma.
- **Intravenous leiomyoma:** A proliferation of benign smooth muscle cells within a vessel wall.
- Fumarate-hydratase deficient leiomyomas-Hereditary, associated with renal cell carcinoma.

Complications/Sequelae

- **Frequency of malignant transformation:** Highly rare (0.5% of all leiomyomas).
- **Torsion:** This is often seen in myomas having a stalk (pedunculated myomas).
- Superadded infection.

Pathological Changes

Secondary changes: Numerous changes have been described in leiomyomas which are long standing:
- **Atrophy:** Reduction in size of the tumor due to a reduced vascularity which is common after menopause/postpartum.
- **Red degeneration:** Seen in pregnancy, causes severe abdominal pain and fever. The leiomyoma assumes a red color possibly due to blood pigment diffusion from thrombosed vessels.
- Hyaline/fatty/cystic degeneration can occur in any leiomyoma where the blood supply is compromised.
- **Calcification:** In leiomyomas of considerable duration.

Gross appearance: Leiomyomas are well circumscribed, variably sized gray-white tumors with a pseudocapsule. The consistency is firm and on cut surface, a characteristic "whorled" appearance is noted. The lesions may be solitary or multiple (Fig. 16.15A).

Histological changes: The tumor is comprised of interlacing fascicles of spindle cells with uniform size, an abundant pink cytoplasm and cigar shaped nuclei. Necrosis/conspicuous mitotic activity is not a feature of the classic benign leiomyoma (Fig. 16.15B).

Immunohistochemical markers positive in leiomyoma include SMA, Desmin, h-caldesmon.

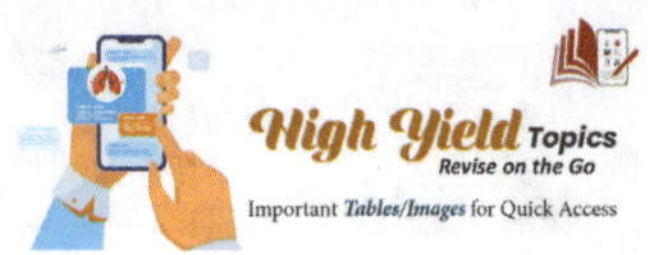

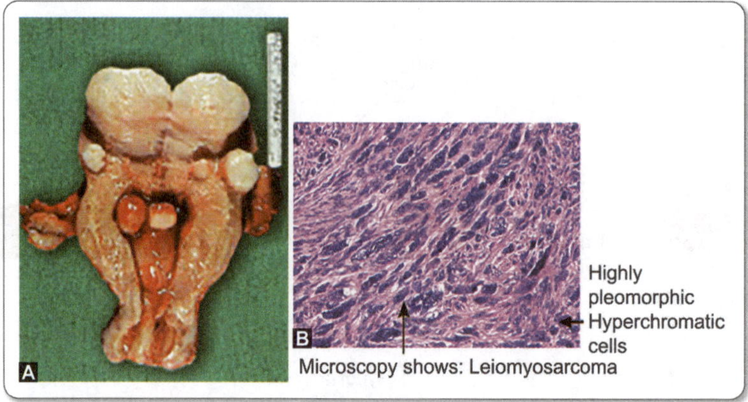

Figures 16.15A and B: Uterine leiomyomas: **A.** gross; **B.** histology

OVARIAN TUMORS

Ovarian tumors usually occur in the age group of 20–40 years. Most of the tumors are benign.

Ovarian tumors are classified as follows (Table 16.5). The mnemonic to remember classes of the ovarian tumors is:

Surface Epithelium Tumors

Surface epithelial tumors are the most common tumors with serous cystadenoma being the common tumor. Benign serous cystadenomas occur in women in between the third and fourth decade.

Gross appearance: These tumors can be of varying sizes and can be up to 10 cm in size. The cyst is unilocular, has a smooth wall and has clear fluid. No solid areas or papillary excrescences can be appreciated.

Histological changes: The cyst wall is lined by a single layer of low cuboidal cells devoid of atypia.

MNEMONIC

My **S**ister **B**egan **E**xperiencing **C**ancer
Doctor **E**xamined **T**he **C**ancer **Y**oung
She **F**elt **G**ood

Table 16.5: Classification of ovarian tumors

Surface epithelial tumors	Germ cell tumors	Sex cord stromal tumors
Mucinous	Dysgerminoma	Sertoli-Leydig cell
Serous	Embryonal	Fibroma
Brenner	Teratoma	Granulosa theca cell
Endometrioid	Choriocarcinoma	
Clear cell	Yolk sac tumour	

Mucinous Tumors or Mucinous Cystadenoma

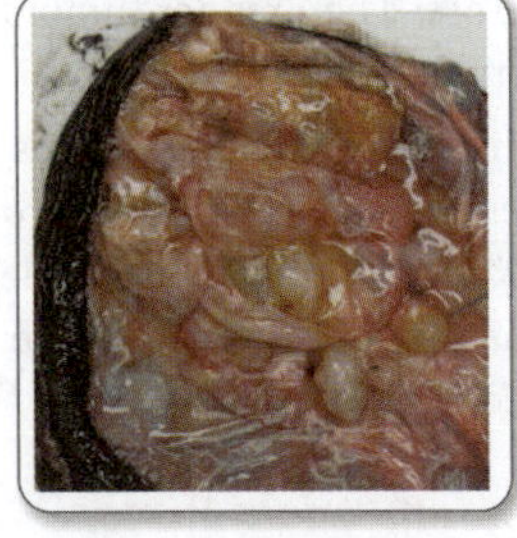
Figure 16.16: Mucinous cystadenoma

Mucinous tumor is a benign ovarian lesion that is usually unilateral and multilocular (Fig. 16.16). The patient presents with a pelvic mass and is often in the fifth to sixth decade. Molecular features associated with mucinous cystadenocarcinoma include TP53 and KRAS mutations and copy number loss of CDKN2A gene.

Borderline mucinous tumor: stratification of lining epithelium without stromal invasion

Gross appearance: The tumor is usually unilateral and is cystic, solid areas may be seen focally. Cysts are multiloculated with the locules being filled with mucinous content.

Histological Changes: The malignant tumor shows stratification and heaping up of the epithelium. Solid areas may be seen. Malignant tumors have thickened areas. The cyst wall is lined by tall columnar epithelial cells filled with mucin referred to as the "picket fence" appearance.

Serous Tumors

Serous tumors vary in size from small and nearly imperceptible to large. Serous tumors can further be of the following types:

- Serous cystadenoma (Fig. 16.17A)
- Benign serous cystadenoma (Fig. 16.17B)
- Serous borderline (Fig. 16.17C). These tumors are usually seen in the perimenopausal age group.

Gross appearance: These lesions are largely cystic and show papillary excrescences and occasional solid areas. The cyst is lined by a single layer of columnar epithelium.

Histological changes: Papillary projections; invasion into the stroma in cases of carcinoma.

- In malignancy: loss of nuclear polarity, epithelial multilayering, stromal invasion.
- In borderline tumors: stromal invasion is absent.

Brenner Tumor

The Brenner tumor (Fig. 16.18) occurs in females in the fifth to seventh decade of life and it occurs by chance frequently detected. Metaplastic transformation of the coelomic epithelium into transitional lining epithelium occurs.

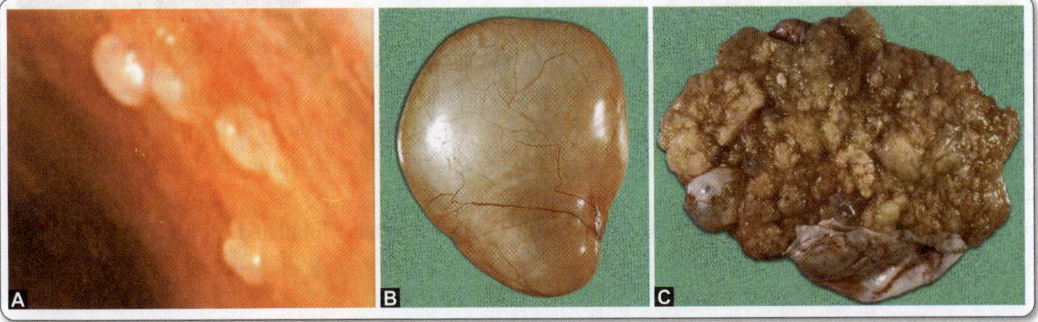

Figures 16.17A to C: **A.** Serous ovarian tumor; **B.** Benign serous cystadenoma of ovary; **C.** Serous borderline tumor of ovary

Gross: The Brenner tumors are usually small, firm whitish yellow and have a rubbery consistency.

Histological changes: This tumor comprises nests of transitional epithelial cells in a dense fibrotic stroma. Tumor cells are ovoid, having coffee bean-like nuclei, opened up nuclear chromatin. In between the tumor cells, small microcystic spaces are identified which may be filled with eosinophilic secretions.

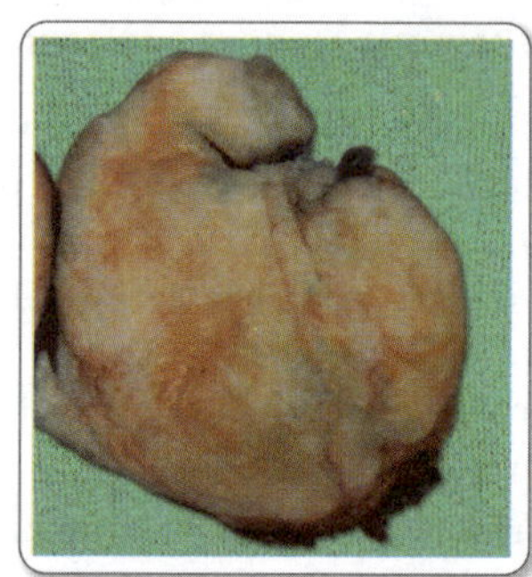

Figure 16.18: Brenner tumor

Endometrioid Tumor

As the name suggests endometrioid tumor shows histomorphology reminiscent of the endometrium. Most tumors are malignant though like other surface epithelial tumors, categories of benign and borderline are also seen (Fig. 16.19). Endometrioid tumors of the ovary are seen in the 5th to 6th decade and are associated with endometriosis. About one fourth of patients have concurrent endometrial carcinoma (endometrioid type) or endometrial hyperplasia. These tumors are also associated with β-catenin mutations (CTNNB1). Endometrioid tumors have the following features:

Gross appearance: Solid-cystic with areas of hemorrhage and necrosis.

Histopathologic changes: Characterized by back-to-back confluent glands. Foci of squamous differentiation may also be seen.

Immunohistochemistry: Tumor cells are positive for PR and vimentin and are negative for napsin A and WT1.

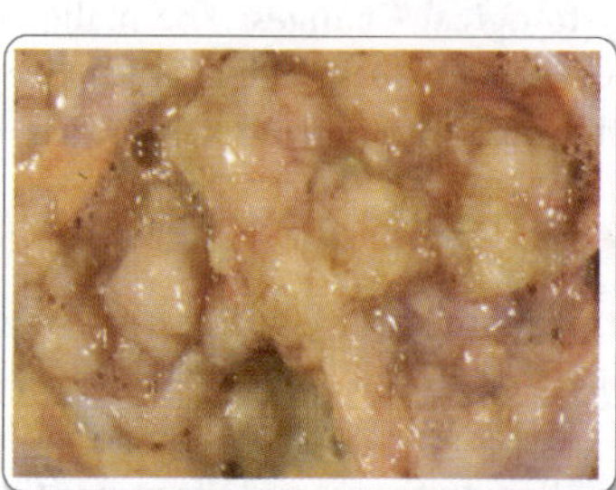

Figure 16.19: Endometroid tumor of ovary

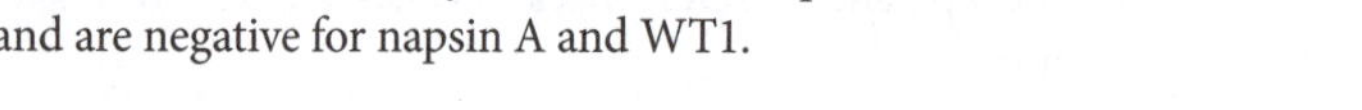

Clear Cell Tumor

Clear cell tumor (Fig. 16.20) is usually seen in the fifth to sixth decade of life. Endometriosis is an important predisposing factor. The tumor is arranged in the form of tubules, papillae and sheets of cells and the cells may deceptively look small and bland but have a conspicuous clear cell change.

Tumor cells are positive for IHC markers PAX8 and napsin and negative for WT1.

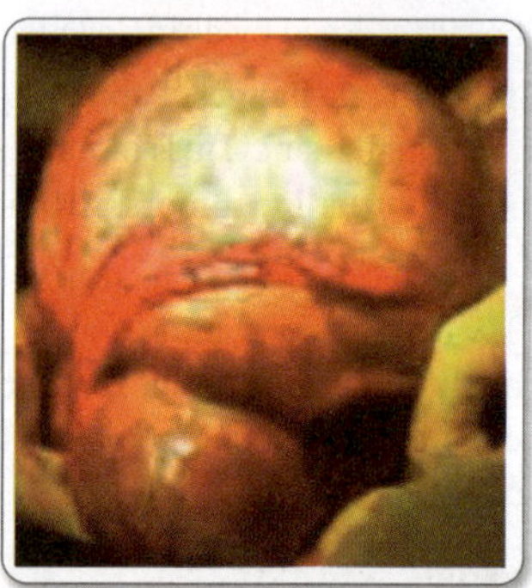

Figure 16.20: Clear cell ovarian tumor

Germ Cell Tumors of Ovary

Germ cell tumors generally occur in the younger age group.

Dysgerminoma

Dysgerminoma (Fig. 16.21A) is the counterpart of teratoma. It occurs in young females and is usually malignant and highly radiosensitive.

Gross appearance: Usually solid appearance; gray-white in color and has a lobulated appearance

Histological changes: Tumor cells are arranged in the form of nests and sheets separated by fibrovascular stroma.

- Tumor cells are moderate in size, round to ovoid and have a moderate amount of clear cytoplasm indicative of the presence of glycogen.
- The fibrovascular stroma is rich in lymphocytes.

Note: Choriocarcinoma and endometrial carcinoma have already been discussed in this chapter.

Teratoma

Teratoma is derived from all three germ cell layers - ectoderm, mesoderm and endoderm. The mature benign teratoma is benign and has a solid cystic appearance.

Gross appearance: Uninoculated cyst. On opening, the cyst reveals the presence of pultaceous material; Rokitansky protuberance (the formation of a solid area). An important prognostic factor is the proportion of neural tissue present in the lesion.

Histological changes: Under microscope, tissues of all germ cell lines are seen including immature components; immature/malignant teratoma is rare. It is histologically characterized by immature tissue, most frequently, neuroepithelial tissue, variegated, with hemorrhage and necrosis.

Monodermal Teratoma

This is also called a specialized teratoma (Fig. 16.21B). This has further categories which include struma ovary in which thyroid follicles are seen; and have carcinoids.

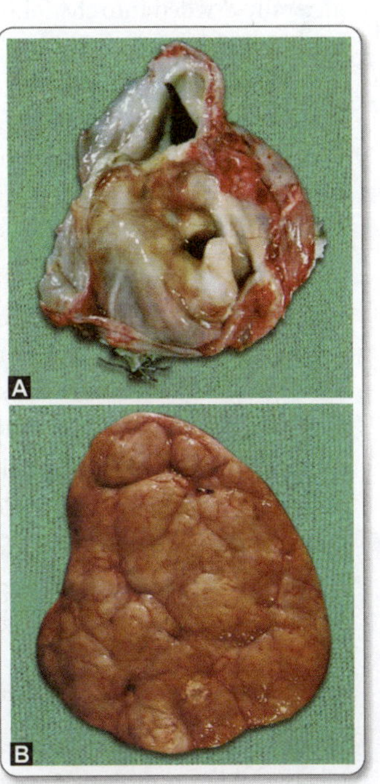

Figures 16.21 A and B: **A.** Dysgerminoma; **B.** Monodermal teratoma

Yolk Sac Tumor (Endodermal Sinus Tumour)

Characteristically secretes AFP. The tumor is usually solid and has focal cystic areas. Papillary projections can be seen around a central lumen—also known as the Schiller-Duval body.

The presence of PAS positive hyaline globules is of diagnostic value.

Sex Cord-Stromal Tumors

Sex cord-stromal tumors are groups of tumors composed of granulosa cells, theca cells, Sertoli cells, Leydig cells, and fibroblasts of stromal origin. These cells are present singly or in various combinations, in the tumor. The clinicopathological features vary along with biologic behavior.

Sertoli-Leydig Cell Tumor

Sertoli-Leydig cell tumor is a rare cancer of the ovaries (Fig. 16.22). The cancer cells produce and release a male sex hormone called testosterone. Patients with Sertoli-Leydig cell tumor often have an abdominal pain and a series of symptoms of defeminization and progressive masculinization such as amenorrhea, deepening of the voice, hirsutism, a male pattern hair growth, and clitoromegaly.

Immunohistochemical markers of Sertoli-Leydig cell tumor include alpha-inhibin, calretinin, and melan-A.

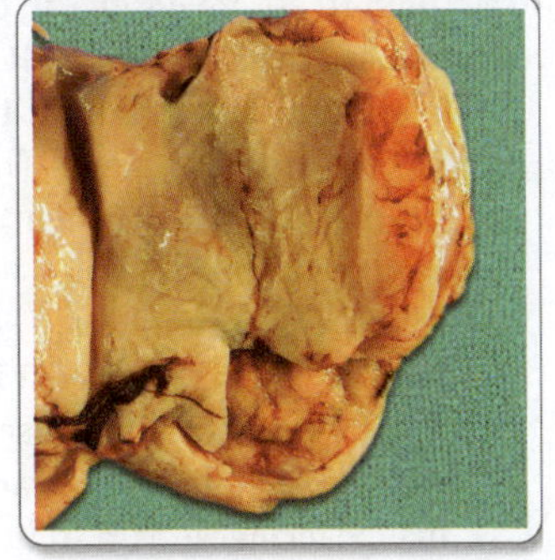

Figure 16.22: Sertoli-Leydig cell tumor

Gross appearance: Almost always unilateral; tumor size ranges widely from <1 cm to 35 cm.

There are variable combinations of Sertoli cells and Leydig cells, among other possible components. They are generally divided into the following histologic subtypes:

- Well-differentiated.
- Moderately differentiated.
- Poorly differentiated.
- With heterologous elements and retiform and mixed.

Fibroma

Fibroma is a growth or tumor that appears near a woman's ovaries and is typically benign (not cancerous). Most instances of ovarian fibroma (Fig. 16.23) develop gradually and have no symptoms. In many cases, a benign ovarian fibroma does not cause the patient any trouble and may not require fibroid treatment.

Gross appearance: They usually present as a solid mass and may be associated with ascites and elevated serum CA-125 levels. Ovarian fibromas are benign neoplasms, and the prognosis is extremely good.

Figure 16.23: Fibroma

Histological changes: Benign stromal tumor composed of fibroblastic cells within a variably collagenous stroma.

Granulosa Theca Cell Tumor

Granulosa theca cell tumors are tumors of sex cord origin (Fig. 16.24). Metastases from ovarian tumors are usually seen in the elderly age group. These ovarian tumors consist of granulosa cells, theca cells, and fibroblasts in various combinations. Granulosa cells in the sex cords produce sex steroids, and peptides needed for folliculogenesis and ovulation.

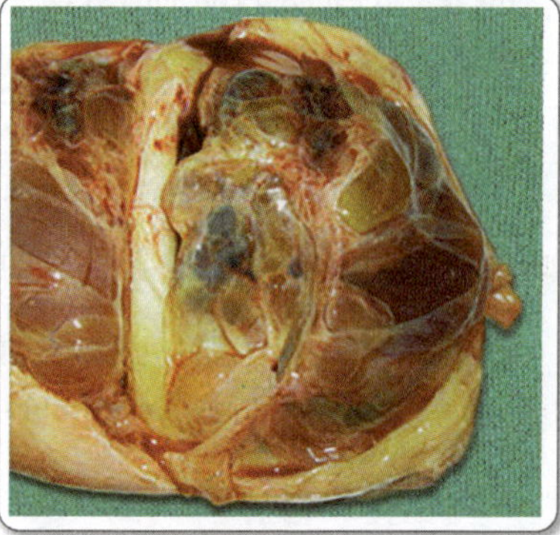

Figure 16.24: Granulosa theca cell tumor

Gross appearance: A large, unilateral, cystic ovarian mass that is tan-yellow in appearance on cross-section.

Histological changes: Microfollicular pattern with Call-Exner bodies and coffee bean nuclei are the most common diagnostic points. Tumor markers are alpha-inhibin and calretinin (these are positive in granulosa theca cell tumor).

Granulosa cell tumor (GCT): GCTs are the most common type of sex cord-stromal tumor. These can be noncancerous (benign) or cancerous (malignant).

- **Juvenile granulosa cell tumor (JGCT) of ovary:** JGCT represents a small fraction of all primary ovarian malignancies. It is a subtype of granulosa cell tumor that is almost always found during the first three decades of life. Histologically, it differs from the typical adult type of granulosa cell tumor.

MUST KNOW

Krukenburg tumor is a metastatic malignancy of the ovary characterized by mucin-rich signet-ring adenocarcinoma that primarily arises from a gastrointestinal site in most cases and less commonly from other sites. The metastasis to the ovary is bilateral. Trans coelomic spread, commonly from gastric carcinoma. Other sites of metastasis include colon, breast, appendix.

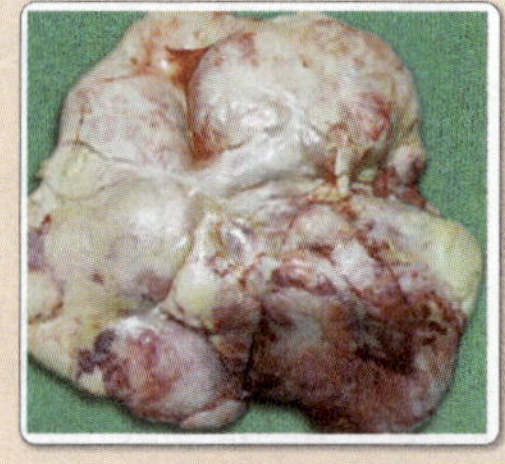

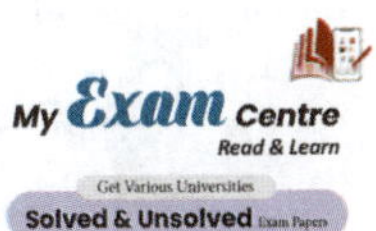

- **Solid cystic tumor:** These are defined as a cyst with thick walls (>0.5 mm), thick septa (>0.5 mm), an intra-cystic mass, or a cyst demonstrating >50% solid components. Benign ovarian tumors are slow-growing solid masses in or on a woman's ovary.

Histopathological changes:
- Grayish white multinodular masses.
- Mucin filled signet string cells.

SUMMARY

- Carcinoma cervix is the most common malignancy in women after breast malignancy and is commonly seen in women between the fourth and fifth decades.
- The most common histological type of cervical carcinoma is squamous cell carcinoma (SCC).
- Type 1 endometrial carcinomas occur in a younger age group.
- Type 2 endometrial carcinomas occur in postmenopausal females.
- TCGA has proposed four subtypes of endometrial cancer based on the tumor molecular profile.
- The most common benign tumor of the uterus is uterine fibroid or leiomyoma.
- Leiomyomas are known to be dependent on the presence of estrogen.
- Leiomyomas are well circumscribed, variably sized gray-white tumors with a pseudocapsule.
- Unlike hydatidiform mole, choriocarcinoma is a malignant and more aggressive form of GTD that spreads into the muscle wall of the uterus.
- The choriocarcinoma may also occur in the ovaries/testis at which time it is called nongestational choriocarcinoma.
- The cysts are commonly seen in the reproductive age group, derived from the normal follicles.
- Chocolate cysts are characterized by the presence of endometrial stroma and glands outside the uterus, i.e., inside the ovaries.
- Benign serous cystadenomas occur in women in between the third and fourth decade.
- Endometrioid tumors of the ovary are seen in the fifth to sixth decade and are associated with endometriosis.
- The mature benign teratoma is benign and has a solid cystic appearance.
- Metastases from ovarian tumors are usually seen in the elderly age group.

ASSESS YOURSELF

Long Answer Questions

1. Discuss ovarian tumors in detail.
2. What are the features of endometrial carcinoma? Discuss the classification of endometrial carcinoma.

Short Answer Questions

1. What is fibroid?
2. Write about leiomyoma.
3. Write short notes on:
   i. Vesicular mol
   ii. Choriocarcinoma

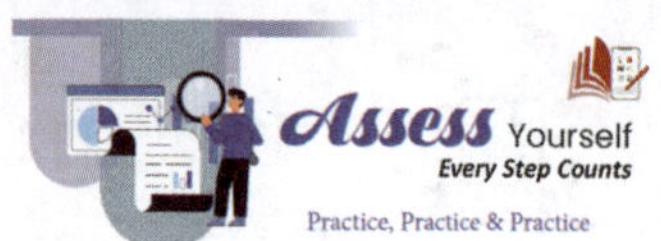

Multiple Choice Questions

1. **The following statements refer to uterine fibroids (leiomyomata). Determine which are true.**
   a. Uterine fibroids are benign tumors of the myometrium present in 25% of women.
   b. Uterine fibroids are more common in Caucasian women, those with a family history, parous women and those using combined oral contraceptive or injectable progestogens.
   c. 25% are asymptomatic.
   d. Around 1% of fibroids are leiomyosarcomata which may result in malignant change.
   e. Complications of fibroids in pregnancy include premature labor, malpresentations, transverse lie, obstructed labor, pain related to red degeneration and postpartum hemorrhage.
   f. None of the above.
2. **Endometrial carcinoma is now the most common genital tract cancer. Identify the statements which are true.**
   a. Prevalence is highest at age 60, with only 15% of cases occurring premenopausally and <1% in women under 35 years of age.
   b. The most common pathology after adenocarcinoma is adenosquamous carcinoma.
   c. Adenocarcinoma of the columnar endometrial gland cells accounts for >90%.
   d. Risk factors include obesity, PCOS, nulliparity, late menopause, tamoxifen use, unopposed estrogen therapy.
   e. Postmenopausal bleeding is the most common presentation and qualifies a 10% risk of carcinoma.
   f. Stage 2 disease is confined to the uterus and includes the cervix, but not the vagina.
   g. None of the above.
3. **Referring to benign conditions of the uterus, identify the statements which are true.**
   a. Adenomyosis, also known as endometriosis interna, is the presence of myometrium within the endometrium.
   b. Amenorrhea is a common symptom of adenomyosis.
   c. Endometritis may occur secondary to STI, as a complication of surgery, including cesarean section and intrauterine surgery, or related to foreign tissue, i.e., IUD and RPOC.
   d. Intrauterine polyps are common in women aged 40–50 years and when estrogen levels are low.
   e. Outflow obstruction may lead to accumulation of menstrual blood in the uterus. This is known as hematometra.
   f. None of the above.
4. **Benign ovarian masses include tumors and functional cysts. Which of the following is a correct statement about functional cysts?**
   a. They are uncommon after menopause.
   b. They do not develop in nulliparous women.
   c. They frequently become malignant.
   d. They require oophorectomy.
5. **The most common presentation of vesicular mole is:**
   a. Vomiting
   b. Abdominal pain
   c. Explusion of grape-like vesicles from vagina
   d. Vaginal bleeding

Answer Key

1. e **2.** e **3.** c, e **4.** a **5.** d

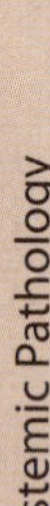

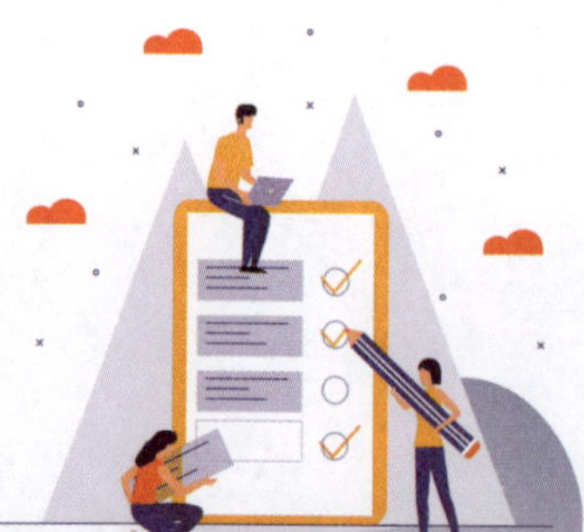

Chapter 17

Breast Diseases

LEARNING OBJECTIVES

After the completion of the chapter, the readers will be able to:

- Discuss fibrocystic changes in the breast.
- Know about fibroadenoma and carcinoma of breast.

CHAPTER OUTLINE

- Introduction
- Fibrocystic Disease
- Breast Fibroadenoma
- Phyllodes Tumor
- Breast Carcinoma

KEY TERMS

Adenocarcinoma: A cancer that develops in gland-forming tissue. Most breast cancers are adenocarcinomas.

Aspiration: The withdrawal (as by suction) of fluid or tissue from the body.

Benign: A condition, tumor or growth that is not cancerous.

Biopsy: The removal of a sample of abnormal tissue that is microscopically examined for cancer cells.

Bone scan: A picture of the bones using a radioactive dye that shows any injury, disease or healing. This is a valuable test to determine if cancer has spread to the bone, if anticancer therapy has been successful, and if affected bony areas are healing.

Chemotherapy: A treatment for cancer that works by killing all rapidly reproducing cells, but also has side effects on normal cells.

CT scan: "Computed tomography scan" in which radiations are used to create cross-sectional pictures of the body.

Fine-needle aspiration (FNA): Procedure in which cells are removed from a lump by needle and syringe, then tested to see if cancer cells are present.

Mammogram: A low dose X-ray of the breast.

Metastasis: The spread of cancer beyond the primary site of the cancer, and beyond the axillary nodes.

Tumor: An abnormal mass of tissue.

INTRODUCTION

Fundamental features of breast anatomy and histology are as follows:

- Normal human breast is a unique modified apocrine gland responsible for milk secretion.
- Breast overlies the 2nd–6th ribs.

- Pectoralis major muscle forms the base of the breast which extends from the second to sixth rib early in life but may extend to below the sixth rib as the breast matures and sags.
- It is comprised of 15–20 lobes of glandular tissue which lie within fatty tissue and the lobes are drained to the nipple via the lactiferous duct.

  Terminal Duct Lobular Units (TDLU)
  - Each lobe is further comprised of 20–40 terminal duct lobular units (TDLU), which represents the basic functional unit of the breast.
  - TDLU unit comprises a lobule attached to the extralobular terminal duct which connects the lobule to the rest of the ductular system.
  - Within the lobule, 10–100 small glandular sacs are called acini and the intralobular terminal duct.
- The ducts and acini are lined by epithelial cells resting on a layer of myoepithelial cells. Anatomically, thus, the breast has both epithelial and stromal compartments.
- The stroma can be within the lobule (intralobular) or in between lobules (interlobular).

Common diseases of the breast, that will be discussed in this chapter include fibrocystic disease of the breast, breast fibroadenoma, phyllodes tumor and breast carcinoma.

FIBROCYSTIC DISEASE

Fibrocystic disease represents the most common form of benign breast disease worldwide and affects women in the reproductive age group (Fig. 17.1). It is rarely observed in the postmenopausal stage unless the female is on hormone therapy.

Clinical Features

- Patient presents with a feeling of a breast that is uneven to touch (lumpy, bumpy breast).
- Sensation of pain and tenderness in the breast (mastalgia), especially in the premenstrual phase.
- Clear or dark brown secretion from the nipple.

Etiology

- Estrogen predominance and progesterone deficiency play an important role.
- Genetic predisposition.
- Breast trauma.
- Hypothyroidism.
- Methylxanthine.
- Due to repeated cycles of menstruation.

Risk Factors

- Early menarche including obesity.
- Late pregnancy.
- Nulliparity.

Pathogenesis

Pathogenesis of fibrocystic disease is shown in Figure 17.2.

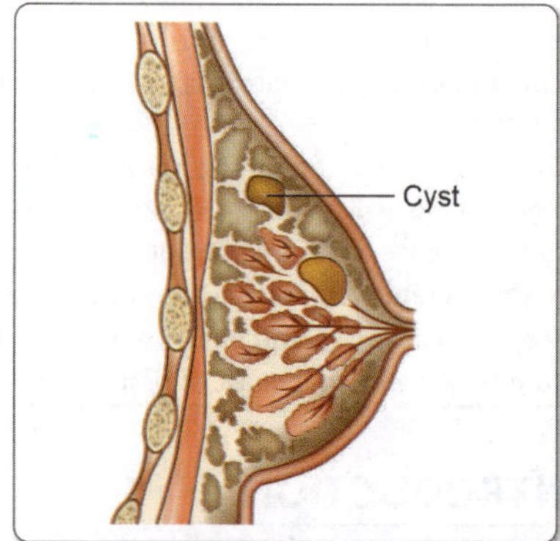

Figure 17.1: Fibrocystic disease with cyst

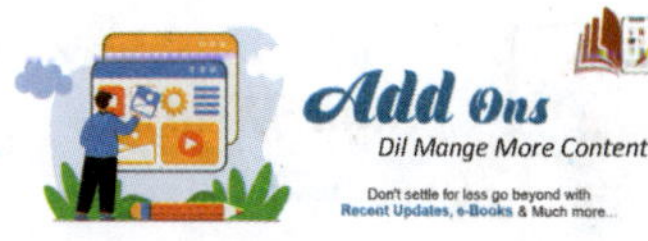

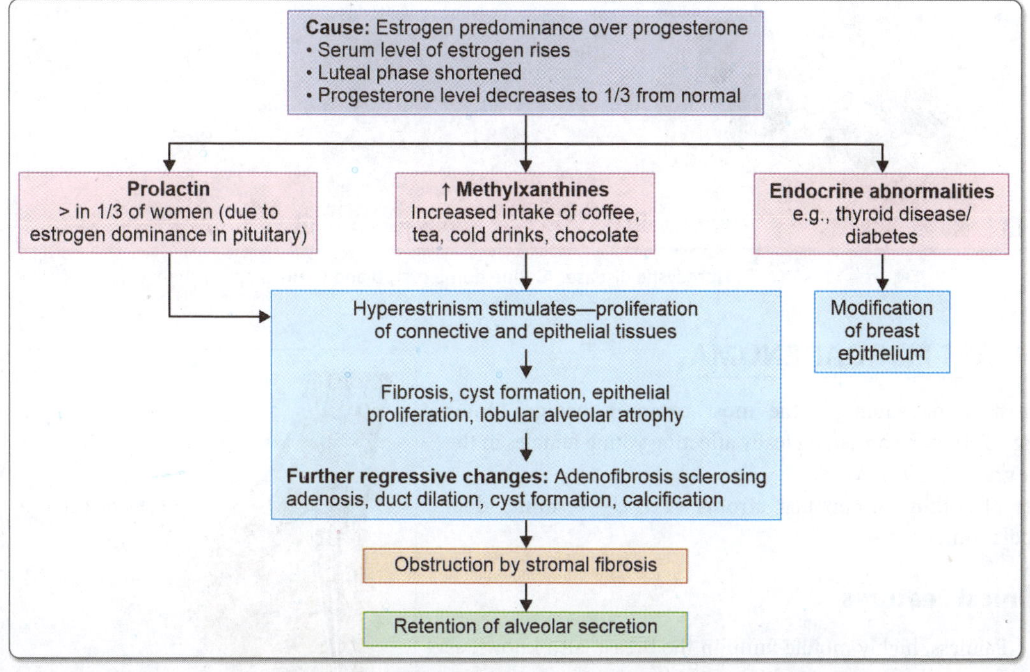

Figure 17.2: Pathogenesis of fibrocystic disease

Pathological Changes

Gross Appearance

Cyst formation: The cysts are formed of variable sizes varying from millimeters to few centimeters. Cysts are usually seen in both the breasts. The cysts are filled with straw-colored to dark brown fluid. These cysts, when large appear to be externally blue in color, giving rise to the term "blue-domed cyst of bloodgood" (Fig. 17.3A).

Histological Changes

- **Glandular changes**
  - Ducts are dilated cystically, with the duct lumina showing inspissated secretions (Figs 17.3B and C).
  - Glands may show lining epithelium that is flattened or displaying epithelial hyperplasia and reactive atypia.
  - The lining cells may show apocrine metaplasia.
- **Fibrosis:** Increased fibrosis around the cysts, of varying degrees
- **Inflammation:** Accompanying inflammatory cells (chronic inflammation comprising lymphocytes, macrophages) again in varying numbers. This is increased when the cyst ruptures.
- **Other changes:** Foci of calcification.

In cases where epithelial hyperplasia is not seen, this disease represents as an example of nonproliferative change in the breast.

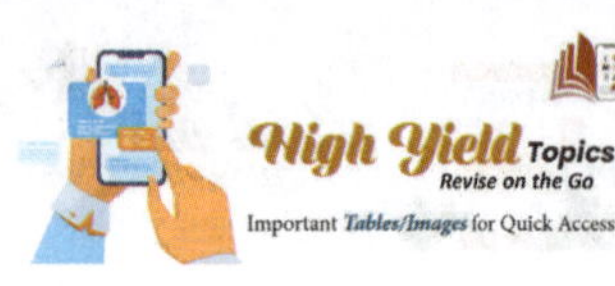

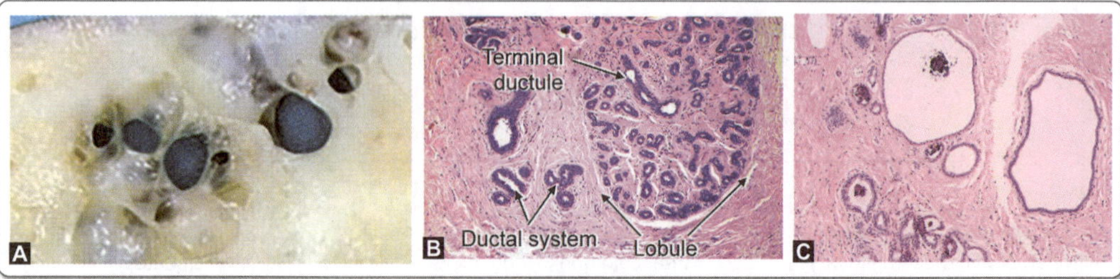

Figures 17.3A to C: Fibrocystic disease: **A.** Blue dome cyst; **B** and **C.** Histological changes

BREAST FIBROADENOMA

Breast fibroadenoma is the most common benign tumor (Fig. 17.4) of the breast, typically affecting young females in the age group of 20–40 years.

Site of origin: Intralobular stroma (TDLU—Terminal duct lobular unit).

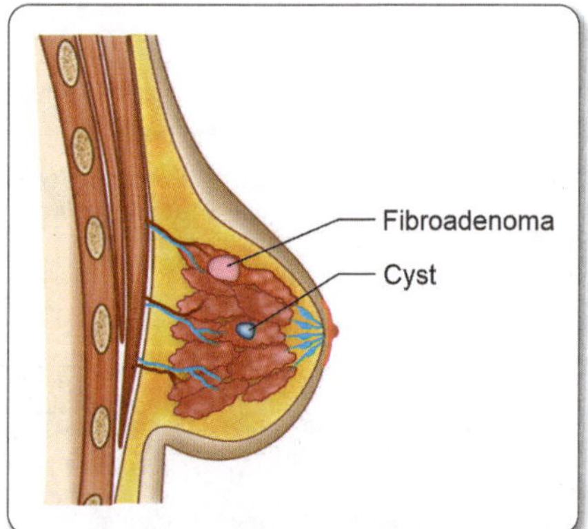

Figure 17.4: Breast fibroadenoma

Clinical Features

- Painless, highly mobile lump in the breast, also known as **"mouse"**, because of its high mobility.
- Firm, rubbery, smooth, masses with well-defined border.
- Generally, solitary mass but may be multiple and bilateral.

Etiology

- The pathogenesis is linked to the hormone estrogen. Fibroadenomas often regress after menopause.
- MED12 gene mutations are also associated with it.

Risk Factors

- Prior history of benign breast disease.
- Young age (<35 years).
- Family history of multiple fibroadenomas.
- Obesity.
- Consumption of oral contraceptives before the age of 20.

Pathogenesis

Pathogenesis of breast fibroadenoma is shown in self-explanatory Figure 17.5.

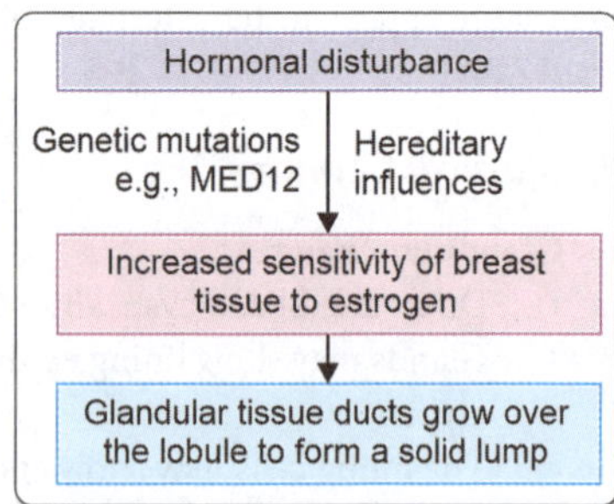

Figure 17.5: Pathogenesis of breast fibroadenoma

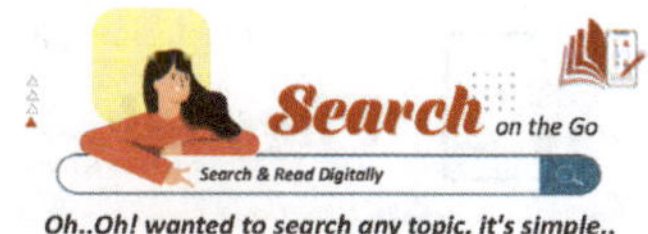

Pathological Changes

Gross Appearance

- Well-circumscribed, gray white in color, encapsulated lesion displaying a whorled /lobulated appearance and at times, slit like spaces (Fig. 17.6).
- Variable size—usually not exceeding 3–4 cm.
- **Mammographic features:** A round well-circumscribed mass.

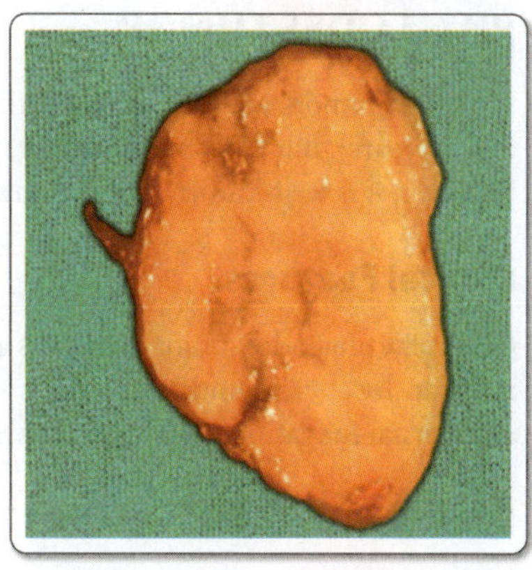

Figure 17.6: Breast fibroadenoma—Gross

Histological Changes

Microscopic examination: Fibroadenomas show a biphasic histological pattern in which duct structures are enmeshed in a fibrous stroma. According to the configuration of the ducts two histological types of fibroadenoma are described as:

- Intracanalicular in which the glands are compressed by the surrounding stroma so that they become narrow and slit like (Fig. 17.7A).
- Pericanalicular in which the ductal lumina are round and patent (Fig. 17.7B).

These histological types do not have any clinical implications. Glandular lining epithelium is cuboidal and the glands show both epithelial and myoepithelial cells. Stroma is dense and may show increased cellularity/myxoid change.

EXTRA EDGE

Cellular fibroadenoma: Fibroadenoma with stromal hypercellularity.
Juvenile fibroadenoma: Fibroadenoma in young age group.
Complex fibroadenoma: Fibroadenoma + calcification + sclerosing adenosis + cysts >3 mm in size + papillary apocrine metaplasia.

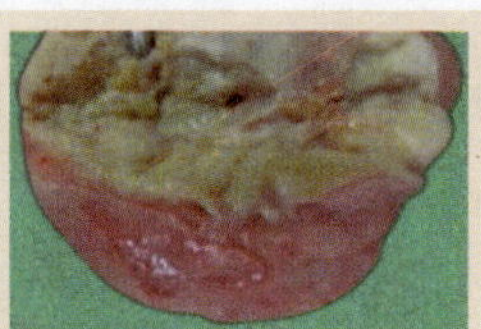

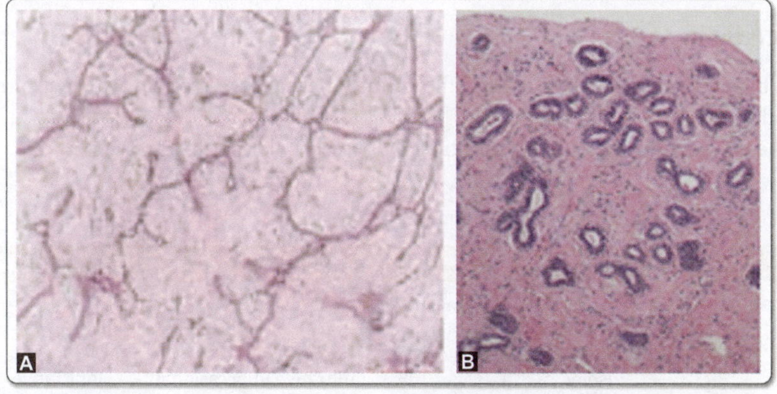

Figures 17.7A and B: Histological types of fibroadenoma: **A.** Intracanalicular; **B.** Pericanalicular

PHYLLODES TUMOR

Phyllodes tumors are less common than fibroadenoma and occurs more frequently in the elder age group (40–60 years). It has been historically referred to as cystosarcoma phylloides implying a malignant condition. However, it is well-known that the phyllodes tumor can be either benign, borderline or malignant.

Clinical Features

Generally, phyllodes tumor manifests as larger masses and display rapid growth. Overlying skin may be shiny and translucent and underlying veins are revealed. A very large tumor may erode through skin and present as an external fungating breast mass. Physical findings resemble those of fibroadenoma.

Etiology

The etiology is unknown.

Risk Factors

- Most common in women in their 40s.
- Women with Li-Fraumeni syndrome (a rare, inherited genetic condition) have an increased risk for phyllodes tumors.

Pathogenesis

Pathogenesis tumor is characterized by stromal proliferation or overgrowth is given in Table 17.1.

Pathological Changes

Gross Appearance

The cut surface of the lesion is firm and white in color. The striking feature looks like fronds on gross examination, hence giving the name of phyllodes tumor (phyllodes in Greek means leaf. It is also seen cleft-like spaces and foci of hemorrhage and necrosis in large/malignant phyllodes.

Histologic Changes

- **Stromal hypercellularity:** More around the epithelial elements—areas in which stroma predominates and glandular elements are not seen.
- **Stomal heterogeneity:** Areas of hyalinization and hypocellularity can also seen.

Table 17.1: Comparative features of phyllode tumors

Parameters	Benign	Borderline	Malignant
Stromal cellularity	↑	↑↑	↑↑↑
Mitotic activity/10 HPF	0–4	5–9	>10
Margins	Pushing	Infiltrative in occasional foci	Infiltrative
Stromal overgrowth	↑	↑↑	↑↑↑

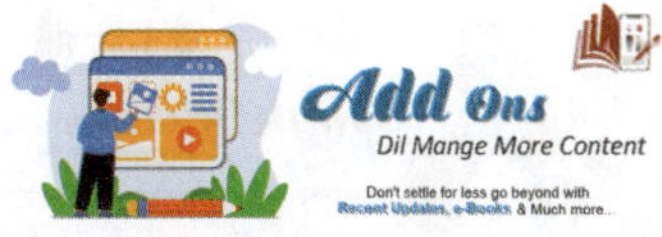

- **Tumor border:** Pushing borders are seen in case of benign tumors whereas infiltrative margins are seen in malignant phyllodes.
- **Mitotic activity:** Another important feature to assess in distinguishing among benign versus borderline versus malignant phyllodes is the presence of mitotic figures (Table 17.2).

Table 17.2: Types of phyllodes according to mitotic count

Mitotic count	Types of phyllodes
0–4 mitoses/10 HPF	Benign phyllodes
5–9 mitoses/10 HPF	Borderline phyllodes
>10 mitoses/10 HPF	Malignant phyllodes

Complete excision, with accurate histologic examination is the treatment of choice.

BREAST CARCINOMA

Breast carcinoma represents the most common carcinoma among females in India and worldwide.

Clinical Features

- Enlargement of breast.
- Breast lump and pain.
- **Nipple retraction:** "Peau d orange" appearance, discharge from nipple.
- **Skin ulceration:** The overlying skin may be red as in inflammatory carcinoma. This may be accompanied by enlarged axillary lymph nodes in the case of tumor spread to the regional lymphatics.

Risk Factors

A number of risk factors have been postulated behind the development of breast cancer which include:
- Female predilection, only 1% cases occur in males.
- Positive family history, i.e., first-degree relatives with breast cancer.
- Advancing age.
- Early menarche and late menopause.
- Age >35 years at first delivery.
- Patients on hormone replacement therapy.
- Obesity.
- Exposure to radiation, pesticides.
- Smoking.

Classification of Breast Tumors

According to status of the basement membrane: *In situ*; and invasive breast carcinoma.
According to molecular tests:

- Luminal A: ER+ & PR +ve
  HER2 –ve
  Ki-67: Low (<14%)
- Luminal B: **1. HER2 Positive**
  ↓
  ER+ & PR +ve
  Ki 67-Any value
  HER2-amplified

	2. HER2 –ve ER+ &/PR +ve Ki 67 ≥14% HER2 –ve
• HER 2 enriched	ER- PR- HER2-amplified
• Triple negative (basal)	ER- PR- HER2-

According to occurrence:

- **Sporadic:** Breast carcinoma may develop for the first time in a patient without any family history.
- **Hereditary:** It may be running in families and genetic predisposition may be the reason.

According to histological type:

- Invasive ductal
- Invasive lobule

According to the sites involved: The most common site is the upper outer quadrant (50%), followed by the upper inner quadrant and followed by the lower outer and inner quadrants. Malignant breast lesions may be *in situ* or invasive. Invasive breast carcinoma is of the following major subtypes are as follows:

- No special type
- Invasive lobular carcinoma
- Medullary carcinoma
- Mucinous carcinoma
- Tubular carcinoma
- Metaplastic carcinoma
- Apocrine carcinoma

The most common site: Upper outer quadrant, fixed to the underlying skin.

TNM Staging of Breast Cancer

One of the ways in which breast cancer is based on an assessment of anatomical spread using three key parameters—tumor size (T), nodal spread (N) and the presence or absence of metastases (M). A brief overview of the must know points of this staging system are presented in following Table 17.3.

Table 17.3: TNM staging of breast cancer

Primary tumor (T)	
TX	Primary tumor cannot be assessed
T0	No evidence of primary tumor
Tis	Carcinoma *in situ*
Tis (DCIS)	Ductal carcinoma *in situ*
Tis (Paget)	Paget disease of the nipple NOT associated with invasive carcinoma and/or carcinoma *in situ* (DCIS) in the underlying breast parenchyma
T1	Tumor ≤2 cm in greatest dimension
T2	Tumor >2 cm but ≤5 cm in greatest dimension
T3	Tumor >5 cm in greatest dimension
T4	Tumor of any size with direct extension to the chest wall and/or the skin

Contd...

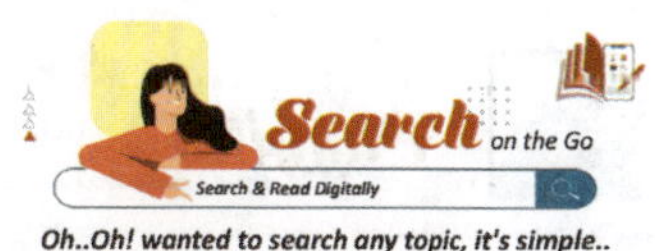

Primary tumor (T)	
N - Nodal spread assessment	
N0	No lymph nodal metastases
N1	Metastases in 1–3 axillary lymph nodes
N2	Metastases in 4–9 axillary lymph nodes
N3	Metastases in >10 axillary lymph nodes/infra or supraclavicular lymph nodes
M - Assessment of distant spread (metastases)	
M0	No distant spread (metastasis)
M1	Distant spread present

Pathogenesis

Breast cancer develops due to DNA damage and genetic mutations that can be influenced by exposure to estrogen. Sometimes, there will be an inheritance of DNA defects or procancerous genes like BRCA1 and BRCA2. The family history of ovarian or breast cancer increases the risk for breast cancer development (Fig. 17.8).

Pathological Changes

The salient pathological features of each types are tabulated in Table 17.4.

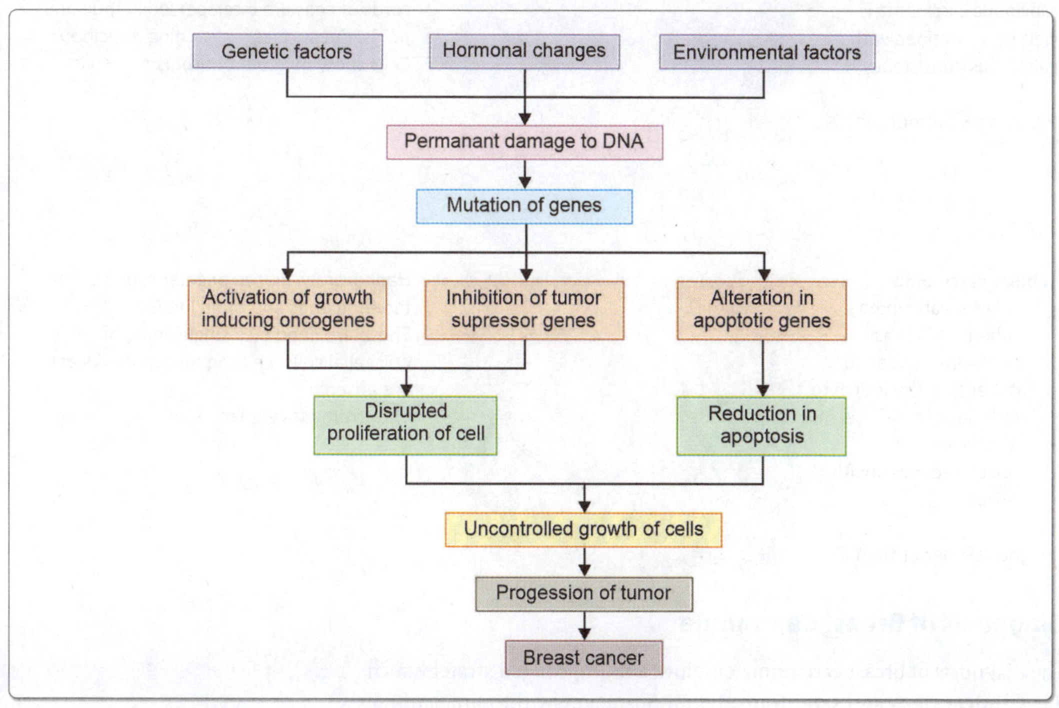

Figure 17.8: Pathogenesis of breast cancer

Table 17.4: Histopathological changes in different types of breast cancer

Type of breast cancer	Histology	Histological changes
Invasive lobular carcinoma		The tumor cells are arranged in cords in a characteristic "Indian file" arrangement. Desmoplastic response is lacking Pleomorphism is mild
Medullary carcinoma • Medullary carcinoma tumor is seen in younger patients and is well-circumscribed. • Unlike other tumors, it is soft and fleshy in consistency. Prognosis—better than invasive ductal carcinoma (IDC).		• Syncytial growth pattern is seen in 75% of the tumor • Lymphoplasmacytic infiltrate • Pushing borders • Pleomorphic nuclei • Lack of glandular differentiation • Lack of fibroblastic response (desmoplasia) • Ductal carcinoma in situ (DCIS)—usually absent • It is a triple negative tumor, i.e., it is negative for ER, PR and Her2/Neu.
Mucinous carcinoma Mucinous carcinoma is well-circumscribed with gelatinous consistency. Prognosis—better than IDC.		• Individual tumor cells, small clusters and cords of cells are interspersed in mucinous pools. Cut surface—glistening, mucinous • Cells show mild pleomorphism.
Tubular carcinoma • Tubular carcinoma subtype of breast carcinoma is seen in patients in the fourth to fifth decade. • It represents a spiculated mass (with spikes). Prognosis—better than IDC.		• Haphazardly, placed angular tubules with tapering ends and open lumina. • These are lined by a single lining of epithelial cells, i.e., the myoepithelial cells are absent. • The stroma is cellular.

Diagnosis of Breast Carcinoma

The diagnosis of breast carcinoma employs a multipronged strategy such as:

- **Clinical signs and symptoms:** Lump-Suspicion by the clinician.
- **Imaging/radiology:** Mammography, USG, MRI.

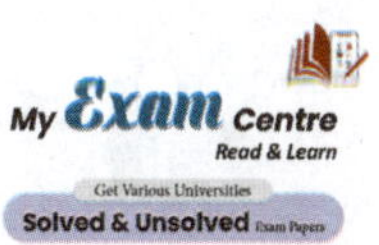

- **Cytology:** Fine-needle aspiration cytology of the breast lump, Nipple discharge cytology, especially in cases of bloody nipple discharge to exclude a papillary lesion of the breast.
- **Histopathology:** Trucut/incisional biopsy, excisional biopsy/histopathological evaluation of resected specimens such as lumpectomy, modified radical mastectomy.
- **Immunohistochemistry**: This is now a routine practice critical for tumor management. Immunohistochemistry analyzes the protein expression of the tumor. A basic panel of estrogen receptor (ER), progesterone receptor (PR), Her2Neu is used for evaluating prognosis of each case.
- Other techniques which are commonly used as:
  - FISH cytogenetics used to analyze Her2Neu gene amplification or the lack of it.
  - DNA microarray may also be used to evaluate the gene expression of the tumor.

SUMMARY

- Fibrocystic disease represents the most common form of benign breast disease worldwide and affects women in the reproductive age group.
- Lumpy, bumpy breast and blue-domed cyst of bloodgood are the characteristic features of fibrocystic disease.
- Fibroadenoma is the most common benign tumor of the breast, typically affecting young females in the age group of 20–40 years.
- The characteristic feature of fibroadenoma is painless, highly mobile lump in the breast, also known as "breast mouse".
- Phyllodes tumors are less common than fibroadenoma and occurs more frequently in the elder age group of 40–60 years.
- The striking feature of phyllodes tumor looks like fronds on gross examination.
- The most common site of development of breast tumor is the upper outer quadrant (50%), followed by upper inner quadrant and the lower outer and inner quadrants.
- Breast cancer develops due to DNA damage and genetic mutations that can be influenced by exposure to estrogen.

ASSESS YOURSELF

Long Answer Questions

1. Explain the pathogenesis of fibrocystic disease.
2. Classify breast carcinoma.
3. Discuss the pathogenesis of breast cancer.
4. Describe histopathological features of breast cancer.

Short Answer Questions

1. What is fibroadenoma?
2. Brief note on diagnostic modalities of breast cancer.
3. Write short notes on:
   i. Phyllodes tumor
   ii. Breast carcinoma

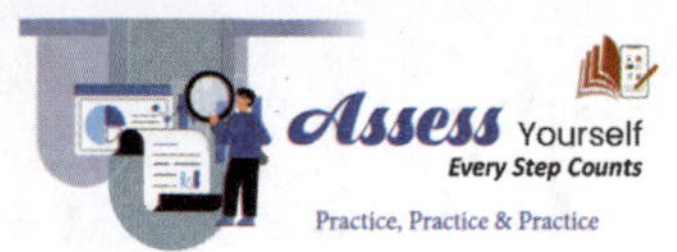

Multiple Choice Questions

1. **Finding breast cancer in early is the key to successful treatment.**
   a. True b. False
2. **Older women are more likely to develop breast cancer.**
   a. True b. False
3. **Most breast lumps are cancer.**
   a. True b. False
4. **Which of the following techniques have been used to screen breast cancer?**
   a. Breast self-examination b. Mammography
   c. Clinical breast examination d. All of these
5. **Most common site of metastases in carcinoma breast:**
   a. Bone b. Lung
   c. Liver d. Brain
6. **True about breast cancer is:**
   a. Doubling time of breast tumor is 1 month
   b. Skip metastasis in level iii lymph nodes is common
   c. Lungs are commonly involved by direct invasion
   d. Dimpling of skin is due to shortening of Cooper's ligaments
7. **Blood stained nipple discharge is seen in:**
   a. Breast abscess b. Fibroadenoma
   c. Fibrocystic disease d. Fat necrosis of breast
8. **Carcinoma of breast is most commonly seen in which quadrant of breast:**
   a. Upper outer b. Upper inner
   c. Lower inner d. Lower outer
9. **TNM staging of breast carcinoma with positive bilateral supraclavicular lymph nodes is:**
   a. N3a b. N3b
   c. N3c d. M1

Answer Key

1. a **2.** a **3.** b **4.** d **5.** a **6.** d
7. c **8.** a **9.** d

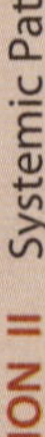

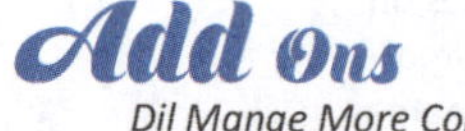

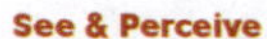

See & Perceive	Recent Update	e-Book
Watch and learn with the selective Important Topic-wise	Regular updates related to Recent advancements & Book Errata	Get PDFs of important chapter/section (Annexures/Appendices) of book *(optional and exclusive for Pro-users and Institutions)*

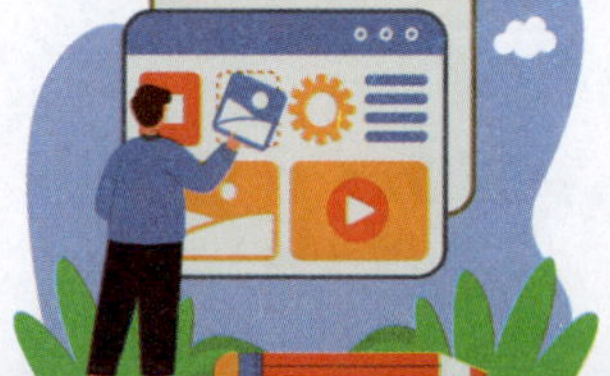

Nursing Next Live
The Next Level of Nursing Education
CBS Phygital Books >
Textbook of Pathology & Genetics PHYGITAL

Chapter 18

Central Nervous System Diseases

LEARNING OBJECTIVES

After the completion of the chapter, the readers will be able to:
- Describe the clinicopathological features of meningitis.
- Distinguish between various types of meningitis (based on lab tests).
- Explain the clinicopathological features of encephalitis.

CHAPTER OUTLINE

- Overview of Central Nervous System
- Meningitis
- Encephalitis
- Stroke
- Tumors of Central Nervous System

KEY TERMS

Encephalitis: Inflammation of the brain parenchyma.

Encephalopathy: Clinical manifestation of disease to the brain parenchyma (altered sensorium), persisting for >24 hours.

Meningoencephalitis: The meninges and brain parenchyma both are inflamed.

Pleocytosis: An increased cell count of CSF. The term is more commonly used when there is both lym-phocytes and neutrophils in the CSF which can be seen both in tubercular and viral meningitis.

OVERVIEW OF CENTRAL NERVOUS SYSTEM

The central nervous system (CNS) is a fundamental component of the human nervous system, playing a crucial role in coordinating and controlling various bodily functions. It consists of two main components: the brain and the spinal cord (Fig. 18.1).

1. **Brain:** It acts as a command center of CNS and is very complex organ. Its parts are:
   - Cerebrum—responsible for conscious thought, memory, and voluntary actions.
   - Cerebellum—involved in coordination and balance.
   - Brainstem—control the basic life functions such as breathing and heart rate.
   - Diencephalon—composed of the thalamus and hypothalamus, regulating various physiological process.
2. **Spinal cord:** The spinal cord is a long, tubular structure that extends from the base of the brain down the vertebral column. It serves as a conduit for nerve signals traveling between the brain and the rest of

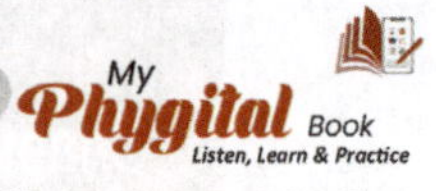

the body. The spinal cord is protected by the vertebral column and is surrounded by cerebrospinal fluid that acts as a cushion.

Nerves: Nerves extend from the spinal cord and brain, forming the peripheral nervous system (PNS). They transmit signals between the CNS and the rest of the body, facilitating communication and control. Motor neurons carry signals from the CNS to muscles and glands, while sensory neurons relay information from sensory receptors to the CNS.

Cerebrospinal fluid: It provides protection to CNS and also helps in the exchange of nutrients and waste products between the blood and nervous tissue.

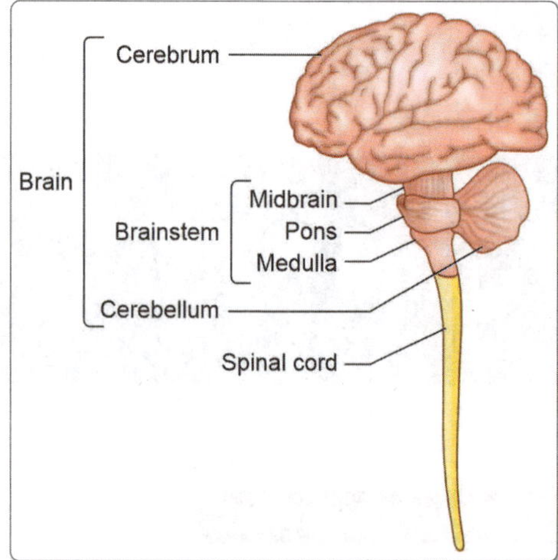

Figure 18.1: Central nervous system

Functions

- The CNS processes and integrates information from various sensory organs, allowing individuals to perceive and respond to their environment.
- Responsible for higher cognitive functions such as learning, memory, language, and problem-solving.
- Motor control, including voluntary and involuntary movements, is coordinated by the CNS.

MENINGITIS

There are three meninges from inner to outer: Pia mater, arachnoid mater and dura mater. Meningitis is inflammation of the meninges which are the protective membranes on the surface of the brain.

- **Pachymeningitis:** Inflammation of the outermost dura mater is called pachymeningitis.
- **Leptomeningitis:** Inflammation of the inner membranes (piamater, arachnoid mater) is called leptomeningitis. Meningitis most often occurs due to an infectious process and must be diagnosed timely for effective management.

Clinical Features

The patient presents with headache, high fever, projectile vomiting with a likely altered mental status, sometimes even leading to seizures, stupor and coma.

Etiology

- Local infection, e.g., mastoid inflammation/otitis media (inflammation of the middle ear).
- Systemic infection: Any infectious agent causing sepsis in the body, can as a complication, produce meningitis.
- Fractures of the head and neck/trauma.
- Immunocompromised states, where fungal meningitis like cryptococcus /viruses like Epstein-Barr Virus (EBV), cytomegalovirus (CMV) may be causative.

Risk Factors

Risk factors for meningitis include:

- Chronic medical disorders (renal failure, diabetes, adrenal insufficiency, cystic fibrosis).
- Extremes of age.

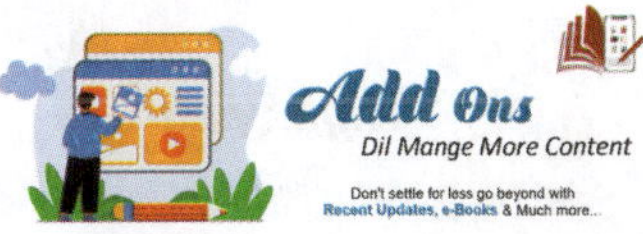

- Under vaccination.
- Immunosuppressed states (iatrogenic, transplant recipients, congenital immunodeficiencies, AIDS).
- Living in crowded conditions.
- Alcohol use disorder.
- Presence of ventriculoperitoneal (VP) shunt.
- Bacterial endocarditis.
- Malignancy.
- Dural defects.
- IV drug use.
- Sickle cell anemia.
- Splenectomy.

Complications of Meningitis

- Seizures
- Hydrocephalus
- Cranial nerve irritation
- Herniation of cerebrum because of increased intracranial pressure
- Empyema (subdural)

Types of Meningitis

Meningitis is commonly classified as follows:

According to duration of symptoms:

- Acute meningitis
- Chronic meningitis

According to etiological agent:

- Infectious meningitis, including disease caused by viral, bacterial, parasitic agents.
- Noninfectious meningitis, including meningitis caused by drugs, immune disorders, chemicals, associated with malignancy (neoplastic), iatrogenic (after lumbar puncture).

According to a clinically relevant perspective:

Three main types of meningitis are important (as given in subsequent subsections), and every nursing professional must be aware of them.

Acute Bacterial Meningitis (Acute Pyogenic Meningitis)

Clinical Features

The patient of acute pyogenic meningitis looks very sick and presents with fever, headache, projectile vomiting, aversion to light (photophobia) and altered mental status manifesting as confusion, drowsiness and in some cases, seizures and even coma.

The patient is visibly irritable and febrile with neck stiffness (nuchal rigidity) which increases when the patient bends forward. Important clinical signs include:

- **Neck (nuchal) rigidity**, aversion to light (photophobia) and sound (phonophobia).
- **Brudzinski sign:** Neck flexion causes flexion of knees and hip.
- **Kernig's sign:** Hip flexion causes pain at the knee joint. These signs are due to motor nerve root irritation as a consequence of the inflamed meninges.

Etiology

Common causative bacteria include Escherichia coli, Streptococcus pneumoniae (adults, children), Haemophilus influenzae in neonates and young children, Neisseria meningitidis (in children and

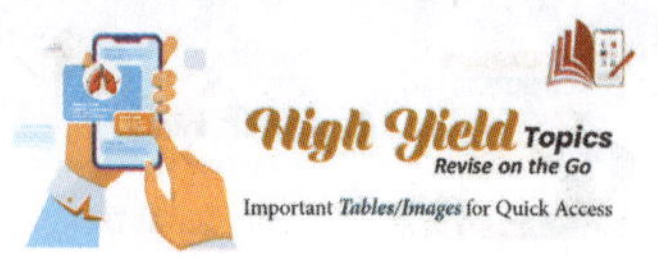

young adults). Neisserial infections may sometimes be associated with adrenal hemorrhage and disseminated intravascular coagulation, known as the Waterhouse-Friderichsen syndrome.

Pathogenesis

Bacteria invade the meninges after crossing the mucosal barrier. Bacteria adhere to the cells of CNS and neuronal apoptosis occurs (Fig. 18.2).

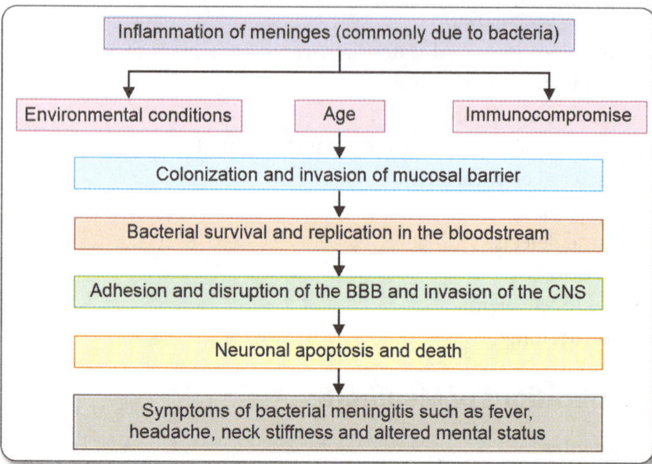

Figure 18.2: Pathogenesis of bacterial meningitis

Pathological Changes

Gross appearance (Fig. 18.3A):

- A purulent, creamy exudate may be noted on the convexities of the brain.
- The cerebrospinal fluid, which is normally clear, becomes turbid and in severe meningitis, pus-like ("purulent").
- The meninges also appear dull and opaque.

Histological changes (Fig 18.3B):

Neutrophils are seen in the meninges and the subarachnoid space. An increased number of neutrophils may be seen around blood vessels. Gram staining is performed to identify the causative bacteria as gram positive or negative.

CSF findings:

- Appearance—turbid.
- WBCs—increased.
- CSF protein—increased (due to secretion by leukocytes and other recruited cells as well as due to disruption of the blood-brain barrier).
- CSF sugar—decreased (due to utilization by bacteria).
- Culture—positivity for a specific bacteria.

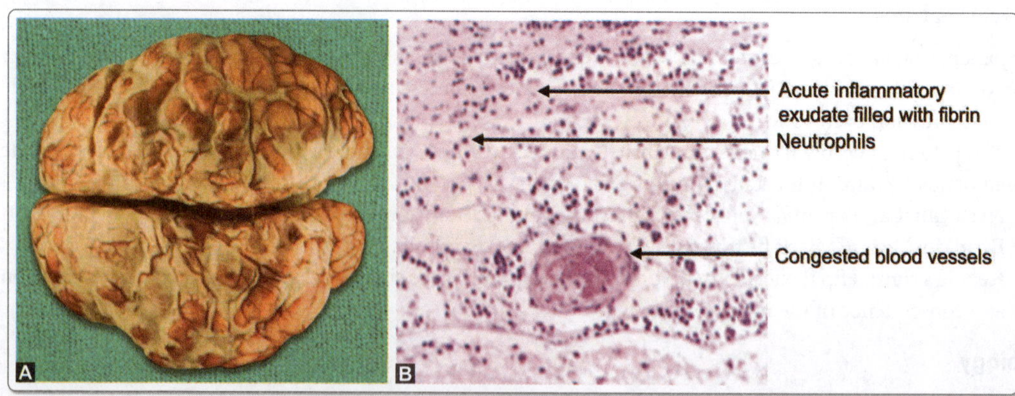

Figures 18.3A and B: Bacterial meningitis: **A.** Gross; **B.** Histology

Acute Viral Meningitis (Aseptic/Lymphocytic Meningitis)

Viral meningitis is commonly seen in children and young adults.

Clinical Features

Clinically, the patient is less sick in comparison to a case of pyogenic meningitis.

Etiology

Common causative viruses include enteroviruses, coxsackie virus, herpes simplex virus (HSV), human immunodeficiency virus (HIV), Mumps virus. It is also known by the name of aseptic meningitis.

Pathological Changes

Gross appearance: No significant abnormality is seen grossly, in some cases however, the cerebral parenchyma may appear edematous.

Histopathological changes: Lymphocytes are seen in the meninges and in the subarachnoid space. Perivascular lymphocytic infiltrates are also noted which extend to the Virchow-Robin spaces.

CSF findings:

- The fluid is clear.
- Protein is slightly elevated.
- Sugar is normal.
- Culture-negative.

Tubercular Meningitis

Etiology

The causative organism here is *Mycobacterium tuberculosis* and is commonly seen in the Indian subcontinent.

Pathogenesis

- Tubercular meningitis is a common form of extrapulmonary tuberculosis. Tubercular meningitis may be contracted through hematogenous spread of foci of tuberculosis elsewhere in the body (frequently in the lungs). It may also be part of miliary tuberculosis. Salient distinguishing features of tubercular meningitis are:
  - Leptomeningeal involvement
  - Presence of basal exudates
  - Subarachnoid space is also inflamed (subarachnoiditis).

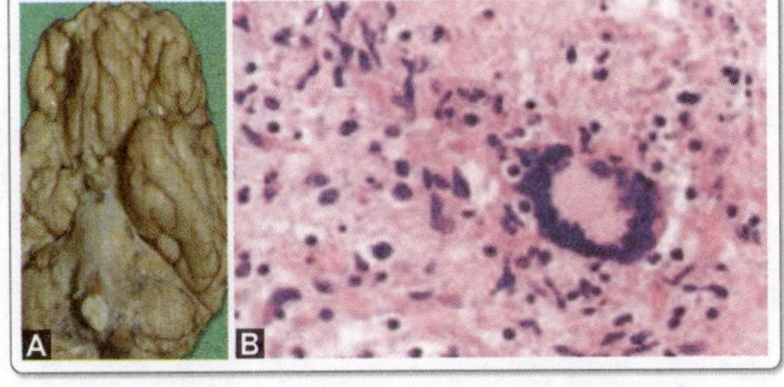

Figures 18.4A and B: Tubercular/tuberculous meningitis: **A.** Gross; **B.** Histology

Pathological Changes

Gross appearance (Fig. 18.4A):

- Thick caseous/cheesy exudate may be seen overlying the basal cisterns.
- Well-defined tubercles, firm in consistency may be noted in the parenchyma.
- The cerebral parenchyma may appear edematous.
- The thick exudate in some cases obstructs the flow of the CSF leading to obstructive hydrocephalus when the CSF accumulates in the lateral and third ventricles.

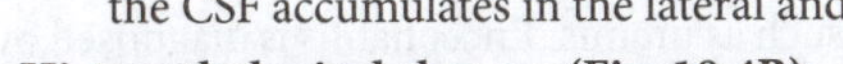

Histopathological changes (Fig. 18.4B):

Features of tuberculosis such as the presence of epithelioid cell granulomas, caseous necrosis, Langerhans giant cells and lymphohistiocytic inflammatory infiltrate are seen.

CSF findings:

- The fluid is straw colored, turbid and characteristically shows a cobweb coagulum due to increased protein content.
- Protein is elevated.
- Glucose is decreased.
- Culture—positive for *Mycobacterium tuberculosis.*

EXTRA EDGE

Parameters of CSF in various types of meningitis

CSF examination is of paramount importance in the investigation of various types of meningitis. This is done by the procedure known as lumbar puncture. This involves inserting a sterile lumbar puncture needle at the intervertebral disk space between vertebral spaces L3-L4/L4-L5 with the patient lying in a lateral recumbent position. The following table highlights the salient differences in parameters of CSF in different types of meningitis.

Parameters of CSF in various types of meningitis

Feature/parameter	Normal person	Acute bacterial meningitis	Acute viral meningitis	Tubercular meningitis
Gross appearance	Clear	Turbid	Clear	• Straw colored • Cob web coagulum on standing
CSF Pressure (mm H_2O)	70–180	>180 (200–300)	Normal to slightly elevated	Elevated
Protein (mg/dL)	15–40	100–500	50–100	100–300
Sugar (mg/dL)	45–100	<40	Normal	<40
Chloride (ug/dL)	116–122 ug/dL	Low	Normal	Very low
Cells (cells/microliter)	<5 (lymphocytes/ mononuclear cells)	100–2000 (mostly neutrophils)	5–100 (lymphocytes >50% with a small proportion of neutrophils)	5–200 (up to 1000) (lymphocytes >80%)
Ancillary tests				
A. Gram's stain CSF sediment	–	+/– as per the type of infecting bacteria	–	–
B. AFB stain CSF sediment	–		–	+ (not always)
C. Culture	–	–/+	–	+ Mycobacterium

ENCEPHALITIS

Encephalitis refers to acute inflammation of the brain parenchyma. This may be due to an infectious or autoimmune process. Encephalopathy is an altered state of consciousness (sensorium) persisting for >24 hours. Encephalitis is one of the causes of encephalopathy which may be due to other causes such as a complication of liver cirrhosis or due to metabolic derangements such as uremia. Encephalitis is diagnosed by CSF examination, imaging (MRI, CT) and EEG.

Clinical Features

Fever, seizures, disorientation/confusion and headache.

Etiology

The most common cause of encephalitis is viral infection. Commonly implicated viruses include enteroviruses, HSV-1 and arboviruses, like Japanese encephalitis. Bacteria/fungal agents may also cause this condition although less frequently.

MUST KNOW

Acute encephalitis is a medical emergency requiring prompt diagnosis and treatment.
Treatment of choice for acute viral meningitis is acyclovir.

Pathological Changes

Gross appearance (Fig. 18.5A)

- Cerebral edema
- Vascular congestion
- Hemorrhage
- Infiltration with leukocytes

Histopathological changes (Fig. 18.5B)

- Dead/degenerate neurons.
- Increased neuronal cytoplasmic eosinophilia.
- Perivascular inflammatory infiltrate (more than lymphocytes, macrophages).
- Necrotic foci
- Surrounding unaffected parenchyma may show reactive gliosis.

CSF findings in viral encephalitis:

- Typically show moderate lymphocytosis.
- Normal glucose levels and moderately elevated protein levels.
- HSV encephalitis is characterized clinically by focal seizures and a frequent right sided hemiparesis.
- MRI shows increased signal intensity in the frontal and temporal lobes.

Figures18.5A and B: Encephalitis: **A.** Gross; **B.** Histology

STROKE

Stroke is the manifestation of reduced blood supply to the brain. It is also known clinically by the terminology cerebrovascular accident (CVA).

Types of Stroke

From a pathological perspective, it is of two types:

1. Ischemic, due to hypoxic injury. Most strokes are ischemic in nature (Fig. 18.6A).
2. Hemorrhagic—characterized by bleeding within the brain parenchyma (intracranial hemorrhage) or into the subarachnoid space (subarachnoid hemorrhage) (Fig. 18.6B).

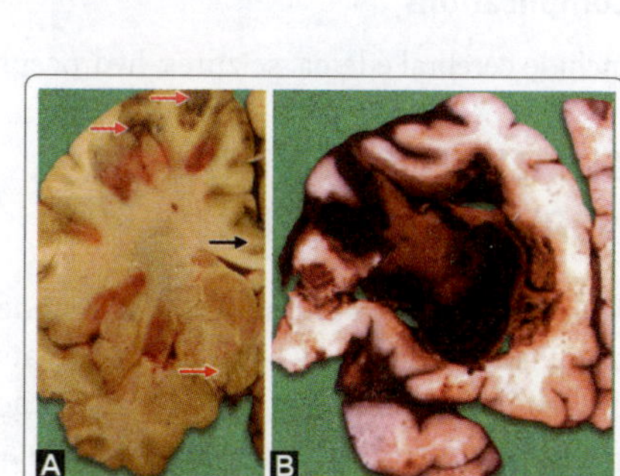

Figures 18.6A and B: **A.** Ischemic stroke; **B.** Hemorrhagic stroke

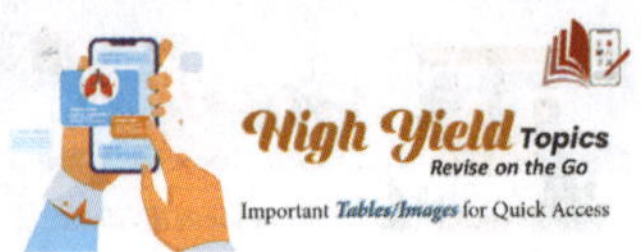

Ischemic Stroke

Etiology

- **Thrombosis:** When clotted blood (thrombus) is seen in the vessels supplying the brain.
- **Embolism:** When clotted blood/debris is accumulated at another site to form a mass which is then transported to vessels supplying the brain.

Thrombotic strokes are usually seen in the elderly and are frequently seen in persons afflicted by atherosclerosis.

MUST KNOW

Transient ischemic attacks (TIAs): They are episodes of ischemia occurring for a short span of time (a few minutes to 24 hours).
Lacunar infarct: Usually seen in elderly individuals suffering from diabetes/hypertension.

Pathological Changes

Histological changes: Features in cases of ischemic stroke:

- The affected (infarcted) area is soft, pale showing liquefactive necrosis.
- Surrounded by neutrophilic infiltrate.

Hemorrhagic Stroke

Usually associated with higher morbidity and mortality and comprises 10–20% of the total stroke cases.

Common sites involved: Basal ganglia, cerebral lobes.

Types of Hemorrhagic Stroke

- **Intracerebral hemorrhage**: Usually seen in patients of hypertension, the episode usually is of rapid onset and bleeding occurs suddenly.
- **Subarachnoid hemorrhage:** When the bleeding occurs in the subarachnoid space. This is frequently due to an arteriovenous malformation /aneurysm/trauma/vasculitis.

Clinical Features

Sudden headache, loss of consciousness.

Complications

Include cerebral edema, seizures, hydrocephalus.

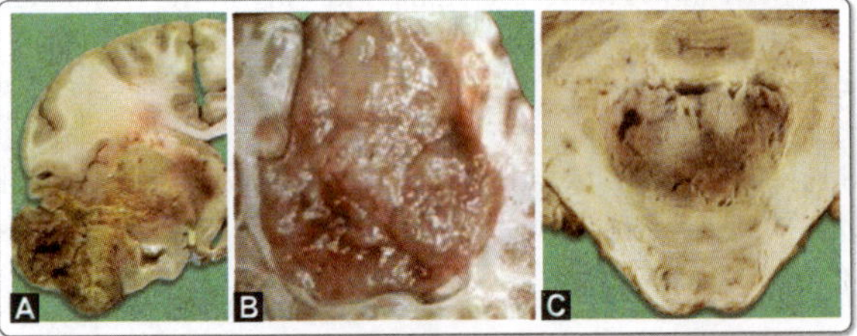

Figures 18.7A to C: **A.** Glioma; **B.** Oligodendroglioma; **C.** Ependymoma

TUMORS OF CENTRAL NERVOUS SYSTEM

The central nervous system (CNS) may undergo malignancy which may be derived from any of the cell lines within the CNS when it is known as primary or frequently as a site of metastasis from other sites when it is called secondary.

Glioma

- Glioma is derived from various cells of the CNS-astrocytes/oligodendroglial cells/ependymal cells (Fig. 18.7A). Accordingly, respective tumors are named as astrocytoma, oligodendroglioma (Fig. 18.7B) and ependymoma (Fig. 18.7C).

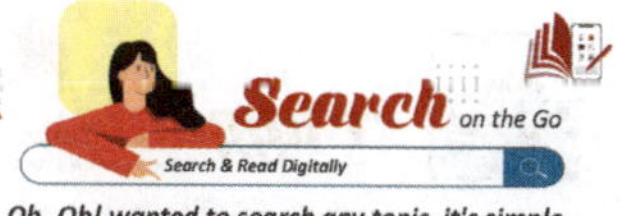

Astrocytoma

Astrocytoma characteristically involves individuals in the fourth to seventh decades and commonly afflicts the cerebral hemispheres.

Categories of astrocytomas—duport system:

This grading system was based on the mitotic activity and presence or absence of atypia, coagulative necrosis and microvascular proliferation (Duport system). Traditionally, astrocytomas were further categorized as:

- **Grade 1:** Pilocytic astrocytoma.
- **Grade 2:** Diffuse astrocytoma.
- **Grade 3:** Anaplastic astrocytoma.
- **Grade 4:** Glioblastoma multiforme.

RECENT UPDATE

WHO classification of tumors of CNS (2021)—molecular basis of adult type diffuse glioma

Recently in 2021, the World Health Organization (WHO) brought in a dramatic change in how CNS tumors were classified. Now, gliomas are classified as per age and molecular characteristics.

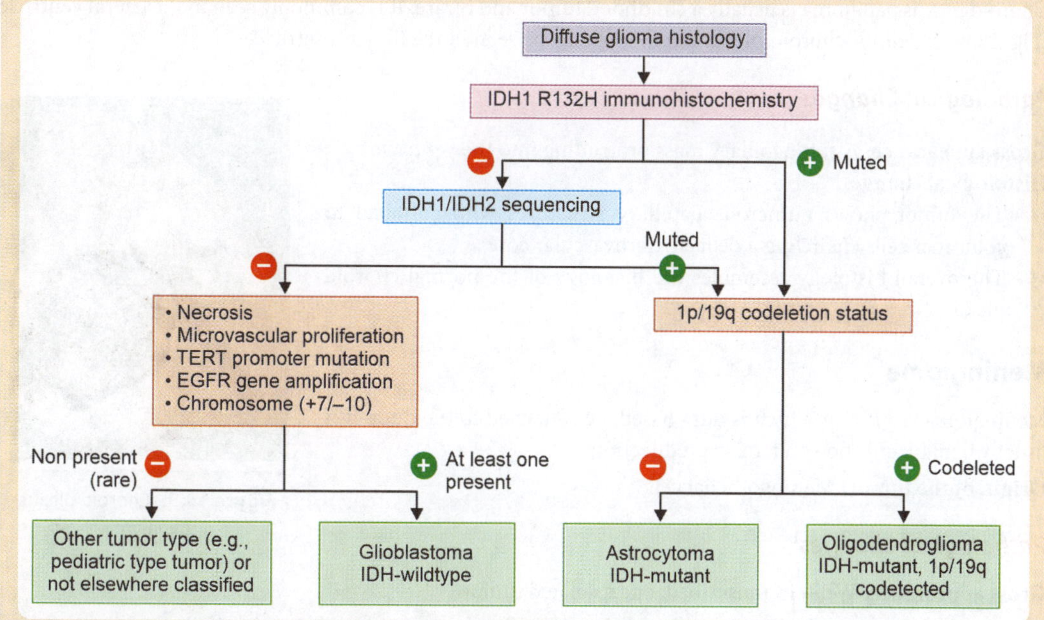

Oligodendroglioma

Oligodendroglioma tumor is derived from oligodendroglial cells.

Gross appearance: The tumor is well-circumscribed and gray-white.

Histopathological changes: Oligodendrogliomas are comprised of sheets of uniform round cells with round nuclei, clear cytoplasm, perinuclear halos and well-defined infiltrative cell margins.

- Chicken-wire vessels are noted throughout the tumor.
- Microcalcifications may also be seen.
- Molecular features:
  - 1p/19q co-deletion
  - IDH1/IDH2 mutation

Ependymoma

As per the WHO classification, grade 2 tumor.

Site: Ependymoma is frequently seen in children commonly seen in an intracranial location, the most common site being the fourth ventricle, while it is seen in the spine (intramedullary) in case of adults.

Gross appearance: Generally, well-delineated tumor

- Tumor cells are round to oval and arranged in the form of pseudo rosettes.
- Nuclei are relatively bland.
- Nucleoli are not prominent. Granular staining quality at the apical zone of the rosette.
- **Immunohistochemistry:** EMA dot positivity.

Anaplastic Ependymoma

Refers to the presence of ependymoma displaying increased cellularity and increased mitotic activity.

Choroid Plexus Papilloma

Choroid plexus papilloma is usually a childhood tumor and is rare. It is commonly seen in the lateral ventricle (Fig. 18.8). In adults, choroid plexus papilloma may be seen in the fourth ventricle.

Pathological Changes

Gross appearance: A soft papillary mass protruding into the ventricle

Histological changes:

- The tumor shows numerous papillary structures with cuboidal to columnar cells encircling a delicate fibrovascular core.
- The overall histology resembles the histology of the normal choroid plexus.

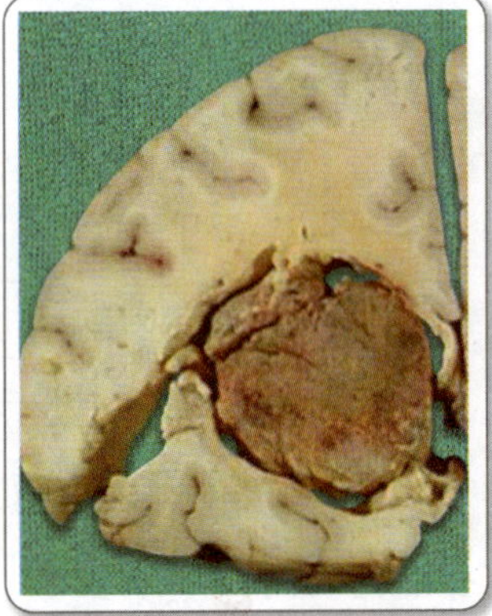

Figure 18.8: Choroid plexus papilloma

Meningioma

Meningioma is a tumor which is dura based, i.e., attached to the dura. It is usually benign and shows a female predilection.

Origin of the tumor: Meningothelial cell.

Pathological Changes

Gross appearance: Well-circumscribed, encapsulated tumor.

Histological changes: The histological types based on the changes in histology are as follows:

- Meningothelial/syncytial.
- Fibroblastic.
- Transitional.
- Psammomatous.
- Papillary.
- Anaplastic.

Immunohistochemical studies: Meningiomas are positive for ER, PR and EMA.

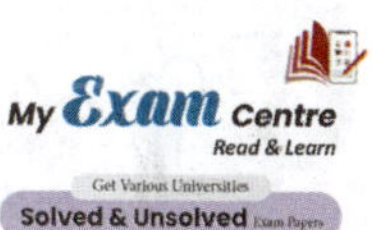

SUMMARY

- Meningitis is inflammation of the meninges which are the protective membranes on the surface of the brain.
- The patient of acute pyogenic meningitis looks very sick and presents with fever, headache, projectile vomiting, aversion to light (photophobia) and altered mental status manifesting as confusion, drowsiness and in some cases, seizures and even coma.
- Tubercular meningitis may be contracted through hematogenous spread of foci of tuberculosis elsewhere in the body.
- CSF examination is of paramount importance in the investigation of various types of meningitis.
- Encephalopathy is an altered state of consciousness (sensorium) persisting for >24 hours.
- Encephalitis is diagnosed by CSF examination, imaging (MRI, CT) and EEG.
- Stroke is the manifestation of reduced blood supply to the brain. It is also known clinically by the terminology cerebrovascular accident (CVA).
- Thrombotic strokes are usually seen in the elderly and are frequently seen in persons afflicted by atherosclerosis.
- Astrocytoma characteristically involves individuals in the fourth to seventh decades and commonly afflicts the cerebral hemispheres.

ASSESS YOURSELF

Long Answer Questions

1. Discuss tumors of CNS in detail.
2. Describe meningitis in detail.

Short Answer Questions

1. Write briefly about different types of stroke.
2. Write in brief about CSF features of types of meningitis.
3. Write short notes on:
   i. Encephalitis
   ii. Meningitis

Multiple Choice Questions

1. **Bacterial meningitis is a condition that results in inflammation of the protective membranes surrounding the ___________.**
   a. Sinus cavity
   b. Spinal cord and brain
   c. Intestinal tract
   d. Heart and lungs
2. **What are the symptoms of encephalitis or acute encephalitis syndrome?**
   a. High fever
   b. Vomiting
   c. Confusion
   d. All of these
3. **What is encephalitis?**
   a. An inflammation in brain
   b. It causes swelling or irritation in brain.
   c. It is also known as Chamki fever
   d. All of these
4. **Classic astrocytoma has which of following microscope features?**
   a. Widespread concentric calcifications
   b. Fibrillary astrocytes in the background of loosely structured microcytes
   c. Cells with rounded vesicular nuclei with small distinct nucleoli, perinuclear halos, chicken wire vessels
   d. Microvascular proliferation and geographic necrosis

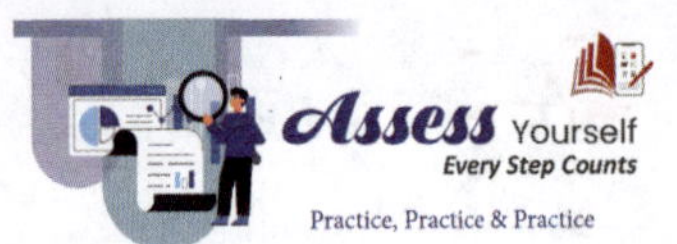

5. **Which of the following features indicate an atypical meningioma (WHO grade II)?**
   a. Meningioma with 4 mitoses per 10 high-power fields
   b. Meningioma with 20 mitoses per 10 high-power fields
   c. Meningioma wtih necrosis but no other worrying features
   d. Meningioma with CEA-immunopositive, PAS-positive secretory globules
6. **Which of the following is true regarding small cell glioblastoma?**
   a. Tumor cells show severe nuclear atypia
   b. Often associated with EGFR amplification
   c. Most of the tumors are IDH-mutated
   d. All of these
7. **All of the following are subtypes of ependymoma; except:**
   a. Clear
   b. Papillary
   c. Tancytic
   d. Giant cell
8. **All of the following are good prognostic markers of glioblastoma multiforme; except:**
   a. Age <50 years
   b. Secondary glioblastoma
   c. MGMT Promotor methylation
   d. Presence of necrosis

Answer Key

1. b	**2.** d	**3.** d	**4.** b	**5.** a	**6.** b
7. d	**8.** d				

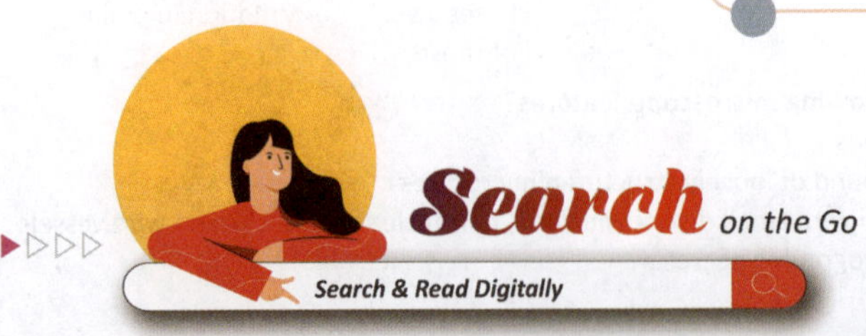

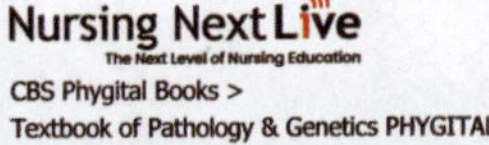

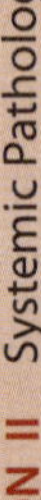

SECTION III

Clinical Pathology

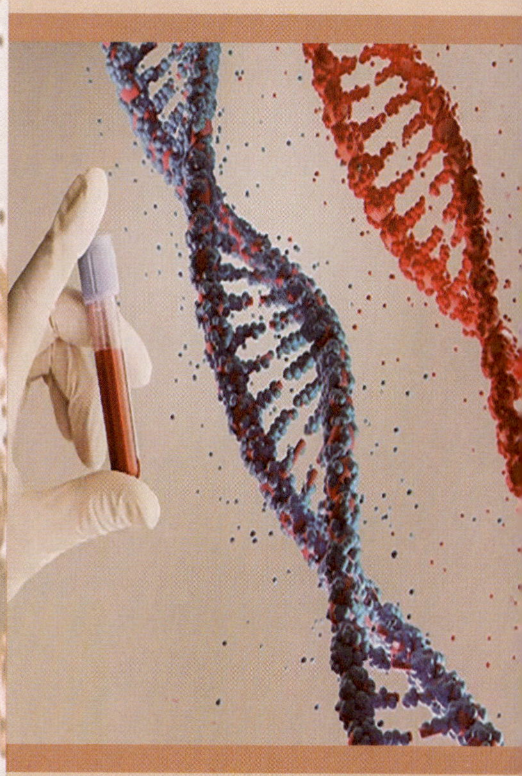

SECTION OUTLINE

Chapter 19

Hematological Tests for the Diagnosis of Blood Disorders

LEARNING OBJECTIVES

After the completion of the chapter, the readers will be able to:

- Explain various types of blood tests and their methods of estimation.
- Describe coagulation tests.
- Demonstrate laboratory tube collection and utilize ideal vacutainers for sample collection.
- Understand common blood biochemistry tests.
- Identify abnormalities in blood gases in clinical settings.
- Interpret bone marrow examination.
- Understand common serological and immunological tests.
- Explain blood grouping and cross-matching.
- Identify various blood components used in the clinical settings.
- Discuss transfusion reactions.

CHAPTER OUTLINE

- Process of Blood Testing
- Anticoagulants
- Blood Collection Tubes or Vacutainers
- Methods of Blood Collection
- Blood Test
- Hemogram
- Determination of Red Blood Cell Indices
- Hemoglobin Estimation
- Erythrocyte Sedimentation Rate
- Coagulation Tests
- Normal Reference Ranges in Hematology and Inference of Data
- Blood Biochemistry
- Blood Culture
- Bone Marrow Examination
- Serological and Immunological Tests

Blood Bank

- Blood Grouping and Crossmatching
- Blood Products
- Pretransfusion Compatibility Testing
- Transfusion Reactions

KEY TERMS

Activated partial thromboplastin time (APTT): The APTT measures the time [ref: 25–35 seconds] taken by plasma to clot when exposed to substances that activate the contact factors, and assesses the 'intrinsic' and 'common' pathways of coagulation.

Bleeding time: Bleeding time is a clinical laboratory test performed to evaluate platelet function. Normal bleeding time is >3 minutes.

Plasma: Plasma appears light-yellowish or straw-colored. It serves as the liquid base for whole blood.

Prothrombin time: The prothrombin time is a measure of the integrity of the extrinsic and final common pathways of the coagulation cascade.

Random donor platelets (RDP): Donated whole blood units are centrifuged and the buffy coats from four donations are separated and platelets are made by recentrifugation.

Single donor platelets (SDP): Pooled in the platelets from one single donor (preferably male) by apheresis technique.

PROCESS OF BLOOD TESTING

Testing of blood is done through three main processes—Preanalytical; analytical; and postanalytical.

Preanalytical phase includes all processes before the start of testing of the blood sample obtained. Blood collection is one such procedure in the pre-analytical phase. It is of utmost importance and improper collection and handling of blood samples can lead to errors in the analytical phase or the 'testing phase'. After the preanalytical phase; all the analysis process/analytical phase (Blood tests, specimen tests, etc) and post-analytical (reporting test results, interpretation, follow up, etc.) is followed.

Preanalytical Variables

Instructions

- A fasting sample is preferred when an optical based instrument is to be used.
- Samples must be collected preferably in the laboratory or must be transported to the lab immediately. For long distance transport plasma needs to be separated.
- Patient must preferably refrain from exercise and stressful activity prior to sampling.
- Venipuncture must be clean, and hemolysis should be avoided especially when an optical based instrument is to be used.
- Sample must be collected within 1 minute of application of tourniquet to avoid venous stasis or tourniquet must be released before sample is collected, as release of tissue thromboplastin may interfere with the results.
- Short-wide bore needle or Infusion set butterfly needle (19–21 G for adults and 22–23 G for children) must be used.
- Sample must be drawn into a plastic disposable syringe.
- The Vacuum tube /container should be filled without frothing. Prompt and adequate mixing with citrate solution should be done by 5-6 gentle inversions.
- The sample must be processed within four hours during which it must be kept at 2–8° C.
- If tests are to be performed later, the sample must be centrifuged at 2,000 g for 15 minutes to produce PPP, discarding a 0.5 mL layer at the bottom while removing the supernatant. A second spin at the same speed for 20 minutes, again discarding a 0.5 mL layer at the bottom is required. A platelet count must be performed on the PPP that must be $<10 \times 10^9$/L. The PPP must be aliquoted into 0.5/1.0 mL Eppendorf tubes, which are ideally "snap frozen" in liquid nitrogen (–196°C) or dry ice-methanol mixture. These can be stored at –70°C for up to 3 months. Storage at –20°C may be permissible in some systems with a maximal storage time of 1 month.

ANTICOAGULANTS

Various anticoagulants are used as suited for the purpose of test (Table 19.1).

Table 19.1: Blood sample collection—anticoagulants and purpose

Color of cap	Anticoagulant used	Purpose
Light blue	Trisodium citrate	Coagulation test
Gray	Sodium fluoride and potassium oxalate	Glucose and lactic acid testing
Green	Heparin	Immediate blood chemistry
Yellow	Sodium polyanethol sulfonate	Culture
Gold	Serum separator and clot activator	Collecting serum for blood biochemistry
Red	Clot activator	Collecting serum for blood biochemistry
Lavender	EDTA	CBC, ESR, PS

Citrate is the preferred anticoagulant.

- The concentration of citrate used is generally 3.2% (0.109 mol/L). The dihydrate salt of trisodium citrate is commonly used. It is dispensed in the liquid form.
- Note, that the ratio of sodium citrate to blood that is traditionally used is 1:9

Effect of other factors

The pH of the assay mixture for PT/APTT based tests should be maintained within narrow limits (7.1–7.35). PT values increase if pH is above or below prescribed limits.

Normally, if blood collection tubes are well stoppered, changes in pH of blood will be minimal. Keeping tubes stoppered prevents loss of CO_2 and the resultant increase in pH.

Citrate concentration must be adjusted in accordance with the hematocrit as follows for a 5 mL blood sample

$C = (1.85 \times 10^{-3})(100\text{-Hct})(V)$

Here,

C = volume of citrate to be added

Hct = hematocrit

V = volume of blood

Drawbacks

In polycythaemia, the relative proportion of plasma is very low. Since citrate is concentrated in the plasma compartment, the concentration of citrate in the plasma of polycythemia patients is high. This citrate complex with the calcium added during PT/APTT measurements, artificially elevating the results.

Samples need to be kept at room temperature and processed within four hours. It has been demonstrated that beyond four hours, coagulation factors get activated or depleted, resulting in shorter PT and APTT values.

BLOOD COLLECTION TUBES OR VACUTAINERS

Testing procedures may require serum or plasma. While performing multiple collections of venous and/or arterial blood samples in a single patient, a color sequence of withdrawing and its indications based on the Clinical and Laboratory Standards Institute (CLSI) is the recommended procedure (Fig. 19.1).

- **Yellow:** The yellow cap color tubes (bottles) contain sodium polyanethol sulfonate (SPS), which serves as an anticoagulant. The primary function of this anticoagulant is to inhibit the activation of complement function.
- **Light blue:** The "citrate tube" is for collecting blood for performing coagulation studies. It contains 3.2% sodium citrate as its anticoagulant. Clotting time differs between specimens and may range from 10 minutes to almost an hour (60 minutes).
- **Green:** The green capped tubes contain heparin (can either be in the form of sodium heparin, lithium heparin, or ammonium heparin), which acts as an

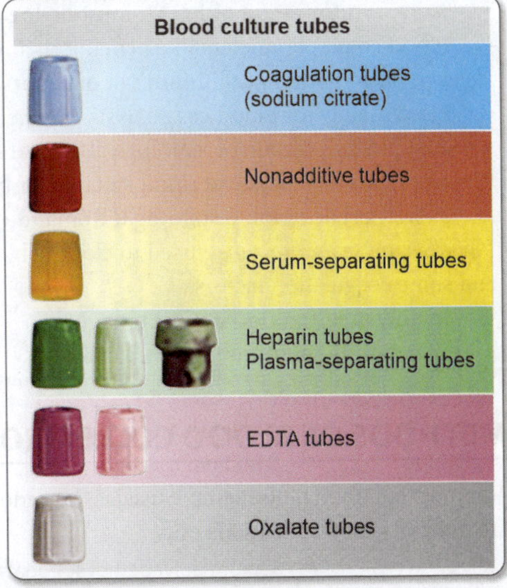

Figure 19.1: Order of draw

anticoagulant (inhibiting thrombin formation). Here plasma component of blood is required for tests. Green capped tubes are frequently used in requesting "stat" or immediate blood biochemistry results in emergency cases.

- **Lavender:** The lavender capped tube is also referred to as EDTA tubes because it uses ethylene-diamine-tetra-acetic acid (acts by chelating calcium ions in the blood to prevent coagulation). Since the blood does not clot, the liquid portion plasma is collected for tests (without the red blood cells). Lavender capped tubes are commonly used to collect blood samples for hematologic assays—CBC, ESR and peripheral smears.
- **Gray:** The gray capped tubes contain potassium oxalate (that binds to calcium, inhibiting coagulation). Another substance, sodium fluoride, is also contained in the tubes, which serve as an antiglycolytic agent, that is why it is used for plasma glucose and lactic acid lactic acid testing.

Order of Draw

The correct application of the "Order of Draw" principle in multiple **blood** tube collection is an essential aspect of ensuring quality laboratory test results.

Points to remember while using vacutainers

Sodium citrate vacuette: Trisodium citrate tubes

- Used to collect blood for coagulation studies like Prothrombin Time (PT) and activated Partial thromboplastic time (APTT).
- Note, commercial tubes provide a mark indicating the amount of blood to be filled in order to maintain a ratio of 9 parts of blood to 1 part of anticoagulant. This crucial step affects analytical phase drastically and must be kept in mind while filling the tubes.

Ethylenediamine-tetra acetic acid tubes:

- EDTA removes calcium which is essential for coagulation and prevents clotting.
- Used for blood cell counts.
- Note, concentration of EDTA must be less than 2 mg/mL which otherwise can lead to changes in the blood count parameters like hematocrit and mean corpuscular hemoglobin concentration.

Heparin tubes: Sodium or lithium salt of heparin at a concentration of 10–20 IU/mL of blood.

- Used mainly for blood gas analysis, biochemistry and emergency tests.
- Also used in certain hematological tests of hemolytic anemia like osmotic fragility test.
- Note, this anticoagulant is not suitable for blood counts as it can cause platelet and leukocyte clumping as well as background staining if Romanowsky dyes are used to stain the smear.

Plain/Serum separator tubes: used to clot the blood and produce serum which does not contain fibrinogen and some coagulation factors.

- Mainly used for biochemical tests.
- Serum is different from plasma in that it.

METHODS OF BLOOD COLLECTION

The most common blood sample used is the venous blood sample. Capillary blood and arterial blood samples are used in specific situations only.

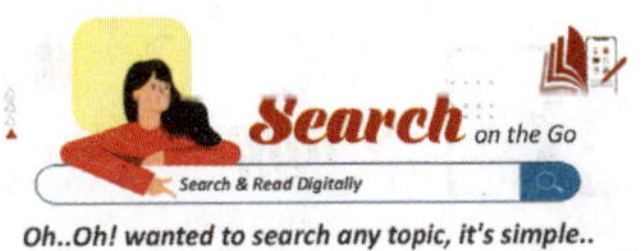

Phlebotomy or Venipuncture Procedure

Phlebotomy: This is the process of obtaining blood sample from a vein using a needle and a suitable device. It is also known as venipuncture.

Phlebotomy Procedure

An adequately trained staff should perform this procedure and before starting the procedure, ensure that the phlebotomy tray has the required equipment.

Equipment: Syringes, needles, tourniquet, appropriate vacutainers/blood culture bottles, alcohol swabs, sterile gauze swabs, adhesive dressings, vacutainer rack and puncture proof disposal containers.

Site of blood sample collection: The preferred site of blood collection is antecubital vein or other prominent veins in the forearm.

Container: Evacuated collection tubes

Additives: As per the requirement of test (refer Table 19.2)

- The tourniquet is placed just above the vein of choice. The skin over the selected vein should be properly cleaned ideally with 70% alcohol and allowed to dry spontaneously to avoid contamination of the cleaned site.
- After the vein is punctured, the tourniquet should be released immediately to avoid hemoconcentration due to stagnation of venous blood within the vein.
- After venipuncture, piston of syringe should be withdrawn only at the pace of blood entering the syringe.
- The collected blood should be transferred to vacutainers in the minimum time possible to prevent coagulation. The order of draw that is proper selection of the sequence in which you will fill the vacutainers also affects analytical phase.

  Note, to not to transfer blood forcefully into the collecting tube (to avoid hemolysis).
- Skin cleaning swab must be moved in concentric rings, from inside to outwards (to minimize infection).
- Invert blood sample containing tube several times, slowly (to mix the additives properly).

Complications of Phlebotomy or Venipuncture Procedure

- **Hematoma formation:** Rapid swelling a puncture site due to blood leaking into tissue.
- **Infection of site:** Due to bacteria present on skin, if site is not cleaned properly.
- **Continuation of bleeding:** Pressure must be applied for a few minutes to promote coagulation.

Skin Puncture

The blood can be collected by skin puncture in adults as well as in infants. This is done to obtain capillary blood to perform a point-of care testing, where only a small drop of blood is required; or in the infants where peripheral vein might not be easily approachable.

Preferred site: In adults, the preferred site is distal portion of 3rd or 4th finger (Fig. 19.2A) on the lateral portion palmer surface while in the infants, lateral portions of the heel (Fig. 19.2B) are the preferred sites.

MUST KNOW

Tying the torniquet for longer than a minute can result in increased hematocrit and falsely elevated hemoglobin and RBC count. This happens due to shift of fluid from intravascular to extravascular compartment due to stagnation in the vein.

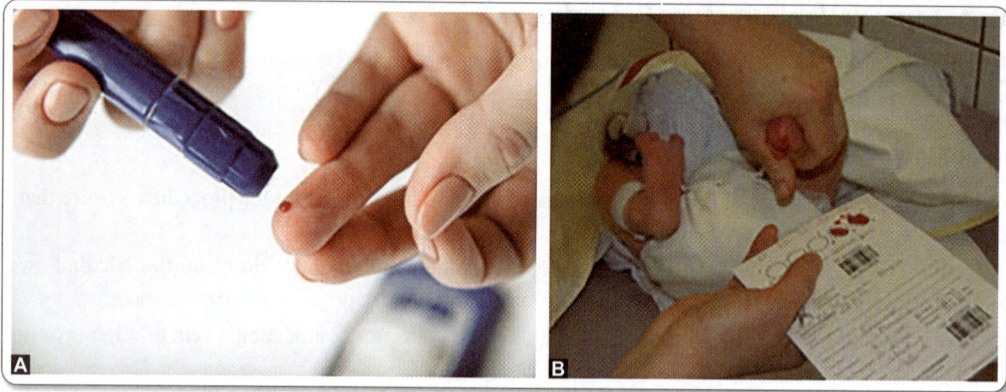

Figures 19.2A and B: **A.** Capillary blood collection in adults and older children; **B.** Heel prick sample in a newborn

BLOOD TEST

Various blood tests are used to determine physiological and biochemical states, such as disease, mineral content, drug effectiveness and organ function.

Blood Cells' Count

There are three types of cells, which need to be tested these are white blood cells, red blood cells and platelets. Let's discuss the morphology of these cells, which will help in their enumeration (Table 19.2).

Table 19.2: Types of blood cells

<table>
<tr><th>Cells</th><th>Normal counts</th><th>Image</th></tr>
<tr><td>Red blood cells (erythrocytes)</td><td>4.5–5.5 million cells/mm</td><td>Size is 6–8 microns</td></tr>
<tr><td>White blood cells (leukocytes)</td><td>4,000–11,000 cells/mm^3</td><td>These are furthur divided into granulocytes and agranulocytes<table><tr><td>Granulocytes</td><td>Agranulocytes</td></tr><tr><td>Neutrophils</td><td>Lymphocytes</td></tr><tr><td>Eosinophils</td><td>Monocytes</td></tr><tr><td>Basophils</td><td></td></tr></table></td></tr>
</table>

Contd...

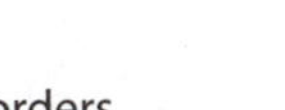

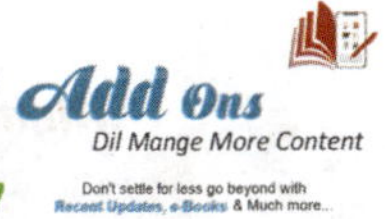

Cells	Normal counts	Image
Platelets and WBC	150,000–450,000 cells/mm^3	Platelets Size is 2–4 microns

Source

- **Most of hematological tests** (complete blood count [CBC] and coagulation tests): Vein.
- **Arterial blood gas analysis:** Artery.
- **Peripheral smear:** From vein or capillary blood.

HEMOGRAM

Hemogram is a group of laboratory tests, which includes hemoglobin measurement, total leukocyte count, red blood cell (RBC) count, platelet count, differential leukocyte count, packed cell volume (PCV), erythrocyte sedimentation rate (ESR) and peripheral smear examination.

Laboratory Determination of Cell Counts

The technique used for counting of blood cells is known as hemocytometry. This method involves manual counting of cells after diluting fluid and the counts are made in special counting chambers with rulings.

RBC Count

- Sample is taken in ethylene diamine tetraacetate (EDTA) or double oxalated blood
- The RBCs can be assessed by manual method using improved Neubauer counting chamber or by automated analyzer (Fig. 19.3).

Manual Method

Determination of Total erythrocyte (Red Blood Cell) Count

Apparatus: Improved Neubauer's counting chamber, RBC pipette, RBC diluting fluid (Hayem's fluid); compound microscope, cover-slips, pricking apparatus.

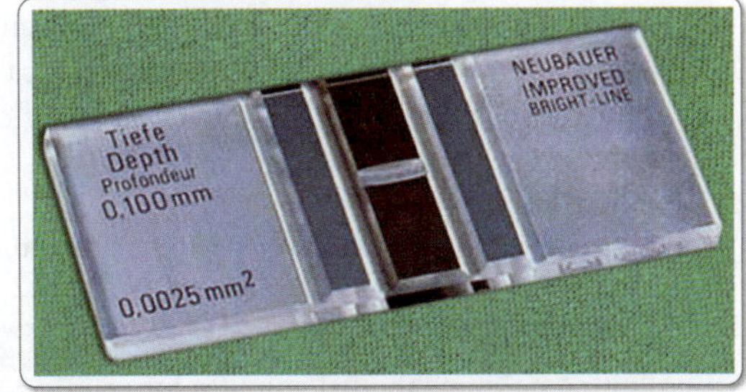

Figure 19.3: Neubauer counting chamber

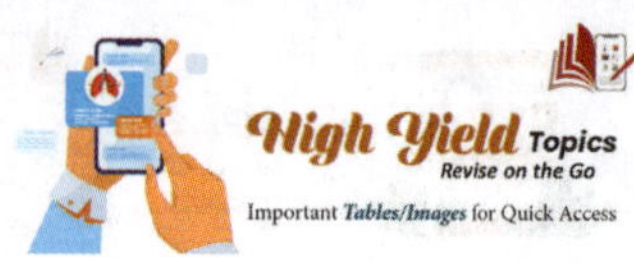

RBC Diluting Fluid (Hayem's Fluid)

Composition: Each 100 mL of fluid contains:

- Sodium sulphate (Na_2SO_4): 2.5 g (to prevent aggregation of RBCs, i.e., rouleaux formation).
- Sodium chloride (NaC1): 0.5 g (to maintain isotonicity of the fluid, therefore, RBCs remain suspended in the solution).
- Mercuric chloride ($HgC1_2$): 0.25 g (preservative: antibacterial and antifungal).
- Distilled water: 100 mL (solvent).

Principle: Since the normal RBC count runs in millions, the count is made possible by diluting the sample of blood before counting and subsequently multiplying the count by the dilution factor.

Procedure:

- Ensure that the improved Neubauer's chamber, cover-slips and the lenses of the microscope are absolutely clean and the RBC pipette is dry and patent.
- Take adequate RBC diluting fluid in a watch glass.
- Prick the finger taking necessary precautions.
- Wipe off the first drop of blood. Suck the next drop of blood in RBC pipette exactly up to 0.5 mark, taking care that there should be no air bubbles. (Any excess of blood drawn in can be removed by tapping the tip of the pipette against the palm of your hand.)
- Wipe of the blood sticking to the tip of the pipette.
- Immediately, thereafter, holding the pipette in a nearly horizontal position, Hayem's fluid is sucked into the pipette exactly up to 101 mark, just above the bulb.
- The pipette is then kept horizontally between the palms and rolled gently for about a minute to ensure thorough mixing of the blood and the fluid. This will give a suspension of RBCs in the bulb of the pipette (dilution: 1/200).
- A clean cover-slip is placed in the Neubauer's chamber so as to cover the ruled area on both sides.
- Focus the RBCs squares of Neubauer's ruling under the low power objective (X10) of the microscope The chamber is than remove from the microscope and placed on the table. The focus of the microscope is not disturbed.
- Discard the first few drops of fluid from the RBC pipette. They constitute the unmixed Hayem's fluid present in the stem of the pipette.

  Charging the Neubauer's chamber

  - A small drop of fluid is allowed to form at the tip of the pipette and this drop is gently brought in contact with the edge of the cover-slip. The fluid is drawn into the chamber by capillary action. Both sides of the Neubauer's chamber are charged.
  - An ideally charged chamber is one which has been charged with a single adequate sized drop which just fills the chamber without leaving any air bubbles. This is learnt by practice.
  - If the fluid overflows into the gutters, it is called over-charging. If it is insufficient to fill the chamber or having air bubbles, it is said to be under-charged.

NOTE

- Should the chamber be over or under-charged, the procedure is repeated after thoroughly cleaning the chamber and the cover-slip with soap and water.
- The chamber should not be charged in parts by two or more smaller drops.

- Allow some time (about 1 minute) for cells to settle down in the counting chamber so that all the cells present will be in the same plane.

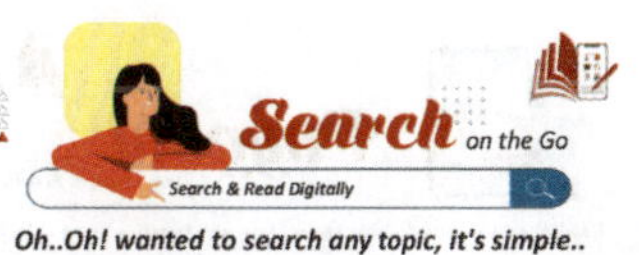

- The charged Neubauer's chamber is now kept under the low power of the microscope (already in focus). Using only the fine adjustments, the cell along the ruled area is brought into focus.
- Check whether cells are uniformly distributed.

Calculation: Calculation is done using following formula:

$$\text{Total number of blood cells/ mm}^3 = \frac{\text{Number of cells counted} \times \text{Dilution factor}}{\text{Volume of the chamber}}$$

$$= \frac{N \times 200}{1/50}$$

Total number of blood cells/mm^3 = N × 10,000.

Number of cells counted = N

Dilution factor = 1 in 200

Area of counting = 80 small squares with an area of 1/400 mm^2

Total area is 80/400 = 1/15 mm^2

Depth of chamber = 1/10 mm

Volume of counting area = 1/5 × 1/10 = 1/50 mm^3

Normal Range of RBC Count

- Adult male: 4.4–6.0 million/mm^3
- Adult female: 3.8–5.0 million/mm^3
- At birth: 6.0–7.0 million/mm^3

The causes of altered red blood cell (RBC) count are presented in Table 19.3.

Table 19.3: Causes of altered red blood cell count

Cause of decreased RBC count	Cause of increased RBC count
Anemia	Polycythemia
Hemodilution	Cyanotic heart disease
Pregnancy	Hemoconcentration (due to burns, cholera, etc.)

WBC Count

Determination of Total Leukocyte (White Blood Cell) Count: TLC

Apparatus: Improved Neubauer's counting chamber, WBC pipette, WBC pipette, WBC diluting fluid (Turk's fluid), compound microscope, cover-slips, pricking apparatus

WBC diluting fluid (Turk's fluid):

Composition: Each 100 mL of fluid contains:

- **Glacial acetic acid:** 3 mL (to lyse/destroy the membrane of blood cells, RBCs and platelets).
- **Gentian violet (1%):** 1 mL (to stain the nuclei of WBCs so that they can be identified easily).
- **Distilled water:** To make 100 mL (solvent).

Principle: Same as in RBC count, however, as the WBC count is much lower than the RBC count, much lesser dilution (1:20) is employed.

Procedure:

- Take WBC diluting fluid (Turk's fluid) in a watch glass.
- After pricking finger, suck the second drop of blood into the WBC diluting fluid by sucking the fluid up to 11 mark (dilution 1 in 20).

NOTE

Take necessary precautions as given under procedure for determination of total RBC count.

- Gently rotate the pipette at least 3–4 minutes.

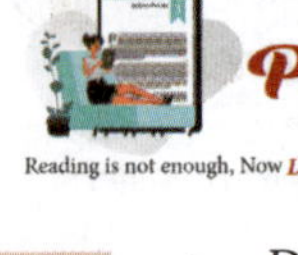
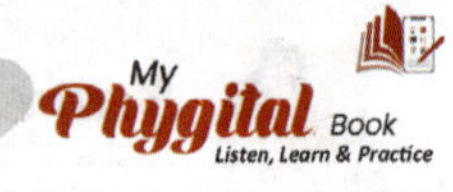

- Discard first few drops of WBC fluid in the stem of the pipette, charge the counting chamber as done during RBC counting and allow the time for settling of cells.
- Under low power objective, identify and check the distribution of WBCs in the four corner WBC squares. Recharge the chamber if distribution is not uniform.

NOTE

WBCs are seen as regular nucleated, rounded bodies with a clear refractility around them.

- Count the number of WBCs in each WBC square preferably under low power objective as per rules observed for counting the cells

Observations: Count the WBCs in 4 corner WBC squares. Enter the observations in the corresponding squares already drawn (Fig. 19.4).

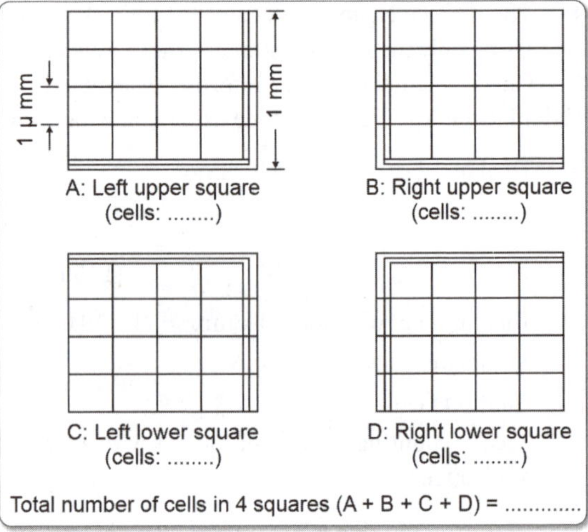

Figure 19.4: Enter the observations after counting the WBCs in the corresponding squares

Calculations:

Dilution factor: $= \dfrac{\text{Final volume achieved (10 parts)}}{\text{Original volume taken (0.5 parts)}} = 20$

Determination of total leukocyte (White Blood Cell) Count: TLC

Calculation of volume of fluid examined:

Area of 4 WBC squares = 4 × 1 mm × 1 mm

= 4 sq. mm

Depth of the chamber = 0.1 mm

Therefore, volume of fluid in the 4 WBC squares

= 4 sq. mm × 0.1 mm

= 0.4 cumm

Eaxmple:

Let 'N' be the total number of WBCs in 4 WBC squares i.e. in 0.4 cumm of diluted blood.

Then total number of WBCs in 1 cu.mm of undiluted blood:

$$= \frac{N \times \text{Dilution factor (20)}}{0.4}$$

$= N \times 50$

Results: Total leukocyte (WBC) count of is:

Comments and discussion: (State whether TLC is within normal range or not; if not, explain)

Normal range of WBC count:

Adults: 4,000–11,000 cells/mm^3.

The causes of altered white blood cell counts are presented in Table 19.4.

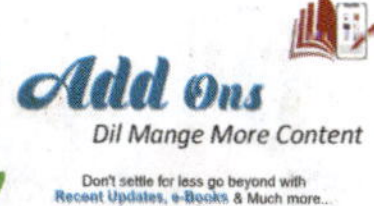

Automated Method

Sample: EDTA or double oxalated blood (preferred one).

Equipment: Neubauer counting chamber, RBC pipette and platelet diluting (contains procaine hydrochloride, sodium chloride and distilled water).

Procedure: The blood sample is drawn up to 0.5 mark and the diluting fluid up to the mark. This makes a dilution of 1 in 200. The sample is mixed well and the sample from stem of the pipette is discarded. The chamber is cleaned and the sample is introduced under the coverslip, the chamber is placed in the petridish with moist filter paper for 15 minutes. The platelets are counted in all the small 25 central squares.

Table 19.4: Causes of altered white blood cell count

Causes of decreased WBC count	Cause of increased WBC count
Aplastic anemia	Physiological-muscular exercise, pregnancy
Drug-induced suppression	Acute infections
Megaloblastic anemia	Chronic infections
Typhoid infections	Leukemoid reactions
Certain viral infections	Leukemia

Calculation

$$\text{Total number of platelets mm}^3 = \frac{\text{Number of cells counted} \times \text{Dilution factor}}{\text{Volume of the chamber}}$$

$$= \frac{N \times 200}{0.1}$$

Total number of blood cells/mm^3 = N × 2,000.

Number of cells counted = N

Dilution factor = 1 in 200

Area of counting = 1 mm^2

Depth of chamber = 1/10 mm

Volume of counting area = 1 × 1/10 = 1/10 mm^3

Platelet Count

Platelets are contractile and adhesive cells, 1–3 µm in diameter, purple colored on standing still with tiny irregular projections on the surface. The function of platelets is clot formation to prevent bleeding. Platelets are rich in intracellular granules, which are released during stimulation· Platelets deliver these to sites of vascular injury, where they contribute to clot formation of the repair process.

Normal range of platelet count:

The normal range is 150,000–400,000/µL or 150–400 × 10^9/L. A deficiency of blood platelets is termed thrombocytopenia. The causes of altered platelet counts are presented in Table 19.5.

Preparation of a Peripheral Blood Smear and Determination of Differential Leukocyte Count (DLC)

Apparatus. 4–5 glass slides, pricking apparatus, compound microscope, cedar-wood oil and Leishman's stain.

Reagents

Leishman's stain: It belongs to Romanowsky group of stains containing an acidic and a basic dye. The remarkable property of this group of stain is:

Table 19.5: Causes of altered platelet count

Causes of decreased platelet count (thrombocytopenia)	Causes of increased platelet count (thrombocytosis)
Immune-mediated destruction	Polycythemia vera, muscular excercises
Aplastic anemia	Postsplenectomy
Megaloblastic anemia	Chronic myeloid leukemia
Acute leukemia	
Hypersplenism	

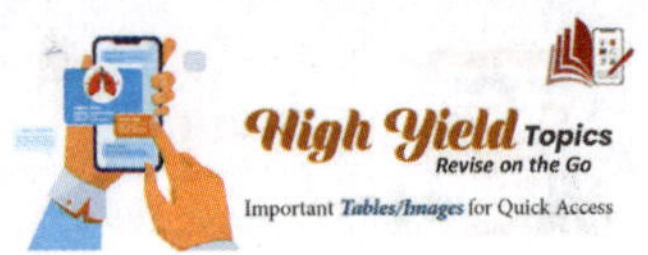

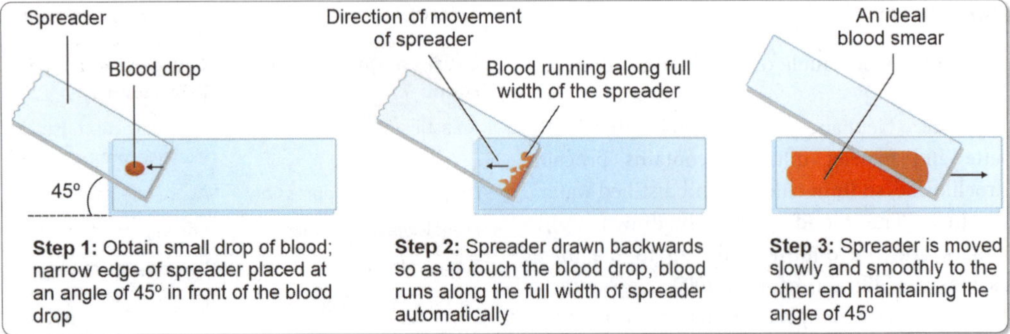

Figure 19.5: Preparation of a blood smear

- Making clear distinction in shades of staining.
- Staining granules differentially.

Eosin: It is an acidic dye (negatively charged) and stains positively charged (basic) particles *viz.*, RBCs and granules of eosinophils.

Methylene blue: It is a basic dye (positively charged) and stains negatively charged (acidic) particles *viz.*, the cytoplasm, nuclei of WBCs and granules of basophils.

Acetone free methyl alcohol. It is a fixative, i.e.:

- It preserves the cells in whatever chemical and metabolic state they are at the time of staining.
- The blood smear also gets fixed to the slide (precipitation of protein in it, by alcohol) so that it cannot be washed off.

NOTE

The methyl alcohol should be acetone free since acetone causes shrinkage of the cells and may even produce crenation and lyses of the cells. It should also be completely water free since water may affect appearance of the film by causing rouleaux formation.

Procedure

Preparation of a blood smear (Fig. 19.5):

- Take 4 or 5 clean, grease-free glass slides with smooth edges; 3–4 to be covered with the blood film and one to be used as a spreader.
- Lay 3-4 glass slides on a table, prick the finger, touch the bleeding point lightly in the centre line about 1 or 2 cm from one end of the slides to obtain a small drop of blood on each.
- Place the narrow edge of the spreader on the surface of slide just in front of the drop of the blood at an angle of 45°. Draw the spreader backwards so as to touch the drop and held there till the blood rungs along the full width of the spreader at the line of junction.
- The spreader is then moved slowly and smoothly to the other end of the slide maintaining an angle of 45°
- Allow the film to dry in air. Repeat the procedure with the other slides.

NOTE

- Rouleaux formation is usually seen in varying degrees in wet preparations of whole blood.
- A properly made blood film will be fairly uniform without uneven streaks or spots/vacuoles in it and neither too thick nor too thin.

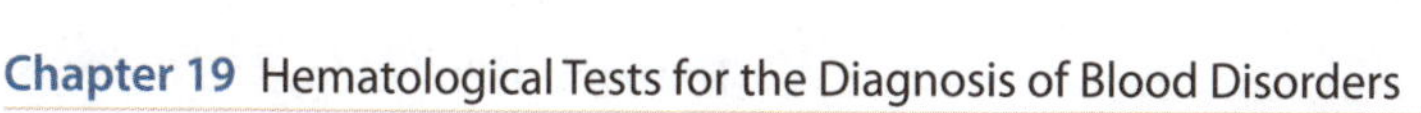

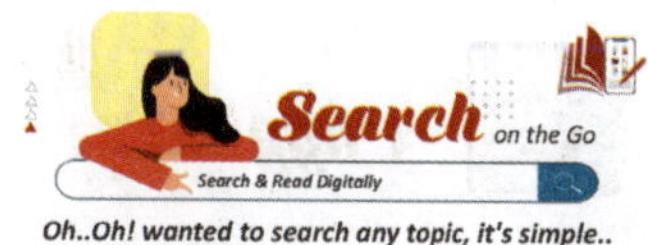

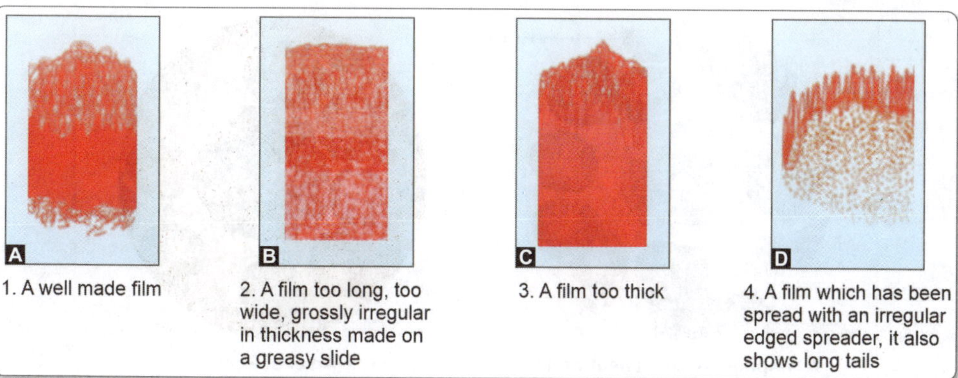

Figures 19.6A to D: Blood films made on glass slides

Criteria of a good blood smear (Figs 19.6A to D)

- It should cover almost entire width and about 3–4 cm length of the slide.
- It is tongue-shaped with no tails at the end.
- It is of uniform thickness, i.e., it is neither too thin nor too chick (a thick smear, when placed on a white background appears red).
- There are no longitudinal/cross striations or air–gaps in the smear.

Fixing and staining of the blood smear

Fixing the smear:

- Place the blood smears across two of the parallel supports on the glass rods, so that the slides are horizontal.
- Pour 8–12 drops of Leishman's stain on each slide, just enough to cover the smear. Note the time. Leave it for about 2 minutes (fixation time).

NOTE

Note the number of Leishman's stain drops poured. In hot weather, the stain should be watched to see that it does not become thick due to the evaporation of the alcohol. If this occurs, the stain will precipitate on the film. This can be avoided by adding more stain to that already on the slide.

Staining the smear

- After 2 minutes, add equal drop of buffered water (pH 6.8) over the stain, taking care that the water is not spilled over

NOTE

Double the number of drops of distilled water may be used in case of non-availability of buffered water]

- Mix the stain and water evenly by gently blowing air intermittently with the help of a dropper.
- If the dilution of the stain is correct, the fluid will be covered by a thin greenish scum. Leave the stain to act for 10 minutes (staining time).

NOTE

Depending on the strength of the Leishman's stain, the fixation time and staining time are variable; they are accordingly specified before the experiment.

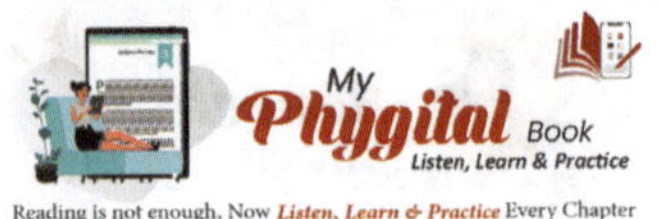

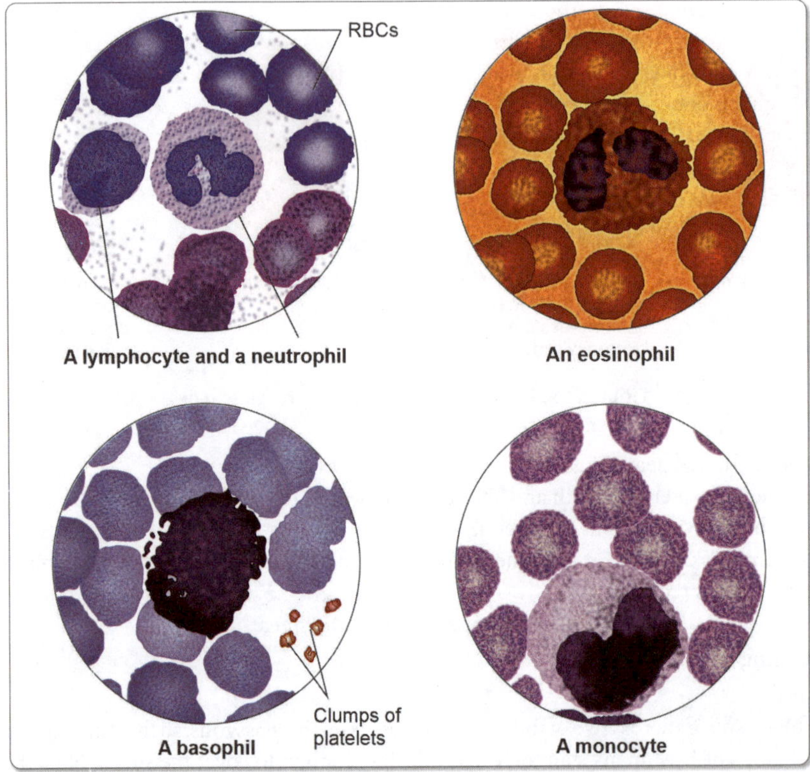

Figure 19.7: Peripheral blood smear showing different types of blood cells (Laishmans stain)

- At the end of 10 minutes, pour off the stain, hold the slide in a slanting position below the tap and the water is allowed to flow over the smear.
- Wash the slide (up to 2 minutes) with tap water gently and thoroughly till the film gets a pinkish tinge. Make sure that:
  - None of the greenish scum settles on the surface of the blood film; and
  - Water stream should not strike the blood smear directly or else it may be washed off
- Wipe, clean the back of the slide and set it upright to dry

Assessment of the quality of the stained smear

Check the staining and thickness of the blood smear (Fig. 19.7) by examining it first under low power objective. A well stained blood smear has the following characteristics:

- The smear is single-cell thick, with not much overlapping of the cells and the cells are uniformly distributed.
- At least one WBC is seen per high power field (x100).
- The RBCs are stained light pink.
- In an over stained smear, RBCs look bluish black and WBCs will take up more methylene blue, hence look totally purple.
- In an under stained smear, RBCs appear very pale and WBCs look almost colorless.

NOTE

If smear is understained, add the stain and repeat the process for a few minutes. If it is overstained, wash the slide for a few-minutes.

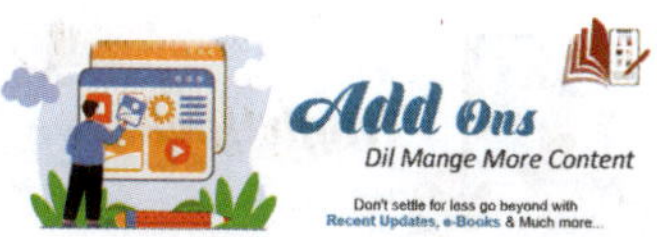

Examination of the stained smear under oil immersion

- Place a drop of cedar-wood oil on the blood film. Swing the oil immersion objective into position. Carefully lower the objective until it just touches the drop oil. Now, raise the objective and focus the cells using fine adjustment.
- Study the distribution (Fig. 19.8) and characteristics of different types of cells in the different parts of the smear
  - The most abundant cell type found anywhere in the smear is, the RBCs. These are seen as light pink, non-nucleated discs of uniform size and shape.
  - At the head end of the smear the RBCs are crowded and superimposed, and the WBCs are poorly stained.
  - At the extreme tail end, the cells are wide apart and the WBCs are distorted.
  - AT the upper and lower edges of the smear, the WBCs are found in plenty but are poorly stained and abnormally rich in granulocytes.

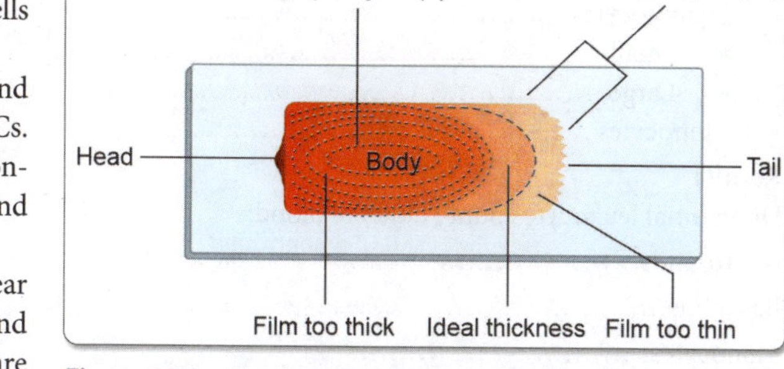

Figure 19.8: Distribution of leukocytes in the different parts of a blood smear

Identification of different types of leukocytes

Identification and counting of different types of leukocytes are done under oil-immersion objective. The WBCs can be differentiated from RBCs by the presence of nucleus and large size. While identifying the WBCs, keep 4 factors in mind:

1. Size of the cells (compare with the surrounding RBCs which are of uniform size, 7.2 µm).
2. Features of the nucleus (color, number of lobes).
3. Features of the cytoplasmic granules (pink or blue; fine or coarse).
4. Nuclear/cytoplasmic ratio.

Observation: Counting of the Different Types of Leukocytes

A minimum of 100 WBCs are identified in a systematic manner (Fig. 19.9) and counting is made using the tally-bar method. Ideally, all the cells should be counted in a single strip running the length of the smear, proceeding from base to apex. Use the mechanical stage to traverse the full length of the film. Move the slide along vertically by a distance equivalent to 2 mm and again traverse the full length of the film, this time in the opposite direction. This method ensures that cells are not counted more than once

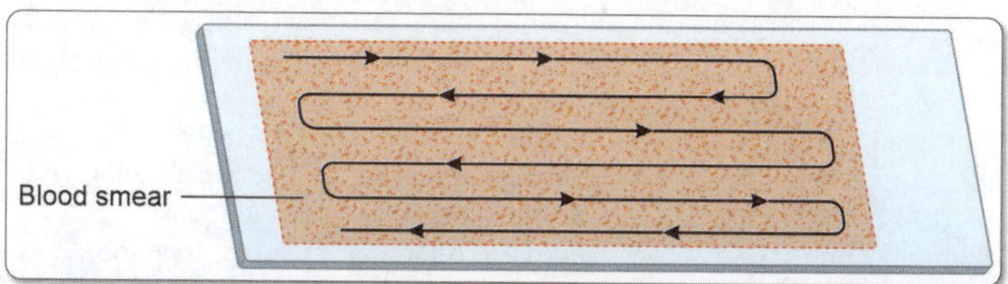

Figure 19.9: Rules for counting the leukocytes. Arrows indicate the directions of movement of the slide

Note: The field move to right/down when the slide is moved to left/up

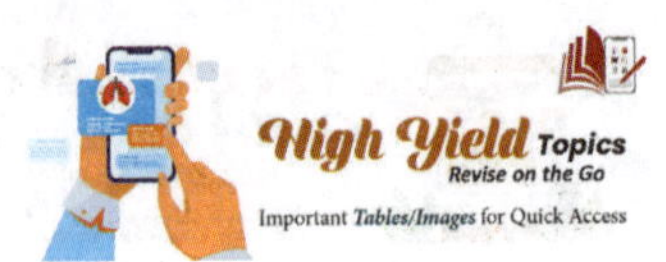

[Keep putting a vertical bar (I) against a cell identified, the 5th bar should be marked obliquely so as to cut all the previous 4 vertical bars (IIII). This will leave you with bundle of five for easy calculation at the end]

- Neutrophils ....
- Eosinophils ....
- Basophils ....
- Lymphocytes ....
  - Small ....
  - Large ....
- Monocytes ....

Results

Differential leukocyte count (DLC) of blood:

Neutrophils................................ %

Basophils................................. %

Monocytes............................... %

Eosinophils......................... %

Lymphocytes.................. %

Characteristic features of the different leukocytes—granulocytes and agranulocytes (Table 19.6 and Figure 19.10)

Table 19.6: Characteristic features of the different leukocytes

Cell type	Cell size (diameter)	Nucleus	Cytoplasm	Granules
Granulocytes				
Neutrophil (50–70%)	10–14 μm (1.5–2 times the size of surrounding RBCs)	Multilobed (1–6 lobes), purple in color	Slight bluish	• Very fine like sand particles • Numerous, reddish brown in color
Eosinophil (1–4%)	-do-	• Usually bilobed (spectacle shape) • Purple in color	Eosinophilic (acidic) light pink, granular	• Large • Coarse • Brick red in color • Do not cover the nucleus
Basophil (<1%)	-do-	• Usually bilobed • Purple in color	Basophilic (basic) appears blue granular	• Large • Coarse • Purple of blue • Overlying the nucleus
Agranulocytes				
Lymphocyte (20–40%)	Small : 7–10 μm (size of RBC) Large: 10–14 μm (1.5–2 times the surrounding RBCs); irregular outline	• Single • Very big occupying whole of the cell • Purple in color • Oval or rounded • Central in position	• Scanty • Sky blue color • Amount: Less than the amount of nucleus	Absent

Contd...

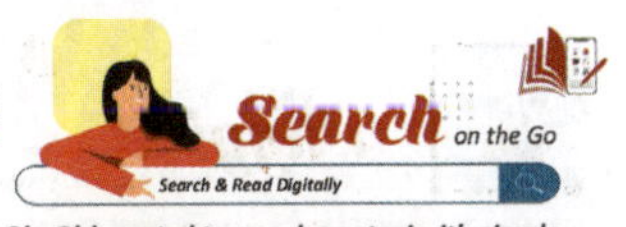

Cell type	Cell size (diameter)	Nucleus	Cytoplasm	Granules
Monocyte (2–8%)	• 10–18 µm (2–2.5 times the size of a RBC) • Irregular outline	• Single; usually indented kidney shape • Pale in color • May be oval or circular • Peripheral in position	• Abundant (amount more than the nucleus amount) • Pale blue in color	Absent

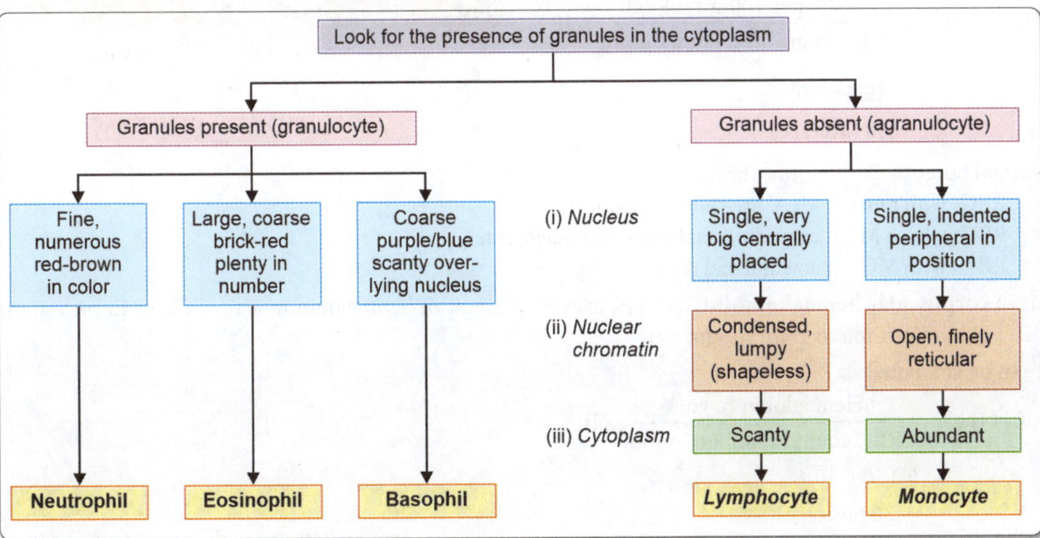

Figure 19.10: Summary of leukocyte identification

Interpretation of Results

Precautions:

- The slides should be clean and grease-free, therefore, these should be cleaned thoroughly with soap and water immediately before use.
- The glass-spreader should be carefully selected. It should have a smooth and clean edge. If a rough-edged spreader is used, many of the leukocytes accumulate at the edges and in the tail of the smear. Also, a gross qualitative irregularity in distribution of cells will occur.
- Make about 4–5 blood films so that at least one is satisfactory.
- Mark the smeared surface with a glass marking pencil.
- Do not heat dry or blot dry the smear.
- Stored blood should not be used for making smear.
- The smear should be stained not later than 2 hours after it has been prepared.
- Assess the quality of the smear, both grossly and microscopically (under low power) before staining it.
- Only properly well stained slide should be examined under the oil-immersion lens.

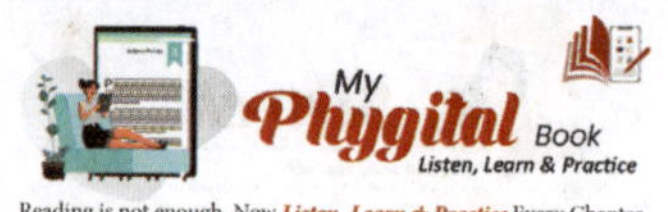

DETERMINATION OF RED BLOOD CELL INDICES

Principle: The values for RBC count. Hemoglobin content and packed cell volume (PCV Table 19.7) can be used to obtain certain EBC indices (also called Absolute Values of Blood index). These indices indicate the size and hemoglobin concentration within the RBC and thus help in diagnosing the type of anemia. The various blood indices are given as under.

Mean corpuscular Volume (MCV), i.e., volume of a single RBC in cubic microns (μm^3). It can be computed as:

$$MCV\ (\mu m^3) = \frac{\text{PVC per 100 mL blood}}{\text{RBC count in million/cumm}} \times 10$$

$$= 45/5 \times 10$$

$$= 90\ (\text{average})$$

Table 19.7: Dilutions of blood and citrate as anticoagulant for PCV test

Dilution for PCV Test	Citrate	Blood
60%	0.4 mL	4.6 mL
70%	0.3 mL	4.7 mL
80%	0.2 mL	4.8 mL

Normal range = 78 – 94 μm^3 (86 $\pm$ 8 μm^3)

- RBCs with normal MCV are called normocytes.
- RBCs whose MCV exceed normal range are macrocytes.
- RBCs with MCV below normal range microcytes.

Mean corpuscular hemoglobin (MCH), i.e., average amount of hemoglobin in a single RBC in pictogram (10^{-12} g) or micro-micro gram ($\mu\mu$gm-$\gamma\gamma$)

It can be computed as:

$$MCH\ (pg) = \frac{\text{Hemoglobin in gm\%}}{\text{RBC count in million/cumm}} \times 10$$

$$= 15/5 \times 10$$

$$= 30\ (\text{average})$$

Normal range = 28–32 pg (29.5 $\pm$ 2.5 pg)

Mean corpuscular hemoglobin concentration (MCHC), i.e., amount of hemoglobin expressed as percentage of the volume of a RBC or it is the hemoglobin concentration in a single RBC.

$$MCHC = \frac{\text{Hemoglobin in gm\%}}{\text{PCV per 100 mL blood}} \times 100$$

$$= 15/45 \times 100$$

$$= 33\ (\text{average})$$

Normal range = 32% – 38% (35 $\pm$ 3%)

- If the MCHC is within normal range, the RBC is normochromic.
- If the MCHC value is below normal range, the RBC is hypochromic. This usually indicates that an individual is suffering from iron deficiency.
- MCHC values never exceed 38% because RBCs cannot hold hemoglobin beyond its saturation point, i.e., metabolic limit of the cell hemoglobin forming mechanism, therefore, anemic can never be hyperchromic.

Clinical Significance

Based on the size and hemoglobin concentration within a RBC, an important morphological classification of anemias can be given in Table 19.8.

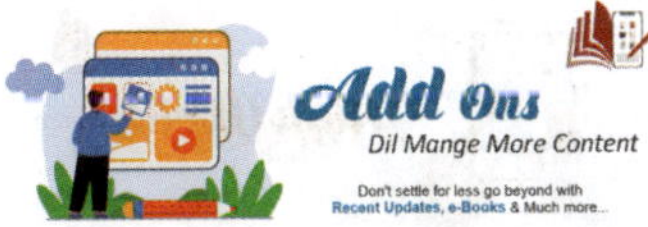

Table 19.8: Morphological classification of anemias

Types of anemia
• Normochromic, normocytic anemia (normal MCHC, normal MCV). These include: ▪ Anemias of chronic disease ▪ Hemolytic anemias (those characterized by accelerated destruction of RBC's) ▪ Anemia of acute hemorrhage ▪ Aplastic anemias (those characterized by disappearance of rbc precursors from the marrow) • Hypochromic, microcytic anemia (low MCHC, low MCV). These include: ▪ Iron deficiency anemia ▪ Thalassemias ▪ Anemia of chronic diseases • Normochromic, macrocytic anemia (normal MCHC, high MCV). These include: • Vitamin B_{12} deficiency • Folate deficiency

HEMOGLOBIN ESTIMATION

Hemoglobin (Hb) is the protein contained in red blood cells that is responsible for delivery of oxygen to the tissues. To ensure adequate tissue oxygenation, a sufficient hemoglobin level must be maintained. The amount of hemoglobin in whole blood is expressed in grams per deciliter (g/dL). The normal Hb level for males is 14–18 g/dL; that for females is 12–16 g/dL. When the hemoglobin level is low, the patient has *anemia*. When hemoglobin level is above normal. it is known as erythrocytosis (Table 19.9).

Structure of Hemoglobin

The hemoglobin molecule is a tetramer consisting of two pairs of globin chains, which are related polypeptide chains. Heme, a compound consisting of protoporphyrin and iron in ferrous form, is affixed to each of the four chains. Adults' primary (96%) form of hemoglobin is known as HbA, and it has two beta and two alpha globin chains ($\alpha_2\beta_2$).

In the early stages of embryonic and fetal development, various forms of hemoglobins predominate. Among them are Gower-1 (found in the early stages of embryonic life), Gower-2, and Hb Portland. Fetal hemoglobin ($\alpha_2\beta_2$) replaces embryonic hemoglobins after the eighth week of development. This makes up 50–90% of all hemoglobin, and is the major hemoglobin until after birth. Its concentration drops to less than 2% by the time the child is 30 weeks old. The predominant hemoglobin is thus HbA.

Table 19.9: Structure and time of occurence of various types of Hemoglobin

Name	Structure	Present in
Adult Hb (HbA)	$\alpha_2\beta_2$	Adults
Fetal Hb (HbF)	$\alpha_2\gamma_2$	Fetal life
Hb Portland	$\zeta_2\gamma_2$	Embryonic life
Gower-1	$\zeta_2\varepsilon_2$	Embryonic life
Gower-2	$\alpha_2\varepsilon_2$	Embryonic life

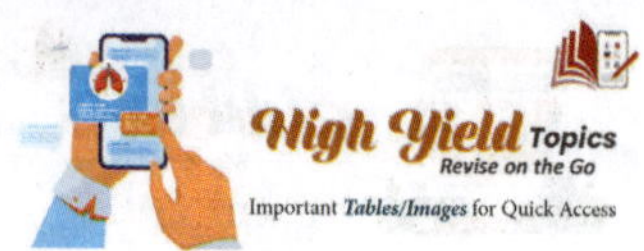

Methods of Hemoglobin Estimation

Colorimetric Methods

Sahli's Method (Fig. 19.11)

Apparatus: Sahli's hemoglobinometer, N/10 HCI, distilled water, pricking apparatus, stirrer, dropper.

Sahli's hemoglobinometer: It consists of:

- A single mark pipette (haemoglobinometer pipette) for measuring 20 cumm (0.02 mL) of blood.
- A round or square haemoglobinometer tube graduated in percentage (10–140) and gram per cent (2 to 22).
- A glass rod, used as a stirrer.
- A rectangular box, comparator fixed with 2 solid standard colored glass rods. The opaque white background provides the necessary contrast for easy comparison.

Principle: The amount of hemoglobin can be estimated by conversion of known volume of blood into acid-hematin by addition of dilute HCI and subsequent calorimetric comparison with a suitable standard.

Procedure:

1. With the help of a dropper, take N/10 HCI in. the graduated hemoglobinometer tube up to its lowest mark (usually 10% or 2 g%).
2. Prick the finger under aseptic precautions. When a drop of reasonable size has collected, hold the pipette horizontally, apply its tip to the drop "and draw exactly 20 cumm of blood into the pipette, taking care that there should be no air bubbles. Take the pipette away and wipe off any blood adhering to the tip.
3. Immediately transfer the blood from the pipette into the N/10 HCl in the graduated hemoglobinometer tube and rinse the pipette several times by drawing the N/10 HCl used for mixing the blood. Avoid foaming.
4. Mix the contents thoroughly and leave the solution to stand for about 10 minutes for maximum conversion of hemoglobin in blood to acid hematin (brown in color).
5. Dilute the acid hematin by adding distilled water in drops. Keep mixing it with the stirrer thoroughly.

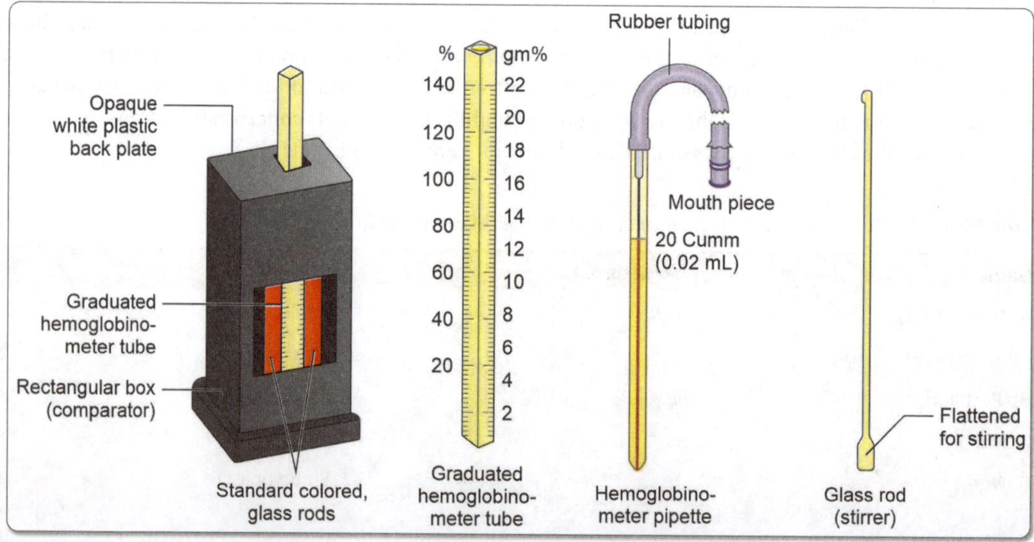

Figure 19.11: Estimation of hemoglobin (Sahli's method)

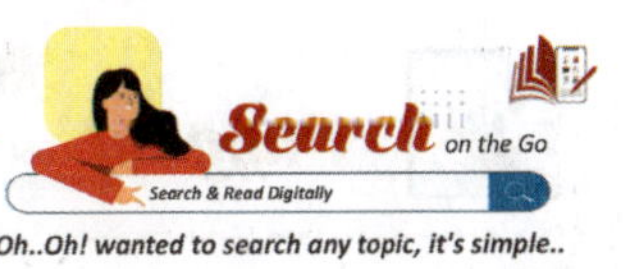

Important note: At no stage the stirrer should be completely taken out of the tube)

- Continue dilution till its color matches with that of the standard. Before comparing the color, the stirrer should be lifted above the solution only.
- Note the reading of the meniscus from the scale provided on the hemoglobinometer tube and express the hemoglobin content as g per 100 Ml of blood.

NOTE

- For colored transparent fluids, lower meniscus need to be read.
- Since the colors may seem to match over a wide range of dilutions, it is advisable to take the average of 2 readings during the course, of dilution; the first when it is just discernably darker and the second when it just gets a shade lighter than the standard.

Precautions:

- The finger should not be squeezed to take out the blood, otherwise tissue fluid might come out, thus giving lower estimation of hemoglobin.
- Blood from the pipette should be transferred quickly into the tube containing N/10 HCI to prevent clotting of blood in the pipette.
- Blood, idler mixing with N/10 HCI, should be left for at least 8–10 minutes for complete formation of acid hematin.
- Distilled water should be added drop by drop to dilute the acid hematin, otherwise over dilution will occur.
- The matching of colors should be done against natural source of light.

Cyanmethemoglobin (HiCN; or Hemiglobincyanide) Method

In this test the blood is diluted in a solution of potassium ferricyanide and potassium cyanide. Potassium ferricyanide oxidizes hemoglobin into methemoglobin (Hi). The cyanide ions (CN^-) of potassium cyanide converts methemoglobin to cyanmethemoglobin (HiCN). The color of this solution is compared against a standard HiCN solution of known Hb value in a spectrophotometer at 540 nm.

Automated Analyzer

Used to measure Hb, packed cell volume and absolute values like mean corpuscular volume (MCV), mean corpuscular hemoglobin (MCH), mean corpuscular hemoglobin concentration (MCHC). In this, RBCs are lysed with the lysate and color is matched against the inbuilt standard colors and Hb value is obtained.

Hemocue Blood Hemoglobin System

It is World Health Organization (WHO) approved test for hemoglobin estimation in blood donors. In this, the hemoglobin is converted into azide methemoglobin by the action of three reagents, i.e., (1) Sodium deoxycholate, (2) Sodium nitrate, (3) Sodium azide.

Haldane Method

In this test, red cells are lysed by adding carbon monoxide, which converts hemoglobin into carboxyhemoglobin and finally, color is compared with the given standard.

Other Methods

- **Copper sulfate specific gravity method:** This test is used to screen the cut-off value of hemoglobin in blood donation camps. In this test the copper sulfate solution with specific gravity of 1.055 for men

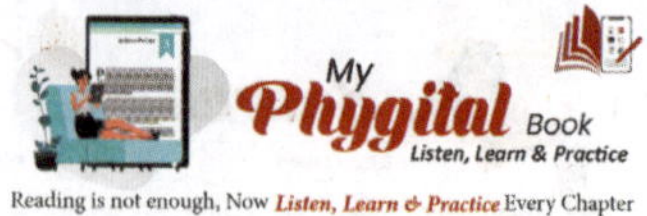

Table 19.10: Method of hemoglobin estimation

Method	Principle
• Colorimetric method: ▪ Visual colorimetric method: ◆ Sahli's method or acid hematin method ◆ Alkaline hematin method ▪ Photocolorimetric method: ◆ Cyanmethemoglobin (HiCN) method ◆ Automated analyzer ◆ Hemocue blood hemoglobin system ◆ Haldane method	These methods are based on measuring the color of hemoglobin or a hemoglobin derivative in the blood either visually or by photocolorimetry; the optical density of color solution is directly proportional to the concentration of the color material in the solution.
• Physical method	Specific gravity
• Chemical method	Iron content of hemoglobin
• Gasometric method	Oxygen-binding capacity

and 1.053 for women is used. A drop of blood is suspended in the solution, if the drop sinks to the bottom, then the hemoglobin value is normal and if the drop floats on the top, it indicates low hemoglobin levels.

- **Gasometric methods:** This test is based on the fact that one molecule of O_2 binds to each iron atom of hemoglobin, which indirectly measures the amount of Hb.

Methods of Hemoglobin estimation have been discussed in Table 19.10.

ERYTHROCYTE SEDIMENTATION RATE

If anticoagulant-added blood is allowed to stand in a tube, the cells settle down at the bottom, leaving clear plasma above. The rate of settling of cells is known as ESR. Changed ESR is a non-specific indicator of chronic diseases. This occurs due to changed levels of plasma proteins, such as fibrinogen and globulin:

Note: ESR is greater in women, increases during pregnancy and is less in infants.

- It is seldom used for diagnostic purpose, but is mainly used for prognosis and monitoring response to treatment. Two methods are commonly used for ESR determination, Westergren method (Figs 19.12A and B) and Wintrobe method.
- Normal values:
  - **Male:** 0–10 mm in 1st hour
  - **Female:** 0–20 mm in 1st hour

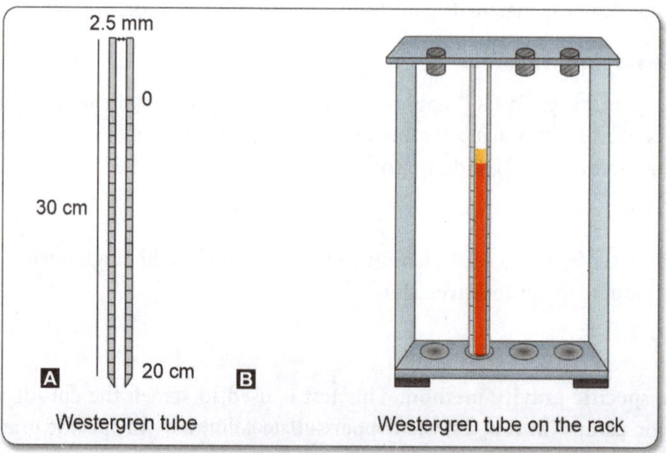

Figures 19.12A and B: **A.** Westergren tube; **B.** Westergren tube on the rack

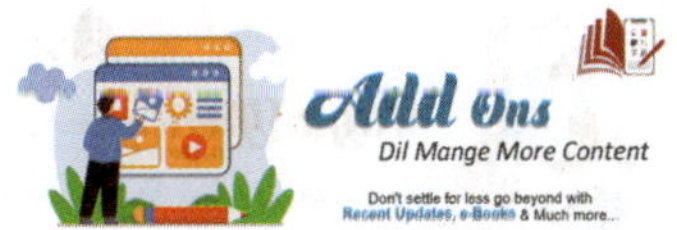

The causes of altered erythrocyte sedimentation rate count are presented in Table 19.11.

Table 19.11: Causes of altered erythrocyte sedimentation rate (ESR) count

Conditions causing increased ESR	Conditions causing decreased ESR
Tuberculosis	Polycythemia
SABE	Spherocytosis
Acute myocardial infarction	Sickle cell anemia
Rheumatoid arthritis	Congestive heart failure
Shock	Newborn infant
Anemia	Hypofibrinogenemia
Liver disease	
Multiple myeloma	
Pregnancy	
Ankylosing spondylitis	

COAGULATION TESTS

The sample collection tubes for coagulation tests are given in Table 19.12.

- **Bleeding time:** It is the time taken form the puncture of the blood vessel to the stoppage of bleeding.
- **Clotting time:** It is the time taken from the puncture of the blood vessel to the formation of a fibrin thread.

NOTE

Assessment of bleeding time is more important than the clotting time; the latter concerns the blood only, i.e. how firm the clot is formed and now no more used, whereas the bleeding time involves the interaction of blood with the injured tissues.

Instructions for sample collection and choice of anticoagulant for various tests

Though the volume of blood required may be less, the volume of blood drawn may be larger since the usual vacuum tubes have a fixed amount of liquid anticoagulant in them. Smaller volume plastic sample tubes can be generated in- house, if required for pediatric cases and other special samples.

Table 19.12: Sample collection tubes for coagulation test

Sl. no.	Tests	Samples	Vacuum tube cap color
1	Prothrombin time	2.7 mL in 0.3 mL citrate in a vacuum tube	Light blue
2.	APTT	2.7 mL in 0.3 mL citrate in a vacuum tube	light Blue

Determination of Bleeding Time (BT)

Apparatus: Pricking apparatus, filter paper, tubes capillary tubes, stop watch.

Procedure

The two methods commonly used for determining the BT are: Duke's method any Ivy's method.

Duke's Method

It is convenient and commonly used method in practice:

- Set the stop watch at 'zero'.
- Clean the tip of a finger thoroughly with spirit and allow it to dry. Make a puncture deep enough (about 3–4 mm) to ensure free flow of blood without squeezing.
- Immediately start the stop watch or note the time. The time of puncture of the finger is referred as "Zero Time".
- Thirty seconds later escaping blood is dried on the edge of a clean piece of filter paper.
- Repeat the procedure in every 30 seconds using a fresh area of the paper on each occasion until bleeding ceases and no further blood spot appears on the filter paper. Therefore, each blot of blood on the filter paper represents 30 seconds flow of blood.
- Count the total number of blood spots on the filter paper and multiply this by ½. This will give the BT in minutes.

Normal bleeding time by this method is 2–6 minutes

NOTE

- Usually, the blood flow is maximum between first 2–½ minutes after pricking; thereafter, the rate is abruptly slowed, but may not cease for a further 2 or 3 minutes
- Do not apply pressure or squeeze the finger at any stage to take out the blood

Ivy's Method

- Clean the anterior surface of the forearm with spirit.
- Apply pressure of 40 mm Hg to the upper arm with a sphygmomanometer and maintain this pressure till the end of the experiment.
- Sterilize the needle and make a puncture deep into the skin on the anterior surface of the forearm. Remove the drop of blood of filter paper as described above.

Normal bleeding time by this method is 3–6 minutes at 37°C

Observations and results

1. Bleeding time by Duke's method is ___________

Comments and discussion ____________________

Precautions

- Finger should be pricked by a single stabbing action to give free flowing blood. At no stage it should be squeezed to obtain the blood.
- Be alert and carefully note the 'zero time'.
- Strictly follow the procedure steps at preferably experiment should be carried out normal body temperature of 37°C.

CLINICAL CORRELATION

Bleeding time is prolonged in:

- Severe liver disease
- Leukemia
- Aplastic anemia
- Thrombocytopenia

Determination of Clotting Time

It is the time required for the formation of solid clot, when blood is removed from vascular system and exposed to a foreign surface.

Procedure (Capillary Method)

- Clean fingertip with alcohol swab and prick deeply so that blood flows freely. After discarding first two drops, fill a capillary tube with blood. Note the time when blood first enters capillary tube. Keep the tube horizontal.
- After 1 minute, break one end of capillary tube and repeat this every 15 seconds till you can see a thread of unbroken clot between two broken ends. Time difference between first and last reading is clotting time.

Normal value: 5–10 minutes at 37°C

Clotting time is increased in:

- Disseminated intravascular coagulation.
- Administration of anticoagulants such as heparin.
- Severe deficiency of coagulation factors.

Prothrombin Time (PT)

The PT test assesses the extrinsic coagulation pathway of coagulation, which consists of activated factor VII (factor VIIa) and the proteins of the common pathway (factors X, V, II, and fibrinogen).

This test also is used to monitor patients on oral anticoagulants. Its result reporting has been modified so that it can be interpreted universally. The internationalized normalized ratio (INR) was developed to standardize the reporting of PT for patients taking oral anticoagulants.

$$\text{INR} = \left\{ \frac{\text{Patients PT}}{\text{Log Mean Normal PT}} \right\} \text{ISI}$$

Where International Sensitivity Index (ISI) for a reagent is a measure of the responsiveness of a given thromboplastin to reduction of the vitamin K-dependent coagulation factors when compared with a reference thromboplastin.

Reagents

- Patient's platelet poor plasma (PPP)
- Control plasma
- Thromboplastin
- $CaCl_2$ solution 0.025 mol/L or (M/40)

Manual Method

- Add 0.1 mL patient plasma to a tube and place in water bath at 37°C.
- Add 0.1 mL thromboplastins to the tube.
- Incubate in the water bath at 37°C for 1–2 minutes.
- Add 0.1 mL of prewarmed $CaCl_2$.
- Start the stop watch.
- Keep mixing the contents.
- Look for the tiny wisps of clotting.
- Stop the stop watch.
- Carry out the test in duplicate.

Note: If thromboplastin contains $CaCl_2$, then take 0.2 mL of thromboplastin and start the stop watch.
Normal range: 12–14 seconds.

If using an automated system, it is necessary to follow the manufacturer's instructions regarding dissolution of lyophilized reagents and mixing times, before loading reagents on the analyzer.

Observations and Results

The common causes of prolonged PTs are as follows:

- Liver disease, particularly obstructive.
- Administration of oral anticoagulant drugs (vitamin K antagonists).
- Vitamin K deficiency.
- Disseminated intravascular coagulation (DIC).
- Rarely, a previously undiagnosed factor VII, X, V, or prothrombin deficiency or defect.

Note: With prothrombin, factor X, or factor V deficiency the APTT will also be prolonged.

Warning

The reliability of INR becomes less with increasing ISI of the thromboplastin as the therapeutic range for PT diminishes. It is provided by each manufacturer based on the degree of variation of the thromboplastin from the World Health Organization (WHO) reference thromboplastin that has an arbitrarily assigned value of 1.0. A common cause of incorrect results is the use of arithmetic mean for calculation of INR. The ISI has to be set for the instrument reagent combination for ideal results. Commercial INR calibrators may help in checking the accuracy of the results.

Activated Partial Thromboplastin Time (APTT)

(It comprises Partial Thromboplastin Time with Kaolin (PTTK) and the Kaolin Cephalin Clotting Time—KCCT) The APTT test measures all the proteins of the so-called intrinsic coagulation protein system (factor XII, prekallikrein, high-molecular-weight kininogen, factor XI, factor IX, and factor VIII) and the proteins of the so-called common pathway (factors X, V, II, and fibrinogen).

The *in vitro* event of factor XII autoactivation in the APTT assay initiates the sequence of reactions of the coagulation cascade.

Reagents

- Patient's platelet poor plasma (PPP).
- Control plasma.

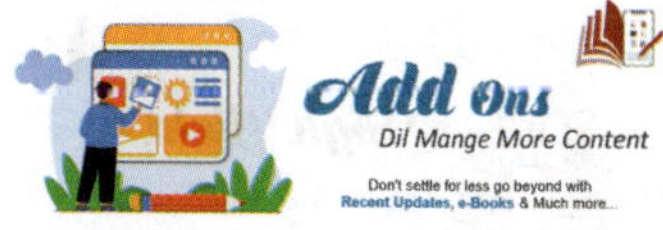

- Kaolin 5 g/L (laboratory grade), in barbitone buffered saline, pH 7.4.
- Phospholipid.
- $CaCl_2$ solution 0.025 mol/L or (M/40).

Manual Method

- Mix equal volumes of phospholipid reagent and kaolin suspension and leave in a glass tube in a water bath at 37°C.
- Add 0.1 mL patient plasma to a new tube and place in water bath.
- Add 0.2 mL kaolin-phospholipid solution or 0.1 mL commercially available APTT reagent.
- Mix contents, and start the stop watch.
- Incubate in the water bath at 37°C for 10mins, with occasional shaking.
- Add 0.1 mL of prewarmed $CaCl_2$. Start a second stop watch.
- Keep mixing the contents.
- Look for the tiny wisps of clotting.
- Stop the stop watch. Note the time.
- Carry out the test in duplicate.

Note: Incubation times on various automated systems are shorter (approx. 3 minutes)

Normal Range: 25–32 seconds.

The time may be longer or shorter or longer for different reagents based on the phospholipid content.

Common Causes of Prolonged APTT

- Disseminated intravascular coagulation.
- Liver disease.
- Massive transfusion with plasma-depleted red blood cells.
- Administration of or contamination with heparin or other anticoagulants.
- A circulating anticoagulant (inhibitor) like Lupus anticoagulant.
- Deficiency of a coagulation factor other than factor VII.

The APTT is also moderately prolonged in patients taking oral anticoagulant drugs and in the presence of vitamin K deficiency. If the patient's APTT is abnormally long, a mixing study is to be performed. To differentiate in deficiency or inhibitor, cases with a long APTT, a 50:50 mixture of normal and test plasma should be tested to distinguish between factor deficiency and the effect of an inhibitor.

NORMAL REFERENCE RANGES IN HEMATOLOGY AND INFERENCE OF DATA

The normal reference ranges (Table 19.13) are laboratory specific as the individual laboratories may use different hematology analyzers and may serve different geographical areas with prominent physiological variations. Hence, it is of importance to establish laboratory specific normal ranges with the analyzer used for patient samples.

A reference range can be established using a blood sample from a small population representative of a larger one called control samples. It is necessary to standardize the conditions in which the test is being performed. For example, if fasting samples are being collected, blood should be collected in the fasting status from all normal controls.

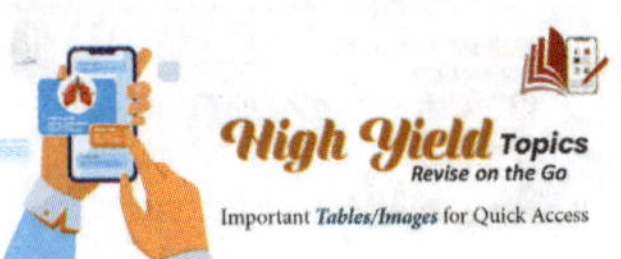

Table 19.13: Normal reference ranges in hematology

	Parameter	Range of reference	Unit
RBC count and indices	**Red blood cell count (RBC)**	Male: 4.52–5.90	x 10^6 per µL
		Female: 4.10–5.10	per µL
	Hemoglobin	Male: 14.0–17.5	g/dL
		Female: 12.3–15.3	g/dL
	Mean corpuscular volume (MCV)	80.0–96.1	fL
	Mean corpuscular hemoglobin (MCH)	27.5–33.2	pg
	Mean corpuscular hemoglobin concentration (MCHC)	33.4–35.5	g/dL
	Red cell distribution width (CV)	11.6–14.6	%
WBC count and differential	**White blood cell counts (WBC)**	4.4–11.3	x 10^3 per µL
	Neutrophils	1.5–8.5	x 10^3 per µL
	Lymphocytes	1.0–4.8	x 10^3 per µL
	Eosinophils	0–0.45	x 10^3 per µL
	Monocytes	0–0.8	x 10^3 per µL
	Basophils	0–0.2	x 10^3 per µL
Platelets	**Platelet count**	172–450	x 10^3 per µL
Coagulation parameters	**Bleeding time (BT)**	2–7 (Ivy method)	minutes
	Prothrombin time (PT)	11–16	seconds
	Activated partial thromboplastin time (APTT)	26–40	seconds
	Thrombin time (TT)	15–19	seconds
	Fibrinogen	180–360	mg/dL

BLOOD BIOCHEMISTRY

This discipline is associated with analysis of body fluids such as serum, plasma, urine cerebrospinal fluid (CSP), pleural fluid, etc. Serum is the most commonly used fluid for analyzing metabolites such as glucose, urea, creatinine, bilirubin, different enzymes, etc. for diagnosis and monitoring of diseases. Some tests are ordered as a panel, such as liver function tests (bilirubin, aspartate aminotransferase, alanine aminotransferase and alkaline phosphatase), which together help in establishing the derangement process and severity.

Sample collection and preparation:

- **Serum:** This is the yellowish fluid, obtained after blood is allowed to clot and centrifuged.
- **Plasma:** This is obtained by centrifuging blood after addition of anticoagulant.

Plasma Glucose Estimation

- Plasma glucose is a commonly ordered test (Table 19.14). The container should contain potassium oxalate, sodium fluoride mixture (3:1 ratio, add 3 mg/mL blood). Sodium fluoride inhibits glycolysis and samples without this preservative may show reduced values for glucose.

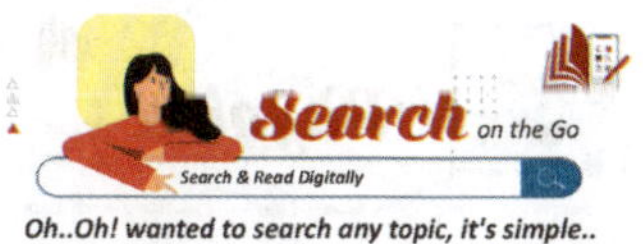

Sample for glucose test: Three types of plasma samples can be collected for glucose estimation:

1. **Fasting sample:** Patient is asked not to eat or drink anything after dinner, except plain water and sample is collected next morning.
2. **Postprandial sample:** After obtaining fasting sample, patient is given glucose orally (75 g commonly used) and blood sample is collected after 2 hours.
3. **Random sample:** Blood sample is collected any time without any relation to meals.

Table 19.14: Normal plasma glucose levels

Fasting	70–110 mg/dL
Postprandial	80–140 mg/dL
Random	<140 mg/dL

- **Using glucometer:** Glucose can also be measured as a bedside test in ward or clinic, by using glucometer. In this test, a drop of blood, usually obtained by finger prick, is placed on special strip impregnated with chemicals and results are read on an electronic device. This method provides immediate blood glucose values.
- **HbA1c:** HbA1c gives average blood glucose (sugar) levels for the last two to three months. The test measures the amount of blood sugar (glucose) attached to hemoglobin. Four basic types of methods are used most commonly to measure HbA1c: immunoassay, ion-exchange high-performance liquid chromatography (HPLC), boronate affinity HPLC, and enzymatic assays.

Serum Urea

- Urea is formed in liver from ammonia, which is a toxic byproduct of amino acid breakdown. Urea is water soluble and is excreted by kidneys in urine.
  The common causes of increased serum urea level is presented in Table 19.15.

Serum Creatinine

- Creatinine is a waste product of creatine, a muscle protein and is produced in constant amount daily. It is excreted in urine and its serum levels are used as an indicator of glomerular filtration. Serum creatinine can be increased in both renal and postrenal causes. Creatinine is considered a better indicator of renal function than urea because its levels are not affected by dietary protein intake.
- Normal values:
  - **Male:** 0.9–1.5 mg/dL
  - **Female:** 0.6–1.1 mg/dL

Table 19.15: Causes of increased serum urea levels

Prerenal causes (reduced blood supply to kidneys)	Dehydration, blood loss, reduced cardiac output
Renal causes	Acute glomerulonephritis, diabetic nephropathy, nephrotoxic drugs
Postrenal causes (obstruction to urine outflow)	Stones in ureter or bladder, tumors, prostate enlargement in males, urethral stricture

Blood Gas Analysis

The pH of blood is normally from 7.36 to 7.42. Patient's acid-base balance and blood gas levels are used for assessment in life-threatening situations. Various metabolic processes lead to production of acids, which are neutralized by buffers present in body, such as bicarbonate-carbonic acid system and hemoglobin. The component of blood gas analysis are given in Table 19.16.

Sample Collection

For blood gas analysis, arterial sample is used, which is usually collected in heparin syringe. Syringe can be heparinized by drawing up a small amount of liquid heparin squirting it out again to remove air bubbles. Most common site for sample collection is radial artery but femoral artery and other sites may also be used. Sample should be processed immediately and exposure to air should be avoided.

Table 19.16: Components of blood gas analysis

Parameter	Normal range
pH	7.36–7.42
PaO_2 (arterial partial pressure of oxygen)	75–100 mm Hg
$PaCO_2$ (arterial partial pressure of carbon dioxide)	35–45 mm Hg
HCO_3^- (Bicarbonate concentration)	22–26 mEq/L

Disturbances in Acid-Base Balance

- **Respiratory acidosis:** Accumulation of H_2CO_3 due to impaired respiration, such as pneumonia, emphysema.
- **Respiratory alkalosis:** Decrease in H_2CO_3 due to voluntary or involuntary hyperventilation.
- **Metabolic acidosis:** This occurs when either body is producing excess acid or kidneys are not removing adequate acid, e.g. lactic acidosis, diabetic ketoacidosis.
- **Metabolic alkalosis:** This is caused due to excessive loss of acids from body, e.g., vomiting.

  Blood gas analysis provides information about the following:
  - Adequacy of ventilation and oxygenation.
  - Assessment of acid-base status by measuring the respiratory and non-respiratory components.

Arterial blood gas monitoring is the standard for assessing a patient's oxygenation, ventilation, and acid-base status. Although ABG monitoring has been replaced mainly by non-invasive monitoring, it is still useful in confirming and calibrating non-invasive monitoring techniques.

MUST KNOW

Reasons for Using Arterial Blood Rather than Venous Blood to Measure Blood Gases

Venous blood in an extremity gives information mostly about that extremity. The metabolic in the extremity can differ from the metabolism in the body as a whole. The differences accentuated in shock when the extremity is cold or underperfused and with local exercise extremity such as opening and closing of the fist.

BLOOD CULTURE

Bacteremia is an important part of any systemic infection and hence, blood culture acquires special significance in specific treatment and may prove to be lifesaving. A diagnosis bacteremia can only be made by growing pathogenic agents on suitable culture media.

Sample Collection

As with other microbiological procedures, strict asepsis is required during sample collection and transportation. Patient's skin is cleaned with spirit alcohol and Betadine applied to the sampling site. Sterile gloves should be used to minimize contamination.

Procedure

A minimum of 10 mL of blood is taken through venipuncture and injected into two or more blood culture bottles (5 mL in each bottle) with specific media for aerobic and anaerobic organisms. It should be ensured that ratio of blood and media is maintained at 1:1. Care needs to be taken that the bottles are not contaminated with bacteria from staff members or other patients.

BONE MARROW EXAMINATION

Bone marrow is the soft, organic, sponge-like material present in the medullary cavities of long bones. It is composed of red and yellow marrow. The red marrow mainly produces erythrocytes, leukocytes and platelets. The yellow marrow is formed of connective tissue and fat cells, which are inactive.

Bone Marrow Aspiration

Bone marrow examination is used in the diagnosis of a number of conditions, including leukemia, multiple myeloma, lymphoma, anemia and pancytopenia.

Sites for taking bone marrow aspirant: Given in Table 19.17.

Table 19.17: Various sites for obtaining bone marrow aspirant

In adults	In children
Sternum	Tibia
Anterior iliac crest	Superior medial surface of the tibia
Vertebral spinous processes	Posterior iliac crest
Posterior superior iliac	Calcaneus

Procedure

After cleaning skin with alcohol and iodine, local anesthetic is injected to make the area numb.

- A needle (Salah and Klima or Jamshidi's marrow aspiration needle) is used to aspirate bone marrow.
- Not >0.2 mL of bone marrow should be taken out at one time.
- After the procedure is complete, the patient should be asked to lie flat for 5–10 minutes to provide pressure over the procedure site.
- Helps to distinguish primary and metastatic tumor.
- Assists in identification, classification and staging of neoplasia.
- Aids in evaluation of the progress and/or response to the treatment of neoplasia.

Contraindications

- Bleeding disorders.
- Infection at site of puncture.

SEROLOGICAL AND IMMUNOLOGICAL TESTS

Serology is the scientific study of blood serum. In practice, the term usually refers to the diagnostic identification of antibodies in the serum. Such antibodies are typically formed in response to an infection, against other foreign proteins or to one's own proteins (in instances of autoimmune disease).

Uses

Serological tests may be used for:

- Early diagnosis of infection such as viral hepatitis and typhoid.
- Detection of infections in which it is difficult to isolate organism, e.g., syphilis.
- In forensic medicine, generally to link a perpetrator to a piece of evidence (e.g., linking rapist to a semen sample).

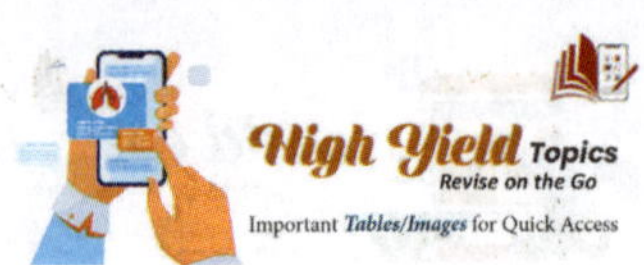

There are several serology techniques that can be used depending upon the antibodies being studied. These include agglutination, precipitation, enzyme-linked immunosorbent assay (ELISA), complement fixation test, immunofluorescence, immunoelectrophore, immunochromatography, etc.

Agglutination Tests

Agglutination is clumping together of cells having surface antigen with its specific antibody. Visible clumps thus formed are known as agglutinates as antigen-antibody complexes formation are insoluble. These are commonly used for detection of antibodies in serum such as widal test for typhoid. Agglutination is usually of two types:

1. Slide agglutination.
2. Tube agglutination.

Precipitation Tests

Antigen and antibody are in soluble form. They react to form insoluble visible precipitate. Weil-Felix test for rickettsial diseases is an example of precipitation test, venereal disease research laboratory (VDRL) test for syphilis is a flocculation test, a modified form of precipitation test.

ELISA Test

The enzyme-linked immunosorbent assay (ELISA) is a biochemical technique used to determine the presence of an antibody or an antigen in a sample. Performing an ELISA involves at least one antibody with specificity for a particular antigen. The antigen antibody complex, which is immobilized on solid support, is detected by detection antibody labeled with an enzyme. Addition of substrate leads to color development due to enzyme action.

Types of ELISA

- **Direct ELISA:** It is used for detection of antigen. The wells of microtiter plate are coated with antibody specific to antigen being tested, e.g., detection of hepatitis B surface antigen (Australia antigen).
- **Indirect ELISA:** It is used for detection of antibodies. Antigen is coated on support and antibodies present in sample bind to it, e.g., detection of anti-HIV antibodies.

Enzymes used in test enzymes commonly used for labeling are horseradish peroxidase (HRP) and alkaline phosphatase (ALP). The intensity of the color produced is proportional to the amount of attached enzyme, and therefore, to the amount of unknown antibody/antigen in the patient's serum.

Hepatitis B Surface Antigen (HBsAg, Australia Antigen)

The detection of HBsAg in serum is the most important diagnostic parameter for a viral hepatitis B. Hepatitis B virus is transmitted through infected body fluids. Acute infection causes hepatitis presenting with jaundice and vomiting, while chronic infection can lead to liver cirrhosis and hepatocellular carcinoma.

This antigen can be detected in the serum 2 or 3 weeks before onset of the disease features and attains a maximum titer on development of characteristic symptoms (icterus, elevated GOT).

The special significance of detection of HBsAg is in the screening of blood donors.

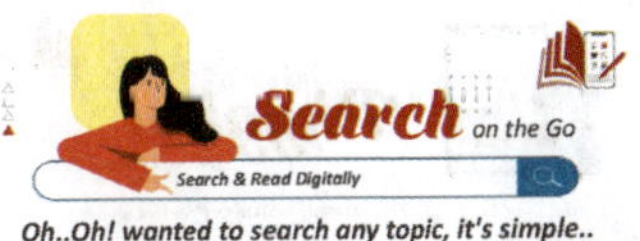

VDRL Test

Venereal Disease Research Laboratory (VDRL) is a blood test for syphilis and is named after Venereal Disease Research Laboratory where it was developed.

Principle:

A phospholipid (cardiolipin), derived from beef heart muscle together with cholesterol and lecithin, is used as an antigen. Antibodies produced by a patient with syphilis react with this antigen, leading to foaming of test tube fluid, known as 'flocculation'. These floccules can be observed with naked eye, hand lens or under a low power objective of a microscope when the reaction is weak.

Widal Test

The Widal test is a serological test for typhoid fever. This test demonstrates the presence of somatic (O) and flagellar (H) agglutinins to *Salmonella typhi* in the patient's serum the recommended method of performing the Widal test is by the tube agglutination technique, but is can be performed by slide method also.

Tuberculin Skin Test

Tuberculin skin test is a screening tool for tuberculosis (TB). Mantoux test, also known as purified protein derivative (PPD) test is the most common form of this test performed.

Procedure

- About 0.2 mL PPD is injected intradermally and read 48–72 hours later. A person who has been exposed to the bacteria is expected to mount an immune response in the skin containing the bacterial proteins.
- The reaction is read by measuring the diameter of induration (palpable raised, hardened area) across the forearm in millimeters. Erythema (redness) should not be measured.
- The induration of more than 10 mm indicates positive tuberculin test and <10 mm, but >5 mm is considered doubtful and test must be repeated. However, in HIV/AIDS or in immunocompromised patients even induration of >5 mm is considered positive test.

  A tuberculin skin test is done in:
  - People who have been in close contact with someone known to have TB
  - Healthcare workers who are likely to be exposed to TB
  - People with TB symptoms, such as an ongoing cough, night sweats and weight loss for no other reasons.
  - People who have had an abnormal chest X-ray.

  A tuberculin skin test should not be done for people who have:
  - Known TB infection
  - Positive tuberculin skin test in the past; a second test may cause a more severe reaction.
  - Skin rash that would make it hard to read the skin test.

BLOOD BANK

BLOOD GROUPING AND CROSSMATCHING

Blood transfusion is a common procedure in hospitals for management of patients with excessive blood/fluid loss. But transfusion is associated with several risks and precautions are necessary to avoid life-threatening complications.

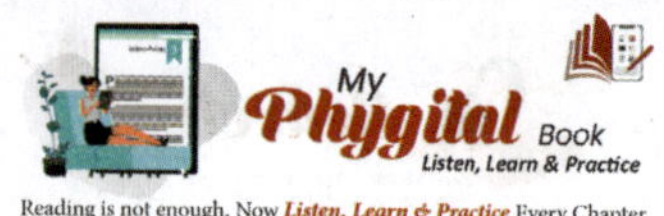

Blood Grouping

Blood group is a classification of blood based on the presence or absence of inherited antigenic substances on the surface of red blood cells. The presence of these antigens is decided by genes from both parents. A total of 29 human blood group systems are now recognized by the International Society of Blood Transfusions:

- The ABO system is the most important blood group system in human blood transfusion. There are three allelic genes A, B and O, which can produce four blood groups A, B, AB and OA, and B genes control the synthesis of enzymes, which modify the red cell membrane glycolipid. These antigens react with their respective antibodies.
- Rhesus blood group system is the second most significant blood group system in human blood transfusion. It is based on presence of another antigen, D and RBCs, which express this D antigen are termed Rh positive. About 85% of population is Rh positive, while 15% is Rh negative.

Determination of Blood Groups (A, B and O System)

The ABO blood group system was first discovered by Landsteiner in 1990. It is based on the presence or absence of blood group specific substances A, B and O in the RBCs. Accordingly, human beings can be divided into 4 main groups viz., A, B, AB and O blood groups.

Apparatus: Antiserum-A, antiserum B, isotonic saline (0.9% NaCl), glass slides, applicator sticks, compound microscope, glass marking pencil and capillary dropper.

Principle: The procedure is based on the principle of agglutination i.e., clumping of RBCs. The phenomenon of agglutination is due to the interaction between the factors—agglutinogen (antigen) present on the RBCs membrane and agglutinin (antibody) present in the plasma. Normal human RBCs possessing a particular antigen will show agglutination in the presence of the corresponding antibody. This may occur quite soon but may not develop for several minutes, if the agglutinin titre of the serum is low.

Procedure:

Preparation of red blood cell suspension

Take 3 mL of isotonic saline (0.9% NaCl) in a clean test tube. Finger is pricked under aseptic precautions so as to assure free flow of blood, the first drop of blood is wiped away with a clean piece of cloth and a drop of blood is added to the test tube. Alternately, red cell suspension may be prepared simply by inverting the test tube over the finger pricked.

Determination of blood groups

- Take and ordinary grease free, clean glass slide and one drop each of antiserum-A (i.e., serum containing α-antibodies) and anti-serum –B (i.e., serum containing β-antibodies) is placed thereon with the help of a dropper. In addition, one drop of isotonic saline (used as control) is also placed on the slide. The slide is accordingly labelled as anti-A, anti-B and control.
- The red cell suspension is drawn from the bottom of the test tube into capillary dropper and a drop of it is added to each of the drops on the slide. (Take utmost care that the nozzle of dropper should not touch any of the drop.) the two are mixed with the help of separate application sticks.
- Wait for 10 minutes, the slide is then gently rocked back and forth and examined for the presence of agglutination (clumping of RBCs). Confirm the findings (Figs 19.13A and B) under the low power of the microscope:

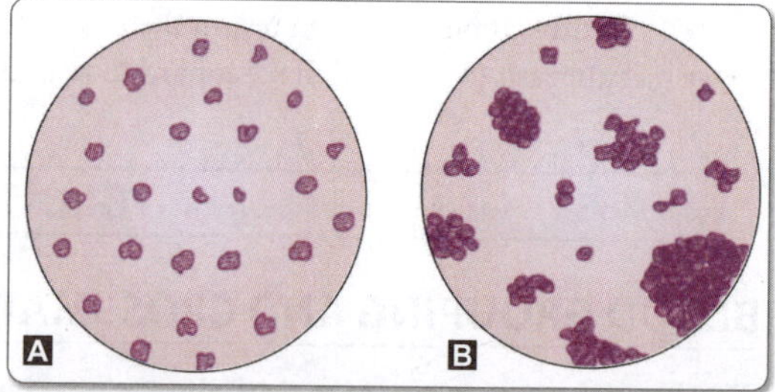

Figures 19.13A and B: RBCs **A.** No agglutination; **B.** Agglutination in incompatible plasma

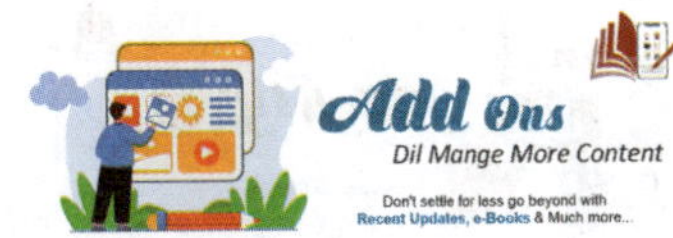

- If there is no agglutination, the RBCs remain separated and evenly distributed
- If agglutination occurs, the RBCs are massed together in clumps and lose their outline

The blood group is determined as indicated in the Table 19.18.

Precautions:

- The slides should be thoroughly cleaned with soap and water.
- The slide should be labelled beforehand after placing the antisera, A and B, and isotonic saline
- There should not be any intermixing of the three drops placed on the slide
- The slide should be examined for agglutination before the solution dries up. Confirm the findings under the low power of the microscope
- Undiluted blood should never be mixed with the antisera directly, otherwise false positive reactions may develop

Table 19.18: Determination of blood group

Group	Reaction		
	Antiserum A	Antiserum B	Antiserum D
AB	+	+	
A	+	–	
B	–	+	
O	–	–	
Rh positive			+
Rh negative			–

Note: '+' : Agglutination i.e. RBCs are clumped together and they have lost their outline; '–' No agglutination, i.e., RBCs remain separate and evenly distributed

Important Note:

- False positive reaction can occur due to use of antisera contaminated with bacterial growth; and
- False negative reaction occurs due to loss of potency of the antisera because of improper storage

Observations:

Reaction of the subject's cells

Antiserum-A	Antiserum-B	Blood Group

'+' : Agglutination present
'–' : Agglutination absent
Results and observations (if any)

Crossmatching

This is a direct test to check compatibility of donor cells and recipient serum. Even if the blood groups have been checked, it is mandatory to do crossmatching before all transfusions. This test is performed in two parts:

- Major crossmatch: Donor's cells are mixed with patient's serum.
- Minor crossmatch: Patients's cells are mixed with donor's serum.

In addition to grouping and crossmatching, blood donors are also screened for various infections, so as to prevent transmission of these infections to person receiving blood transfusion:

- Malarial parasite
- Hepatitis B and C
- Human immunodeficiency virus (HIV)
- Syphilis

Uses of Blood Grouping and Complications of Blood Transfusion

The important uses of blood grouping and complications of blood transfusion is presented in Table 19.19.

Table 19.19: Uses of blood grouping and complications of blood transfusion

Important uses of blood grouping	• Blood transfusion • Organ transplantation • Hemolytic disorder in newborn • Medico-legal cases
Complications of blood transfusion	Early complications: • Hemolytic reactions • Allergic reactions • Circulatory overload • Air embolism • Hyperkalemia Late complications: • Transfusion transmitted infections: Hepatitis B and C, syphilis, malaria, HIV • Transfusion iron overload

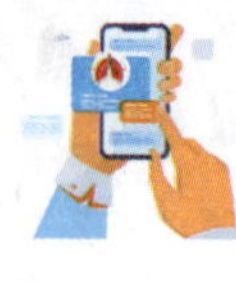
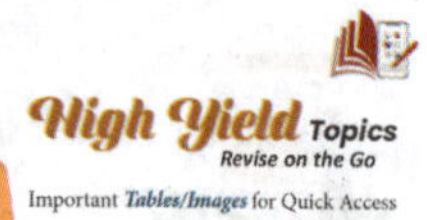

BLOOD PRODUCTS

The use of whole blood for transfusion is taking a back seat now. Specific blood components, like RBCs, fresh frozen plasma, platelets, etc., and plasma derivatives such as albumin, coagulation factors and immunoglobulins are mostly used in clinical practice nowadays. Few commonly used blood components are described here briefly:

Packed Red Blood Cells (PRBC)

Packed red blood cells are made by centrifugation of whole blood. These are used in various conditions, like anemia, acute blood loss, etc. It is better to use PRBC than whole blood to avoid volume overload-related side effects (Fig. 19.14).

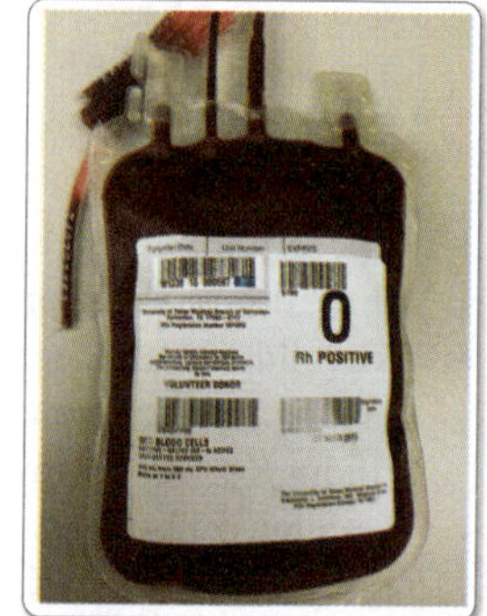

Figure 19.14: Packed red blood cells

Red Cells in Additive Solution

In PRBC preparation, the majority of plasma is removed and replaced by 100 mL saline, adenine, glucose and mannitol additive solution (SAG-M). It reduces the viscosity of PRBCs as well as increases its viability and half-life.

Irradiated Red Cells

Irradiated red cells are indicated for patients at risk of transfusion-associated graft-versus host disease (like post-transplant patients, or aplastic anemia patients who has been treated with ATG, etc.). The component must be irradiated by gamma or X-rays within 14 days of collection and it has a shelf life of 14 days from irradiation.

Washed Red Cells

Indicated for patients with recurrent or severe allergic or febrile reactions to red cells, and severely IgA-deficient patients with anti-IgA antibodies for whom red cells from an IgA deficient donor are not available.

Platelets

Platelet transfusion is indicated for treatment or prevention of bleeding in thrombocytopenia or platelet function disorders. There are two types of platelets, which are transfused: Random donor platelets (RDP) and single donor platelets (SDP).

The ABO antigens are found on the surface of platelets, which may result in decreased survival of transfused platelets if given to an ABO incompatible recipient, however most of the time it is not clinically significant. Anti-A or anti-B antibodies in residual plasma can sporadically lead to hemolysis in infants and young children. So, preferably blood group-matched platelets are better to transfuse (Fig. 19.15).

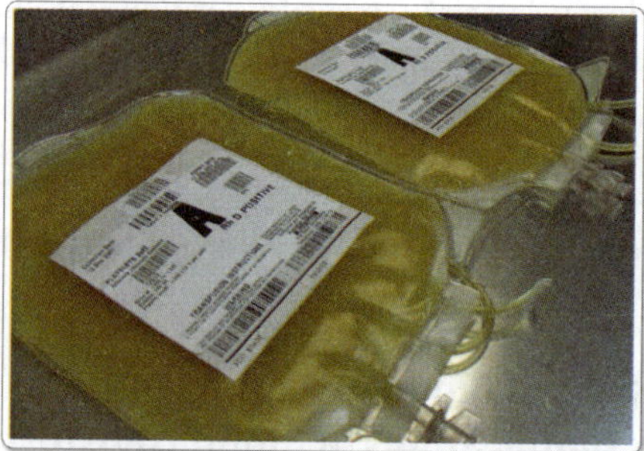

Figure 19.15: Platelets concentrates

Random donor platelets (RDP): Donated whole blood units are centrifuged and the buffy coats from four donations are separated and platelets are made by recentrifugation.

Single donor platelets (SDP): Pooled in the platelets from one single donor (preferably male) by apheresis technique. It reduces the risk of transfusion-related acute lung injury (TRALI) as WBCs are very less in SDPs. The continual agitation and temperature-controlled incubators (20°–24°C) are used to preserve platelets. Platelets should never be kept in freezer.

Fresh Frozen Plasma (FFP)

Most commonly given in cases of coagulation disorder, factor deficiency, acute bleeding, etc. Plasma is frozen soon after collection to maintain the activity of blood-clotting factors. It can be stored for up to 36 months at –25°C or below. Thawed units of FFP can be stored for up to 24 hours at 4°C before transfusion (Fig. 19.16). The recommended dose is 12–15 mL/kg (minimum of four units in a 70 kg adult).

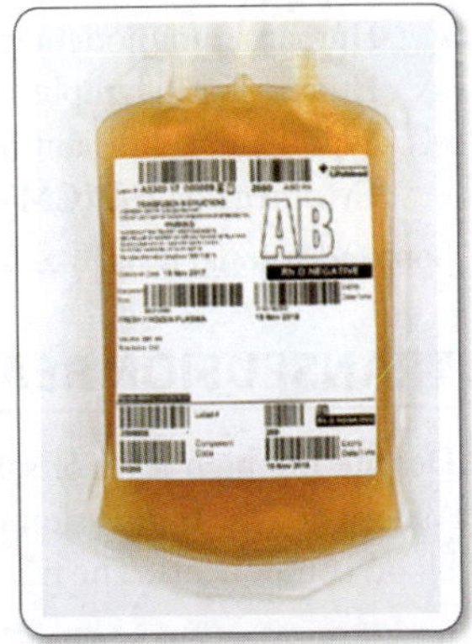

Figure 19.16: Fresh Frozen plasma bag

Plasmapheresis: Plasmapheresis is a therapeutic intervention that involves extracorporeal removal, return, or exchange of blood plasma or components. The underlying mechanism of this procedure is accomplished by either centrifugation or filtration using semipermeable membranes.

Indications

- To treat various autoimmune diseases such as myasthenia gravis, Gullian-Barré syndrome, demyelinating polyneuropathy.
- To treat certain complications of sickle cell disease.
- To treat critically ill with infections and problems such as Wilson's disease and thrombotic thrombocytopenic purpura.
- In patients who received an organ transplant to counter rejection process.

PRETRANSFUSION COMPATIBILITY TESTING

Blood Grouping and Screening

It is of utmost importance to determine the ABO and Rh blood group of recipients before blood transfusion. The plasma is to be screened for antibodies, known as "reverse grouping". Antibody screening is performed using a panel of red cells that contains commonly encountered blood group antigens. ABO and Rh group matched and free from any alloantibodies blood units are selected from the blood bank for transfusion. Grouping can be done in both manual and automated modes. Automated methods are much safer and quicker than manual techniques.

Compatibility Testing

After grouping, serological cross matching is the final step to be done before transfusion as part of blood compatibility testing. Recipient's blood plasma is added to red blood cells of selected blood unit and is looked for any agglutination. This is performed by the indirect antiglobulin test method at 37°C.

Tests on Blood Units

Screening for Infectious Agents

For each donated units infectious screening is mandatory. The following tests are done for each unit:
- Hepatitis B—HBsAg
- Hepatitis C—anti-HCV and HCV NAT
- Human immunodeficiency virus—anti-HIV 1 and 2 and HIV NAT (nucleic acid testing)
- Human T-cell lymphotropic virus—anti-HTLV I and II
- Syphilis—syphilis antibodies.
- Cytomegalovirus (CMV) antibodies

Some additional tests, like malaria, trypanosoma, etc. are also done in special circumstances.

TRANSFUSION REACTIONS

Despite the high level of safety of modern blood transfusions, fatalities and severe morbidity still happen. Majority of the transfusion reactions occur due to identification of patients, blood samples and mismatched blood components. The transfusion reactions can be acute or delayed.

Acute Transfusion Reactions

Acute transfusion reactions (ATRs) can range in severity from mild febrile or allergic reactions to life-threatening events and appear within 24 hours of the transfusion. These include:
- Febrile non-hemolytic transfusion reactions.
- Allergic transfusion reactions—urticaria, angioedema, anaphylaxis, etc.
- Acute hemolytic transfusion reactions—e.g., ABO incompatibility.
- Bacterial contamination of blood unit—fever, chills, septic shock, etc.
- Transfusion-related acute lung injury (TRALI).
- Transfusion-associated circulatory overload (TACO).
- Hypotensive reactions.
- Delayed Hemolytic Transfusion Reactions (DHTRs).
- Transfusion-associated Graft-versus-host Disease (TA-GvHD).

Febrile Nonhemolytic Transfusion Reactions (FNHTRs)

Febrile nonhemolytic transfusion reactions (FNHTRs) is the most common acute adverse reaction of blood transfusion. They can occur up to 2 hours after completion of the transfusion. It commonly presents with fever, chills and rigor, muscle pain, nausea, etc. It occurs mostly due to pyrexic and inflammatory cytokines released from leukocytes in stored blood components. So, transfusion of leucodepleted blood products has lesser chance of developing FNTHRs. The management is mostly symptomatic and conservative.
- Temporarily stopping the transfusion or slowing down the transfusion rate is most of the time enough to control Mild FNHTRs (pyrexia >38°C, but <2°C rise from baseline).
- Anti-pyretic, like paracetamol can also be given, if needed. Keep the blood units outside freeze and wait till its temperature reaches the room temperature before starting the transfusion.
- Moderate FNHTRs (pyrexia >2°C above baseline or >39°C or rigors and/or myalgia) are also managed symptomatically. Stopping the transfusion is mandatory in them.

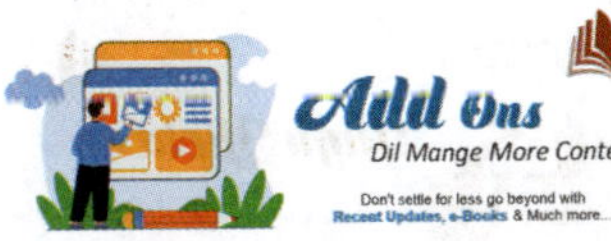

- Close follow up of the patients for any aggravation of symptoms is mandatory not to miss the signs of severe transfusion reactions or any hemolytic reactions.
- Check the blood products for any bacterial growth or discoloration. Send the blood unit to blood bank for further analysis.

Hemolytic Reaction

Acute Hemolytic Transfusion

The ABO-incompatible red cell transfusion is often fatal and its prevention is the most important step in clinical transfusion practice. Anti-A and/or anti-B in the recipient's plasma binds to the transfused RBCs and activates the complement pathway, leading to intravascular hemolysis and the release of inflammatory cytokines that can cause shock, renal failure and disseminated intravascular coagulation (DIC).

Transfusion of ABO-incompatible plasma containing anti-A or anti-B, usually from a group O donor, can cause hemolysis of the recipient's red cells, especially in neonates and small infants with a lesser blood volume. Red cells stored in SAG-M additive solution contain very less residual plasma, so the risk of hemolytic reactions due to SAG-M is very low. Group O red cell components for intrauterine transfusion, neonatal exchange transfusion or large-volume transfusion of infants are screened to exclude those with high-titre anti-A or anti-B. Group O plasma-rich blood components such as fresh frozen plasma (FFP) or platelet concentrates should not be given to patients of group A, B or AB if ABO-compatible components are readily available.

Transfusion-Related Acute Lung Injury (TRALI)

Classical TRALI is caused by antibodies in the donor blood reacting with the patient's neutrophils, monocytes or pulmonary endothelium. Inflammatory cells are sequestered in the lung and get trapped. Plasma leaks into the alveolar gaps and causes non-cardiogenic pulmonary edema. Symptoms are predominantly cough, pink frothy sputum, breathlessness, fever and often hypotension.

Most cases present within 2 hours of transfusion and maximum within 6 hours. TRALI is often confused with acute heart failure due to circulatory overload. Supportive care is provided, along with high-concentration oxygen and ventilatory assistance as needed.

Transfusion-associated Circulatory Overload (TACO)

Transfusion-associated circulatory overload (TACO) is defined as acute or worsening pulmonary edema within 6 hours of transfusion. It frequently presents with acute respiratory distress, tachycardia, and hypertension. TACO causes significant morbidity and mortality. Patients with extremes of age, like neonates, elderly, etc., have higher risks of developing TACO.

Few comorbid conditions which predispose in developing TACO are heart failure, renal impairment, hypoalbuminemia, etc. Inadequate pre-transfusion clinical evaluation and insufficient surveillance during transfusion are frequent characteristics of reported cases. So, a proper medical history is to be taken before transfusion.

If TACO is suspected, transfusion should be stopped immediately, followed by oxygen support and diuretics. Close monitoring and if necessary, assistance for critical care should be taken.

Allergic or Transfusion Reactions

Allergic reaction or shock symptoms may vary from severe hypotension, wheeze, stridor, swelling of face, angiedema to skin changes, like flushing, urticaria, rash, etc. It is an acute, life-threatening emergency.

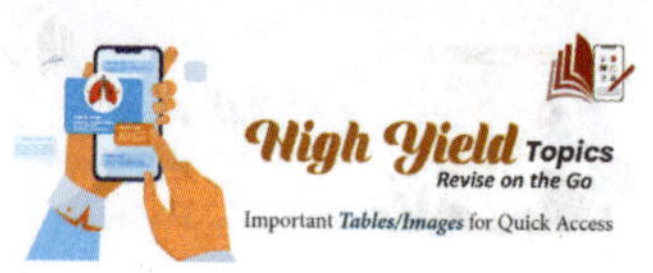

The recipients should be monitored closely during blood transfusion and if any of these symptoms arise, transfusion should be stopped immediately. Anti-allergic drugs like injection Avil can be given.

Intravenous access should be kept patent for further intervention, if needed. All blood components can cause severe allergic and anaphylactic responses; however, they are more frequently recorded with plasma-rich components, like platelets or FFP.

Hypotensive Reactions

An isolated drop in systolic blood pressure of 30 mm Hg or more (to <80 mm Hg) during or within an hour of transfusion without any additional allergic response or hemorrhage is a sign of hypotensive reactions. While they frequently escalate to shock and organ malfunction, the majority are transient. Although, they may be more frequent in people using ACE inhibitors, the majority of these events have an unclear etiology. So, taking a drug history before transfusion and close monitoring for any signs or symptoms of hypotension is of utmost importance. Patient should be kept in "recovery position" (lying flat with leg elevated) and the transfusion to be stopped immediately.

Early recognition of ATRs by careful monitoring of vital signs during transfusion is important. Patients should be asked to report symptoms that arise during the transfusion and for at least the next 24 hours. Few things to note for prevention of ATR:

- Transfusion should be given in clinical set up areas only so that patients can be kept under vigilance of trained staffs and some emergency measurement can be taken when acute reactions like anaphylaxis occur.
- Training of clinical and laboratory staff about the precautions and history to be taken for comorbid conditions and treatment history pre-transfusion and about the presenting symptoms and signs of adverse effect during transfusion, like fever, chills, itching, redness, etc.
- If any symptoms develop, the staff should check vital signs immediately and start appropriate resuscitation.
- Stop the transfusion, and venous access with normal saline should be maintained.
- Patient identification, transfused blood unit's group and details should be checked immediately for any mismatch.
- If the wrong blood has been transfused inform the transfusion laboratory urgently.
- The transfusion pack and IV-set to be sent to transfusion laboratory for investigation.
- Look for any abnormal clumps or discoloration of the transfused product.
- When a patient is getting transfused for acute blood loss and develops hypotension in-between, it may be due to continuation of blood loss. So, careful assessment of these patients is necessary and continuation of blood transfusion in these situations may be proven beneficial rather than stopping the transfusion.
- Inform the critical care and hematology teams urgently. Admission to an intensive care unit may also be necessary.

Delayed Hemolytic Transfusion Reactions (DHTRs)

In a patient who has previously been "alloimmunized" to a red cell antigen via blood transfusion or pregnancy, hemolytic transfusion reaction may occur in them 24 hours after transfusion. The antibody sometimes falls to an undetectable level by pre-transfusion antibody screen.

These patients get re-exposed to red cells of the immunizing group accidentally. Antibodies to the Kidd (JK), Rh antigens are most common offending agents in DHTRs. Treatment is usually supportive and conservative. The offending antibodies must be recorded on the transfusion laboratory and medical records and patients.

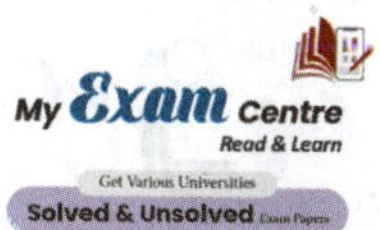

Transfusion-associated Graft-versus-host Disease (TA-GvHD)

When viable lymphocytes from a donor are engrafted in the patient, they launch an immunological attack against the recipient's cells with a different HLA type, it can lead to transfusion-associated graft-versus-host disease. This complication is uncommon and severe and may lead to deadly consequence. Typically, at-risk individuals are mostly having impaired cell-mediated immunity, like, fetuses receiving intrauterine transfusion, patients having an allogenic bone marrow transplant or chemotherapy, like purine analogues, patients with inherited immunodeficiency disorders (most commonly T-cell deficiency, etc.). Patients usually present with fever, skin rash, diarrhea, deranged liver function, etc, classically within 7–14 days post-transfusion. It may also present till day 30 post-transfusion.

SUMMARY

- Bleeding time is the time taken from the puncture of the blood vessel to the stoppage of bleeding.
- Clotting time is the time taken from the puncture of the blood vessel to the formation of a fibrin thread.
- Sample must be collected within 1 min. of application of tourniquet to avoid venous stasis.
- The sample must be processed within four hours during which it must be kept at 2°–8°C.
- The PT test assesses the extrinsic coagulation pathway of coagulation, which consists of activated factor VII (factor VIIa) and the proteins of the common pathway (factors X, V, II, and fibrinogen).
- The APTT test measures all the proteins of the so-called intrinsic coagulation protein system.
- The APTT is also moderately prolonged in patients taking oral anticoagulant drugs and in the presence of vitamin K deficiency.
- Packed red cells are made by centrifugation of whole blood.
- In PRBC preparation, the majority of plasma is removed and replaced by 100 mL saline, adenine, glucose and mannitol additive solution (SAG-M).
- Platelet transfusion is indicated for treatment or prevention of bleeding in thrombocytopenia or platelet function disorders.
- Thawed units of FFP can be stored for up to 24 hours at 4°C before transfusion.
- Plasmapheresis is a therapeutic intervention that involves extracorporeal removal, return, or exchange of blood plasma or components.
- Majority of the transfusion reactions occur due to identification of patients, blood samples and mismatched blood components.
- Acute transfusion reactions (ATRs) can range in severity from mild febrile or allergic reactions to life-threatening events and appear within 24 hours of the transfusion.

ASSESS YOURSELF

Long Answer Questions

1. Explain coagulation tests and method of estimation of bleeding time.
2. Describe various laboratory methods for estimation of hemoglobin.

Short Answer Questions

1. Define blood products.
2. What are transfusion reactions?

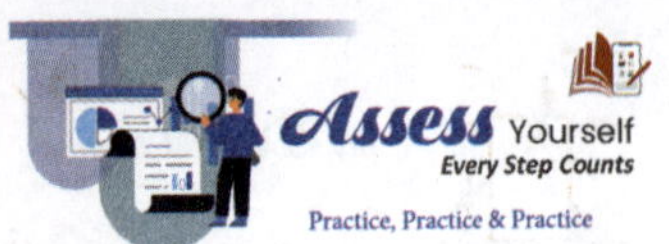

3. Write short notes on:
   i. Blood glucose estimation
   ii. Plasmapheresis

Multiple Choice Questions

1. **Which of the following is the most common complication of transfusion?**
   a. Acute hemolysis
   b. Acute lung injury
   c. Circulatory overload
   d. Fever
2. **All blood components are made from donated whole blood; except:**
   a. Platelets
   b. Plasma
   c. Human insulin
   d. PRBC
3. **What is the maximum time that blood (red cells) can be out of and then returned to temperature controlled storage?**
   a. 15 minutes
   b. 30 minutes
   c. 45 minutes
   d. 1 hour
4. **........ are involved in the formation of antibodies?**
   a. WBCs
   b. RBCs
   c. Platelets
   d. None of these

Answer Key

1. d **2.** c **3.** b **4.** a

Chapter 20

Examination of Body Cavity Fluids

LEARNING OBJECTIVES

After the completion of the chapter, the readers will be able to:

- Explain examination of cerebrospinal fluid.
- Enlist Indications for CSF testing.
- Describe sputum examination.
- Demonstrate collection of sputum.
- Elaborate appearance, microbiological and cytological examination of sputum.
- Explain wound discharge analysis.
- Demonstrate collection of wound sample.
- Explain peritoneal and pleural fluid analysis.

CHAPTER OUTLINE

- Introduction
- Cerebrospinal Fluid Analysis
- Sputum Examination
- Routine Gastric Juice Examination
- Wound Discharge Analysis
- Peritoneal Fluid Analysis
- Pleural Fluid Analysis

KEY TERMS

Cerebrospinal fluid: Cerebrospinal fluid (CSF) is an ultrafiltrate of plasma contained within the ventricles of the brain and the subarachnoid spaces of the cranium and spine.

Exudate: "Exudate" is fluid buildup caused by tissue leakage due to inflammation or local cellular damage.

Gastric juice: A digestive fluid produced by the stomach lining is known as gastric acid, gastric juice, or stomach acid. Gastric acid, which has a pH between 1 and 3, is essential for the digestion of proteins.

Lumbar puncture: Lumbar puncture (LP), also referred to as "spinal tap", is a commonly performed procedure that involves obtaining and sampling cerebrospinal fluid from the spinal cord.

Pleural effusion: It is a collection of fluid in a pleural space.

Sputum: The mixture of saliva and mucus that is coughed up from the respiratory system, usually as a result of an infection or irritation of the mucosa, is "sputum".

Transudate: "Transudate" is fluid buildup caused by systemic conditions that alter the pressure in blood vessels, causing fluid to leave the vascular system.

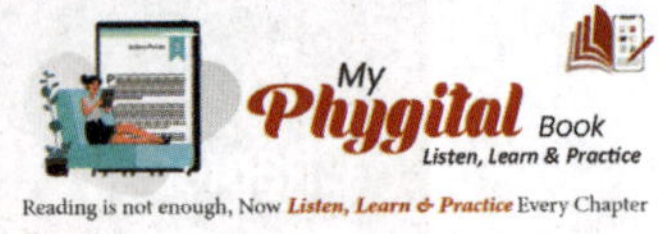

INTRODUCTION

Any kind of fluid that the human body secretes or excretes is referred to as body fluid. The human body is made up of different types of fluids. Each of these fluids plays a crucial role in keeping the body functioning. Examples of bodily fluids include:

- Blood plasma (carries blood cells, nutrients, hormones and others).
- Urine (waste product secreted by the kidney).
- Interstitial fluid (fluid that are located in-between cells).
- Cerebrospinal fluid (fluid surrounding the brain and spinal cord).
- Saliva and intestinal fluid (help in the process of digestion).

CEREBROSPINAL FLUID ANALYSIS

Methods of Collection and Examination of CSF

- CSF is produced in the ventricles of the brain by the choroid plexus—however, the ependymal cells, which line the ventricles, produce a smaller portion. The choroid plexus arises from the walls of the lateral ventricles and the roofs of the third and fourth ventricles. CSF is produced at a rate of around 500 mL/day; there are estimates that there is approximately 125–150 mL of CSF in the body at any given time.
- After production, CSF circulates through the ventricles, subarachnoid space, and parenchyma and is then ultimately reabsorbed into the venous circulation. It is reabsorbed into the blood through structures in the arachnoid mater called arachnoid villi (arachnoid granulations). Importantly, this fluid can be examined clinically through a lumbar puncture. With a lumbar puncture, physicians can look for abnormalities in the CSF, which can help create a differential diagnosis.

Composition

The composition of CSF is clear and colorless, with a density of 1.003–1.008 g/cm.

On average, around 140 mL of CSF is divided between the ventricular system (approx. 35 mL), the spinal canal (~30–70 mL), and the subarachnoid spaces.

Indications for CSF Testing

- CNS infections.
- Autoimmune CNS diseases, like Guillain Barrié syndrome.
- CNS vasculitis.
- CT negative subarachnoid hemorrhage.
- Malignant cells in metastasis.
- For injection of dye, like fluorescein to identify site of CSF leaks.

Therapeutic

- Benign intracranial hypertension.
- Acute communicating hydrocephalus.
- Cryptococcal meningitis in HIV infections.
- For CSF leaks.

Delivery of Intrathecal Drugs

- Delivery of antibiotics.
- Delivery of antineoplastic drugs.

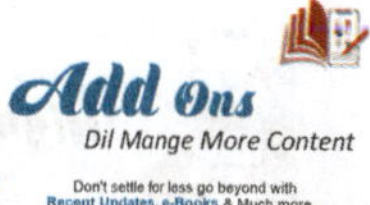

Lumbar Puncture

- An important clinical test that clinicians use to monitor CSF is the lumbar puncture (spinal tap).
- Usually under sterile precautions, 22–24 G spinal needle is inserted after identifying the lumbar L2–3 or L3–4 space and local infiltration.
- Once the spinal subarachnoid space is identified using loss of resistance, controlled removal of stylet is done to prevent excessive drainage of CSF.
- A manometer can be connected if CSF opening pressure measurement is planned. Color of CSF is noted and if blood stained due to traumatic puncture, it may be needed to wait for the blood to be cleared before samples are collected.
- Samples are usually collected in three to four test tubes each of 3-5 mL CSF for analysis. Samples are transported to lab in biohazard bag without refrigeration.

Contraindications for Lumbar Puncture

Relative Contraindications

- Platelet count of <20,000–40,000/cumm.
- Thienopyridines therapy.

Absolute Contraindications

- Noncommunicating obstructive hydrocephalus.
- Uncorrected bleeding diathesis.
- Anticoagulant therapy (timing of LP depends on the stopping of anticoagulant drug).
- Platelet count <20,000/cumm.
- Spinal canal stenosis or spinal cord compression above level of puncture.
- Local skin infections.

Gross Examination

Color

Normally CSF is clear and colorless. The color of CSF is examined by holding the CSF tube against a clean white paper.

The following alternation in CSF color may be observed due to the following conditions:

- A cloudy appearance can suggest an infectious cause.
  Red or xanthochromic color:
  - Following subarachnoid hemorrhage
  - Systemic hyperbilirubinemia (serum bilirubin >10–15 mg/dL)
  - Protein ≥150 mg/dL

Pressure

The first thing to note when doing a lumbar puncture is the opening CSF pressure. A high opening pressure can suggest various conditions, including hydrocephalus, intracranial mass, and intracranial hypertension. When there is an elevated CSF pressure, there is a risk of damage to the brain by reducing the pressure too quickly. For this reason, care is necessary to rule out intracranial space-occupying lesions and significantly associated mass-effect prior to performing this procedure. Intracranial space-occupying masses can be excluded on computed tomography (CT) imaging of the head or magnetic resonance imaging (MRI) of the brain.

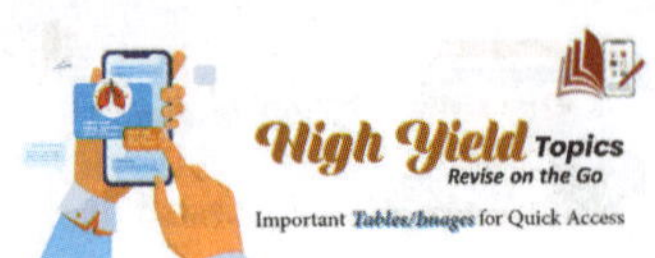

A low CSF pressure can also be clinically significant. This situation can occur in conditions that allow for CSF to leak into surrounding tissues. CSF can leak due to physical trauma, previous lumbar punctures, or without an obvious physical cause (spontaneous cerebrospinal fluid leak).

Microbial Examination

Normal CSF composition is shown in Table 20.1.

Table 20.1: Normal composition of CSF

Features	Normal range
Color	Clear
Specific gravity/pH	1.006–1.007/7.4
Opening pressure	50–200 mm H_2O
RBCs count	Nil
WBC count	0–5 (up to 30 in neonates)
WBC types	Lymphocytes
CSF Proteins	15–40 mg/dL
CSF lactate	1–3 mmol/L
CSF glucose	50–80 mg/dL (Two-thirds of blood glucose
Microbial examination	No microorganism

- Altered CSF findings can be seen in meningitis, findings are documented in Table 20.2.

Table 20.2: Cerebrospinal fluid analysis in various types of meningitis

CSF analysis	Bacterial	Tuberculosis	Viral	Fungal	Aseptic
Pressure	Increased	Increased	Normal to elevated	Normal to mild increase	Increased
Color	Turbid	Turbid	Clear	Clear	Clear to turbid
Glucose	<40 mg%	Low	Normal to mild less	Low to normal	Low
Proteins	Elevated	Greatly elevated	Normal to mild elevation	Normal to mild increase	Elevated
Lactate	Elevated (>6 mmol/L)	Elevated	0-6 mmol/L	Normal	Normal
RBCs	Elevated	Elevated	Normal	Normal	Elevated
WBCS	10–2,000/cumm	Elevated, but <500	>100/cumm	10–50/cumm	Mildly elevated
WBC types	Neutrophils	Lymphocytes	Lymphocytes	Lymphocytes	Neutrophils
Gram stain	Positive	Acid fast bacilli	Negative	Negative India ink for spores/ fungi	Negative
Microbial	Positive	Positive (yield is high in	Negative	Positive	Negative

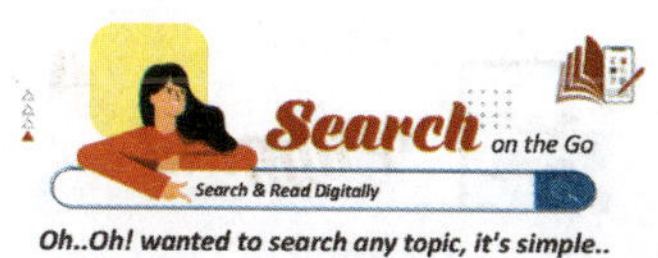

- CSF analysis is a very useful investigations in patients presenting with acute neurological conditions. While it is mandatory for acute meningitis to identify the microbial organisms, it will help as a supporting investigation to establish diagnosis, prognosticate and to assess the effect of various therapies to treat the patient conditions.

SPUTUM EXAMINATION

Matter expectorated from the respiratory system, particularly the lungs, is called sputum. It is mostly made up of mucus, although in certain disease conditions it can also include blood, pus, fibrin, or microorganisms (like bacteria). Precisely defined as the combination of saliva and mucus that is coughed up from the respiratory system, usually as a result of an infection or irritation of the mucosa, is "sputum".

Types of Sputum

1. **Expectorated sputum:** Generated from a deep productive cough.
2. **Induced sputum:** Produced with hypertonic saline if patient is unable to produce sputum on his own.

Indications for Sputum Collection

- To identify the causative agent or organism associated with a particular suspected infection of the lower respiratory tract, e.g., suspected tuberculosis.
- To establish an initial diagnosis of TB.
- To monitor the degree of infection of the patient.
- To determine the effectiveness of treatment.
  - Pneumonia, especially if severe or in an immunocompromised host.
  - Pneumocystic carinii pneumonia in HIV-positive patients.
  - Suspected fungal infection.
  - Infective exacerbation of a chronic disease, like bronchiectasis.
- **Cytological examination** for the investigation of viral infections (viral inclusions in *cytomegalovirus* and *herpes simplex* infections), fungal infection, asbestosis and malignant cells.

Collection of Sputum

- As secretions build up overnight, it is best to collect a sputum sample as soon as possible in the morning, before taking any food or mouthwash.
- A sterile, clean, dry, wide-mouthed plastic container with a screw cover that fits snugly is used to collect sputum samples. To prevent desiccation and aerosol production, the container should be made of unbreakable or break-resistant plastic, be leak-proof, and hold approximately 30 mL.
- It is recommended that the patient inhales deeply two or three times, fills his/her lungs, coughs deeply, and spits into the plastic container. Sputum samples should be ideally between 2 and 5 mL in volume. For laboratory studies, a sample that is only made up of saliva (which has a watery, transparent, and frothy look) is not suitable; instead, another sample needs to be taken. The sputum sample jar is safely sealed and appropriately labeled.

NURSING CONSIDERATIONS

- Receive patient and laboratory form. Make sure the form is complete.
- Specimen collection is an aerosol generating procedure, anyone in the room during specimen collection must wear a particulate respirator type N-95 and be part of the respirator protection plan.
- All mycobacteria specimens are collected into a sealed leak proof container.
- If the patient has come to the TB health facility for the first time, the sputum is examined for diagnosis.
- In this case, 3 sputum samples are examined (SPOT—MORNING—SPOT).
- After a patient is diagnosed as a case of tuberculosis, treatment is started. For follow-up examinations, two samples are obtained (MORNING— SPOT).

Demonstration of Sputum Collection

- Patient should preferably rinse his mouth as food particles may give false positive results.
- The patient is instructed to inhale deeply (2–3 times), which will initiate the cough reflex in most patients.
- The sputum is retained in the mouth and spit into the pre-labelled container without spilling.
- Some patients may not be able to expectorate with deep breathing. In this condition, expectoration should be demonstrated to them how they should place their palms on the waist, squat or sit and continue deep breathing again (Fig. 20.1).
- Tapping or thumping of the back may encourage expectoration. (Sitting and placing hands on the waist fixes the shoulder and pelvic muscles and brings the intercostal muscles of ribcage and diaphragm into action).

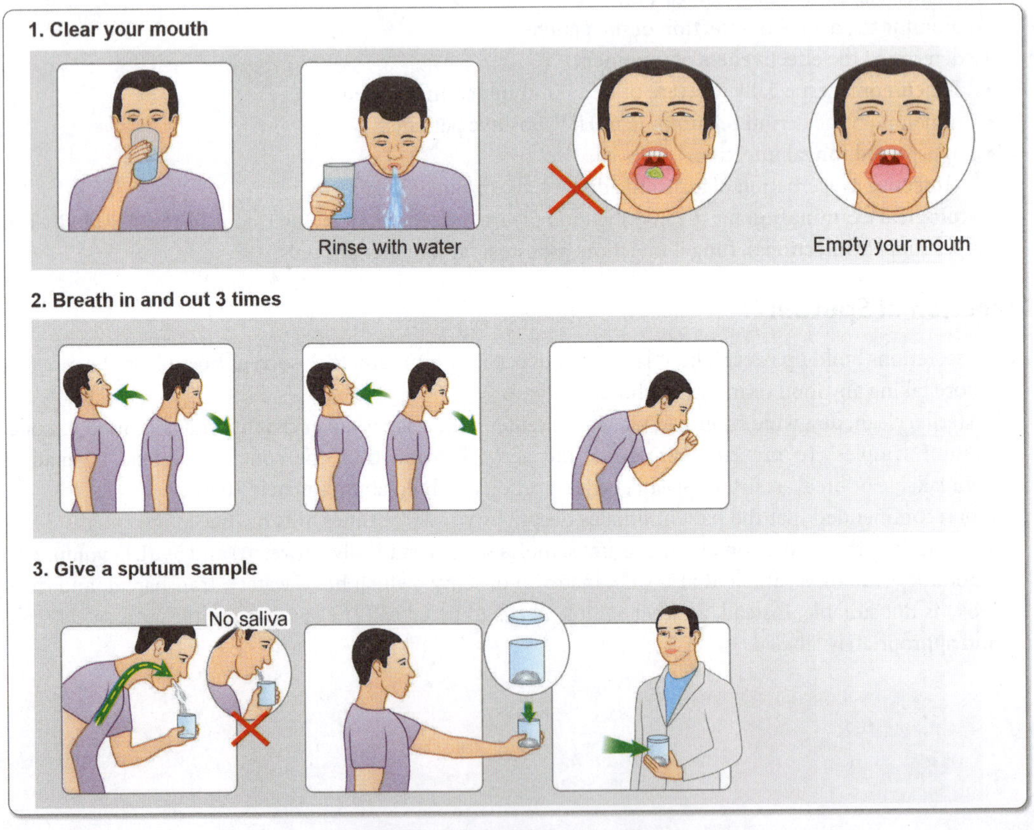

Figure 20.1: Steps of sputum collection

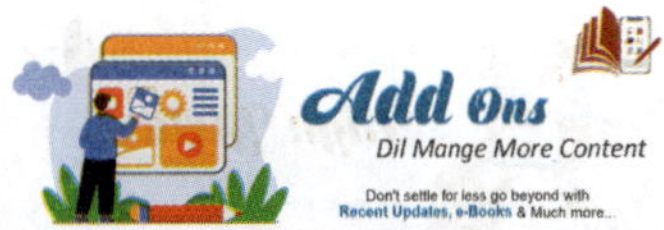

Sputum Quality

Specimens (Fig. 20.2) are thick and contain mucoid or mucopurulent material.

- Ideally, 3–5 mL in volume, although smaller quantities are acceptable if the quality is satisfactory.
- Poor quality specimens are thin and watery. Saliva and nasal secretions are unacceptable.

A good sputum sample is:	A poor quality sputum sample is:
• Thick (semisolid), coughed out deeply from the lungs. • Purulent (yellowish mucus) • Sufficient in amount.	• Contains only saliva (watery) or nasal mucus. • Small in quantity (<2 mL).

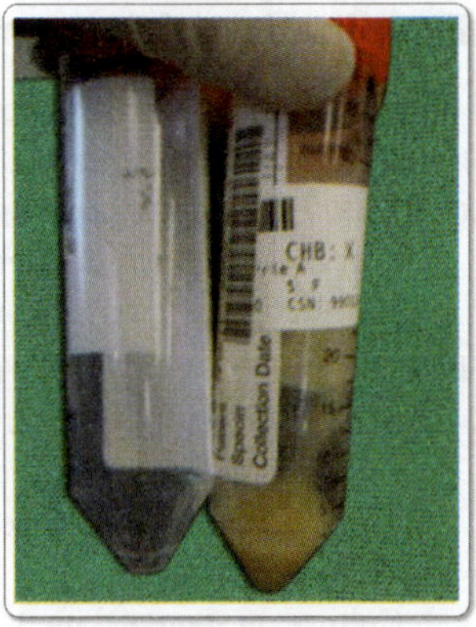

Figure 20.2: Sputum sample

Appearance of Sputum

Physical appearance of sputum is often indicative and symptomatic of the underlying pathologic process as follows:

- **Bloody:** Hemoptysis (pulmonary tuberculosis, bronchogenic carcinoma, bronchiectasis, lung abscess, pulmonary infarction, mitral stenosis).
- **Bloody and gelatinous (red currant jelly):** *Klebsiella* pneumonia.
- **Rusty:** Pneumococcal lobar pneumonia.
- **Purulent and separating into 3 layers on standing:** Lung abscess, bronchiectasis.
- **Copious amounts of purulent sputum:** Bronchopleural fistula, lung abscess, bronchiectasis.
- **Green:** *Pseudomonas* infection.
- **Pink, frothy (air bubbles):** Pulmonary edema.

Microbiological Examination of Sputum

Sputum sample is usually adulterated and contaminated with normal flora of the pharynx and oral cavity.

Pathogenic organisms found in sputum include:

- **Gram-positive:** *Staphylococcus aureus, Streptococcus pyogenes, Streptococcus pneumoniae.*
- **Gram-negative:** *Klebsiella pneumoniae, Moraxella catarrhalis, Haemophilus influenzae, Yersinia pestis, Pseudomonas aeruginosa.*

Sputum samples for bacterial analysis should be processed in the lab one hour after collection. Sputum is thinned down and placed on a sterile petridish, where its physical characteristics are recorded. Using a clean stick, make a thin smear from the purulent component of the sputum on the grease-free sterile glass slide. After fixing, air-drying, and applying Gram's stain, the slide is stained. Samples that are completely watery, mucoid, white, or frothy frequently exhibit squamous epithelial cells coated in bacterial clusters; this characteristic suggests that the sample is primarily made up of secretions from the mouth and throat. These samples are unacceptable for analysis by microbiologists.

Culture

Sputum sample is considered unsuitable for the bacterial culture if it contains >25 squamous epithelial cells/low power field.

An ideal sputum sample for bacterial culture contains bronchial epithelial cells, numerous neutrophils (>5/high power field), alveolar macrophages, and few squamous epithelial cells (<10/high power field).

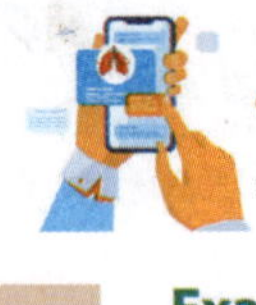
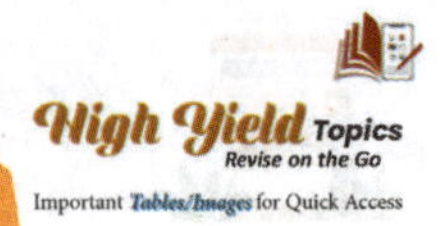

Examination of Sputum for Mycobacterium Tuberculosis

Tuberculosis is a crucial public health problem in developing countries. Early diagnosis of pulmonary tuberculosis will lead to early induction of treatment facilitating cure, and also inhibiting the spread of disease to others. There are two main approaches for the identification tuberculosis.

1. **Direct test:** It includes detection of *M. tuberculosis* or its components.
2. **Indirect test:** It consists of detection of cellular or humoral immune response to tuberculosis infection.

Direct tests for the detection of tuberculosis on sputum sample are as follows:

- Examination of sputum smear.
  - Ziehl-Neelsen technique.
  - Fluorescence microscopy.
- Molecular method.
- Culture on standard media.
- Commercial automated culture system.

Prepare the Slide for Examination of TB Bacilli

- The next step regarding preparing, staining, examining and reporting a sputum smear are summarized here.
- Label the slide with the laboratory serial number.

Explanation of step in the preparation and staining of slides have been depicted in Table 20.3.

Table 20.3: Explanation of step in the preparation and staining of slides

Illustration	Steps of the staining procedure	Reasons for/comments on each step
	• Spread sputum on the slide using a broomstick. • Smear preparation should be done near a flame. This is required as approximately 6 inches around the flame is considered a sterile zone which coagulates the aerosols raised during smear preparation.	• If sample are spread too thickly or too thinly, staining and microscope examination will not be accurate. • A different broomstick is used for each smear so that one patient's sputum is not mixed with another patient's sputum mixed with another patient's sputum.
3 2 4	Allow the slide to air dry for 15–30 minutes.	Heating the slide while it is wet could result in bubbling of TB bacilli into the air.
	Fix the slide by passing it over a flame 3–5 times for 3–4 seconds each time.	• Fixation makes the sputum stick to glass slides. • Fixation preserves the shape of the bacilli. • Heating for too long a period could change the shape of bacilli and also cause the slide to break. • Heating for too short a period can result in a false-negative outcome because the TB bacilli will not be well preserved on the slide.
	Pour filtered carbol fuchsin to cover the entire slide.	• Carbol fuchsin stains the TB bacilli red. • The carbol fuchsin solution must be filtered before use. If it is not filtered before use. If it is not filtered, small particles (sediments) get poured onto the slide and can appear red like the TB bacilli under the microscope.

Contd...

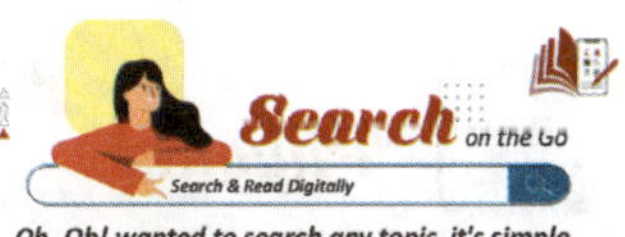

Illustration	Steps of the staining procedure	Reasons for/comments on each step
	Gently heat the slide with carbol fuchsin on it until vapor rises. DO NOT BOIL.	• Carbol fuchsin solution must not be allowed to boil or to dry on the slide, otherwise it will form small particles resulting in a false-positive reading. These particles may look like TB bacilli. • When the slide is heated to 80°–90°C, the carbol fuchsin on the slide penetrates the wall of the TB bacilli to stain the bacilli red. • Allowing the carbol fuchsin to boil, will change the shape of the TB bacilli and may result in a false-negative reading.
	Leave carbol fuchsin on the slide for 5 minutes.	The wall of the TB bacillus is thick and waxy. It is essential to give the carbol fuchsin sufficient time to penetrate the wall so that it can stain the bacilli.
	Rinse GENTLY with tap water until all free carbol fuchsin stain is washed away.	If water is poured too vigorously, the smear itself will be washed off the slide.
	Tilt the slide to drain off excess water.	If water is not drained off, it will dilute the next stain/ reagent that is poured, reducing the effectiveness of the next step.
	Pour 25% sulphuric acid onto the slide.	Sulphuric acid removes the carbol fuchsin stain from all of the contents of the sputum expect the TB bacilli. For this reason, TB bacilli are known as AFB, or Acid-Fast Bacilli, because the red color of the AFB from the carbol fuchsin remains after they are decolorized with sulphuric acid.
	Let the slide stand for 2–4 minutes.	• Allowing the slide to stand gives sulphuric acid time to wash out the stain from everything except the TB bacilli. • If insufficient time is given, bacteria and sputum contents other than TB bacilli may retain their stain, giving a false-positive result.
	Rinse GENTLY with tap water.	• Rinsing too strongly can wash the smear itself off the slide. • Sulphuric acid burns the skin. Do not let it splash. • If the slide is still stained red, you may apply sulphuric acid for a second time, letting the slide stand for 1-3 minutes this time. • It is helpful to use sulphuric acid to clean the bottom of the slide, on the opposite side of the smear. This makes it easier to examine the slide under the microscope.

Contd...

Illustration	Steps of the staining procedure	Reasons for/comments on each step
	Pour 0.1% methylene blue onto the slide.	• Methylene blue is the counterstain. It colors everything on the smear blue except the AFB. • The contrast between the AFB which are stained red by the carbol fuchsin and the rest of the smear stained blue by the methylene blue, makes it easier to view the TB bacilli.
	Leave methylene blue on the slide for 30 second.	It takes about 30 seconds for methylene blue to stain the material on the slide.
	Rinse GENTLY with tap water.	Always rinse gently so that the smear is not washed off the slide.
	Allow the slide to dry and then examine it under the microscope.	• Examining a slide when it is still wet may damage the microscope. • Examining a wet slide will also make it difficult to focus the microscope and read the slide correctly. • Do not dry the slides by blotting.

- If the sputum contains 5,000–10,000 tubercle bacilli/mL, the Ziehl-Neelsen stained sputum smear is considered positive. It is reported that the procedure has a sensitivity of 60–80%.
- Using a bleach concentration technique or examining multiple sputum samples increases the likelihood of finding tubercle bacilli.
- The sputum sample is mixed with a concentrated sodium hypochlorite (NaOCl) solution in the bleach concentration procedure, which liquefies the mucus and kills mycobacteria.
- The sample is kept for overnight sedimentation (or centrifugation), from the sediment of sputum a thin smear is prepared, stained and examined.
- Against a green or blue background, mycobacteria stained with Ziehl-Neelsen stain appear as bright red, straight or slightly curved rods (0.2–0.5 μ in width and 2–4 μ in length). Acid-fast bacilli (AFB) are mycobacteria that are both acid- and alcohol-fast.
- A minimum of 100 fields are examined before the smear being reported as negative. The number of acid-fast bacilli should be reported if they are observed.
- A negative sputum smear does not always mean that tuberculosis cannot be diagnosed because the sample may not have been taken correctly, the smear may be of low quality, or the organisms may be few in number.

Examination of Sputum for Organisms Other Than Tubercle Bacilli

- **Paragonimus:** Saline wet mount of sputum for eggs.
- **Histoplasmosis:** Giemsa smear.
- **Pneumocystis carinii:** Bronchoalveolar lavage fluid stained with Giemsa stain and silver stain.
- **Yersinia pestis (pneumonic plague):** Giemsa smear.
- **Aspergillus:** Potassium hydroxide wet mount of sputum.
- **Yeast-like organisms on Gram's smear:** Sabouraud dextrose agar.

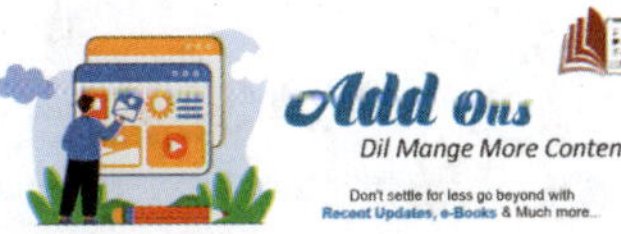

Cytological Examination of Sputum

- Early morning sputum collection is preferred for cytological examination. To increase the likelihood of detecting malignant cells in lung cancer samples, it is recommended to collect sputum samples every day for the first five successive days.
- The sputum sample should be sent to the laboratory immediately following collection without the addition of any fixative. If the sample is to be transported to a remote laboratory, pre-fixation of sputum with Saccomano's fixative is advised. This entails collecting sputum in a mixture of 2% carbowax and 50% ethyl alcohol.

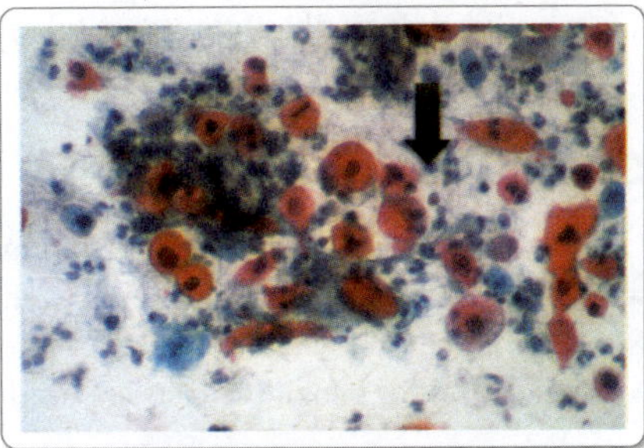

Figure 20.3: Image shows malignant squamous cells in sputum

When it comes to sputum examination, the average sensitivity for finding malignant cells is roughly 65%. Under the following circumstances, sensitivity increases:

- Size of tumor is large.
- The lesion lies in the center of the lung as opposed to the outer regions.
- Unlike adenocarcinoma or small cell carcinoma, the histologic form of carcinoma is squamous (Fig. 20.3).

ROUTINE GASTRIC JUICE EXAMINATION

Gross Examination

- **Amount:** Normal fasting amount is 50–100 mL.
- **Color:**
  - **Normally:** Pale gray.
  - **Abnormal hues:**
    - **Yellow green:** Indicates presence of bile.
    - **Brown and granular:** Flecks/streaks of blood, seen in minor trauma during intubation, characterized by coffee ground appearance.
  - **Odor:** Odorless or faintly pungent or slightly sour.
    - **Foul:** Infection or necrotic lesion.
    - **Fecal:** Intestinal obstruction.
  - **Absence of food particles:** Normally food particles are absent in gastric fluid. Presence of food particles suggests delayed gastric emptying and pyloric obstruction.
  - **Character:** It is translucent and slightly viscous.
  - **Reaction:** Normally, acidic.

Microscopic Examination

- Normal components in stomach:
  - RBC and WBC in small amounts
  - Yeast cells in small amount
  - Bacterial normal flora- Escherichia coli
- Abnormal components in stomach
  - Increased number of WBC: Indicates infection or inflammation

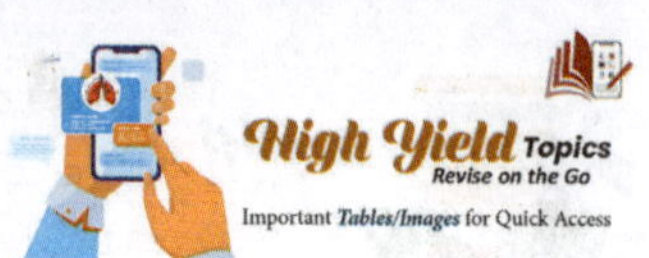

- Increased number of yeast cells: Indicates pyloric obstruction
- Protozoan and parasites: Ova of ascaris lumbricoides or hookworm
- Tubercle bacilli: Pulmonary tuberculosis or tuberculosis in other locations
- H. Pylori bacilli: Strong urease producing bacilli which is an indication of gastritis.

Chemical Examination

Collected gastric fluid must be free from mucus and food particles for chemical examination:
- **To measure the overall H^+ (hydrogen ion) concentration:** To 5 drops of gastric juice in an evaporating dish, add dimethylaminobenzene. Cherry red color appearance with HCl.
- Guaiac test or benzidine tests are used for the chemical evaluation of blood in gastric fluid.

WOUND DISCHARGE ANALYSIS

General Considerations

- Preferably collect specimen prior to institution of therapy and only from wounds that have clear signs of clinical infection, are deteriorating, or that fail to heal over a long period. Indiscriminate submission of a wound specimen, especially from a superficial site, may provide useless information that leads to unnecessary antibiotic treatment.
- Always cleanse/debride the skin or mucosal surface to be sampled. *Do not skip this step. Proper preparation of the wound can minimize contamination.*
- Sample viable tissue rather than superficial debris.
- Obtain aspirates or biopsy samples rather than swabs. *Note, however, that because of variability in numbers and types of organisms present in different parts of chronic wounds, the validity and value of a single biopsy specimen is debatable.*
- Gram stain will be done on specimens of sufficient quantity, even if it is not ordered. *Note: if specimens are collected on swabs, always submit two.* The quality of the specimen and determination of extent of workup will be based on Gram stain results. The presence of epithelial cells indicates contamination of the specimen with skin or mucous membrane microbiota while the presence of leukocytes is a good indicator of infection.
- Information regarding the type of wound (surgical, traumatic pressure ulcer, etc.) and location of the wound is important and should be indicated when ordered.
- Tissues and aspirates are acceptable for anaerobic culture, if indicated.

Method of Collection

- Aspiration of fluid-for obtaining sample from deeper site.
- Swab stick method to collect cells or pus from superficial wound site (Fig. 20.4).

Appearance

Wound drainage is described by type, color, amount, and odor. Drainage can be:
- **Serous:** Clear and thin; may be present in a healthy, healing wound.
- **Sero sanguineous:** Containing blood; may also be present in a healthy, healing wound.
- **Sanguineous:** Primarily blood.
- **Purulent:** Thick, white, and pus-like; may be indicative of infection and should be cultured.

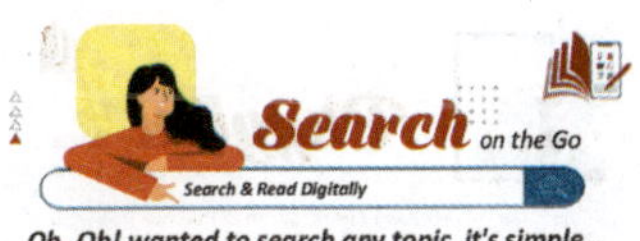

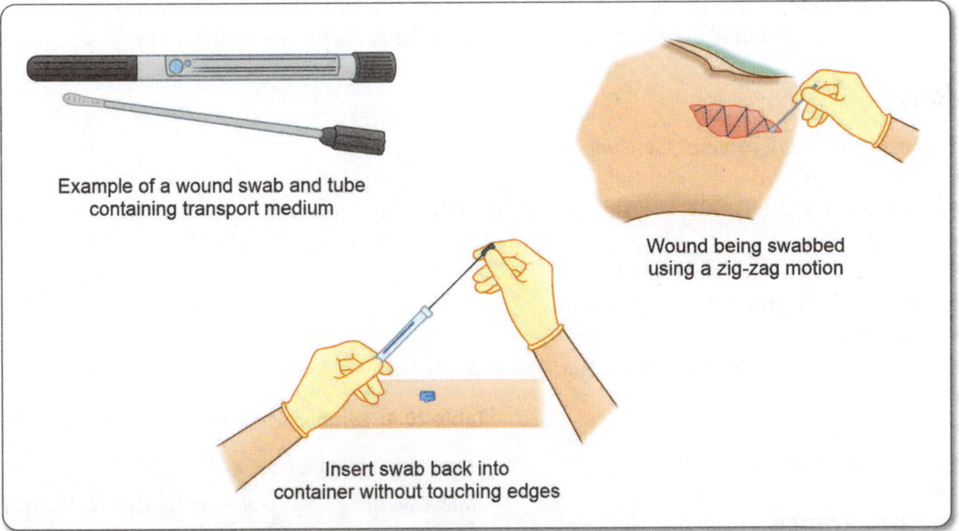

Figure 20.4: Method of taking wound swab

Color: Generally clear to pale yellow (normal)

- **Red:** Indicates fresh blood.
- **Brown:** Dried or old blood.
- **Blue-green:** Usually indicative of *Pseudomonas* infection and should be cultured.

The amount of drainage is generally documented as absent, scant, minimal, moderate, large, or copious.

- A large amount of drainage can indicate infection, whereas a reduction in the amount of drainage can indicate an infection that is resolving or inadequate arterial circulation.
- The presence and degree of odor can be documented as absent, mild, or foul. Foul odors can be indicative of an infection.

Chemical Examination

Investigations, such as electrolytes, lactate, glucose and protein analyses, and enzyme lactate dehydrogenase levels.

Microbiological Examination

- **Gram stain:** It is done to determine the type of bacteria.
- **Bacterial wound culture and sensitivity:** To identify the bacteria that cause infections in a wound.

PERITONEAL FLUID ANALYSIS

Peritoneal fluid lubricates the abdominal cavity. It is present in trace amounts in the spaces between the peritoneal layers. Mesothelial cells in the membranes create peritoneal fluid, which moistens the organs' exteriors and reduces friction when the organs move during digestion.

A variety of conditions can cause accumulation of peritoneal fluid (ascites). The most common cause by far is cirrhosis of the liver.

In addition to the patient's history and physical examination, laboratories use a preliminary set of assays (cell count, albumin, and fluid appearance) to help identify the cause for the fluid buildup.

Etiology

- Transudate (<30 g/L protein) (*systemic disease*)
  - Liver (cirrhosis)
  - Cardiac, e.g., RHF, CCF, SBE right heart valve disease and constrictive Pericarditis
  - Renal failure
  - Hypoalbuminemia (nephrosis)
- Exudate (>30 g/L protein) (*local disease*)
  - Malignancy
  - Venous obstruction, e.g., Budd-Chiari, schistosomiasis
  - Pancreatitis
  - Lymphatic obstruction
  - Infection (especially TB)

Table 20.4: Peritoneal fluid analysis—gross appearance

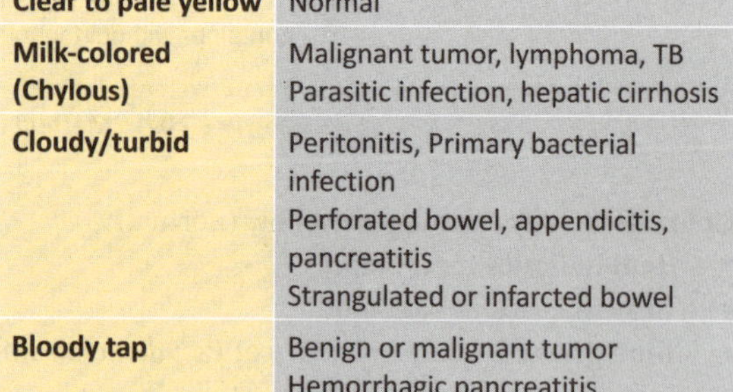

Clear to pale yellow	Normal
Milk-colored (Chylous)	Malignant tumor, lymphoma, TB Parasitic infection, hepatic cirrhosis
Cloudy/turbid	Peritonitis, Primary bacterial infection Perforated bowel, appendicitis, pancreatitis Strangulated or infarcted bowel
Bloody tap	Benign or malignant tumor Hemorrhagic pancreatitis, perforated ulcer

Gross Appearance

It is clear, serous and light yellow.

Abnormal appearances may give clues to conditions or diseases present and may include (Table 20.4):

- **Yellow** with liver disease, milky from obstruction of the lymphatic system, and greenish from bile
- **Reddish** peritoneal fluid may indicate the presence of blood, most often due to trauma.
- **Cloudy** peritoneal fluid may indicate the presence of microbes and/or white blood cells (WBCs), pointing to an infection. It may also indicate lymph system blockage or trauma.

Infectious disease tests—tests may be performed to look for microbes if an infection is suspected.

- **Gram stain:** Ideally, no germs should be found in peritoneal fluid; this is necessary for the direct examination of bacteria or fungi under a microscope.
- **Bacterial susceptibility testing and culture:** If bacteria are detected, susceptibility testing can be carried out to direct antibiotic treatment. The absence of bacteria does not rule out infection; they could be there in trace amounts or may be inhibited in growth as a result of prior antibiotic treatment.
- **Fungal tests:** If a culture is positive, the report will identify the fungus or fungi that are causing the infection, and susceptibility testing may be done to guide therapy.
- **Adenosine deaminase:** When a person exhibits symptoms suggestive of tuberculosis, there is likely a Mycobacterium tuberculosis infection in that region of the body, as indicated by a noticeably elevated amount in the peritoneal fluid. This is particularly true if the person lives in an area where tuberculosis is highly prevalent.

Chemical Tests

- **Albumin:** Albumin levels can either be much lower or comparable to those of plasma albumin. The differential between the albumin concentrations in the ascitic fluid and serum is known as the Serum Ascites-Albumin Gradient, or SAAG.

- Glucose levels are normally comparable to blood glucose levels, although they can be lower in cases of infection.
- Amylase/lipase levels are higher in pancreatic disease.
- Although total protein cannot be utilized in the SAAG calculation, it may be requested instead of albumin.
- Lactic dehydrogenase higher levels (>200 IU/L) is seen in inflammatory effusions.

Microscopic Examination

It may be carried out if cancer or an infection is suspected. White blood cells (WBCs) are present in normal peritoneal fluid in small amounts, but neither red blood cells (RBCs) nor bacteria are present.

- **Total cell counts:** The number of WBCs and RBCs in the sample. Infections and malignant diseases can cause elevated WBCs.
- WBC difference is the calculation of the proportions of various WBC types. Bacterial infections may cause an increase in neutrophil counts.
- **Cytology:** A sample that has been cytocentrifuged is stained with a particular dye and inspected under a microscope to check for aberrant cells and the differentiation of white blood cells. The differential can assist in identifying if the cells are the consequence of a tumor or an infection.

PLEURAL FLUID ANALYSIS

Pleural fluid serves a physiologic function in respiration, while also being a useful measure to diagnose and assess disease, trauma, and other abnormalities. A healthy human body contains 10–20 mL (about four tablespoons) of pleural fluid in the pleura. Other parameters are:

The accumulation of fluid usually occurs due to:

- **Transudate:** An imbalance pressure within blood vessels or low blood protein concentration causes fluid to leak inside the pleural space. This condition is normally due to heart failure or cirrhosis.
- **Exudates:** Injury or inflammation of the pleurae that causes excess amount of fluid inside pleural space. Exudates effusion usually occurs in cases, like pneumonia, tuberculosis and cancer.

Appearance

- **Color:** Clear, straw-colored fluid suggests a transudate:
  - Frankly purulent fluid indicates an empyema (an anaerobic empyema is likely if the fluid has a putrid odor).
  - A milky fluid suggests chylothorax or pseudochylothorax. This is most often caused by lymphatic obstruction secondary to malignancy, chronic inflammation or thoracic duct injury by trauma or a surgical procedure.
  - Grossly bloody fluid is usually associated with trauma. Less common causes include tuberculosis (TB), aortic dissection, ruptured aortic aneurysm and malignancy.
  - Straw-colored fluid with the distinctive smell of ammonia is indicative of urinothorax.
  - The presence of food particles suggests esophageal rupture.
- **Cholesterol:** 3.5–6.5 mmol/L.
- **Protein:** <2% (1–2 g/dL).
- **White blood cells (WBC):** <1,000/mm^3.
- **Glucose:** A low pleural fluid glucose level (<3.4 mmol/L) may be found in empyema, rheumatoid pleuritis and pleural effusions associated with TB, malignancy and esophageal rupture.A very low pleural glucose concentration (<1.6 mmol/L) is indicative of empyema and rheumatoid disease.

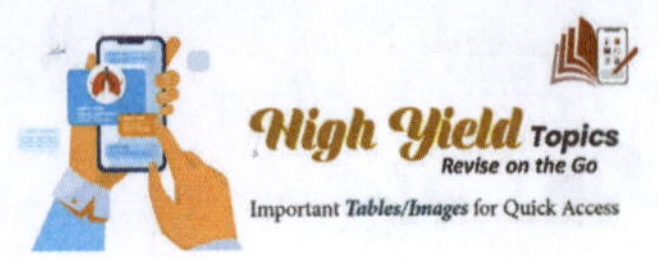

- **LDH:** Levels >1,000 IU/L are suggestive of empyema, malignancy or rheumatoid effusion.
- **Pleural pH:** A pleural fluid pH of <7.3 is associated with the same pathologies that cause low pleural fluid glucose levels. In malignant effusions, a pleural fluid pH of <7.3 has been associated with more extensive pleural involvement and shorter life expectancies.
- **WBC:** Results generally are not diagnostic, but most transudates have WBC counts <1,000 cells/µL, whereas exudates generally have WBC counts >50,000 cells/µL. Pleural fluid lymphocytosis suggests TB, sarcoidosis or malignancy. Neutrophil dominant effusions are associated with empyema or pulmonary embolism. Pleural fluid eosinophilia (PFE) is usually caused by the presence of air or blood in the pleural space.
- **Amylase:** 30–110 U/L.
- **Cholesterol and triglycerides:** Pleural fluid triglyceride levels >1.24 mmol/L with a cholesterol level of <5.18 mmol/L is diagnostic of chylothorax. A triglyceride level of <0.56 mmol/L with a cholesterol level of <5.18 mmol/L is associated with pseudochylothorax.

MUST KNOW

The Light Criteria

The light criteria are used to determine if an effusion is exudative or transudative.

- Pleural fluid protein/serum protein >0.5.
- Pleural fluid LDH/Serum LDH >0.6.
- Pleural fluid LDH >2.3 Serum LDH upper limit of the reference range.

Biochemistry Tests

The biochemistry tests related to pleural fluid analysis are total protein, albumin and LDH level.

Transudate

- Total protein, albumin and LDH level will be low.
- Value of SAAG above 1.1 g/dL is considered evidence of a transudate condition.

Exudate

- Total protein, albumin and LDH level will be high.
- Value of SAAG below 1.1 g/dL is considered evidence of the occurrence of exudates.
- Glucose level will be low.

SUMMARY

- Cerebrospinal fluid (CSF) is produced in the ventricles of the brain by the choroid plexus.
- The composition of CSF is clear and colorless, with a density of between 1.003 and 1.008 g/cm.
- An important clinical test that clinicians use to monitor CSF is the lumbar puncture.
- Normally CSF is clear and colorless.
- CSF analysis is a very useful investigations in patients presenting with acute neurological conditions.
- Sputum is a discharged material from the bronchial tree, with minimal amounts of oral or nasal material.
- Sputum sample is ideally collected in the morning (since secretions accumulate overnight), soon after awakening and before taking any mouthwash or food.

Contd...

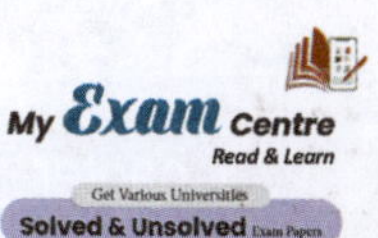

- Ziehl-Neelsen stained sputum smear is considered positive, if 5,000–10,000 tubercle bacilli/mL are present in the sputum
- A large amount of drainage can indicate infection, whereas a reduction in the amount of drainage can indicate an infection that is resolving.
- Peritoneal fluid is clear, serous and light yellow in appearance.
- Cloudy peritoneal fluid may indicate the presence of microbes and/or white blood cells (WBCs) indicating infection.
- WBCs are present in normal peritoneal fluid in small amounts.
- Transudate occurs due to an imbalance pressure within blood vessels or low blood protein concentration causing fluid to leak inside the pleural space. This condition is normally due to heart failure or cirrhosis.
- Exudates occurs due to an injury or inflammation of the pleurae that causes excess amount of fluid inside pleural space.
- Clear, straw-colored fluid suggests a transudate.
- Black pleural fluid is extremely rare, indicative of only a few diseases, such as Aspergillus Niger infection.
- Pleural fluid lymphocytosis suggests TB, sarcoidosis or malignancy.

ASSESS YOURSELF

Long Answer Questions

1. Explain pathological analysis of peritoneal fluid in detail.
2. Discuss sputum examination and its types.

Short Answer Questions

1. Write about wound discharge examination.
2. What is microbiological examination of sputum.
3. Write shot notes on:
   i. Examination of pleural fluid
   ii. Transudates and exudates

Multiple Choice Questions

1. **Wound discharge appears greenish in which of the following condition?**
   a. Klebsiella infection
   b. Staphylococcus infection
   c. Pseudomonas infection
   d. Proteus bacteria
2. **Method of peritoneal fluid collection is known as:**
   a. Thoracentesis
   b. Paracentesis
   c. Lumbar puncture
   d. Bone marrow aspiration
3. **Increased amount of amylase in ascetic fluid indicates:**
   a. Bronchitis
   b. Pancreatitis
   c. Gastritis
   d. Meningitis
4. **Brownish red or coffee color gastric juice is seen in which condition:**
   a. Pyloric obstruction
   b. Presence of fresh bile
   c. Presence of old bile
   d. Presence of large amount of blood

Answer Key

1. c **2.** b **3.** b **4.** d

Chapter 21

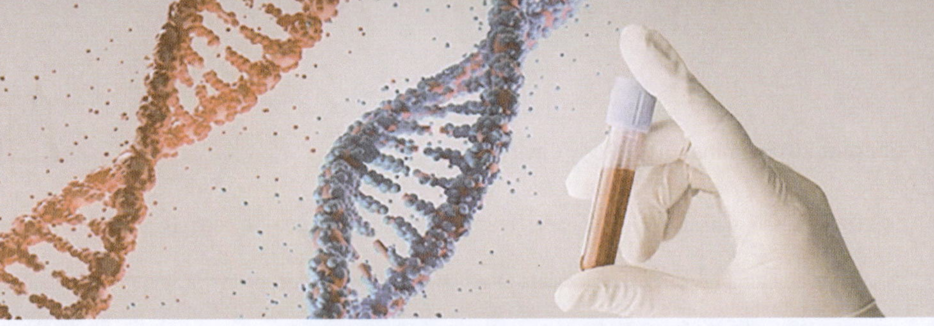

Examination of Semen

LEARNING OBJECTIVES

After the completion of the chapter, the readers will be able to:

- Explain indication of semen analysis.
- Describe special requirement and procedure for collection of semen sample.
- Conduct examination of seminal fluid.
- Describe clinical significance of semen analysis.

CHAPTER OUTLINE

KEY TERMS

Asthenozoospermia: An infertility condition in males in which they produce sperms with low motility. It's the most frequent seminal alteration.

Azoospermia: Lack of sperm cells in semen.

Infertility: Inability to achieve spontaneous pregnancy within one year of regular unprotected sexual intercourse.

Oligozoospermia: When sperm cell concentration is <20 million per cc, or when a whole ejaculated matter has <40 million spermatozoids.

Teratozoospermia: It's the presence of an abnormally high proportion of morphologically altered sperm cells.

INTRODUCTION

Semen analysis is a laboratory test used to evaluate male fertility. The inability to conceive following a year of unprotected sexual activity is known as *infertility*. Infertility affects 15% of all couples who are of reproductive age. A thorough physical examination, a detailed medical and sexual history, and semen assays are used to diagnose infertility in men. Approximately, half of all cases of infertility have a male element which accounts for 30% of the cases.

Infertility is defined as the "inability to achieve spontaneous pregnancy within one year of regular unprotected sexual intercourse."

During ejaculation, boluses of semen are released. They are composed of spermatozoa which are produced in the testes, processed in the epididymides, and combined with secretions from the prostate, bulbourethral glands, seminal vesicles, and the epididymides, among other male accessory sex organs. The overall quantity of spermatozoa, the fluid volume, the concentration of sperm, and the type of spermatozoa—including their viability, motility, and shape—as well as the discharge composition can all be used to evaluate semen. A thorough examination of these factors will help in determining the cause of the male factor's infertility.

INDICATIONS OF SEMEN ANALYSIS

- Investigation of infertility.
- For checking effectiveness of vasectomy.
- Paternity testing.
- Rape cases.
- Selection of donors for artificial insemination/assisted reproductive technology.

MUST KNOW

In order to ensure the accuracy and dependability of the results, two sperm analyses are required to prove sterility or fertility. A person's reproductive health may not be fully represented by a single analysis because sperm count and quality can change over time. Two analyses provide for a more accurate assessment of sterility or fertility by more effectively identifying any potential abnormalities or fluctuations.

SPECIMEN REQUIREMENTS AND PROCEDURE

- The male collects the semen sample at home or in close proximity to the lab by self-masturbating. It is advised that semen be extracted following a minimum of three days and a maximum of seven days without sexual activity.
- The sample needs to be collected in a clean, wide-mouthed container that is not toxic for spermatozoa. The ideal temperature range for the sperm container to be maintained in, is between 20°C and 37°C.
- To prevent sperm quality from being impacted by temperature fluctuations and dehydration, the semen should be sent to the lab within an hour of collection.
- To liquefy the specimen, place it on a bench or in an incubator set at 37°C for the first five minutes. Semen becomes more uniform and fluid, with only small patches of coagulation, when liquefaction is given time. Spermatozoa acquire the ability to move when they become immobile in the coagulum. It may take up to 60 minutes for liquefaction.
- It is necessary to measure the volume of semen. The pH of the semen is then determined, and wet preparations are made. The appearance, motility, and dilution necessary to accurately determine the quantity of spermatozoa are evaluated with the aid of wet preparations.
- Sperm vitality is evaluated, particularly if the amount of sperm is low.
- Sperm motility is best analyzed within an hour of collection. Determining the viability of immotile sperms depends on the condition of their cell membranes.
- To determine the number of sperm, the semen is diluted.
- After four hours, smears are ready to examine the morphology of the sperm.

MUST KNOW

The semen analysis is performed every 2–4 weeks. This implies that in order to track any changes or improvements in the quality of the semen, the analysis should be carried out every 2–4 weeks. At this point, routine testing enables a more accurate evaluation of the person's reproductive health and fertility.

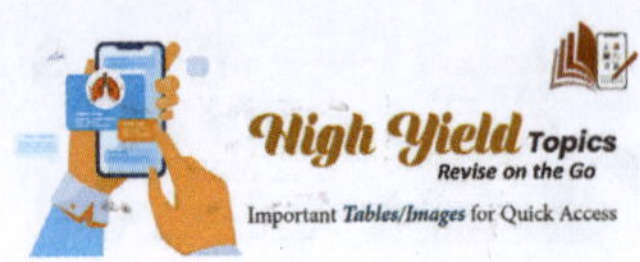

EXAMINATION OF SEMINAL FLUID

Physical Examination

- Visual appearance
  Opaque: Grayish-white, after abstinence it is slightly yellow.
- Viscosity
  Normal semen will fall drop by drop, if droplets form thread >2 cm long, it indicates that the viscosity is increased. Normal semen liquefies in 30 min, if liquefaction does not occur in 60 minutes, there is an abnormal increase in viscosity.
- Volume
  Normal ≥1.5 mL.
- pH
  Normal ≥7.2 mL.

Microscopic Examination

- **Motility:** It is an ability of sperm to move, three types of motility can be noted:
  - Rapidly progressive—moving fast and forward in a straight line.
  - Slowly progressive—crooked, curved and slow forward movement.
  - Nonprogressive—movement of tail only.
  - Normal finding: >32% progressive motility, >40% progressive + nonprogressive motility.
- **Vitality**
  - Number of live sperms are called viable.
  - Viable sperms are characterized by intact cell membrane and they won't take up eosin Y dye.
  - Normal finding: >58% normally viable.
- **Count**
  - Sperms can be counted following their liquefaction with diluting fluid (sodium bicarbonate).
  - Normal finding: >15 million/mL.
- **Morphology**
  - Sperm morphology refers to the size, shape, and structure of sperm cells. Aberrant sperm morphology can have a major impact on a couple's ability of conceiving.
  - Normal sperm have an oval head with a long tail.
  - Abnormal sperm morphology has the following types:
    i. **Head abnormalities:** The head of the sperm can be unusually larger than normal, affecting its ability to penetrate the female egg. It can also be abnormally small affecting its genetic material. Other abnormalities of sperm head include: doubled head or pointed head.
    ii. **Mid-piece abnormalities:** Mid-piece of the sperm contains mitochondrion required as an energy source for motility. When the mid-piece of the sperm is abnormally thick, it can cause motility impairment.
    iii. **Tail abnormalities:** These abnormalities include: Short tail, no tail or coiled tail. Abnormalities of tail can affect sperm motility and its ability to reach egg.
  - Normal finding: >4% spermatozoa should show normal morphology.

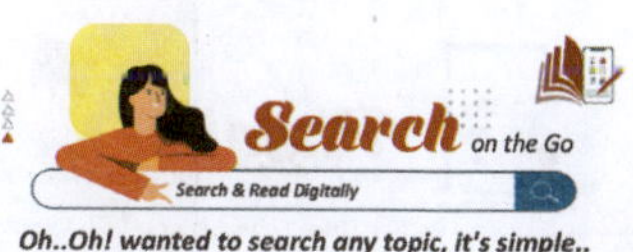

Figures 21.1 and 21.2 show the normal and abnormal morphology of sperm.

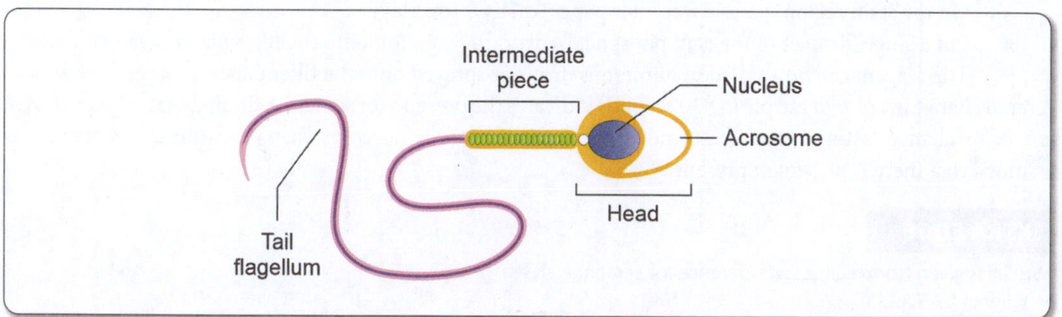

Figure 21.1: Normal morphology of sperm

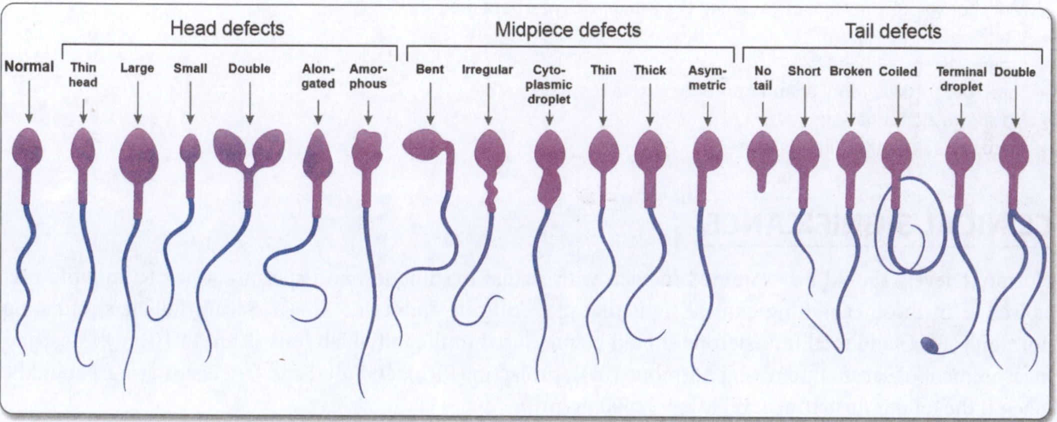

Figure 21.2: Abnormal morphology of sperm

Chemical Examination

Chemical analysis of semen consists of the following tests:

- **Fructose test:** It determines androgen deficiency or ejaculatory obstruction to semen. It has been demonstrated that decreased fructose levels correlate with both testosterone levels and androgen insufficiency. The fructose test should be performed on a postejaculate urine sample to assess for retrograde ejaculation when azoospermia and low semen volume are present.

  Procedures:
  - Semen is heated in a strong acid in the presence of resorcinol in order to quantify the amount of fructose present.
  - A photometer can read the red color that fructose produces (the Seliwanoff reaction).
  - The average fructose level is 315 mg/dL.
  - **Acid phosphatase test:** The purpose of this process is to ascertain whether semen may be present on evidentiary material.

  Procedures:
  - Locate stain areas by a visual examination
  - Swab stain areas with a moistened swab

- Small cutting placed on filter paper or other appropriate clean surface
- On the stain region, press a wet filter paper (diH_2O) (overlay)
- Put a single droplet of the acid phosphatase working solution onto the filter paper, swab, or cutting. The reagent can be applied in numerous drops or sprayed onto the filter paper for larger overlays.

A rapid change in color to purple in >30 seconds indicates the presence of semen. A finding that is inconclusive is a color change lasting between 31 and 59 seconds. If there is no color change within 60 seconds, it is assumed that there is no semen present.

EXTRA EDGE

WHO has given Normal limits of reference for semen analysis:

- Volume ≥1.5 mL
- pH ≥7.2
- Total sperm number = 39 million sperm per ejaculate or more
- Morphology ≥4% normal forms using the Kruger or Tygerberg method
- Vitality ≥58% live sperm
- Progressive motility ≥32%
- Total (progressive motility and non-progressive motility) ≥40%
- No sperm agglutination
- Viscosity ≤2 cm after liquefaction

CLINICAL SIGNIFICANCE

Hormone levels should be examined in men with sexual dysfunction and sperm count <10 million/ mL, as well as in those exhibiting clinical signs that may indicate endocrine illness. Serum follicle-stimulating hormone (FSH) and total testosterone should be measured in the initial lab tests (8 am to 10 am). A second measurement of serum luteinizing hormone (LH), prolactin (PRL), and total and free testosterone should be taken if the total testosterone level is low (<300 ng/mL).

SUMMARY

- Failure to conceive after 1 year of unprotected sex is considered infertility.
- A semen analysis is a routine test for infertility.
- Azoospermia refers to the condition where there is no measurable amount of sperm present in the semen.
- Two sperm analyses are needed to confirm sterility or fertility.
- The interval for the semen analysis is 2 to 4 weeks apart.
- Semen collection after a period of sexual abstinence is recommended in order to allow for the build-up of sperm in the male reproductive system.
- The ejaculate volume should be at least 1.5 mL and not >5.5 mL.
- Sperm concentration refers to the number of sperm cells present in a given volume of semen.
- The liquefaction time for semen refers to the time it takes for semen to change from a gel-like consistency to a more liquid state.
- Semen viscosity refers to the thickness or stickiness of semen.
- Sperm motility refers to the ability of sperm to move and swim effectively.

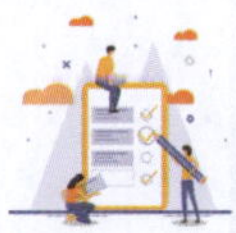

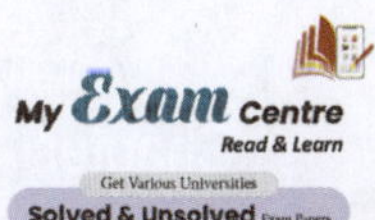

ASSESS YOURSELF

Long Answer Question

1. Define semen analysis and explain examination of seminal fluid in detail.

Short Answer Questions

1. Write about acid phosphatase test.
2. What do you understand by abnormalities in morphology of sperm?
3. Write short notes on:
   i. Semen analysis
   ii. Semen collection

Multiple Choice Questions

1. **Lack of sperm cells in semen is called.......**
   a. Polyspermia
   b. Azoospermia
   c. Oligospermia
   d. Asthenospermia
2. **What is a semen analysis?**
   a. A seldom test done for infertility
   b. A routine test for fertility
   c. A routine test for infertility
   d. A detailed scan of sperm
3. **How many sperm analyses are needed to confirm sterility or fertility?**
   a. 2
   b. 4
   c. 1
   d. 3
4. **What is the interval for the semen analysis?**
   a. 2–6 weeks apart
   b. 3–6 weeks apart
   c. 2–4 weeks apart
   d. 2–3 weeks apart
5. **What is the liquefaction time for semen?**
   a. 5–35 minutes
   b. 10–20 minutes
   c. 5–30 minutes
   d. 30 minutes–1 hour

Answer Key

1. b **2.** c **3.** a **4.** c **5.** c

Chapter

22

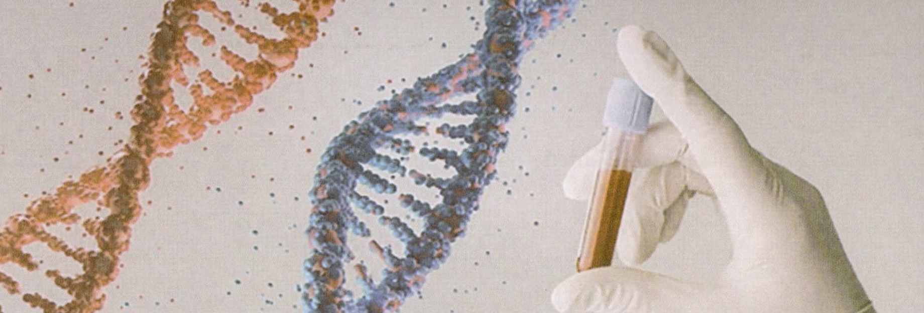

Urine Examination

LEARNING OBJECTIVES

After the completion of the chapter, the readers will be able to:

- Explain components of routine urinalysis and specimen collection and evaluation.
- Describe physical examination of urine.
- Understand chemical characteristics of urine.
- Describe examination of urine sediments.

CHAPTER OUTLINE

- Introduction
- Components of Basic (Routine) Urinalysis
- Urine Dipstick Test
- Urine Culture and Sensitivity Test

KEY TERMS

Oliguria: Oliguria is defined as urinary output >400 mL/day or <20 mL/hr and is one of the earliest signs of impaired renal function.

Polyuria: Polyuria is excessive or abnormally large production or passage of urine. Polyuria is urine output of >3 L/day.

Ultrafiltration: Ultrafiltration (UF) refers to the process of movement of fluids through a membrane caused by a pressure gradient.

Urine-specific gravity: Urine specific gravity (USG) is a comparison of the density of urine to that of water. It is an estimate of urine osmolality (the solute concentration of a solution).

Urobilinogen: Urobilinogen is a product of hemoglobin metabolism and is formed by bacterial degradation of bilirubin in the colon.

INTRODUCTION

In the normal adult, approximately 1,200 mL of blood perfuses the kidneys each minute, which accounts for about 25% of the cardiac output.

The glomeruli (normally numbering at least 1 million per kidney) receive blood through afferent arterioles, and an ultrafiltrate of the plasma passes through each glomerulus into the Bowman space. From here, the filtrate is passed through the tubules and collecting ducts, where reabsorption or secretion of various substances and the concentration of urine can occur.

Urine is an unstable fluid; as soon as it is removed *via* micturition, its composition changes. For the sample to remain intact, precise handling, storage, and collection are essential.

The best representative urine samples for testing are those that are taken from the first void, also known as "morning urine". Because the urine that is accumulated in the bladder over-night is more concentrated, it may provide information about the kidneys' ability to concentrate as well as reveal traces of substances that might not be present in more diluted samples.

Urine specimens can be obtained by non-invasive or invasive approaches. The primary non-invasive method is spontaneous voiding, while children who are still unable to control their urination may benefit from other methods (e.g., bag urine). On the other hand, the two invasive procedures that have been documented to date are suprapubic bladder puncture and urethral catheterization. The fundamental principle of methods is to acquire a specimen free from outside contamination.

COMPONENTS OF BASIC (ROUTINE) URINALYSIS

The basic (routine) urinalysis consists of four parts:

1. Specimen collection and evaluation.
2. Gross/physical examination.
3. Chemical characteristics.
4. Examination of urine sediment.

Specimen Collection and Evaluation

The patient should be explained the correct way of sample collection:

- Instruct the female patient to clean the local area with wet cotton swab, separating the labia with fingers and urinate.
- Males should be instructed to withdraw the foreskin, and clean the urethral meatus and glans with wet cotton swab.
- Discard initial 10–20 mL of urine. Then clean catch midstream sample in a wide mouthed, sterile plastic container. Types of urine sample have been depicted in Table 22.1.

Table 22.1: Types of urine specimen

Types	Description
Random specimen	This can be collected at any time of the day, it is the most effective method for assessing WBC or RBC.
First-morning sample	The first-morning sample is defined as urine that has been in the bladder for eight hours. This will have a higher analyte and cellular element concentration.
Postprandial 2 hours	The postprandial 2 hours sample is collected after 2 hours of a high carbohydrate diet.
Midstream clean catch urine	It is required for determining culture and sensitivity of urinary infections. After cleaning the urethra, the patient is instructed to discard the first few milliliters of urine. Urine is collected midstream and is placed in a sterile container.
24-hour of a urine sample	Urine is timed and collected for a 24-hour urinalysis, which is used to evaluate proteinuria, estimate residual renal function in end-stage renal disease using urea and creatinine clearance. The first morning sample that the patient voids is discarded. The laboratory provides containers for collecting the urine produced over the next 24 hours, including the first specimen to be voided in the morning. In order to stabilize the urine sample for subsequent analysis, a preservative solution is added during collection. Urine is collected for a full day and then the total volume is noted. After that, a representative sample is sent to the lab for examination out of the entire collection.

- Close the screw cap of the container.
- Considerations include proper labeling, proper specimen for the requested examination, and proper preservative, visible signs of contamination.
- Properly-labeled specimen must have the patient's full name and the date and time of collection.
- For routine urinalysis, the first voided morning urine, which is the most concentrated, is considered the best one.
- Sometimes, there is a need to obtain a catheterized specimen or suprapubically collected urine specimen.
- If a single specimen is sent for several investigations, the bacteriologic investigation should be performed first, provided that the urine should be collected correctly.
- Only a limited amount of urine may be available for processing in pediatric patients and those experiencing acute renal failure. In these situations, the measurements that are most relevant to the diagnosis should be completed first.
- Timed urine collection (12- or 24-hour collection) is favored over random specimen collection for quantitative measures.

Gross/Physical Examination of Urine

Urine Color (Fig. 22.1)

- **Normal:** Yellow (light/pale to dark/deep amber)
- **Amber:** Bile pigments
- **Brown/black (tea-colored):** Bile pigments, fava beans, homogentisic acid (alkaptonuria), levodopa, melanin or oxidized melanogen, methemoglobin, methyldopa, myoglobin, nitrofurantoin, primaquine, rhubarb, riboflavin.
- **Dark yellow:** Concentrated specimen (dehydration, exercise).
- **Green/blue:** Amitriptyline, biliverdin, cimetidine, methylene blue, propofol, pseudomonal UTI, triamterene.
- **Orange:** Bile pigments, carrots, coumadin, nitrofurantoin, phenothiazines, phenazopyridine, rifampin, vitamin C.
- **Pink/red:** Beets, blackberries, chlorpromazine, food dyes, hematuria, hemoglobinuria, menstrual contamination, myoglobinuria, phenolphthalein, porphyrins, rifampin, rhubarb, uric acid crystals.

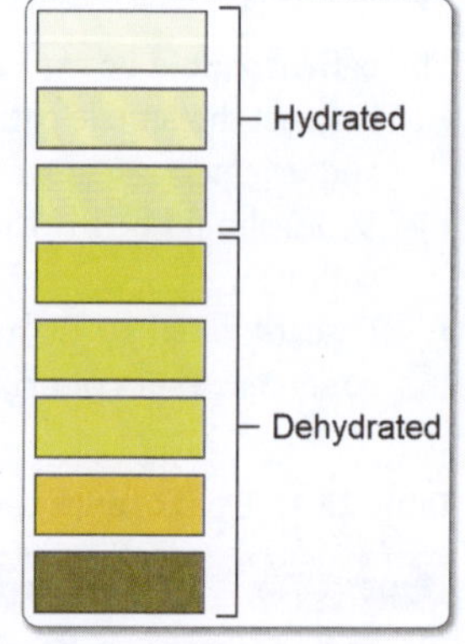

Figure 22.1: Urine color on the basis of hydration status

Appearance

- **Normal:** Clear or translucent
- Presence of bacteria, blood clots, contrast media, mucus, lymph fluids, small calculi, precipitation of cells such as WBC's, RBC's, epithelial cells, casts or crystals can cause turbidity in the appearance of urine.

Volume

The volume of urine varies greatly. 1–2 L/day is considered the normal range. To get rid of wastes, the kidneys need to produce at least 500 mL of urine per day. A lower output than this is known as oliguria and can be caused by severe dehydration or renal illness. Urine output almost completely absent is known as anuria. Polyuria, or the overproduction of urine, can result from either diabetes insipidus or diabetes mellitus. Daily urine collection is about 600–1200 mL in normal adults. Volume of urine can be measured by collecting 24-hour urine samples.

Conditions associated with urine volume have been depicted in Table 22.2.

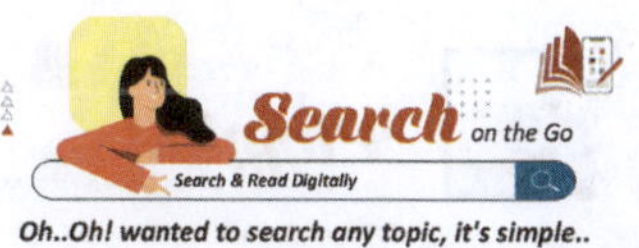

Table 22.2: Urine volume

Volume condition	Volume	Causes
Normal	1–2 L/day	
Polyuria	>2.5 L/day	Diabetes mellitus; diabetes insipidus; excess caffeine or alcohol; kidney disease; certain drugs, such as diuretics; sickle cell anemia; excessive water intake
Oliguria	300–500 mL/day	Dehydration; blood loss; diarrhea; cardiogenic shock; kidney disease; enlarged prostate
Anuria	<50 mL/day	Kidney failure; obstruction, such as kidney stone or tumor, enlarged prostate

Clarity (Character)

Cloudy urine can be attributed to the presence of various cellular elements. Leukocytes may form a white cloud similar to that caused by phosphates, but the cloud remains after acidification. Likewise, bacterial growth may cause a uniform opalescence that is not removed by acidification or filtration. It has been suggested that turbidimetric assessment using a double-beam turbidimeter may be useful for urine infection screening.

Odor

Urine normally will have a faint, aromatic odor of undetermined source. Specimens with extensive bacterial overgrowth can be recognized by an ammoniacal, fetid odor. Urine odor is not normally reported.

MUST KNOW

- Cystine decomposition: Sulfuric smell.
- Dehydration/prolonged room temperature: Strong smell.
- Diabetes mellitus: Honey.
- Diabetic ketoacidosis: Fruity/sweet.
- Gastrointestinal-bladder fistula: Fecal smell.
- Maple-syrup urine disease: "Burnt sugar".
- Prolonged bladder retention: Ammoniacal.
- Urinary tract infection: Pungent or fetid.
- Medications and diet: Onions, garlic, asparagus.

Normal pH

Because of metabolic activity, urine typically has a mild acidity. When systemic acidemia (serum pH <7.35) is present, a urine pH >5.5 indicates renal dysfunction due to a failure to eliminate hydrogen ions. Conversely, a stale urine sample that has allowed bacteria to proliferate and urea to break down, releasing ammonia, is the most common cause of alkaline urine. Urine pH can be used to diagnose and manage urinary tract infections and calculi formation.

Normal Urine pH: 4.5–8 (usually 5.5–6.5)

Acid Urine

Acid urine may be produced by a diet high in meat protein and with some fruits, such as cranberries. Dehydration, diabetes mellitus, diabetic ketoacidosis, diarrhea, emphysema, medications (methionine, mandelic acid, etc.) can cause acidic urine.

Alkaline Urine

The urine tends to become less acidic following a meal (the so-called alkaline tide). In metabolic alkalosis, an alkaline urine with higher levels of urinary bicarbonate is produced, and ammonia production is decreased. It is seen in conditions, such as: hyperventilation, renal tubular acidosis, vomiting, etc.

Methods for PH measurements:

- Reagent Strip
- pH Electrode

Specific Gravity

Normal adults with adequate fluid intake will produce urine of specific gravity 1.016 to 1.022 over a 24-hour period.

When the specific gravity of the urine is <1.007, it is referred to as **hyposthenuric urine**. The loss of concentrating ability associated with diabetes insipidus causes large amounts of urine to be produced, with a specific gravity as low as 1.001 (water has a specific gravity of 1.000).

Pyelonephritis and glomerulonephritis are two renal abnormalities that can also be associated with prolonged urine excretion of low specific gravity.

Excessive water loss/dehydration, adrenal insufficiency, hepatic illness, or congestive heart failure can all result in high specific gravity. **Isosthenuria** is the state in which there is little to no variation found among multiple specimens from a patient and the specific gravity remains constant at roughly 1.010. This suggests significant kidney injury with impaired concentrating and diluting capacities.

Chemical Characteristics

Protein in Urine

The glomerular capillary wall is permeable to molecules smaller than 20,000 daltons under normal circumstances. The majority of the tiny portion of filtered proteins are taken up again by the proximal tubule cells, where they are metabolized. Thus, trace levels of proteins are typically found in urine.

About one-third of the total urine proteins are albumin, another third are Tamm-Horsfall glycoproteins, which are released by tubular cells, and the remaining portion are plasma proteins such as globulins.

Normally, up to 150 mg of protein is excreted in the urine daily, with the average urine protein concentration varying from 2 to 10 mg/dL depending on urine volume.

Albumin and transferrin, two types of proteins are not typically filtered, through a damaged glomerular capillary walls. Therefore, low blood albumin, subsequent widespread edema, and elevated serum lipids—as in nephrotic syndrome may be associated with this pattern. Protein excretion ranges from 3.0 g/day to 3.5 g/day on average.

Proteinuria Quantification

Sulfosalicylic Acid (SSA) Method

Qualitative: This method depends on formation of a precipitate for determination of the presence of protein.

Procedures

- Specimens should be centrifuged and a clear supernatant used.
- Take approximately 3 mL of supernatant urine in a clean test tube, aliquot an equal amount of 3% SSA.
- Invert to mix. Let stand exactly 10 minutes.
- Invert again twice.
- Using ordinary room light (not a lamp), observe the degree of turbidity and/or precipitation, and grade the results according to the following descriptions:
  Negative- No turbidity (.5 mg/dL or less)

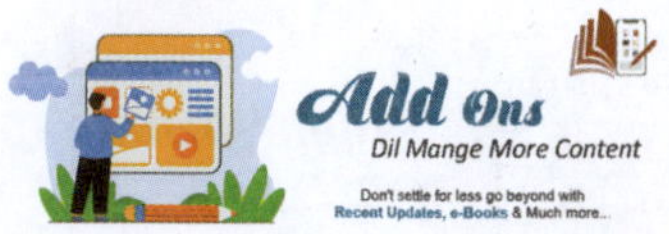

Trace - perceptible turbidity (.20 mg/dL)
1+ - Distinct turbidity, but no discrete granulation (.50 mg/dL)
2+ - Turbidity with granulation, but no flocculation (.200 mg/dL)
3+ - Turbidity with granulation and flocculation (.500 mg/dL)
4+ - Clumps of precipitated protein or solid precipitate (.1.0 g/dL or more)

This method will detect about 5–10 mg/dL. Albumin, globulins, glycoproteins, and Bence-Jones proteins are all detected.

NOTE

Bence-Jones globulin associated with multiple myeloma, lymphoma and macroglobulinaemia is **NOT** detected by dipstick urinalysis.

EXTRA EDGE

Type IV collagen and laminin are basement membrane markers which can be demonstrated immunohistochemically, loss of these markers points to...INVASION

Blood Cells in Urine

The primary activity of erythrocytes' peroxidase is detected by the blood dipstick test, however, hemoglobin and myoglobin can also catalyze this process. As a result, hematuria, myoglobinuria, or hemoglobinuria are indicated by a positive test result.

Normal: Negative (typically) or less than or equal to five RBCs per milliliter (lab-dependent value).

- **Hematuria:** Renal calculi, glomerulonephritis, pyelonephritis, tumors, anticoagulants, etc.
- **Hemoglobinuria:** Hemolytic anemia, transfusion reaction, severe burn, infections.
- **Myoglobinuria:** Muscle trauma, muscle wasting diseases, prolonged coma.

EXTRA EDGE

Benzidine test: It is used for the determination of blood (RBC's or hemoglobin) in urine.

Procedure

- Add 2 mL of urine in a test tube.
- Add 2 mL of 1% Benzidine solution in acetic acid. Shake well.
- Add 2 mL of hydrogen peroxide.
- Mix well and observe change in the color.

Interpretation: Appearance of green or blue color indicates hematuria.

Glucose and Other Sugars in Urine

Various sugars may be found in the urine under certain circumstances, both pathologic and physiologic. These include glucose, fructose, galactose, lactose, maltose, pentose, and sucrose. The presence of detectable amounts of glucose in urine is termed **glycosuria**.

Glycosuria typically occurs when the serum glucose content is 180 mg/dL. This condition occurs whenever the glucose level in the blood surpasses the renal tubule capacity for reabsorption, example diabetes mellitus.

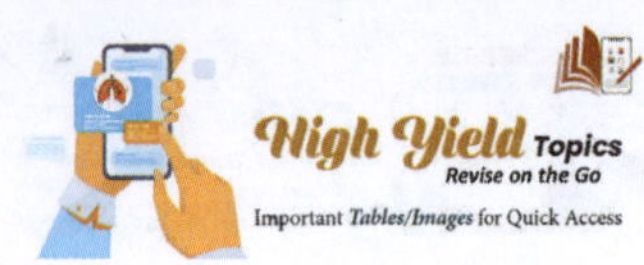

Glycosuria with concomitant hyperglycemia is seen in several endocrine disorders. These include pituitary and adrenal disorders such as acromegaly, Cushing syndrome, hyperadrenocorticism, functioning alpha cell pancreatic tumors, hyperthyroidism, and pheochromocytoma.

Method for Testing

Copper reduction tests: An early technique for determining the presence of glucose in urine. The test is based on the concept that compounds in the presence of heat and an alkali, convert copper sulfate to cuprous oxide would change color, indicating the presence of glucose.

The copper reduction method will detect sufficient quantities of any reducing substances in the urine, including reducing sugars such as lactose, fructose, galactose , maltose, and the pentoses. It includes: Benedict's test and Fehling's test.

Benedict's Test

Reducing sugars (monosaccharides and some disaccharides) with free ketone or aldehyde functional groups can be identified by the Benedict's test. Urine can be tested for the presence of glucose using Benedict's solution.

Principle of Benedict's Test

Benedict's solution turns orange or brick red when heated in the presence of simple carbohydrates. The reducing property of simple carbohydrates triggers this reaction. The color shift in Benedict's solution is caused by the reduction of copper (II) ions to copper (I) ions.

Procedure of Benedict's Test

- Add 5 mL of Benedict's reagent in a test tube.
- Add 8 drops of urine to the Benedict's reagent.
- Heat it carefully on a flame of gas burner.
- Cool and observe the color change and precipitate formation and analyze the result.

Interpretation of Results (Figure 22.2)

- There will be 0.5–1 g% sugar in solution if the color becomes green when it boils.

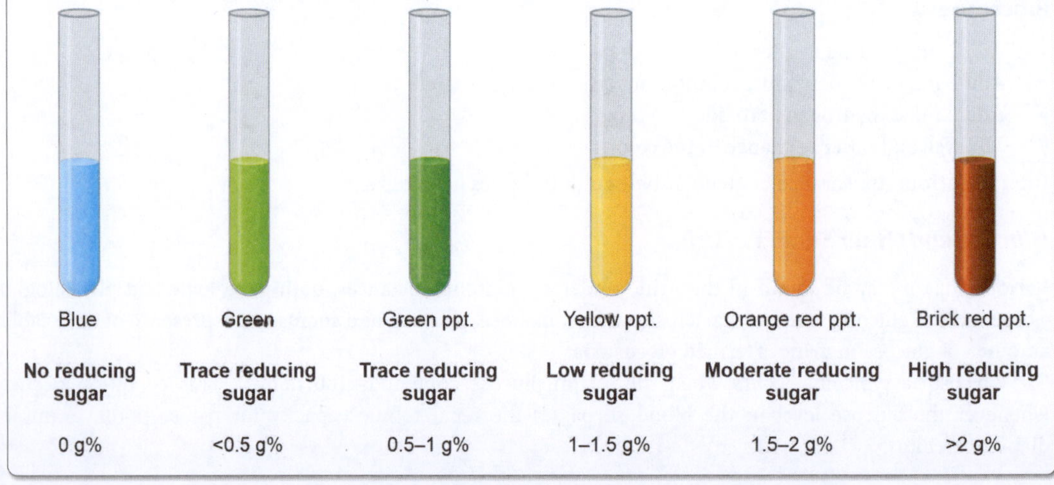

Figure 22.2: Interpretation of Benedict's test result

- Yellow color indicates 1–1.5 g% sugar in the sample.
- Orange color indicates the presence of 1.5–2 g% sugar.
- If the color turns red, there is between 1.5 and 2.0 g% sugar in the mixture.
- Additionally, brick red color indicates, the solution contains more sugar than 2% g percentage of sugar.

Ketones in Urine

The body makes up for any deficits in the metabolism or absorption of carbohydrates, or for any insufficiency in the amount of carbohydrates consumed, by breaking down fatty acids in greater proportion. Ketone bodies, byproducts of incomplete fat metabolism, begins to appear in the blood and are eliminated through the urine when this increase is significant. The three ketone bodies found in the urine of people with ketonuria are 3-hydroxybutyrate (20%), acetone (2%), and acetoacetic (diacetic) acid (20%).

Methods for examining urine sediment depending on the methods used, total ketone bodies (as acetone) can range as high as 17–42 mg/dL.

Method of Testing

Rothera's Test

A complex with a purple color is created when acetoacetic acid and acetone react with an alkaline sodium nitroprusside solution. Acetoacetic acid above 1–5 mg/dL and acetone above 10–20 mg/dL can be detected using this approach. There is no trace of beta-hydroxybutyrate.

Procedures

- Transfer about 5 mL of urine into a test tube.
- Add 1 g of the powdered Rothera mixture, and stir well.
- Add 1–2 mL of pure ammonium hydroxide in the urine.
- Observe pink-purple ring at the interface.

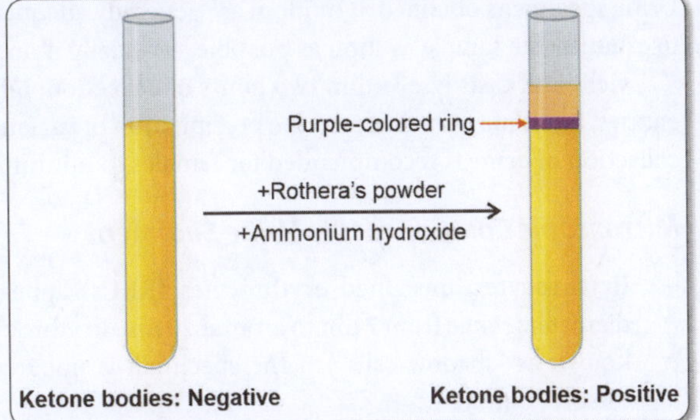

Figure 22.3: Rothera's test for detection of ketones in urine

Interpretation

- At the contact, a purple permanganate-colored ring forms immediately, indicating the presence of ketone bodies (positive) [Fig. 22.3].
- Absence of ketone bodies at the interface: no production of a purple permanganate-colored ring (negative) [Fig. 22.3].

Nitroprusside Test

The nitroprusside reaction serves as the basis for the ketone body test. In an alkaline media, acetoacetic acid, sodium nitroferricyanide, and glycine combine to form a complex that is violet to purple in color. Acetoacetic acid in urine can be found in as little as 5 mg/dL using the reagent strip method.

Ketones can be reported as negative, 1+, 2+, 3+, or 4+, or as small, moderate, or large amount.

Bilirubin in Urine

Bilirubin is not found normally in the urine. It can be seen in conditions, such as: Liver dysfunction, biliary obstruction, congenital hyperbilirubinemia, viral or drug-induced hepatitis, cirrhosis.

Fouchet's test is done for the detection of bilirubin in urine. The reagent oxidizes yellow bilirubin to green biliverdin. Green color indicates the presence of bilirubin.

NOTE

Only conjugated bilirubin can be excreted as bilirubinuria. A positive test for urine bilirubin confirms conjugated hyperbilirubinemia

Urobilinogen

It is a normal constituent of urine. The degradation product of bilirubin metabolism from bacteria in the intestine. Normal value is: 0.1–1 mg/dL in random samples or up to 4 mg/day. The majority of urobilinogen is either returned to the liver or transformed into bile, or it is eliminated in the feces. The remaining urobilinogen (<1%) is excreted in urine.

It is elevated in hemolysis, liver disease, sickle-cell disease, and thalassemia.

Ehrlich's test is done for the detection of urobilinogen in urine.

Examination of Urine Sediment

Microscopic examination of urine, in conjunction with dipstick chemical analysis, has been used for decades to assist in the detection of renal and urinary tract disease processes.

Methods for Examining Urine Sediment

Urine specimens obtained at random are generally adequate for microscopic analysis; however, it is advisable to examine the sample as soon as possible, especially if no preservative has been added.

Cells and casts lyse within two hours of collection; refrigeration (2°–8°C) inhibits the lysis of pathologic entities, but it may also increase the precipitation of various amorphous and crystalline materials. Midstream collection of urine is recommended for females to minimize contamination from vaginal elements.

Microscopic Components in Urine Sediment

- **Erythrocytes:** unstained erythrocytes (RBCs) appear as pale, biconcave disks at high power. Their diameters range from 7 µm to around 20 µm. Erythrocytes may look as weak, colorless circles (sometimes known as "shadow cells") if the specimen is not fresh when it is examined, as the hemoglobin may dissolve out.
- **Polymorphonuclear leukocyte (neutrophil):** The most common form of leukocyte (white blood cell, or WBC) seen in urine is the polymorphonuclear leukocyte, also known as a neutrophil. These cells have multilobated nuclei and resemble granular spheres with a diameter of around 12 m when magnified greatly. Occasionally, isolated, tiny, spherical nuclei may be observed within nuclear segments.
- **Epithelial cells:** The most common and least significant type of epithelial cells found in normal urine are squamous epithelial cells. Squamous epithelial cells, which line the distal portion of the urethra, are large, flat cells with small, rounded central nuclei and an abundance of cytoplasm in urine.
- **Casts:** The kidney is the sole location where casts, which are formed components of urine, originates. The glycoprotein known as Tamm-Horsfall protein, which makes up roughly one-third of the total protein in urine in healthy persons, is released by the thick section of the ascending loop of Henle (and potentially the distal tubule). The casts preserve the cylindrical shape of the tubule in which they were formed. In healthy conditions, just a small number of hyaline or finely granular castings may be seen. Depending on the urine sample's pH, cellular casts can disintegrate within 30 to 10 minutes, therefore prompt testing is essential for appropriate testing. Refer to Table 22.3 to know about various types of casts.
- **Cells:** Various types of cells present in urine are depicted in Table 22.4.

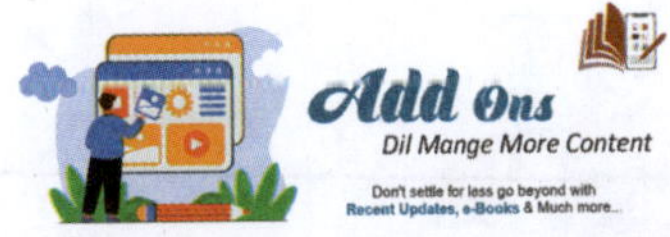

Table 22.3: Types of casts and its associated condition/disease

Type of casts	Associations/conditions
Red blood cell casts	Glomerulonephritis, vasculitis, intrinsic renal disease (tubulointerstitial nephritis, acute tubular injury/necrosis)
White blood cell casts	Pyelonephritis, interstitial nephritis, glomerulonephritis, renal inflammatory processes
Epithelial cell casts	Acute tubular injury/necrosis, interstitial nephritis, glomerulonephritis, eclampsia, nephritic syndrome, transplant rejection
Granular casts	Glomerular or tubular disease, pyelonephritis, advanced renal disease, viral infections, stress/exercise
Waxy casts	Advanced renal failure (dilated tubules with decreased flow)
Hyaline casts	fever, exercise, diuretics, pyelonephritis, chronic renal disease
Fatty cast	Heavy proteinuria (nephrotic syndrome), renal disease, hypothyroidism, acute tubular necrosis, diabetes mellitus

Table 22.4: Types of cells present in urine

Cells	Normal levels	Associations
Red blood cells	0–5 cells/high-power field	UTI, inflammation
Eosinophil	Absent	Interstitial nephritis, acute tubular necrosis, UTI, kidney transplant rejection, hepatorenal syndrome
White blood cells	0–5 cells/high-power field	UTI, inflammation
Epithelial cells	Less than or equal to 15–20 squamous epithelial cells/high-power field	Heavy metal poisoning, drug-induced toxicity, viral infections, pyelonephritis, malignancy, acute tubular necrosis
Bacteria, fungi and parasites	Absent	UTI, contamination

Crystals

Urine contains a significant amount of metabolic end products, which can precipitate as crystals. Although some types of crystals are linked to specific diseases, the presence of crystals is not always related with pathological conditions. Leucine and tyrosine crystals are linked to severe liver illness, whereas cholesterol crystals are observed in polycystic renal disease and nephrotic syndrome.

Uric Acid

Yellow to orange-brown, diamond or barrel-shaped crystals. These are associated with uric acid nephropathy, hyperuricosuria and acidic urine (Fig. 22.4).

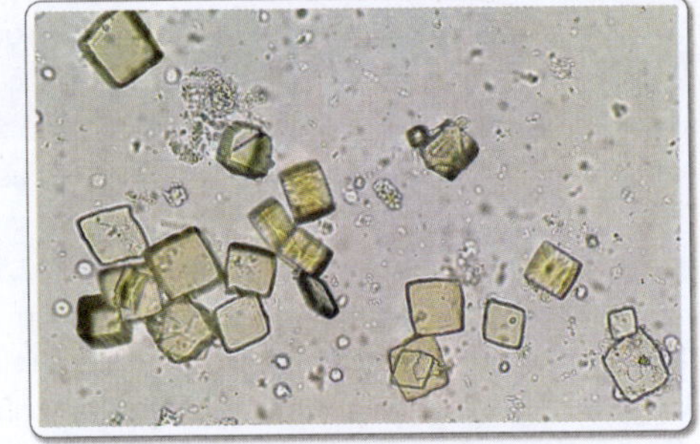

Figure 22.4: Uric acid crystals

Calcium Oxalate

It is the most commonly seen crystal in human urine. It is seen in acidic urine, ethylene glycol poisoning and hyperoxaluria. It is refractile square or 'envelope'-shaped (Fig. 22.5).

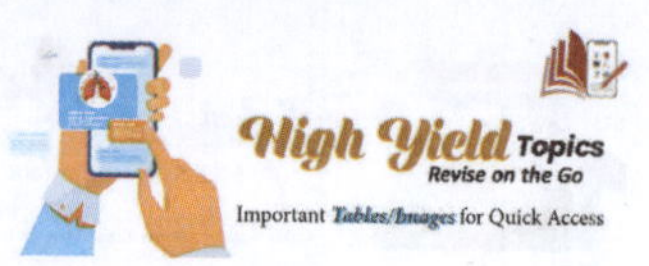

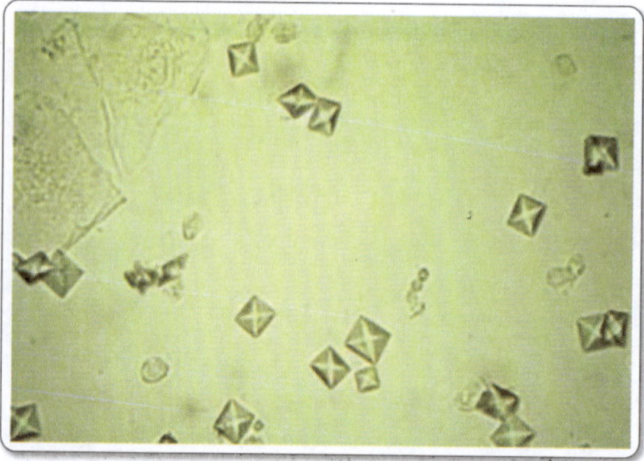
Figure 22.5: Calcium oxalate crystal

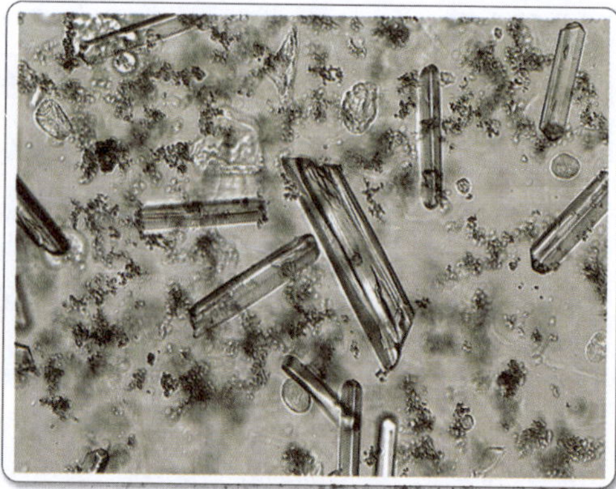
Figure 22.6: Struvite crystal

Calcium and Magnesium Phosphate

It is associated with alkaline urine, intake of diet rich in calcium, prolonged immobilization and bone metastasis.

Triple Phosphate (Struvite)

These are 'coffin lid'-shaped crystals, seen in conditions such as: alkaline urine, UTI from urease producing bacteria (Proteus, Klebsiella) (Fig. 22.6).

Cysteine

These are colorless crystals with hexagonal shape. It is associated with cystinuria (Fig. 22.7).

Figure 22.7: Cystein crystal

URINE DIPSTICK TEST

It is a screening and/or diagnostic technique used to detect materials or biological material in the urine associated with renal failure, metabolic diseases, or urinary tract infections (UTI). The presence of normal and abnormal chemical components in the urine can be detected using a dry reagent strips called dipsticks. These strips are impregnated with chromogen and reagents (Figs 22.8 and 22.9).

The test strips are dipped in the urine, following which the reagents are activated and a chemical reaction occurs. The chemical reaction results in a specific color change, which is then compared with the available color codes.

Dipstick testing is quite helpful; it can be used as a definitive test for certain disorders and as a screening test for others. Dipstick testing should be correlated with microscopy and clinical indicators in complicated cases or serious diseases.

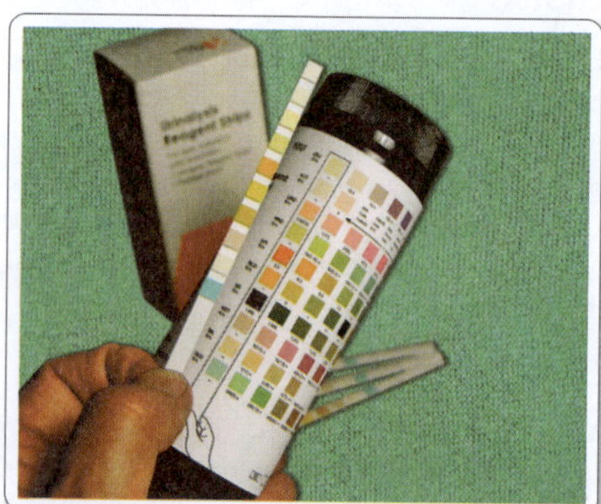
Figure 22.8: Urine dipstick test kit

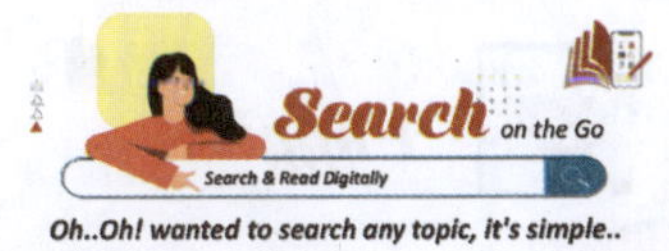

Specific gravity densidad densidade 60 sec/seg.	1.000	1.005	1.010	1.015	1.020	1.025	1.030	
pH 60 sec/seg.	5.0	6.0	6.5	7.0	8.0	9.0		
Leukocytes leucocitos 60–120 sec/seg.	Neg.	ca.15	ca.75	ca.125	ca.500 Leuko/μL			
Blood/hemoglobin/ sang(re)(ue)/ hemaglobina 60 sec/seg.	Neg.	ca. 5–10	ca. 10	ca. 25	ca. 25	ca. 50	ca. 50	ca. 250 Ery/μL
Nitrite/nitrito/nitritos 60 Sec/seg.	Neg.	+	++					
Ketones/ C. cetonicos 60 sec/seg.	Neg.	5 (0.5)	15 (1.5)	50 (5)	150 (15) mg/dL (mmoL/L)			
Bilirubin/bilirrubina 60 sec/seg.	Neg.	+	++	+++				
Urobilinogen(0)/ urobilinogênio 60 sec/seg.	Normal	1 (17)	4 (70)	8 (140)	12 (200) mg/dL (μmol/L)			
Protein/proteinas/ proteinas 60sec/seg.	Neg.	15 (0.15)	30 (0.3)	100 (1)	300 (3)	1000 (10) mg/dL (g/L)		
Glucose/glucosa/ glicose 60 sec/seg.	Normal	100 (5.5)	300 (17)	1000 (55) mg/dL (mmol/L)				

IVD

+30° C

+2° C

2011-02

23054941

LOT

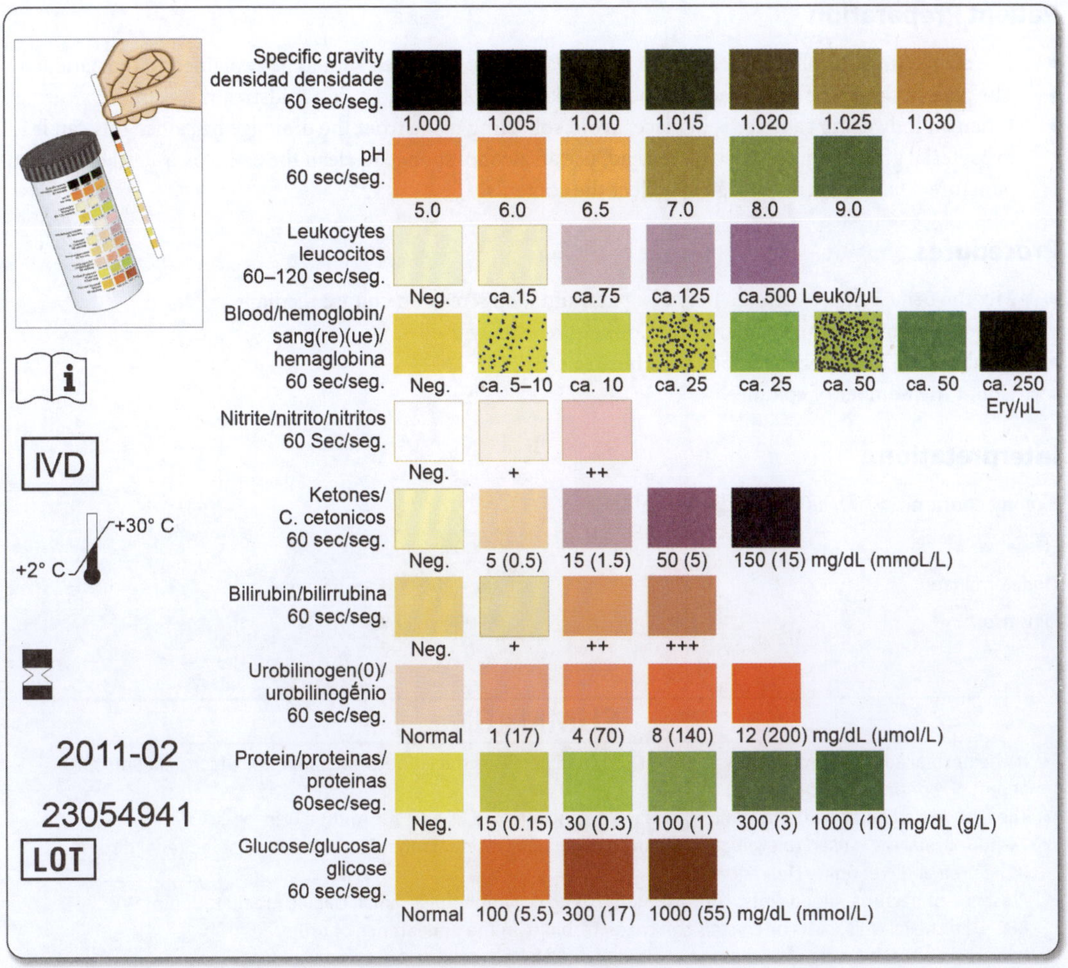

Figure 22.9: Dipstick urinalysis chart

URINE CULTURE AND SENSITIVITY TEST

Urine culture test is done to cultivate and identify organisms that may cause a urinary tract infection (UTI), primarily bacteria and fungus. Urine is typically sterile and organism-free when it is in the bladder. Compared to adult males, females and children are more likely to get urinary tract infections.

When a person exhibits symptoms, like painful and frequent urination, urine culture and sensitivity are used to diagnose and test for diseases or medical conditions associated with urinary tract infections.

The term "sensitivity" describes an antibiotic's ability to effectively inhibit microorganisms. Clinical response can vary, even though it usually follows therapy that is directed by sensitivity testing.

Type of Sample

Clear catch midstream collection. The best specimens are those obtained early in the morning after the bladder has been incubated overnight and have the highest bacterial counts.

Patient Preparation

- The correct way to collect a clean catch midstream urine specimen should be explained to the patient.
- The patient should be explained to wipe their skin completely and take a midstream specimen.
- When an indwelling catheter is in place, avoid collecting urine from the drainage bag since this can lead to bacterial growth within the bag. Instead, use an alcohol sponge to clean the catheter, a sterile needle to puncture it, and a sterile syringe to collect the contents.

Procedures

- Mix the urine sample with the help of a platinum loop streak on culture media
- Standard nutrient agar, standard MacConkey are usually used
- Incubate at 37°C aerobically for 24–28 hours
- Count the number of colonies.

Interpretation

Colony count no. >100,000/mL indicates infection

Negative	<10,000 colonies/mL
Indeterminate	10,000–100,000 colonies/mL
Positive	>100,000 colonies/mL

SUMMARY

- In the normal adult, approximately 1,200 mL of blood perfuses the kidneys each minute, which accounts for about 25% of the cardiac output.
- The first voided morning urine, which is the most concentrated, is best for routine urinalysis
- 24-hour urinalysis is used to evaluate proteinuria, estimate residual renal function in end-stage renal disease using urea and creatinine clearance.
- Presence of bacteria, blood clots, contrast media, mucus, lymph fluids, small calculi, precipitation of WBC's, RBC's, epithelial cells, casts or crystals can cause turbidity in the appearance of urine.
- Polyuria can result from either diabetes insipidus or diabetes mellitus.
- Cloudy urine can be attributed to the presence of various cellular elements.
- Urine normally will have a faint, aromatic odor of undetermined source.
- Acid urine may be produced by a diet high in meat protein and with some fruits, such as cranberries.
- Normal adults with adequate fluid intake will produce urine of specific gravity 1.016–1.022 over a 24-hour period.
- Benzidine test is used for the determination of blood (RBC's or hemoglobin) in urine.
- The presence of detectable amounts of glucose in urine is termed glycosuria.
- Reducing sugars (monosaccharides and some disaccharides) with free ketone or aldehyde functional groups can be identified by the Benedict's test.
- Tamm-Horsfall protein is the glycoprotein secreted by the thick part of the ascending loop of Henle (and possibly the distal tubule), which constitutes about one-third of the total urinary protein in normal individuals.
- Urine contains a significant amount of metabolic end products, which can precipitate as crystals.
- Struvite crystals are 'coffin lid'-shaped crystals which are seen in conditions such as: alkaline urine, UTI from urease-producing bacteria (Proteus, Klebsiella).
- In urine dipstick test, presence of normal and abnormal chemical components in the urine can be detected using a dry reagent strips called dipsticks.

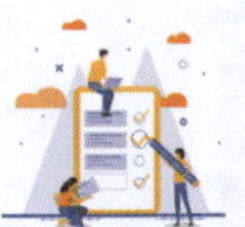

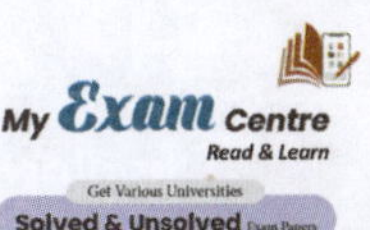

ASSESS YOURSELF

Long Answer Questions

1. Explain various types of urine sample and procedure for collection of 24-hour urine sample.
2. Discuss physical examination of urine in detail.

Short Answer Questions

1. What is Benedict's test?
2. Write about types of urine crystals.
3. Write short notes on:
   i. Examination of urine segment
   ii. Urine culture and sensitivity test

Multiple Choice Questions

1. **Which test is done to detect ketones in urine sample of a diabetic patient?**
   a. Rothera's test
   b. Heat coagulation test
   c. Benedict's test
   d. Benzidine test
2. **Fruity odor of urine is present in:**
   a. Bacterial decomposition
   b. Diabetic ketoacidosis
   c. UTI
   d. Phenylketonuria
3. **Benzidine test is used to identify _______________ in urine.**
   a. Proteins
   b. Occult blood
   c. Bile salts
   d. Ketones
4. **False positive tests for hematuria on urinalysis may occur due to:**
   a. Myoglobin
   b. Glomerulonephritis
   c. Urinary tract infection
   d. Renal cell carcinoma
5. **A possible contraindication for performing urinalysis on a sample is:**
   a. Late menstruation
   b. Urinary frequency
   c. Aged sample
   d. Fever
6. **Oliguria refers to urine output less than _______________.**
   a. 150 mL/day
   b. 500 mL/day
   c. 400 mL/day
   d. 200 mL/day

Answer Key

1. a **2.** b **3.** b **4.** a **5.** c **6.** c

Chapter 23

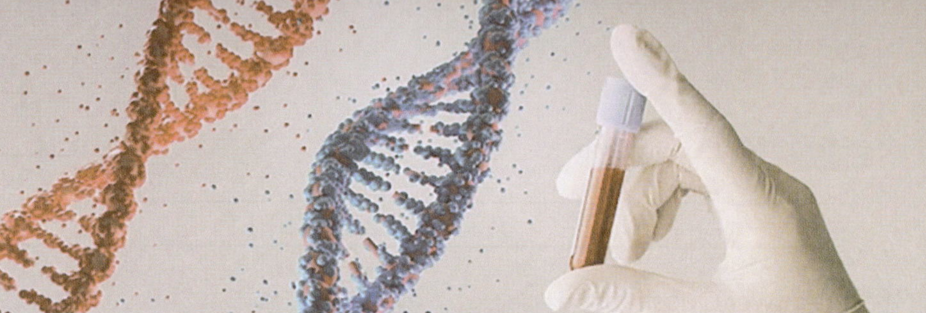

Examination of Feces

LEARNING OBJECTIVES

After the completion of the chapter, the readers will be able to:
- Explain indications and sample for stool examination.
- Describe macroscopic or gross examination of feces.
- Discuss microscopic examination of feces.
- Analyze chemical examination of stool.
- Describe procedure for taking stool culture.

CHAPTER OUTLINE

- Introduction
- Indications for Stool Examination
- Sample for Stool Examination
- Macroscopic or Gross Appearance of the Stool
- Microscopic Examination of the Stool
- Chemical Examination of the Stool
- Stool Analysis
- Stool Culture
- Other Stool Tests

KEY TERMS

Bristol stool chart: It is used to evaluate the consistency of stool. It is used to classify the form of human feces into seven categories.

Cellophane tape test: It is used to pick up the ova of *Entrobius vermicularis* from the perianal area.

Steatorrhea: Steatorrhea is an increase in fat excretion in the stools. It is one of the clinical features of fat malabsorption and noted in many conditions such as exocrine pancreatic insufficiency (EPI), celiac disease, and tropical sprue.

INTRODUCTION

Stool investigations provide vital information regarding conditions affecting the gastrointestinal tract. Stool can be investigated macroscopically, microscopically, chemically and immunologically, and microbiologically. The stool samples that will be tested should to be collected as soon as possible, stored in a clean container or both.

INDICATIONS FOR STOOL EXAMINATION

- To assess the gastrointestinal tract's integrity and functionality.
- To exclude the possibility of white blood cells (WBCs) and red blood cells (RBCs).

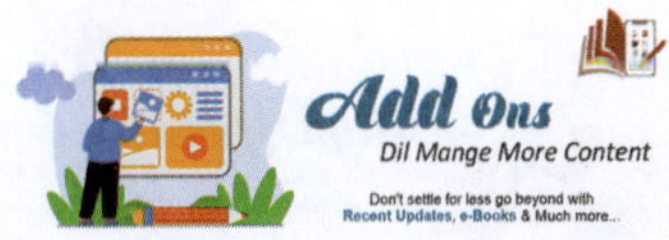

- To identify parasites or ova.
- To check for fat if malabsorption syndrome is present.
- For the purpose of colon cancer screening.
- For GI tract ulceration that exhibits no symptoms.
- Examining illnesses when constipation and diarrhea are present.

SAMPLE FOR STOOL EXAMINATION

- The fresh stool should be examined for moving organisms.
- Helminths and protozoa can be treated with stool in 10% formalin.
- The stool is concentrated using a formalin-ethyl acetate stool.
- Two to five grams of stool is the minimum amount required for the examination.
- For ova and parasites, there are three methods:
  - Direct stool examination.
  - Concentration method.
  - The permanent stain of the stool.
- The patients should be given the following information for at least 48 hours prior to the stool collection.
  - Avoid mineral oils.
  - Do not take bismuth.
  - Don't take antibiotics, like tetracyclines.
  - Anti-diarrheal drugs are nonabsorbent.
  - Avoid anti-malarial drugs.
  - The patient should not have a barium swallow examination before the stool examination.
  - Stop iron-containing drugs, meat, and fish 48 hours before the collection for occult blood.
- For the ova and parasites, warm stools are preferable.
- Storing feces in the refrigerator can cause ova and parasites.
- Formalin and polyvinyl alcohol can be used to collect stool samples for parasites and ova. These have a fixative purpose.
- Since the majority of pathogens are found in blood or mucus, these materials should be included in the stool, if they are present.

MACROSCOPIC OR GROSS APPEARANCE OF THE STOOL

Samples need to be examined as soon as they are collected. Long-standing samples will deteriorate helminthes, ova, other parasites, and increase the number of bacteria and monilia, which will produce inaccurate results. Nevertheless, the following features of stool should be examined.

Stool samples should be evaluated macroscopically in terms of color, consistency, quantity, form, odor, and presence of mucus.

- **Quantity:** Normally, the body eliminates waste products once or twice daily. An adult human excretes between 100 and 250 g (3 and 8 ounces) of feces every day. The typical composition of feces is 25% solid matter and 75% water.
- **Consistency and form:** Stool consistency is considered a good predictor of bowel function since it has a high correlation with both stool transit time and frequency of bowel movements. Recurrent passages of firm or loose stools and irregular bowel movements (too frequent or infrequent) can suggest irritable bowel syndrome (IBS) or functional constipation. Modified Bristol chart is used to evaluate the stool consistency (Fig. 23.1).

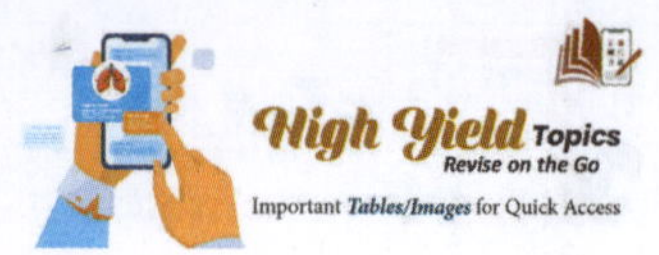

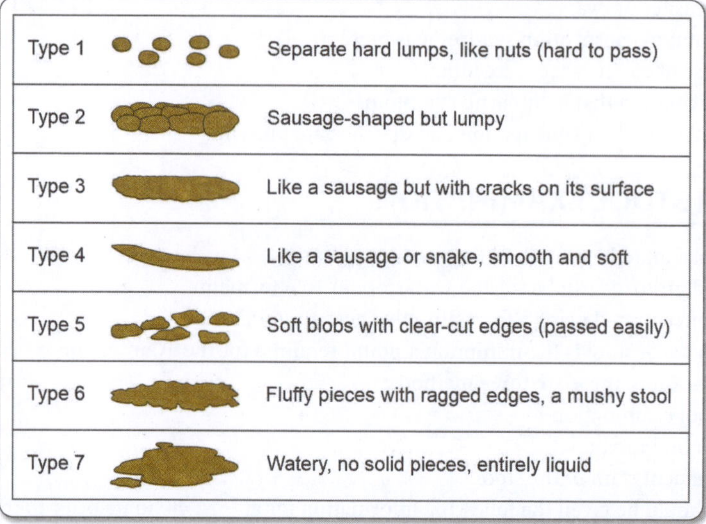

Type 1		Separate hard lumps, like nuts (hard to pass)
Type 2		Sausage-shaped but lumpy
Type 3		Like a sausage but with cracks on its surface
Type 4		Like a sausage or snake, smooth and soft
Type 5		Soft blobs with clear-cut edges (passed easily)
Type 6		Fluffy pieces with ragged edges, a mushy stool
Type 7		Watery, no solid pieces, entirely liquid

Figure 23.1: Bristol stool chart for assessing the stool consistency

A typical stool is well-formed. However, the stool is solid (hard) in constipation (dehydration) and semi-solid (soft or loose) in response to some drugs and laxatives. Stool appears liquid or watery in instances of abnormality such as diarrhea and dysentery. Stools from cholera appear like rice water. Stools from fat malabsorption are often pale, thick, and semi-solid.

Thus, regular bowel movements and a normal condition of stool are desirable for good health.

- **Color:** Stools often range in color from light brown to dark brown because of the presence of bile pigments.
  - **Dark black:** If the bleeding is occurring in the small intestines, the stools will appear dark and tarry as a result of the production of acid hematin. Stool may appear brilliant red in cases of bleeding in the large intestines or the rectum, because it contains fresh blood.
  - **Red:** Stool appears red after consuming some colorful foods, such as red beets.
  - **Clay color:** If there is a biliary tract blockage, the stool may have a clay color because of the absence of stercobilinogen.
- **Odor:** The combination of Indole and Skatol produced the typical feces odor. Stool odor might become offensive in conditions such as intestinal amebiasis. Due to the lack of fecal matter, stools in cholera and bacillary dysentery cases do not smell bad.
- **Blood:** The blood is present on the outer surface of the feces and this caused either by contamination from menstrual cycle blood in women or bleeding hemorrhoids from the blood vessels. Blood should be noted in stools if present as it is indicative of ulceration or presence of any other pathology, like malignancy.

  Stool color varies greatly depending on diet. Clay-colored or putty colored stool is observed in biliary obstructions. If more than 100 mL blood is lost from the upper gastrointestinal system, black, tarry stool is observed. Besides bleeding, black-colored stool may also be observed due to iron or bismuth treatment. Red-colored stool is observed in lower gastrointestinal tract bleeding.
- **Mucus:** The presence of a small amount of mucus in stool is normal. However, the presence of copious mucus or bloody mucus is abnormal.

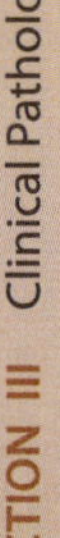

- **Parasite:** Stools may contain adult helminthes. Nematodes, like Ascaris are easily visible as their size is large. Hookworms and Proglottids of cetodes may also be present. These may be visible to the naked eye (Fig. 23.2).

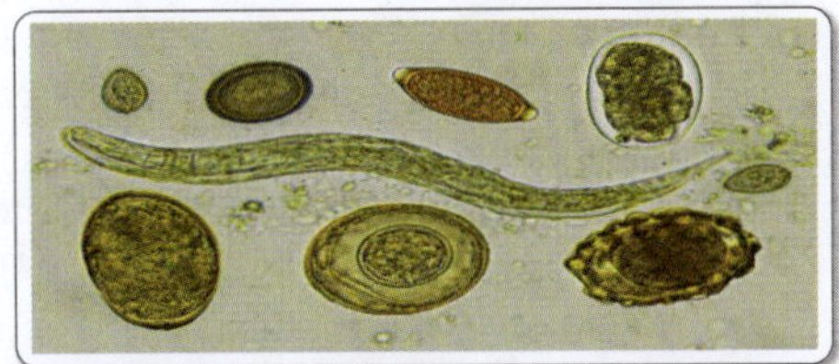

Figure 23.2: Morphology of common helminthes ova found in stool specimen

- **Detection of fat in the stool:** <6 g of fat is excreted daily in the feces by healthy humans, and this amount does not change even if they consume 100–125 g of fat each day. In people without fat malabsorption who have diarrhea, there may be a slight increase in the excretion of fat in the stool. Stool fat quantification is the gold standard for diagnosing steatorrhea. In order to achieve this goal, the patient is placed on a daily diet containing 100 g of fat, and the feces is collected for 72 hours. The Sudan III stain and acid steatocrit tests are used for detection of fat in the stool.

MICROSCOPIC EXAMINATION OF THE STOOL

Microscopic examination of feces is the most crucial step in the diagnosis of intestinal problems and stool abnormalities. Microscopic analysis is a diagnostic method used to identify helminths, protozoa, and fecal leukocytes. The stool can be examined by the following techniques:

- **Saline wet mount examination:** A large drop of the feces is emulsified in normal saline, put on a glass slide, and then covered with a cover slide. After that, the specimen should be inspected under a light microscope. To view large molecules, cells, ova, and helminthes, firstly observe it through a 10x objective lens. Then adjust it to a 40x objective.
- **Iodine examination:** Iodine stains the glycogen in ova and cysts, it improves visibility of their morphological characteristics. Nevertheless, method has the drawback since the iodine kills the live trophozoites of Entamoeba histolytica and other live parasites, they cannot be observed. For the iodine test, the same examination instructions as for the normal saline must be followed.
- **Buffered methylene blue stain:** It is used for the Nuclear stain in Entamoeba histolytica
- **Cellophane tape test:** NIH swab (National Institute of Health) is used to pick up the ova of *Entrobius vermicularis* from the perianal area.

MUST KNOW

- It is possible to analyze fresh feces right away for moving organisms.
- For helminths and protozoa, the feces may be preserved in 10% formalin if examination is not possible immediately.
- Two to five grams of feces is the minimum amount needed for testing.
- To examine parasites, at least three consecutive stool samples are needed.

Microscopic examination includes the following:

Examine fecal specimens using a light microscope with 10x and 40x objectives, noting any:

- **Pus cells:**
  - **Excessive amounts of pus cells:** Shigellosis is characterized by clusters of pus cells that exceed 50 cells per high power field, erythrocytes, and macrophages.
  - Infections caused by invasive *E. coli* and salmonellosis are associated with fewer pus cells—less than 20 per high power field.
- RBCs
- Monilia

- **Protozoa:** *Giardia*, *Cryptosporidium* spp., *Dientamoeba fragilis*, *Entamoeba* spp. (including nonpathogenic species), *Blastocystis* spp., and *Cyclospora cayetanensis* are the most common pathogenic protozoa reported in stool samples.
  - ***Entamoeba histolytica*:** To investigate the vegetative phase (trophozoite) and cyst, causing amoebic dysentery disease (Figs 23.3 and 23.4).
  - ***Entamoeba coli*:** Trophozoite + cyst
  - ***Giardia lamblia*:** Trophozoite + cyst (Figs 23.5 and 23.6), cause watery diarrhea disease in children, especially. Giardiasis is a common gastrointestinal parasitic infection associated with diarrhea, stomach cramps, upset stomach, and excessive gas.
  - ***Balantidium coli*:** Trophozoite + cyst, causing Balantidiasis in colon.

CLINICAL CORRELATION

Entamoeba histolytica (*E. histolytica*) cysts and trophozoites are examined under a microscope in order to diagnose intestinal amoebiasis. To search for trophozoites, staining with iron hematoxylin and/or Wheatley trichrome is recommended. With *E. dispar*, phagocyted erythrocytes can also be observed.

Microscopy examinations are unable to distinguish between strains of *Entamoeba histolytica*, *Entamoeba dispar*, and *Entamoeba moshkovskii*. Due to the fluctuating excretion of cysts and trophozoites, it may be necessary to send three samples on different days in order to detect infection. To find cysts, the samples are intensified and stained with iodine.

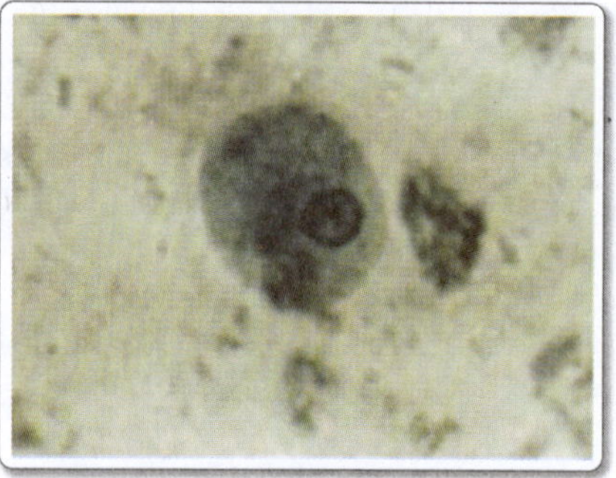

Figure 23.3: Entamoeba histolytica (trophoziot)

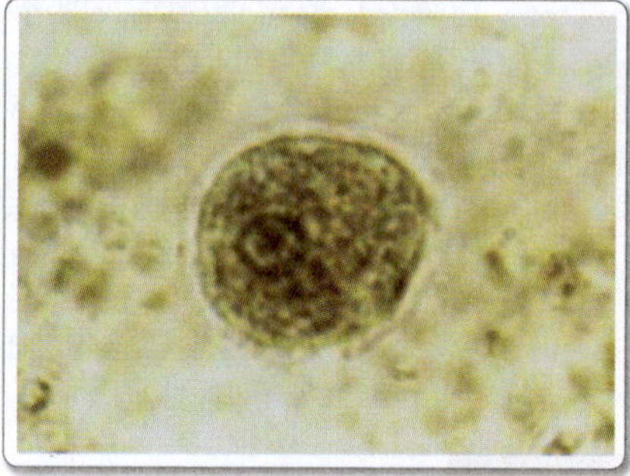

Figure 23.4: Entamoeba histolytica (cyst)

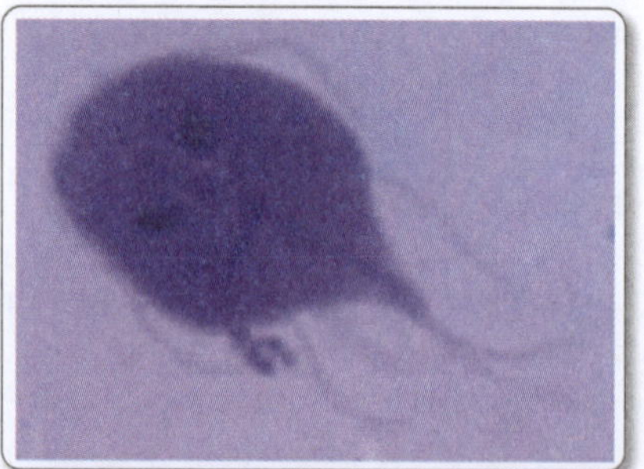

Figure 23.5: Giardia lamblia (trophoziot)

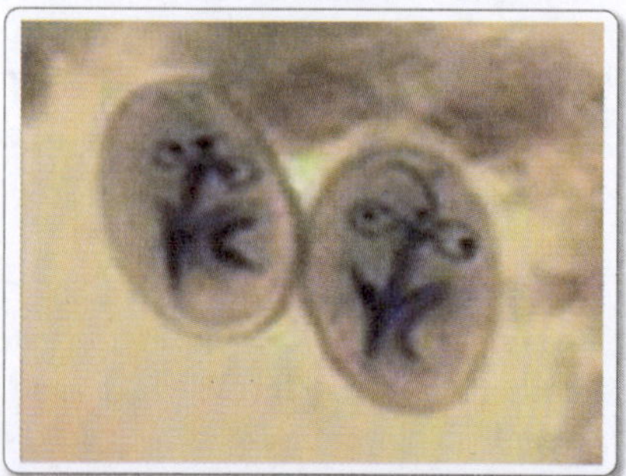

Figure 23.6: Giardia lamblia (cyst)

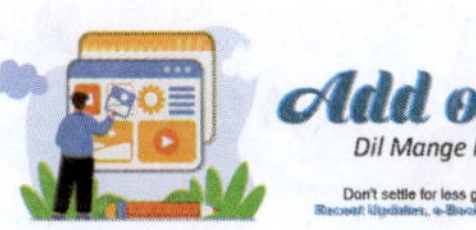

- **Worms**
  - ***Enterobius vermicularis* (pinworm):** Investigating the eggs that are of convex and flat surface and a pointed end.
  - ***Ascaris lumbricoides*:** Investigating for eggs which is characterized by the content of granular yellow to brown irregular albumin membrane.
  - **Hookworm (*Ancylostoma duodenale*):** Investigating the eggs where the egg yolk is divided and surrounded by a thin membrane.
  - **Tapeworms, (*Taenia solium*):** Investigating the worm pieces called gravid segments or Proglottids that come out with the feces.
  - ***Schistosoma mansoni*:** Investigating the eggs distinct by lateral spin.

CHEMICAL EXAMINATION OF THE STOOL

- **pH:** This pH of stools is acidic in amoebic dysentery and is alkaline in bacillary dysentery.
- **Occult blood:** A number of diseases, including gastrointestinal tract cancer, can present with occult blood. Powdered benzidine is the reagent used. A test tube is filled with a pinch of benzidine powder, one or two drops of glacial acetic acid, and thorough mixing. One milliliter of hydrogen peroxide is added to this and is stirred well. After that, place a clean glass slide on top of a tiny amount of feces. Apply one or two drops of the previously made benzidine mixture to the stool specimen that was placed on the glass slide, then watch for a color change. A change in color from green to blue indicates that there may be occult blood in the stool sample.
- **Reducing factors:** Mono- and di-sucrose levels in stool (0.25 mg/dL); any increase in these levels suggests a disruption in the enzymes lactase and sucrase, which are responsible for breaking down sugar (e.g., Lactase, sucrase).

STOOL ANALYSIS

Characteristics of normal and abnormal stool is depicted in Table 23.1.

Table 23.1: Characteristics of normal and abnormal stool

Normal	The stool appears brown, soft, and well-formed in consistency.
	The stool does not contain blood, mucus, pus, undigested meat fibers, harmful bacteria, viruses, fungi, or parasites.
	The stool is shaped like a tube.
	The pH of the stool is 7–7.5.
	The stool contains <0.25 (g/dL) of reducing sugar.
	The stool contains 2–7 g of fat per 24 hours.
Abnormal	The stool is black, red, white, yellow or green.
	The stool is liquid or very hard.
	There is too much stool.
	The stool contains blood, mucus, pus, undigested meat fibers, harmful bacteria, viruses, fungi or parasites.
	The stool contains low levels of enzymes, such as trypsin or elastase.
	The pH of the stool is <7.0 or g >7.5.
	The stool contains 0.25 g/dL or more of sugars (reducing factors).
	The stool contains more than 7 g/24 hours of fat (if your fat intake is about 100 g a day).

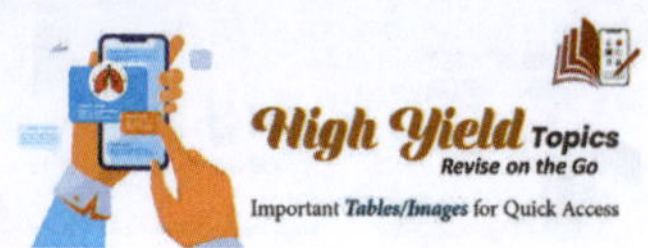

STOOL CULTURE

- A minimum of 4 mL or 4 cm^3 of feces specimen is collected and placed in a dry, clean container with a tight-fitting cover.
- Avoid leaving the sample out for an extended amount of time; ideally, it should be examined within an hour of the sample being taken in order to prevent eccentric parasite death.
- The optimum time to collect a sample is early in the morning because there is a higher likelihood of complicated parasites and eggs emerging due to the stool being present all night.
- To avoid contaminating the stool sample with urine, it is preferable for children to urinate prior to collecting a stool sample.
- Menstrual blood, water, soil, or urine shouldn't contaminate stool. Water and urine kill trophozoites, while dirt introduces foreign organisms and prevents thorough investigation.
- The sample container needs to be labeled with the patient's name, date, time, and number.
- As soon as the stool is received at the laboratory, it should be tested (ideally, within an hour after collection).
- Samples should be refrigerated if a delay in investigation is expected, as warm, recently passed feces are the ideal environment for parasite detection.
- The patient cannot use laxatives before obtaining a stool sample.

Procedures

Stool is cultured by looping a sample and culturing it on various culture media types based on the type of bacteria or case diagnosis being examined.

- If the patient is suspected to have cholera, it is grown on Thiosulfate citrate bile salts sucrose agar medium.
- If the patient is suspected of having gastrointestinal tuberculosis, it is cultured on Lowenstein-Jensen medium for *Mycobacterium tuberculosis*.
- If *Staphylococcus aureus* infection is suspected, it is cultivated on blood agar because it is hemolytic.
- To find lactose fermentation bacteria in pink colonies, such as *Enterobacter, Klebsiella*, and *E. coli*, it is cultivated on MacConkey agar medium. However, if it's not a lactose fermenter, it's either pseudomonas, which can be determined by the pyocynin test, or Proteus, which may be determined by the diffusion phenomenon. Additionally, to differentiate between Salmonella and Shigella through the use of biochemical and serological testing.

OTHER STOOL TESTS

- **Rotavirus rapid test:** The rotavirus test is a stool test used to diagnose a rotavirus infection. Rotavirus affects the intestines and causes vomiting and diarrhea. This infection is especially common in young children, but it can affect adults, too. A rotavirus infection causes a condition called viral gastroenteritis. To perform the Rotavirus rapid test, an aliquot of diluted stool sample is added to the sample well of the Rotavirus rapid test cassette. The sample flows through a label pad containing rotavirus antibody. If the sample on the Rotavirus rapid test contains rotavirus antigens, the antigen will bind to the antibody coated on the colloidal gold particles to form antigen-antibody-gold complexes.
- ***H. pylori* antigen stool test:** *Helicobacter pylori* (*H. pylori*) bacteria are a common cause of peptic ulcers (sores in the lining of the stomach, small intestine, or esophagus). In this test (Fig. 23.7), a stool (feces) sample is used to determine if *H. pylori* antigens are present in the gastrointestinal (GI) system.

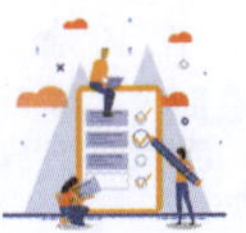

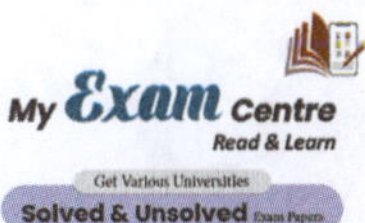

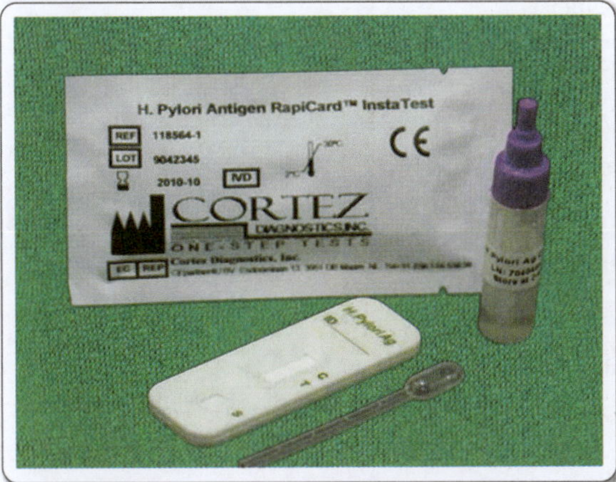

Figure 23.7: *H. pylori* antigen stool test kit

SUMMARY

- Stool examination is carried out in laboratories for various diagnostic purposes.
- A clean container which does not contain any detergent or disinfectant is sufficient for all types of stool examinations including stool culture.
- Physical examination of the stool for the following aspects of stool should be examined for its quantity, Consistency and form, color, odor, blood, mucus, parasite.
- The laboratory diagnosis of most parasitic infections is by the demonstration of ova of the parasite in the stools of the infected person.
- The stool can be examined by the following techniques, namely wet Mount examination, Iodine preparation, Buffered methylene blue stain, Cellophane tape test: NIH swab and concentration techniques.

ASSESS YOURSELF

Long Answer Questions

1. Explain the techniques used for stool examination.
2. Discuss stool culture.

Short Answer Questions

1. What is Bristol stool culture?
2. Write about chemical examination of stool.
3. Write short notes on:
   i. Iodine examination
   ii. Occult blood

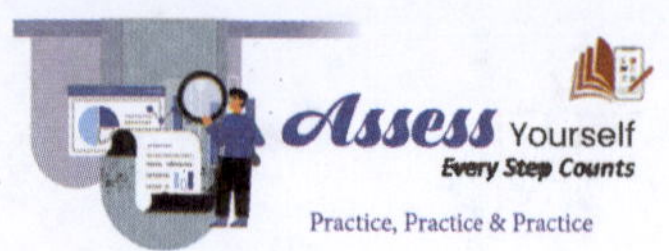

Multiple Choice Questions

1. **Stool sample is collected:**
   a. On fasting
   b. Randomly
   c. At night
   d. Early morning
2. **Which fecal test requires a 3-day specimen?**
   a. Fecal occult blood
   b. APT test
   c. Elastase I
   d. Quantitaive fecal fat testing
3. **Stools from persons with steatorrhea will contain excess amount of:**
   a. Barium sulfate
   b. Blood
   c. Fat
   d. Mucus
4. **A black tarry stool is indicative of:**
   a. Upper GI bleeding
   b. Lower GI bleeding
   c. Excess fat
   d. Excess carbohydrate

Answer Key

1. d **2.** d **3.** c **4.** a

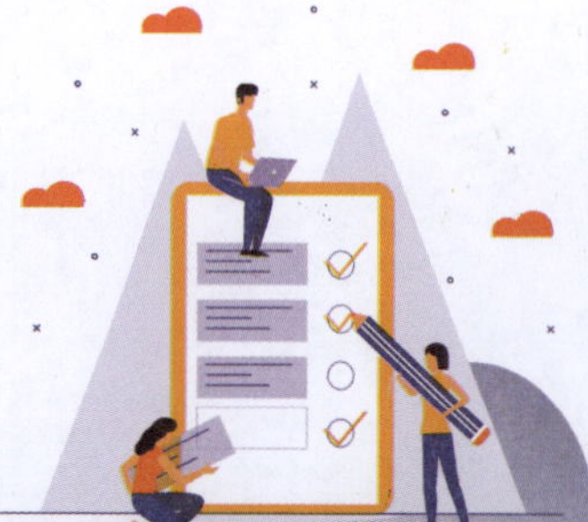

SECTION IV

Genetics

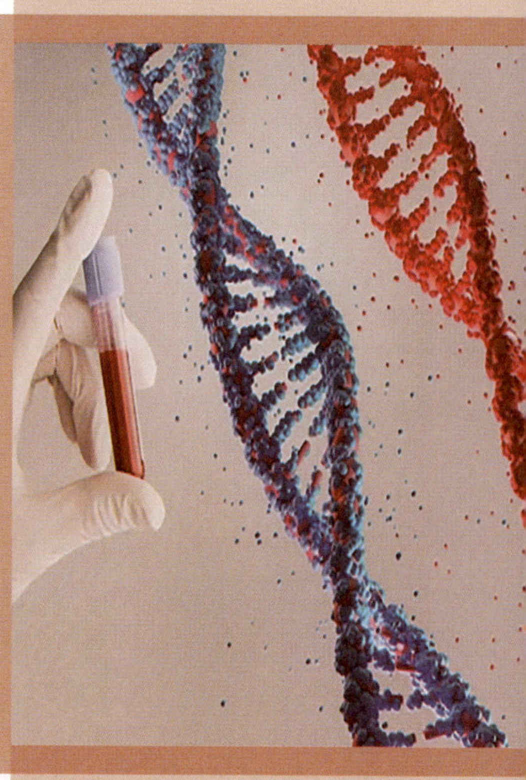

SECTION OUTLINE

Chapter 24

Basics of Genetics

LEARNING OBJECTIVES

After the completion of the chapter, the readers will be able to:
- Discuss basic concepts of genetics.
- Explain the practical applications of genetics.
- Understand the pattern of inheritance.

CHAPTER OUTLINE

- Introduction
- Branches of Genetics
- Practical Applications/Role of Nurses in Genetics
- Impact of Genetic Condition in Families
- Factors Impacting Genetic Conditions in Families
- Basic Structures Involved in Genetics
- Review of Cell Division: Mitosis and Meiosis
- Chromosomes: Sex Determination
- Gene Mutations/Errors in Transmission
- Chromosomal Aberrations
- Patterns of Inheritance
- Mechanism of Inheritance
- Multiple Alleles and Blood Groups

KEY TERMS

Allele: One of the two or more versions of DNA sequence (a single base or a segment of bases) at a given genomic location. An individual inherits two alleles, one from each parent, for any given genomic location where such variation exists.

Di hybrid cross: A cross between two individuals differing in two characteristics.

Dominant: Allele that is always expressed when present, regardless of whether the organism is homozygous or heterozygous for that gene.

Gene expression: Process by which information from a gene is used in the synthesis of a functional gene product. These products are often proteins.

Genes: The basic physical and functional unit of heredity. Genes are made up of DNA.

Genetics: The study of heredity is called genetics.

Genotype: The genetic make-up of an individual.

Heredity: The process of passing of traits from one generation to another.

Heterozygous: Possessing a pair of different alleles for a particular locus (Tt).

Homozygous: Possessing a pair of identical alleles for a particular locus (TT/tt).

Hybrid: An offspring resulting from the mating between individuals of two different genetic constitutions.

Locus: Location of allelic genes on the chromosome.

Mono hybrid cross: A cross between two individuals differing in one characteristic.

Phenotype: The outward expression of genotype is called phenotype.

Contd...

Recessive: An allele that is only expressed when the organism is homozygous and not expressed when heterozygous (when paired with a dominant allele).

Trait: A specific characteristic of an individual that can be passed from parent to offspring.

INTRODUCTION

Human genetic diseases are not related to gender, age, race, religion, economic or social status. Although many relate it to infancy or childhood. Genetic disease can be manifested at any time in the life cycle. Contribution of genetics to diseases such as cancer and Alzheimer disease is well established. The improved detection, testing methods and evolved clinical practices have resulted in patient survival with genetic disease.

- Heredity describes how some traits are passed from parents to their children.
- The traits are expressed by genes, which are small sections of DNA that are coded for specific traits.
- Genes are found in chromosomes.
- Humans have two sets of 23 chromosomes one set from each parent.

BRANCHES OF GENETICS

The following are the branches of genetics:

- Cytogenetics
- Molecular genetics
- Biochemical genetics
- Cancer genetics
- Immunogenetics
- Developmental genetics
- Behavioral genetics
- Population genetics

PRACTICAL APPLICATIONS/ROLE OF NURSES IN GENETICS

Nurses need to understand and distinguish the adult genetic disorders from childhood genetic disorders. The role of nurses differs based on the type of genetic disorders and the needs of the patient and his/her family. The following are some of the roles and responsibilities played by the modern nurses while handling the patient suffering from genetic disorders.

Understanding Genetic Basis of Disease

Early diagnosis of genetic disorders may contribute toward health promotion with genetic aspects. It also helps to prevent genetic conditions, their management and care of genetic disorders. Understanding genetic basis of diseases depends on:

- Planning, implementing, and evaluating genetic disorders.
- Screening or testing programs.
- Managing home care therapy.
- Developing an individual plan of care.

Genetic Information and Counseling

A nurse must keep a neutral opinion about genetically acquired issues. Genetics information and counseling starts with taking family histories that are comprehensive and relevant to genetic disorders. It involves:

- Interviewing clients.
- Applying fundamental skills learnt in the nursing courses.
- Following up on newborn screening.

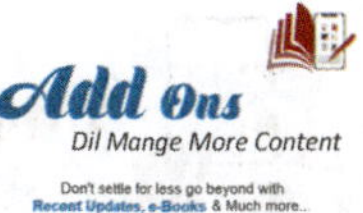

Referral Services

- Assessing the needs and interactions in clients and his/her family.
- Working with families under stress of genetic disorders.
- Remaining resourceful about the referral options.

Handling Social and Ethical Issues Related to Genetics

- Advocating and supporting for genetic disorders patients and their families.
- Monitoring and evaluation of patients with genetic disorders on ethical grounds.
- Maintaining respect, confidentiality and trust while working on issues related to genetics.

Understanding Genetic Basis of Disease

Knowledge of genetics helps to:

- Understand the genetic basis of a noncurable disease.
- Understand the role of genes in causing genetic defects and its consequences.
- Know the effects of abnormal cell division and genetic regulation on the disease manifestation.
- Know the way of progression of genetical diseases from one generation to the next.
- Understand the role played by genetic factors in an individual's health.
- Analyze the basic mechanisms of inheritance and transmission genes.

Early and Effective Diagnosis of Genetic Disorders

The early and effective diagnosis of genetic disorders helps in:

- Having information about genetic risk, genetic testing and the implications.
- Interpreting the results of genetic tests in meaningful manner.
- Creating awareness of the possibility of an inherited or genetic component for a client condition and knowledge of cardinal features of familial predisposition.
- Preventing of diseases with early diagnosis and treatment. For example, phenylketonuria (PKU)-related mental retardation could be prevented with early newborn screening, diagnosis and diet management.

Understanding Correlation between Environment and Genetical Changes

- To understand how structural changes at gene level can bring big transformations and cause diseases such as diabetes Type 1.
- To promote healthy prenatal environment to ensure minimal risk of genetic defects among newborns.

Applying Genetic Approach While Caring Patients with Genetic Disorders

Knowledge of genetics empowers a nurse with skills to manage and care patients with genetic disorders with understanding of complex mechanisms.

IMPACT OF GENETIC CONDITION ON FAMILIES

Cognitive impact: This involves information processing, applying intelligence, reasoning, memory and language development. Cognitive disabilities produce physical restrictions to:

- Inability to interpret the information.

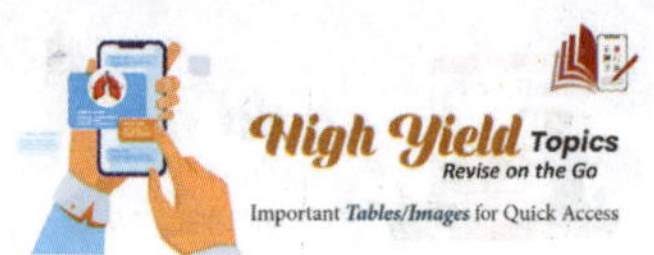

- Difficulties with spoken and written languages.
- Difficulties with coordination and self-control.
- Difficulties with learning.

Psychological impact: Every genetic diagnosis does not eventually develop into genetic disorder, however it will impact the psychology of the individual and the other family members.

- It will cause tension in the family when the diagnosis is made after birth of baby, and if it is made during pregnancy, it may create a difference of opinion to have a child or not.
- It makes one to feel low.
- Family may feel profound grief, guilt and shame.
- The sufferer and the family members may undergo depression and fear due to anticipated survival outcome of the disorder.

Social impact:

- Genetic disorder will pose a social stigma on the family members.
- Fear of society's opinion and acceptance makes families hesitant disclose the diagnosis results.
- It becomes difficult to select marriage partners.
- Normal relationship between parents and child gets impacted.

Economic impact: The economic impact of genetic disorders is terrible on families with low socioeconomic status.

- The cost of diagnosis of genetic disease is unaffordable for some families.
- Most of the genetic diagnostic tests are costly so the family cannot afford the cost.
- Genetic treatment and health management become a burden.
- Loss of job and job discrimination.

Emotional impact: Patient and family both go through the following emotional impact:

- Anxiety
- Guilt
- Anger
- Sadness and uncertainty about future

FACTORS IMPACTING GENETIC CONDITIONS IN FAMILIES

Genetic disorders can be caused by mutation in one gene (monogenic disorder), by mutations in multiple genes (multifactorial inheritance disorders), by a combination of environmental factors and gene mutations, or by damage to the chromosomes which changes the number or/and structure of whole chromosome.

- **Mutations:** Some diseases, caused by mutations are inherited from the parents and are present in an individual at birth, like sickle cell disease. Other diseases are caused by acquired mutations in a gene or group of genes that occur during a person's life.
- **Environment:** Some harmful environmental factors can change a gene's nucleotide sequence. For example, UV radiation can break DNA strands. Certain chemicals, like those in plastic or cigarette smoke, change the chemical behavior of DNA bases, which can cause one DNA base to substitute for another.
- **Migration of small founding populations followed by population expansion**: It depends on whether the genetically affected child with inherited mutated genes survives to adulthood and reproduces and whether that child's children survive to reproduce, and so on.

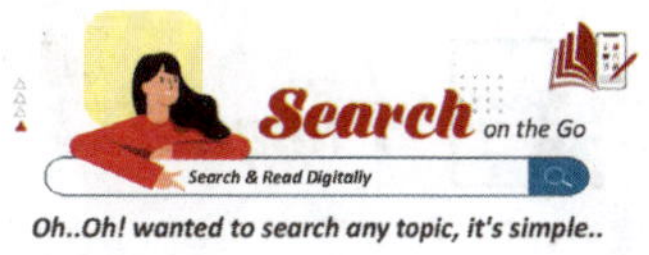

BASIC STRUCTURES INVOLVED IN GENETICS

Genes are the basic units of hereditary transmission. Basic structure involved in genetics has been depicted in Figure 24.1.

Nucleosome

Structurally strands of DNA coil around each other to form a double-stranded helical structure, that is left-handed coil. These double-helical structures with DNA binding proteins (histones or non-histone proteins) form the nucleosomes, which are connected by the small segment of linker DNA. These eventually leads to the formation of chromatin structures. Nucleosomes are the basic units of chromatin.

Chromosome

Many chromatin structures together form a chromosome that can be seen under the light microscope and appear as thread-like structures. The shape of these chromosomes varies depending on the stages of cell division. Chromosomes (Fig. 24.2) have a centromere. The centromere plays an important role in cell division, (to which the spindle fibers attach) and aid in segregation of chromosomes. Chromosomes also have specialized structures called telomeres located at each end - DNA sequences with tandem repeats. These telomeres play important function in cell aging and cancer.

There are 46 chromosomes in a somatic cell and in zygote (Figs 24.3A and B). This is known as the diploid (2N) number. In normal conditions, chromosomes appear in pairs, one of each pair is derived from mother and another from father.

- **Somatic cells:** In a somatic cell, there are 22 pairs of autosomes or homologous (chromosomes common for both sexes) and one pair of sex chromosomes. The female has two X chromosomes (XX), whereas in a male, there is one X chromosome and one Y chromosome (XY) in a normal condition.

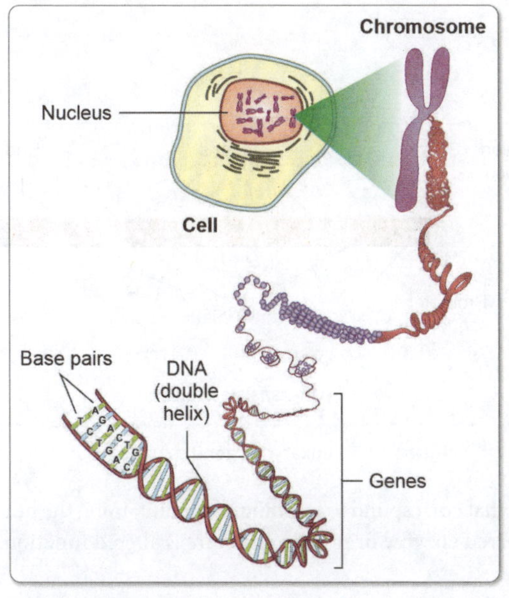

Figure 24.1: Basic structure involved in genetics

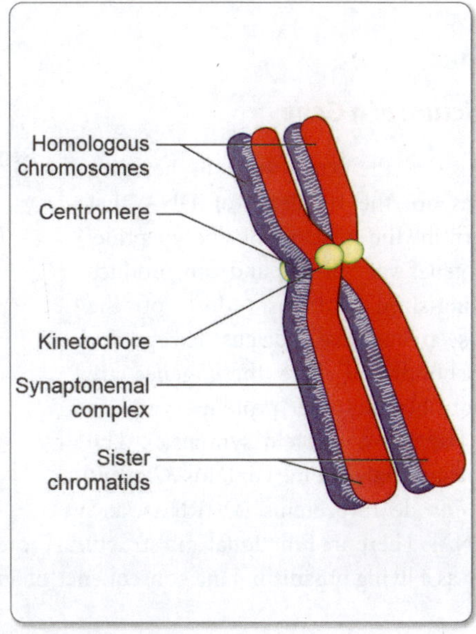

Figure 24.2: Structure of a chromosome

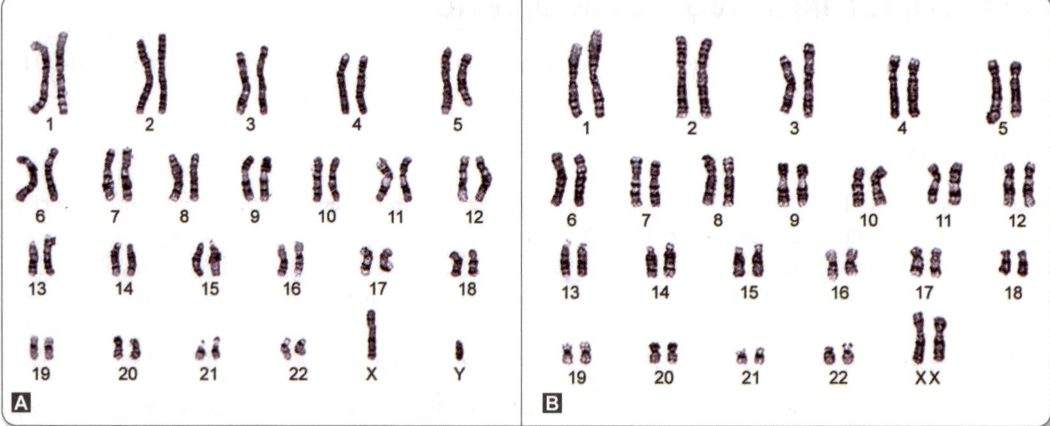

Figures 24.3A and B: Set of 46 chromosomes in humans; **A.** Male; **B.** Female

- **Gametes:** In contrast to somatic cells, gametes (ova and sperm) contain one member of each chromosome pair, that is total of 23 chromosomes (22 autosomes and one sex chromosome). This is called haploid (N) number.
- **Zygote:** The fusion of male and female gametes during fertilization restores the diploid number of chromosomes in the zygote in a normal condition. The homologous chromosomes have identical number of arrangements for genes, whereas it is not true for sex chromosomes.

MUST KNOW

After the successful completion of the human genome project, it is believed that there are 30,000–35,000 genes in a human genome. About 99.9% of humans have a common DNA sequence.

Genes

Structure of a Gene

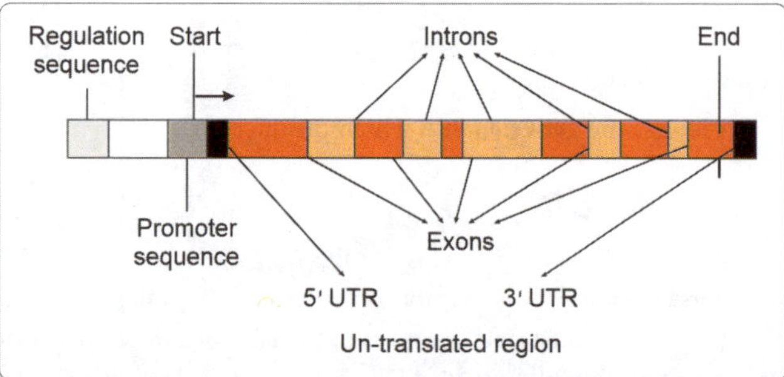

Figure 24.4: Eukaryotic gene structure

Genes are the basic units of heredity. Genes are the segments of DNA that determine the structure of a polypeptide. The genes vary in size and can produce varying-sized proteins. Most of the genes are in the nucleus except for mitochondria, (where these genes are responsible for the protein synthesis and the rate of protein synthesis). The mitochondrial genome contains 37 genes that encode 13 proteins, 22 tRNAs, and 2 rRNAs. There are functional and structural proteins that correspond to building and maintaining the human body as a living organism. One consequence of an altered enzyme or protein structure is altered function.

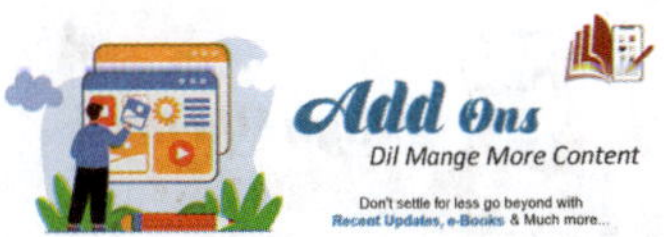

Genes are complex structures (Fig. 24.4) composed of the following regions:

- **Exons:** Code the sequence transcribed and translated for amino acids in the polypeptide chain.
- **Introns:** Coding sequence is separated by noncoding sequences called introns. All introns share the base sequence GT in the 5' end and AG in the 3' end.
  Significance of introns: Introns encode RNAse which regulate the gene expression.
  - Contains regulatory sequences that control transcription and mRNA processing.
  - Allows exons to be joined in different combinations (alternative Splicing) resulting in the synthesis of different proteins from the same gene.
  - Plays an important role in evolution by facilitating recombination between exons of different genes (exon shuffling).
- **Promotor sequence:** It is regulatory region of DNA located upstream controlling gene expression.
  - **Core promoter:** Transcription start site (-34).
  - **Proximal promoter:** Contains primary regulatory element responsible for binding of RNA polymerase.
- **Upstream sequence:** mRNA transport and initiation of translation; and stabilization of mRNA.
- **Downstream sequence:** 3' UTRs serve to add mRNA, stability and attachment site for poly A-tail.
- **Terminator:** Recognized by RNA polymerase as a signal to stop transcription.
- **Enhancers and silencers:**
  - **Enhancers:** Enhance the transcription of a gene up to few thousand 'bp' upstream.
  - **Silencers:** Reduce or shut down the expression of a nearby gene.
- **Signals:** (Upstream sequence signal for addition of 'cap', downstream sequences signal for addition of 'poly' a tail).

Types of Genes

Based on the behavior, the genes are categorized into the following types:

- **Basic genes:** The fundamental genes that bring about expression of a particular character.
- **Lethal genes:** Bring about the death of their possessors.
- **Cumulative gene:** Genes that have additive effects on the action of other genes.
- **Multiple genes:** When two or more pairs of independent genes act together to produce a single phenotypic trait.
- **Inhibitory gene:** Gene which either suppresses or inhibits the expression of another gene.
- **Modifying gene:** Gene which cannot produce a character by itself but interacts with other genes to produce modified effect.
- **Pleiotropic genes:** Genes which produce changes in more than one character.

Functions of Genes

- Genes control the functions of DNA and RNA.
- Protein synthesis is mainly controlled by the genes.
- Genes instruct a particular set of instructions or specific functions. For example, globin gene instructs to produce hemoglobin.
- Genes can affect a specific trait.
- Genes may interact with an individual's environment and change the function that it dictates and brings genotypic or phenotypic variations.

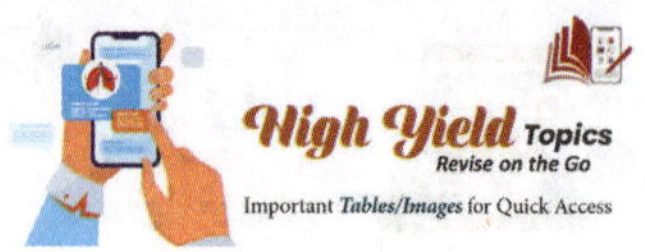

EXTRA EDGE

Historical Background

- **Gregor Mendel:** Discovered the fundamental Laws of Inheritance (1900)
- **Wilhelm Johannsen:** Coined the term Gene (1909)
- **William Bateson:** Coined the term Genetics (1905)

Concepts of Genes

- **TM Morgan theory:**
  - Chromosomes are bearers of hereditary units
  - Genes are arranged on the chromosomes in the linear order and on the special regions or locus.
- **Classical concept:**
  - Introduced by Sutton (1902) and was elaborated by Morgan (1913), Bidge (1923), Muller (1927) and others.
  - Genes are discrete particles inherited in Mendelian fashion that occupies a definite locus in the chromosome and responsible for expression of specific phenotypic character.
  - Several genes are located on each chromosome.
  - Genes may exist in several alternate formed called alleles.
  - Genes may undergo sudden changes in position and composition called mutation.
  - Each gene occupies specific position called locus. If the position of gene changes, character changes.
  - Genes are capable of self-duplication producing their own exact copies.
- **Modern concept:**
  - Benzer (1957) coined different terms for different nature of gene and genetic material.
  - Genes as unit of transmission or cistron. The part of DNA specifying a single polypeptide chain is termed cistron. A cistron can have 100 nucleotide pairs in length to 30,000 nucleotide pairs.
  - Genes as unit of recombination or recon. A recon consists of not more than two pairs of nucleotides.
  - Gene as unit of mutation or muton.

REVIEW OF CELL DIVISION: MITOSIS AND MEIOSIS

Some of the cells remain for the entire life of a human (neurons) whereas others replace those that die (hepatocytes). The new diploid cells are generated from the division of the existing diploid cells involve mitosis (nuclear division) and cytokinesis (cytoplasmic division).

Mitosis

Mitosis is the division of the nucleus, followed by the division of cytoplasm, into two new cells of similar sizes. Mitosis usually requires about 1–2 hours to complete.

Interphase

During this phase of pre-processing, the cells duplicate their content including DNA, this phase is called interphase. When mitosis and interphase reoccur in alternate, then it is referred to as cell cycle (Fig. 24.5). Interphase is divided into three phases, namely, G_1, S, G_2, and M phase.

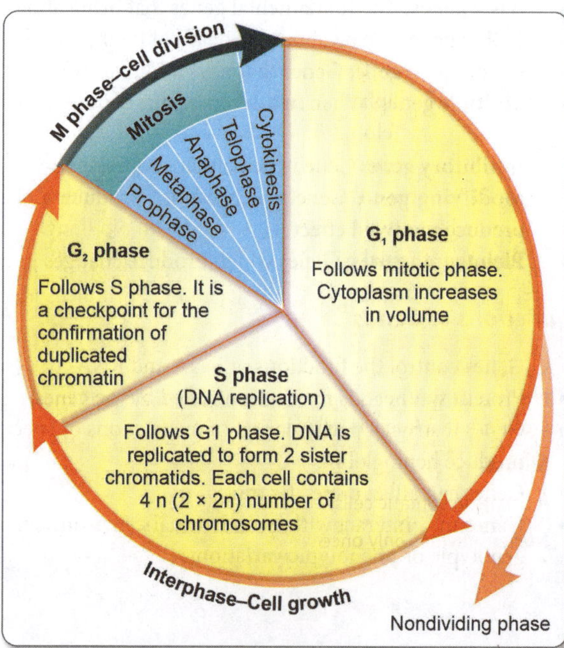

Figure 24.5: Phases of cell cycle

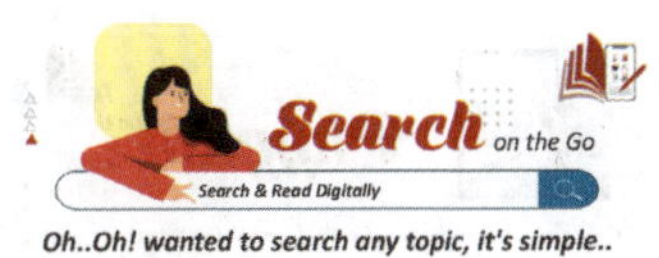

The duration of cell cycle varies considerably from one cell type to another cell type, some cells divide in <10 hours whereas few cells divide once a year whereas others lose the property of cell division.

- **G_1 Phase:** Among all the phases, the longest phase of cell cycle is G_1 phase (Gap 1), and if the cell stops dividing for long time, then cells are in the G_0 phase also referred to as quiescent phase. During the G_1 phase, synthesis of RNA and proteins occurs.
- **S Phase:** During the S phase, DNA synthesis occurs and DNA content doubles in quantity. Currently the cells have 46 chromosomes.
- **G_2 Phase:** In the G_2 phase cell has two identical copies of each 46 chromosomes and these chromosomes are referred to as sister chromatids.
- **M Phase:** A cell to enter a cell cycle requires internal or external signals, for example, DNA replication must be accurately completed. Among all signals, the most important ones are the cyclin dependent kinases (CDKs) that regulate important regulatory proteins by phosphorylation. The CDKs form a complex with various cyclins that are synthesized at specific cell cycle stage otherwise CDKs will degrade if not needed.

Phases of Mitosis

Mitosis is divided into four phases, those are prophase, metaphase, anaphase, and telophase (Figs 24.6A to D).

1. **Prophase:** During the prophase chromosomes get condensed and coiled. Both the sister chromatids are attached to each other through the centromere. By now the centrioles move to both ends of the cells. Spindle fibers start appearing and connecting the centromere to centrioles and aid in pulling apart the sister chromatids to the opposite ends.
2. **Metaphase:** During the metaphase, chromosomes get highly condensed and can be easily visualized. By now the spindle fibers start contracting and pulling the centromeres of the chromosomes. In this phase, the chromosomes are arranged as a plate (metaphase plate) along the middle of the cell also referred to as equatorial plane of the cell.
3. **Anaphase:** During the anaphase, centromeres of the chromosomes split and the two sister chromatids are separated. Now the spindle fibers pull the sister chromosomes to the opposite side of the cell. During the end of the anaphase, cell has 92 separated identical chromosomes, half on each end of the cell.
4. **Telophase:** Telophase is initiated with the appearance of nuclear membrane around each of the 46 chromosomes. Further spindle fibers start disappearing, and chromosomes become decondensed. With telophase the nuclear division ends and the cytokinesis starts, where the cytoplasm is roughly divided into two equal cells and two diploid daughter cells are formed. These daughter cells are identical with the original cell.

   Division of somatic cells under mitosis, produces identical daughter cells with 46 chromosomes.

MUST KNOW

Mitosis is known as equational division and meiosis is known as reduction division. Differences between meiosis and mitosis are tabulated as follows:

Mitosis	Meiosis
It occurs in somatic cells	It occurs in germ cells
Nucleus divides only once	Nucleus divides twice

Contd...

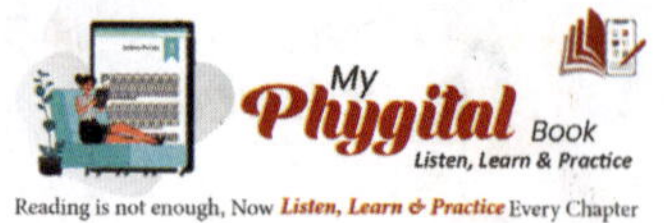

Mitosis	Meiosis
It is divided into prophase, metaphase, anaphase and telophase	Meiosis I and II divided into prophase I and II, metaphase I and II, anaphase I and II and telophase I and II
Daughter cells are diploid	Daughter cells are haploid
No crossing over takes place	Crossing over takes place
Increased number of normal cells	Produces egg and sperm cells
Involved in healing and growth	Involved in genetic variations
2 daughter cells are produced	4 daughter cells are produced
Malfunction results in cancer	Malfunction results in genetic disorder such as Down's syndrome, Klinefelter's syndrome and Turner's syndrome.

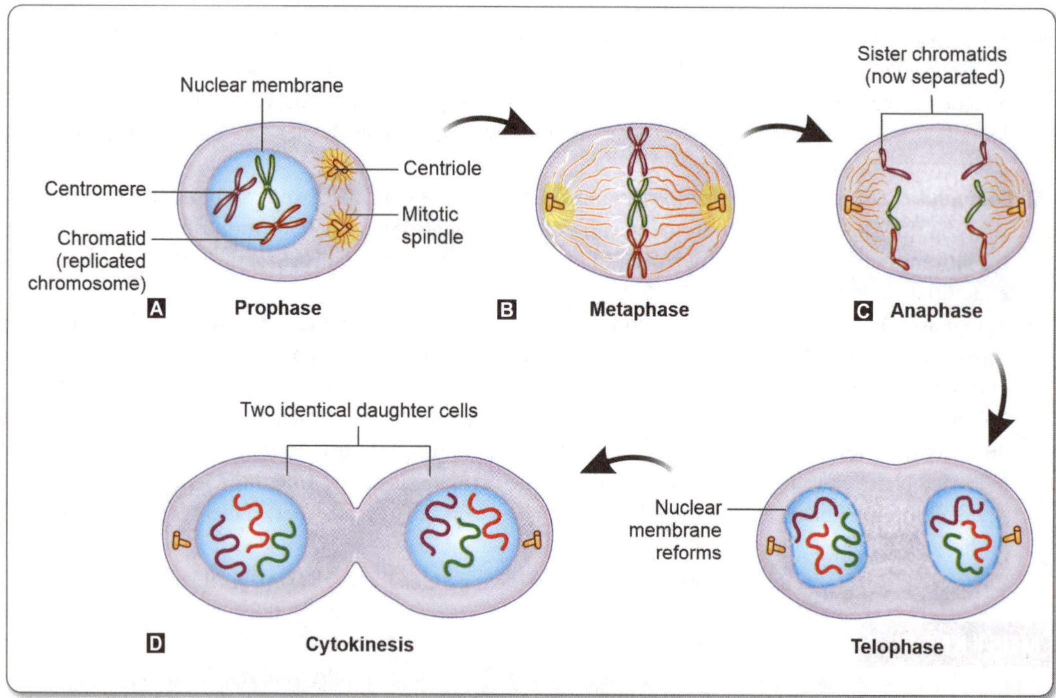

Figures 24.6A to D: Different phases of mitotic cell division

Meiosis

Meiosis is a special type of cell division (Figs 24.7A and B) that forms the gametes. The gametes are formed by meiosis in the oogonia in females and spermatogonia in males. Gametes are haploid (n) in nature and fuse to form a zygote that is diploid (2n) in nature.

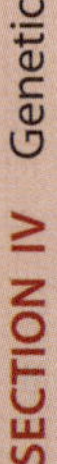

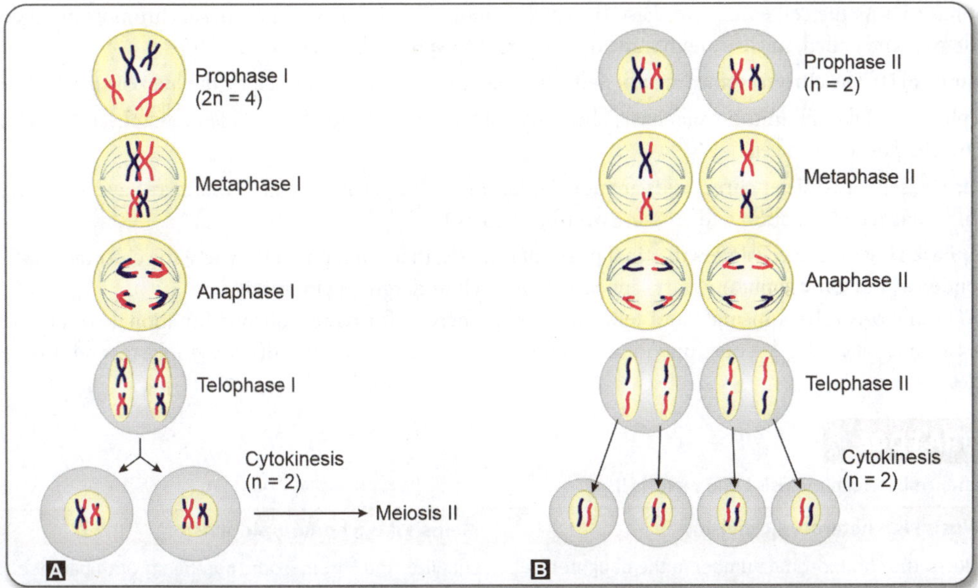

Figures 24.7A and B: Different phases of meiosis: **A.** Meiosis I; **B.** Meiosis II

Meiosis I–First Meiotic Division

Interphase I: Meiosis I starts with interphase I. During this phase replication of DNA takes place and prepares the cells for the next phase.

Prophase I: The second phase of meiosis I is prophase I. It is more complex phase that involves the coiling and condensation of chromosomes. During prophase I, the homologous chromosomes form a process called synapsis, wherein they align side by side.

- **Synapsis formation:** As the prophase I progresses the homologous chromosomes intertwine with each other and the pair of chromosomes are formed, called bivalent (two chromosomes) or tetrad (four chromatids).
- **Formation of chiasmata:** It is attachment of sister chromatids which facilitate the exchange of genetic material known as crossing over.

Metaphase I: The spindle fibers appear and align the bivalent chromosomes on the equatorial plane of the cell. The bivalents are still attached at the chiasmata and centromeres lie on the opposite side of the plane.

Anaphase I: In the anaphase I, chiasmata disappears and the chromosomes are pulled toward the opposite poles. In this stage, the centromeres do not divide, instead each set of chromosomes (22 autosomes and one sex chromosome) migrate toward each pole.

Telophase I: In the telophase I chromosomes reach opposite poles, they start to decondense, and a nuclear membrane starts to appear.

Meiosis II–Second meiotic Division

Interphase II: This is a very brief phase compared to interphase I and mitotic interphase as it lacks DNA replication.

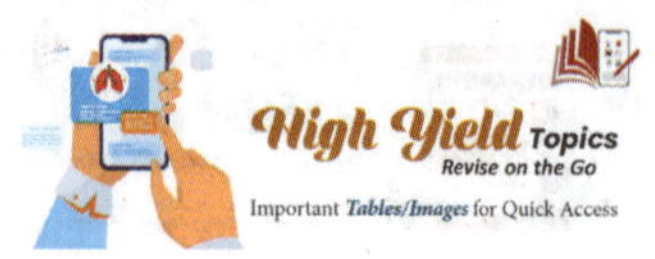

Prophase II: As the cell enters prophase II, which is more like the mitotic prophase, chromosomes become condensed and coiled, nuclear membrane disappears, and spindle fibers appear.

Metaphase II: The chromosomes are aligned at the equatorial plane of the cell by the help of spindle fibers.

Anaphase II: Like the mitotic anaphase, chromosomes segregate into chromatids in anaphase II and move toward the pole of each cell.

Note: The separated sister chromatids are not similar due to the genetic material that may have been changed during chiasmata formation and crossing over in Meiosis 1.

Telophase II: Now the cell enters the final phase of meiosis, that is telophase II, where the chromatids start to decondense, nuclear membrane starts appearing, and cell undergoes cytokinesis.

The meiosis differs in male and female. In male there is formation of four functional daughter cells; whereas in females, there is one functional daughter cells formed with most of the cytoplasm, and three polar bodies.

EXTRA EDGE

Difference between meiosis I and meiosis II

Meiosis I is a heterotypic division	Meiosis II is a homotypic division
Reduces the chromosome number in the daughter cell	Equalizes the chromosome number of both parent and daughter cells
Homologous chromosomes are present at the beginning	Individual, bivalent chromosomes are present at the begining
Prophase I, metaphase I, anaphase I and telophase I are the four phases	Prophase II, metaphase II. anaphase II and telophase II are the four phases
Individual chromosomes are present in the daughter nuclei	Sister chromosomes are present in the daughter nuclei
Chromosomal cross- over occurs during prophase I	No chromosomal cross-over occurs during prophase II
A complex division and takes more time	Comparatively less simple and takes less time
Preceded by interphase	No interphase takes place
Cohesin protein complexes at the arms of the homologous chromosomes are cleaved	Cohesins at the centromeres are cleaved in order to separate the two sister chromatids

CHROMOSOMES: SEX DETERMINATION

The sex determination in mammals is governed by the chromosomes and is not influenced by the environmental factors. Humans have 46 chromosomes. Half of them come from the mother and the other half from the father. Out of these 46 chromosomes, 44 are autosomes and 2 are sex chromosomes. The sex chromosomes are not always a perfect pair (Fig. 24.8).

In females—there are 44 autosomes and two X chromosomes (44+XX),

In males—there are 44 autosomes, one X chromosome and one Y chromosome (44+XY). A male produces two types of sperms-one type has 22+X composition and the other type has 22+Y. For example, in every 100 sperms, 50 have Y chromosomes and 50 have X chromosomes.

The gonad carrying X chromosome will produce a female offspring and Y carrying gonad will produce a male offspring. Female has XX chromosomes and can produce gametes with only X chromosomes, whereas male has XY chromosome and can produce two kinds of gametes carrying X or Y chromosome in it.

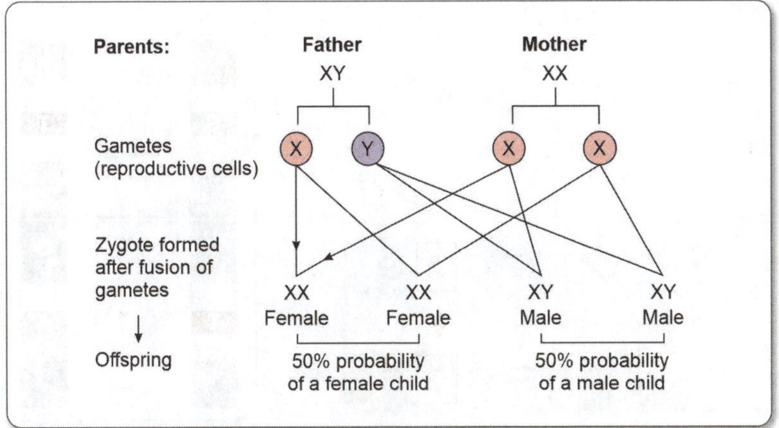

Figure 24.8: Sex determination in humans

When a male gamete carrying X chromosome fertilizes the egg, the offspring will be a female; if it carries the Y chromosome then offspring will be male.

EXTRA EDGE

The Y chromosome is crucial in determining sex in humans, as person having more than one X chromosome and one Y chromosome can be male; whereas a person having one X and no Y chromosome (XO) becomes female with ovaries whereas ovarian follicles will not be maintained.

GENE MUTATIONS/ERRORS IN TRANSMISSION

A mutation is a change in the DNA sequence of an organism. Mutations can result from errors in DNA replication during cell division, exposure to mutagens or a viral infection (Figs 24.9 to 24.11).

Effects of Mutations

- Mutations can cause genetic disorders by affecting one or more genes. For example, cystic fibrosis which is caused by the mutation in one or more genes.
- Mutation may be one of the contributing factors causing cancer.
- Mutations can result in new versions of proteins and help the organisms to adapt to changes in the environment—called evolution.
- Mutations can make bacteria more antibiotic-resistant so that they can survive in the presence of antibiotics.

A mutation is a sudden, heritable modification in an organism's traits. The term "mutant" refers to a person who exhibits these heritable alterations. Mutations usually produce recessive genes.

Classification and Types of Mutations

Based on the molecular changes, the mutations can be classified as point mutation, chromosomal mutation and copy mutation.

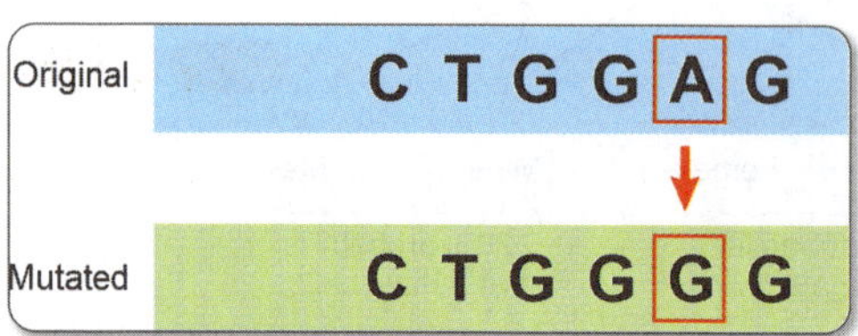

Figure 24.9: Substitution mutation

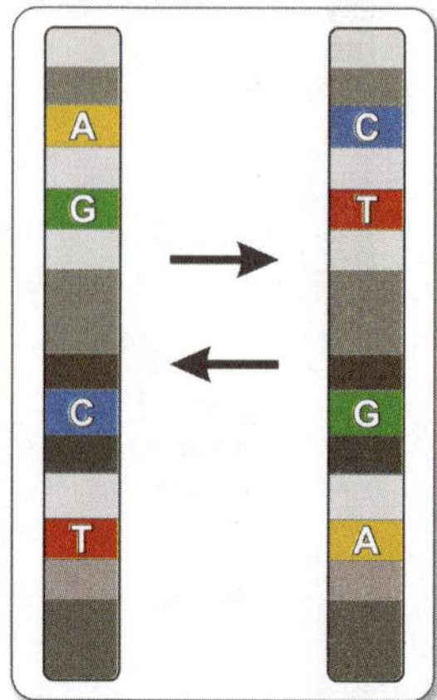

Figure 24.10: Transversion mutation

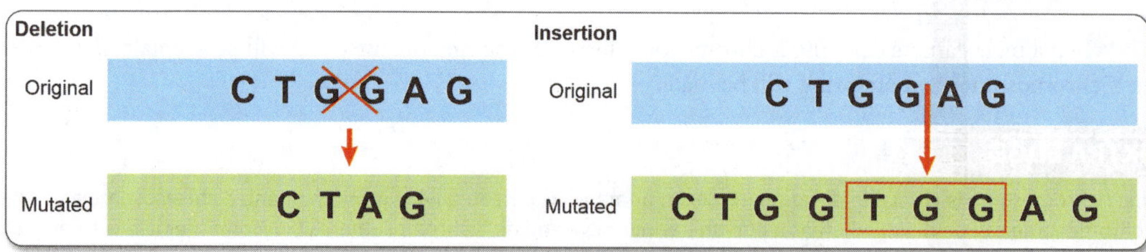

Figure 24.11: Deletion and insertion mutations

Point Mutation

- **Substitution:** During replication, one base is incorrectly inserted at the place of a correct base also called mismatch mutation (Fig. 24.9). For example, sickle cell anemia.
- **Insertion leading to frameshift:** While replicating, one or more additional nucleotides are added in the DNA, frequently causing a frameshift (Figs 24.11 and 24.13). For example, β-thalassemia.
- **Deletion leading to frameshift:** During replication, one or more nucleotides may be "skipped" or get deleted, which usually causes a frameshift. For example, cystic fibrosis.

Chromosomal Mutation

- **Deletion:** When a chromosome segment is lost, all the genes in that segment are also gone, e.g. Cri du chat syndrome (Fig. 24.11).
- **Inversion:** The flipping and reinserting of a single chromosomal region, for example, Opitz-Kaveggia syndrome.
- **Translocation:** A section of one chromosome is inappropriately joined to another chromosome (Fig. 24.12). For example, leukemia.
- **Duplication:** A chromosomal segment is repeated, increasing the concentration of the genes in that area, e.g., some cancers.

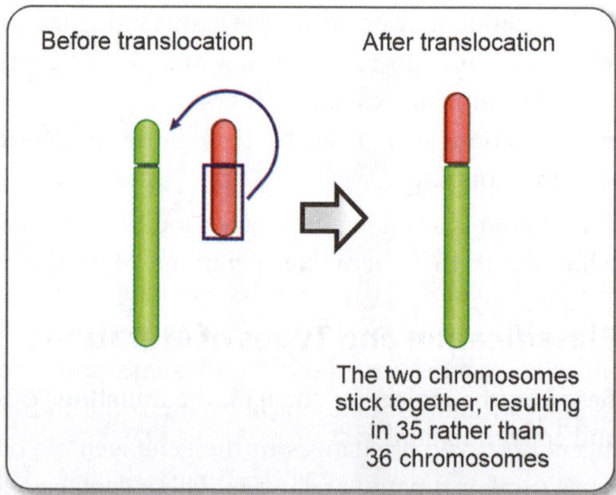

Figure 24.12: Translocation—Robertsonian

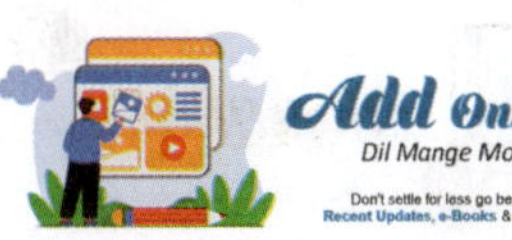

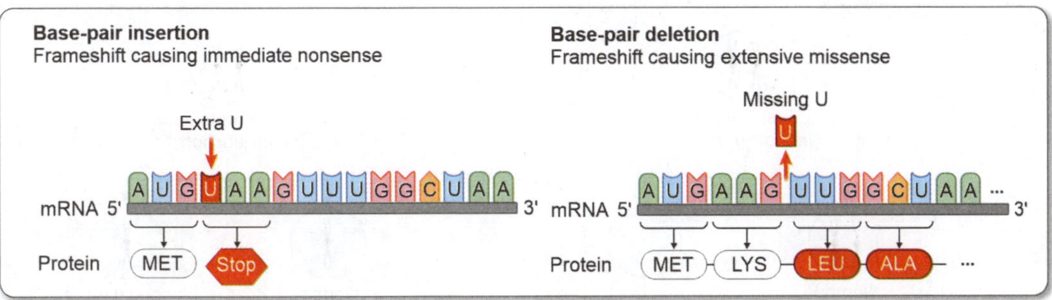

Figure 24.13: Frame shift mutations by insertion and deletion

Figure 24.13 exhibits frame shift mutations using insertion and deletion.

Copy Mutation

- **Expanding trinucleotide repeat:** There are more repeating trinucleotide sequences than usual. For example, Fragile X syndrome, Huntington's disease.
- **Gene amplification:** An increase is made in the tandem copies of a locus, For example, breast cancers.

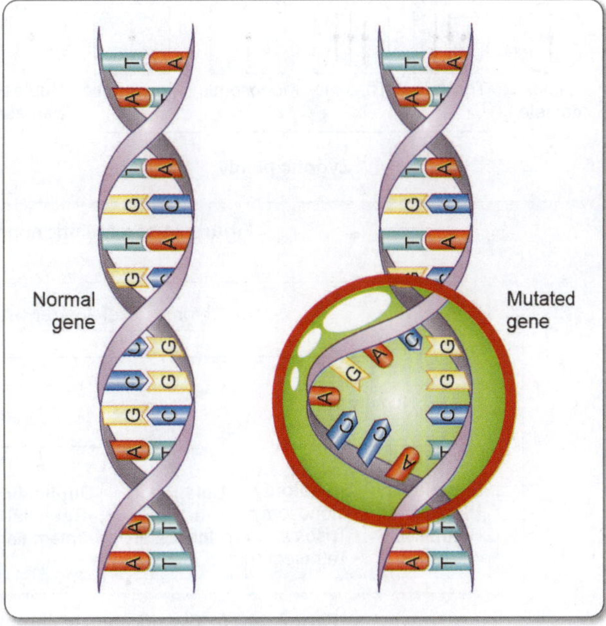

Figure 24.14: DNA mutation

Causes of Mutation

The mutation is caused due to the following reasons:

Internal causes: Such mutations occur when the DNA fails to copy accurately during cell division.

External causes: DNA breaks down when exposed to certain chemicals or radiations. The ultraviolet radiations cause the thymine dimers to break resulting in a mutated DNA (Fig. 24.14).

CHROMOSOMAL ABERRATIONS

Any change in the genetic component leads to variation in phenotypic characters. Depending on the extent of the aberration, these effects can range from being lethal to being harmless variations. Chromosomal aberrations typically affect multiple genes (loci). These chromosomal aberrations occur due to errors in cell division (nondisjunction of chromosomes and chromatids), and are affected by maternal age or environment. Single or multiple mutations in a gene are due to environmental agents or heredity. Based on the environmental agent and type of changes in the gene, genetic background, type of tissue affected, the outcome can be a structural or functional damage. These damages can lead to various abnormalities in biochemistry, immune function, growth, development, reproduction, behavior, or combination of these.

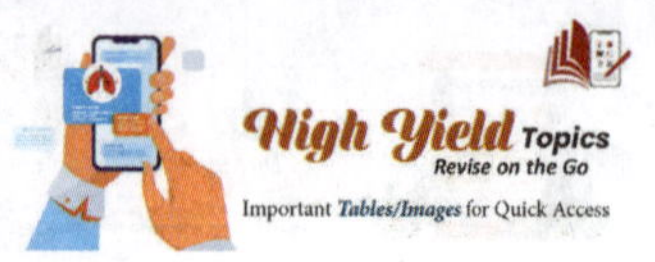

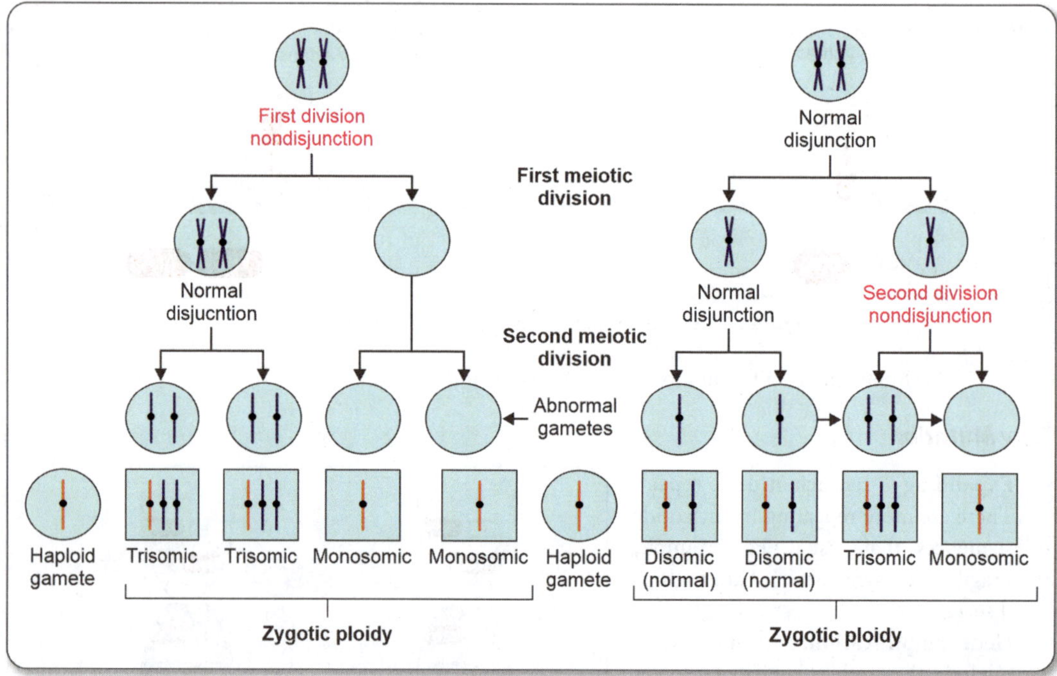

Figure 24.15: Meiotic nondisjunction

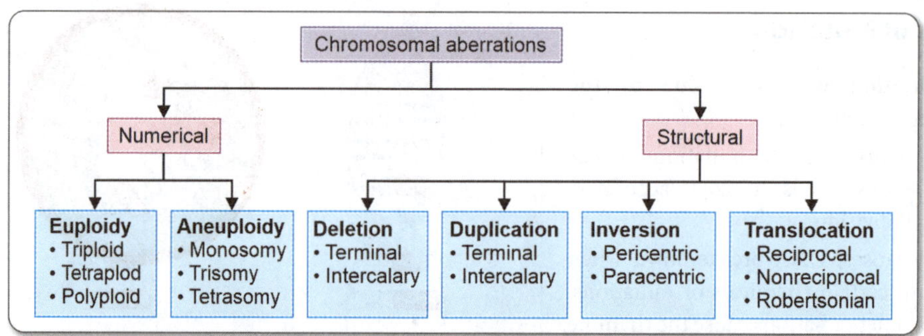

Figure 24.16: Classification of chromosomal aberrations

Relation between age and aneuploidy: Older mothers are more likely to produce aneuploid eggs because of meiotic non-disjunction during oocyte maturation which produces abnormal gametes (Fig. 24.15).

Types of Chromosomal Aberrations

Chromosomal aberrations are broadly classified as numerical and structural aberrations (Fig. 24.16).

Numerical Aberrations

Numerical aberrations cause a change (addition or deletion) in the number of chromosomes. They are further classified as:

- **Euploidy:** A complete set of 46 chromosomes without any defects in the chromosomes can be referred to as euploidy. In a rare natural incident euploidy can delineate by quantitative or qualitative. The quantitative aberrations include the changes in the correct set of chromosome numbers (less than or more than 46), for example, triploid (3n), tetraploid (4n) etc. In humans, euploidy conditions do not exist because the extent of abnormality is too large to sustain life. Most of the triploids and tetraploids have live birth but fail to survive for few days.
  - **Polyploidy:** This condition involves an extra exact set of haploid chromosomes, for example, 3n, having total of 69 chromosomes. Polyploidy is commonly observed in plants, and is incompatible with human life. These can be:
    - Triploid (3n)
    - Tetraploid (4n)
    - Pentaploid (5n)
- **Aneuploidy** is the condition when an organism gains or loses one or more chromosomes and not the entire set. For example, trisomy (2n + 1), monosomy (2n – 1). Aneuploidy conditions, are more common and are manifested in disorders, such as Down syndrome, Klinefelter syndrome and Turner syndrome. There is no extra exact set of haploid chromosomes, instead there will be:
  - **Trisomy:** an extra chromosome (2n + 1) is gained and is referred to as trisomy (total of 47 chromosomes)
  - **Monosomy:** There will be a loss of chromosome (2n – 1) which is referred to as monosomy (total of 45 chromosomes).

Structural Aberrations

The qualitative aberrations are variations in the chromosome structure also referred to as heteromorphism. These aberrations are observed specifically in chromosomes 1, 9 and Y chromosomes. The alterations in the chromosomes can be classified into four groups (Fig. 24.17). These are as follows:

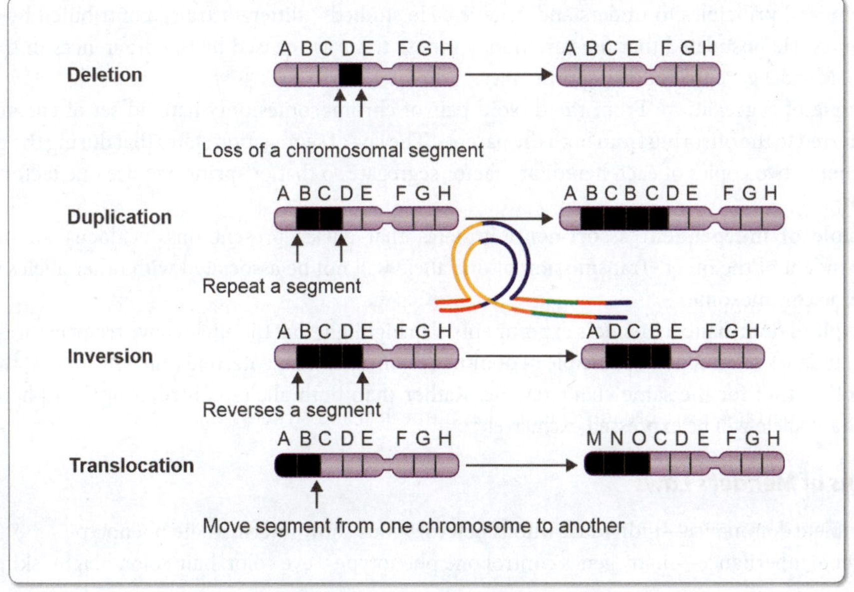

Figure 24.17: Alterations in chromosomes

- **Deletions or deficiencies:** Loss of a part of chromosome is called deletion. A deletion can at the end of chromosome referred to as terminal deletion or if the deletion is within the body of chromosome, then referred to as interstitial deletion. Examples of human chromosome deletion aberrations are 5p- (cri-du-chat) and 4p- (Wolf-Hirschhorn syndrome).
- **Duplications**: If a segment of chromosome happens to be more than the normal number of times in the same chromosome, it is called duplications. Duplications can alter the normal chromosome structure and affect the crossing over. Duplication results in extra copy of genes.
- **Inversions and Translocations:**
  - **Inversions:** These are the structural defects in the chromosome in which a segment of chromosomes is rearranged in reverse order. In humans, inversion can occur during the crossing over and mostly involves chromosomes 9.
  - **Translocations:** During translocation, a segment of chromosome is transferred from one region to another region. The translocation may be nonreciprocal, or it may be reciprocal. In reciprocal translocation, chromosome segments are exchanged randomly between the same chromosome or between two different chromosomes.

NOTE

Mosaicism: If different cells are derived from the same zygote and bear variation in chromosome or gene number or structure, are referred to as mosaicism.

PATTERNS OF INHERITANCE

To understand the cause of transmission of genetic disease it is important to know the basic laws of inheritance.

Mendelian Theory of Inheritance

John Gregor Mendel is regarded as "The Father of Genetics". His well-planned studies on green pea gave a few fundamental principles to understand genetics. He studied 7 different traits, contributed by 7 different chromosomes. He postulated that the variations in these traits are caused by the differences in the alleles at each locus. Mendel gave the following principles:

- **Principle of segregation:** From the diploid pair of chromosomes only haploid set of chromosomes is transferred to the offspring from both the parents. The law of segregation states that during the production of gametes, two copies of each hereditary factor segregate so that offspring acquire one factor from each parent.
- **Principle of independent assortment:** It states that alleles present on one locus are transmitted independent of the other. Transmission of one allele will not be associated with other alleles present on the same chromosome.
- **Principle of dominance:** Mendel's experiments also highlight that the alleles have recessive and dominant characteristics referred to as principle of dominance. In a heterozygote, one trait will conceal the presence of another trait for the same characteristic. Rather than both alleles contributing to a phenotype, the dominant allele will be expressed exclusively.

Variations of Mendel's Laws

- Incomplete dominance—individual who is heterozygous show intermediate phenotype.
- Polygenic inheritance—many genes control one phenotype—eye color, hair color, height, skin color.

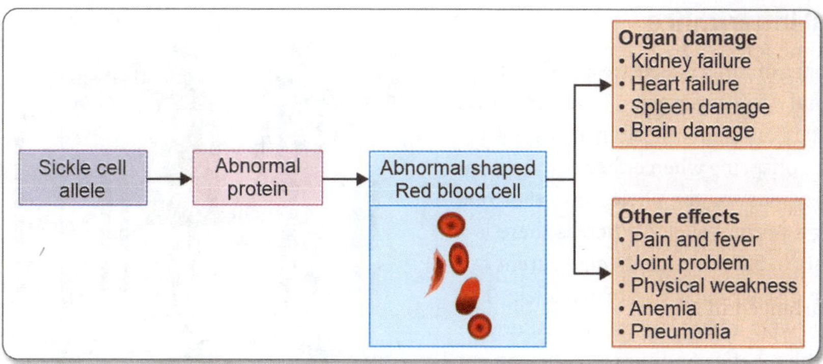

Figure 24.18: Pleiotropy

- Codominance—two different alleles are fully expressed in phenotype.
- Pleiotropy—one gene has many effects (Fig. 24.18).

MUST KNOW

Pedigree Analysis

To predict genetic disease using the pattern of inheritance, family history is necessary. Regarding the normal allele, an allele carrying a mutation can have characteristics of dominance, codominant or recessive.

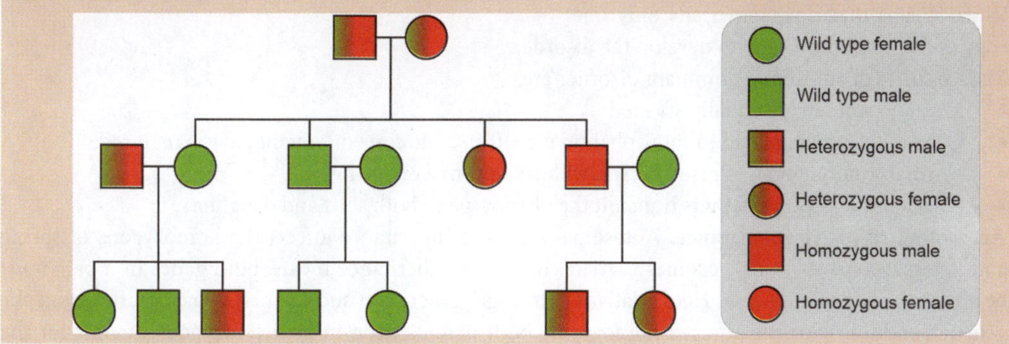

MECHANISM OF INHERITANCE

The inherited traits are determined by genes that are passed from parents to children. A trait may not be observable, but its gene can be passed on to the next generation. Each person has two copies of every gene—one copy from mom and a second copy from dad. These copies may come in different variations, known as alleles, that express different traits. For example, 2 alleles in the gene for freckles are inherited from mom and dad:

Allele from mom = has freckles (F)

Allele from dad = no freckles (f)

Now the child will inherit gene pair as Ff (F allele from mom and f allele from dad).

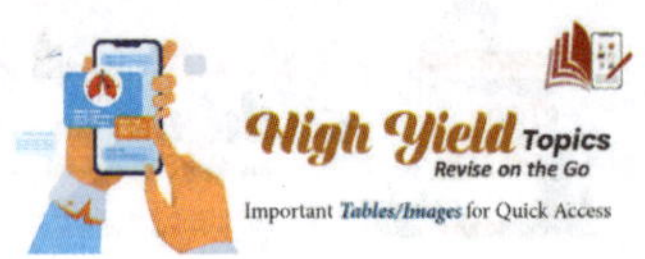

Autosomal Inheritance

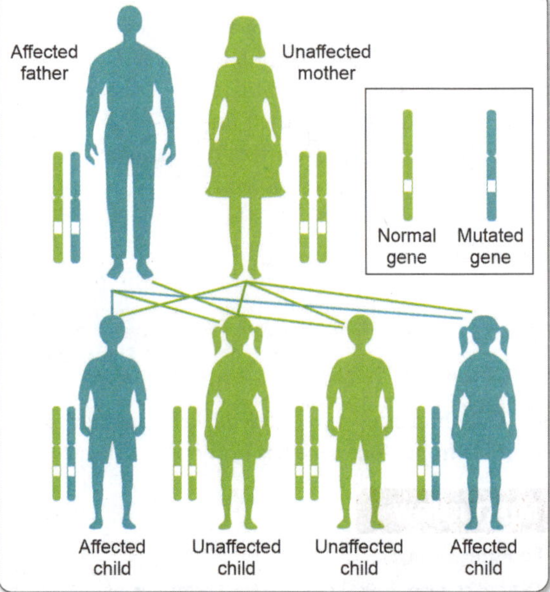

Figure 24.19: Autosomal dominant inheritance

The basic modes of inheritance are as follows:

- **Autosomal dominant inheritance:** Autosomal dominant inheritance (Fig. 24.19) affects the offspring when either of the parent is heterozygous for the allele and other one is having a normal allele. Whereas there is a probability of 50% that an effected parent can transfer a disease allele or normal allele. The offsprings who inherit normal genes, do not develop the genetic condition and they do not pass the disease to their children. The clinical characteristics in a genetically affected person may vary from no symptoms to mild symptoms. The person who has acquired a mutated gene has again 50% probability of passing mutated gene to his offsprings. The effect of mutated genes may not appear in one generation and skip it. Huntington's disease is an autosomal dominant disorder, which means that a person needs only one copy of the nontypical gene to develop the disorder.
  Main features of autosomal dominant disorder are:
  - Men and women are equally affected.
  - Gene is an autosome and to show phenotypic effects, one copy of mutant gene is required.
  - Normal children of an affected person will have normal offsprings.
  - Affected mothers and fathers transmit the phenotype to both sons and daughters.
- **Autosomal recessive inheritance:** Autosomal recessive inheritance affects the homozygous offspring and heterozygous offspring becomes carriers. Recessive inheritance means both genes in a pair must be abnormal to cause disease. Here relatives of a single generation such as first cousins suffer from the genetic condition. For the affected homozygote both parents need to be heterozygous carriers for the disease allele. When carriers have children together, there is 25% chance that each child may inherit mutated gene from each parent, for example, cystic fibrosis and albinism (Fig. 24.20).

Sex-Linked Inheritance

X and Y are the two sex chromosomes present in humans. In a female offspring, there are two X chromosomes, one derived from the maternal side and one from paternal side. Whereas in a male offspring there is X chromosome from maternal side and Y chromosome from paternal side. The X chromosome encodes for 2000 genes, whereas Y chromosomes is one of the smallest chromosomes and encodes for fewer genes. As most of the genes are present on the X chromosomes but there is no counterpart allele for these genes present on the Y chromosomes. Whether a gene is dominant or recessive, it has only one copy on the X chromosome in males as the Y chromosome lacks most of the genes.

In X-linked recessive inheritance, female partner is heterozygous carrier for the mutant gene and a male is normal, then four possible outcomes for an offspring are possible.

1. A female carrier like mother.
2. A normal female without the mutant gene.
3. A normal male without the mutant gene.
4. A male who is affected with the disease.

The risk for male offspring is high as he has 50% chances of being affected. In this condition both male and female are affected, and both can transmit the gene to next offspring.

- **X-linked dominant inheritance:** It is associated with X chromosome and defects in one X chromosome are capable to cause the disease. All the male offspring carrying this defect will be affected, whereas the female offspring homozygous for X chromosome will not be affected and will be a carrier. Affected males pass the disorder to all daughters but to none of their sons. Affected heterozygous females married to unaffected males pass the condition to half their sons and daughters. For example, hemophilia A, fragile X syndrome, hypophosphatemic rickets.

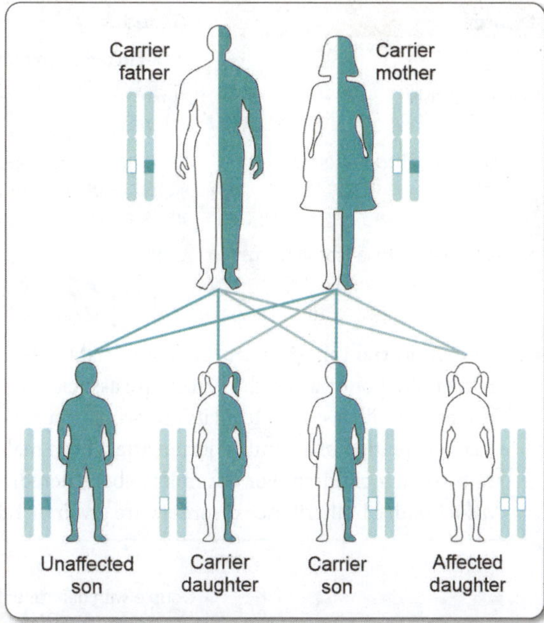

Figure 24.20: Autosomal recessive inheritance

- **X-linked recessive inheritance:** It is associated with X chromosome carrying a defective allele that is recessive. Many more males than females show the disorder. All the daughters of an affected male are "carriers". None of the sons of an affected male shows the disorder or are carriers. For example, hemophilia A (Table 24.1).

Table 24.1: X-linked disorder inheritance

Disorder	Genetics	Characteristics
	X-linked recessive inheritance	
Duchenne muscular dystrophy	Mutation in dystrophin gene	Early life muscle degeneration; eventual death
Fragile X syndrome	Expansion of CGG trinucleotide repeat on X chromosome	Most widespread single-gene cause of autism and inherited cause of intellectual disability, especially among boys
Hemophilia A	Mutant allele; ~70% of the time X- linked recessive trait, 30% of cases arise from mutations.	Deficiency in clotting factor VIII, causes increased bleeding; usually affects males
Red-green color blindness	Absence or mutation of genes for red or green color receptors	Difficulty in discriminating red and green hues
Rett syndrome	Mutations in gene MECP2 located on X chromosome	Typically no verbal skills, 50% of individuals affected do not walk. Scoliosis, growth failure, constipation very common

Contd...

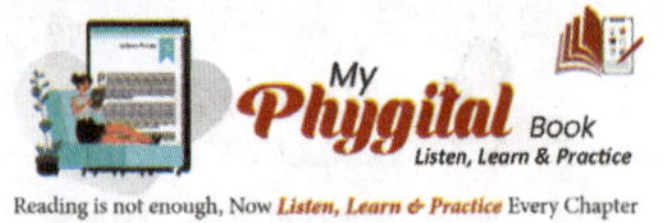

Disorder	Genetics	Characteristics
X-Linked Dominant Inheritance		
Hypertrichosis	Unknown	Abnormal amount of hair growth over body
X-linked hypophosphatemia	Mutation in PHEX gene sequence (Xp.22); subsequent inactivity of PHEX protein	Can cause bone deformity including short stature and genu varum (bow leggedness).
Retinitis pigmentosa (some forms)	Unknown	Degenerative eye disease; causes severe vision impairment; often blindness

- **Mitochondrial inheritance:** Mitochondrial inheritance (Fig. 24.21) is associated with the genes present in the mitochondria and the defects are associated with female offspring. A defective mitochondrial gene in a female will pass it on to all its offspring, whereas male will not. Mitochondrial disorders can appear in every generation of a family and can affect both males and females, but fathers do not pass mitochondrial traits to their children. For example, Leber's hereditary optic neuropathy (LHON).
  Mitochondrial inheritance disorders are given in Table 24.2.

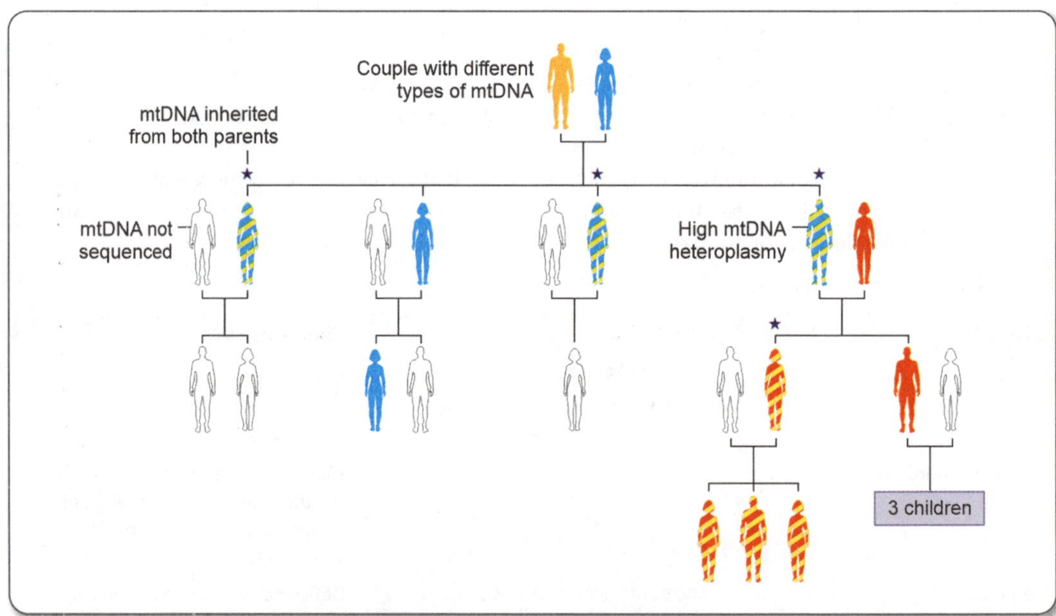

Figure 24.21: Mitochondrial inheritance

Table 24.2: Mitochondrial inheritance disorders

	Types of DNA defect	Examples of disorder	Protein/mechanism involved
Sporadic	Major rearrangements of mtDNA	KSS, CPEO, Pearson's	mtDNA protein synthesis
Maternal	Point mutations of mtDNA	MELAS, MERRF, NARP, LHON, familial duplications	mtDNA protein synthesis In LHON complex I activity reduced

Contd...

	Types of DNA defect	Examples of disorder	Protein/mechanism involved
Autosomal dominant	mtDNA homeostasis	Multiple deletions mtDNA depletion	POLG, ANT1, Twinkle TK2, DGUOK
Autosomal recessive	Deficiencies in specific MRC subunits	Complex I	Flavoproteins: NDUFV1 Iron sulphur protein: NDUFS4 Electron transfer proteins: NDUFS7 and NDUFS8
		Complex II	Flavoprotein SDHA
	Assembly defect mtDNA homeostasis	Complex IV/COX deficiency	SURF-1
		mtDNA depletion	TK2, DGUOK
		MNGIE	Thymidine phosphorylase
X-linked		Pyruvate dehydrogenase deficiency	Pyruvate dehydrogenase complex

Abbreviations: COX, cyclooxygenase; CPEO, chronic progressive external ophthalmoplegia; DGUOK, deoxyguanosine kinase; KSS, Kearns-Sayre syndrome; LHON, leber hereditary optic neuropathy; MELAS, mitochondrial encephalomyopathy, lactic acidosis and stroke-like episodes; MERF, myoclonic epilepsy with ragged red fibers; MNGIE, mitochondrial neurogastrointestinal encephalopathy; NARP, neuropathy ataxia retinitis pigmentosa syndrome

EXTRA EDGE

Codominant pattern disorders: Two different versions (alleles) of a gene can be expressed, and each version or mutated gene makes a slightly different protein. Both alleles influence the genetic trait or determine the characteristics of the genetic condition. For example, blood type.

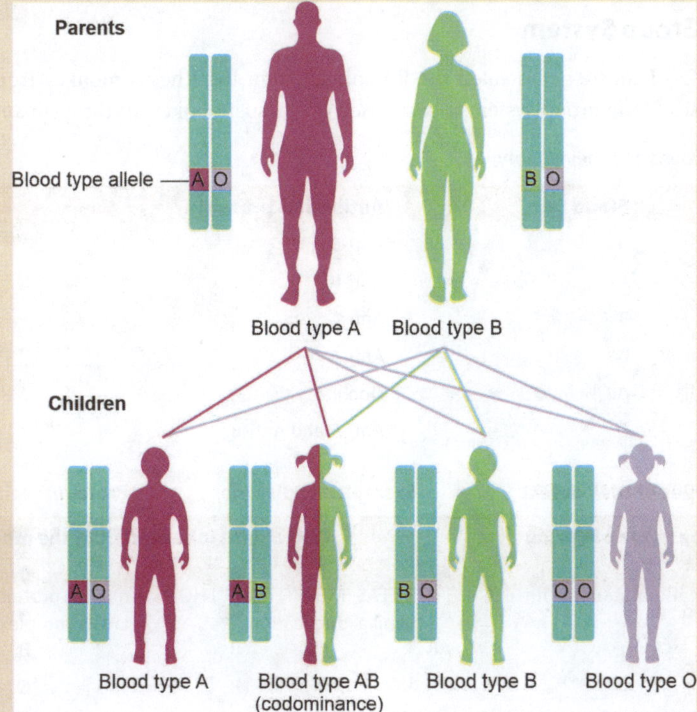

MULTIPLE ALLELES AND BLOOD GROUPS

There are a few different types of blood groups defined based on the different antigens present on the red blood cells. The different antigens are the result of the presence of differences in the gene sequences. There are two blood group systems that have special significance in biology – ABO and Rh systems.

ABO System

The ABO system was discovered by Karl Landsteiner in the year 1901. In the ABO system, the RBCs have either A or B antigen or neither antigen (O group). Based on the presence and absence of these antigens, there are four different blood groups A, B, AB, and O. This system has two major antigens labeled as A and B. If a person has an A antigen on his RBCs, then the person will also have antibodies against B antigen and vice versa. This is the reason why a person with blood group A cannot receive blood with group B, hence it will provoke a severe antibody reaction. The ABO system is encoded by the single gene present on the chromosome 9, and it has three important alleles and these are I^A, I^B, I^O (Table. 24.3).

The I^o allele does not produce any antigens, individuals having homozygous for I^o will have O blood group whereas individuals who are heterozygous for I^AI^o and I^BI^o have blood group A and B, respectively.

Encoding of blood groups: The ABO locus encodes specific glycosyltransferases that synthesize A and B antigens on RBCs. Under the influence of H precursor, synthesis of A or B antigen occurs. In RBCs, the enzyme that synthesizes the H antigen is encoded by the H locus (FUT1). If H antigen is not produced, the ABO blood group antigens are also not produced. This can be misleading in paternity cases.

The ABO blood group antigens are encoded by one genetic locus, the ABO locus, which has three alternative (allelic) forms—A, B, and O. A child receives one of the three alleles from each parent, giving rise to six possible genotypes and four possible blood types (phenotypes) (Table 24.4).

Rhesus Blood Group System

In the year 1930, Karl Landsteiner isolated the Rh antigen from the Rhesus monkey from where it got its name Rh. The Rhesus blood group system is comprised of Rhesus monkey erythrocyte antigens such as the

Table 24.3: Blood groups and their genotypes

Genotype	Blood type	Antibodies present
I^AI^A	A	Anti-B
I^AI^O	A	Anti-B
I^BI^B	B	Anti-A
I^BI^O	B	Anti-A
I^AI^B	AB	Non
I^OI^O	O	Anti-A and Anti-B

Table 24.4: ABO blood group antigens

ABO genotype in the offspring		ABO alleles inherited from the mother		
		A	**B**	**0**
ABO alleles inherited from the father	**A**	A	AB	A
	B	AB	B	B
	0	A	B	O

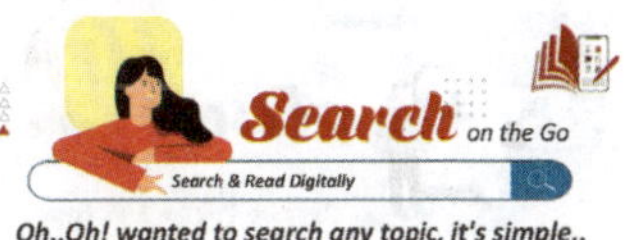

D antigen that is found on the red cells of most humans, who are Rh+. This system is quite complex, and the rare Rh alloantigens are still not characterized biochemically. The Rh factor varies considerably among the population and has a significant role in assessing the genetic variation. Both ABO system and Rh system play an important role in resolving the complications related to blood transfusion and tissue graft transplantations.

MNS Blood Group System

It was first discovered in 1927, following the discovery of the ABO system. The MNS system, named after the first two antigens discovered, M and N, is complex. It currently consists of 46 antigens; however, the most important of these in terms of clinical relevance are M, N, S, s, and U.

The MNS antigens are produced by two co-dominant alleles, located on chromosome 4. These genes code for GYPA and GYPB proteins, which are the carriers of MNS antigen.

MNS and malaria: There is a link between the MNS system and resistance or susceptibility to malaria. The absence of the Glycophorin A gene (which carries the M antigen) has been associated with resistance to the *Plasmodium falciparum* parasite, which causes malaria.

Kell Blood Group System

The Kell blood group system is complex and contains many antigens that are highly immunogenic. These antigens are the third potent antigen after the ABO and Rh blood groups, at triggering an immune reaction. The Kell blood type system is highly polymorphic because there are about 25 different Kell alleles, different forms of a gene. The most common are the K (Kell-positive) and k (Kell-negative). Kell-negative alleles are more common. Kell antigens are important determinants of blood type and are targets for autoimmune diseases which destroy red blood cells.

Duffy Blood Group System

The Duffy blood group system is a complex of highly immunogenic glycoprotein antigens that are present on the surface of red blood cells (RBC), alveolar epithelial cells, endothelial cells, collecting tubules of the kidney, and on the surface of Purkinje cells in the brain. Duffy blood group is rare in Whites. This is the reason that Duffy antigen is used to find genetic admixture among people from Black African descent.

Kidd Blood Grouping System

The Kidd blood group system is simple, and has only three antigens, Jk^a, Jk^b, and Jk^3. Jk^a and Jk^b are antithetical alleles, and the Jk^3 is a high-prevalence antigen. Jk^a and Jk^b differ from each other in a single amino acid in the extracellular domain. The Kidd antibodies are generally difficult to detect, making them hazardous in transfusion medicine, where they are suspected to be a common cause of delayed hemolytic transfusion reactions (DHTRs).

SUMMARY

- The modern nurses should be able to take the family history of a patient up to three generations.
- A nurse must keep a neutral opinion about genetically acquired issues.
- Harmful environmental factors can change a gene's nucleotide sequence.
- Nucleosomes are the basic units of chromatin.
- During the metaphase, each chromosome can be identified based on the size and shape.

Contd...

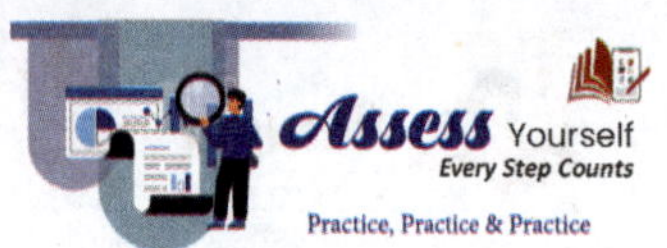

- Chromosomes appear in pairs, one of each pair is derived from mother and father.
- The female has two X chromosomes (XX), whereas in a male there is one X chromosome and one Y chromosome (XY) in a normal condition.
- One consequence of an altered enzyme or protein structure is altered function.
- Genes may interact with an individual's environment and change the function that it dictates and bring genotypic or phenotypic variations.
- The duration of cell cycle varies considerably from one cell type to other cell type, some cells divide in less than 10 hours, whereas few cells divide once a year.
- Mitosis is divided into 4 phases, those are prophase, metaphase, anaphase, and telophase.
- Meiosis is a special type of cell division that forms the gametes with haploid number of chromosomes starting from diploid cell.
- In male, there is formation of four functional daughter cells; whereas in females, one functional daughter cells is formed with most of the cytoplasm, and three polar bodies.
- Chromosomal aberrations are substantial changes in chromosome structure which typically affect multiple genes (loci).
- In humans, euploidy conditions do not exist because the extent of abnormality is too large to sustain life.
- Aneuploidy conditions, are more common and are manifested in disorders such as Down syndrome.
- Polyploidy is commonly observed in plants, and is incompatible with human life.
- The qualitative aberrations are variations in the chromosome structure also referred to as heteromorphism.
- From the diploid pair of chromosomes only haploid set of chromosomes is transferred to the offspring.
- Law of independence says that alleles present on one locus are transmitted independent of the other.
- Mendel's experiments also highlight that the alleles have recessive and dominant characteristics referred to as principle of dominance.
- Regarding the normal allele, an allele carrying a mutation can have characteristics of dominance, codominant or recessive.
- Mutations are of four types, substitution, deletion, insertion, and translocation.
- The genetic disorders due to inheritance may be recessive or dominant.
- There are different patterns of inheritance, these are autosomal, and sex-linked inheritance.
- Mitochondrial disorders can appear in every generation of a family and can affect both males and females, but fathers do not pass mitochondrial traits to their children.
- Two different versions (alleles) of a gene can be expressed, and each version or mutated gene makes a slightly different protein.
- There are two blood group systems that have special significance in biology are the ABO and Rh systems.
- The ABO system is encoded by the single gene present on the chromosome 9, and it has three important alleles and these are IA, IB, IO.

ASSESS YOURSELF

Long Answer Questions

1. Discuss genetics and heredity. Explain laws of inheritance.
2. What is impact of genetic disorders on a family? Explain.
3. Describe the role of a nurse in genetics.

Short Answer Questions

1. Write down the difference between mitosis and meiosis.
2. Mention the characteristics and structure of genes.
3. Write short notes on:
   i. Chromosomal disorders
   ii. Limitations of NIPT

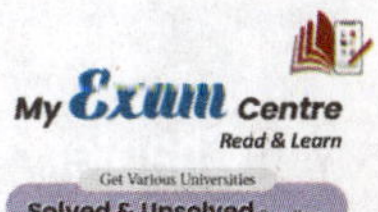

Multiple Choice Questions

1. **Down's syndrome is caused due to:**
   a. Monosomy of 21st chromosome
   b. Disomy of 21st chromosome
   c. Trisomy of 21st chromosome
   d. An extra X chromosome in female
2. **What type of allele produces its effects only in homozygous individuals?**
   a. Recessive
   b. Dominant
   c. Incomplete recessive
   d. None of the above
3. **When alleles move into different gametes, it shows the:**
   a. Dominance
   b. Incomplete dominance
   c. Segregation
   d. Crossing over
4. **The ABO blood group in human is the example for:**
   a. Dominance
   b. Recessive
   c. Incomplete dominance
   d. Codominance
5. **Turner's syndrome is caused due to:**
   a. Presence of extra X chromosome in male
   b. Absence of one of the X chromosome in male
   c. Absence of one of the X chromosome in female
   d. Presence of one extra chromosome in female.
6. **Female has____chromosomes.**
   a. XX
   b. XY
   c. XXY
   d. YYY
7. **Genetics is the study of:**
   a. Variation
   b. Inheritance
   c. Both a and b
   d. None of these
8. **Genetic constitution of an organism is:**
   a. Phenotype
   b. Genotype
   c. Dihybrid
   d. Monohybrid
9. **Different forms of gene are:**
   a. Chromosome
   b. Alleles
   c. Linkage
   d. All of these

Answer Key

1. c	**2.** a	**3.** c	**4.** d	**5.** c	**6.** a
7. c	**8.** b	**9.** b			

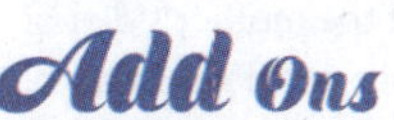

Dil Mange More Content

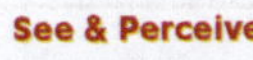

See & Perceive	Recent Update	e-Book
Watch and learn with the selective Important Topic-wise	Regular updates related to Recent advancements & Book Errata	Get PDFs of important chapter/section (Annexures/Appendices) of book *(optional and exclusive for Pro-users and Institutions)*

Nursing Next Live
The Next Level of Nursing Education
CBS Phygital Books >
Textbook of Pathology & Genetics PHYGITAL

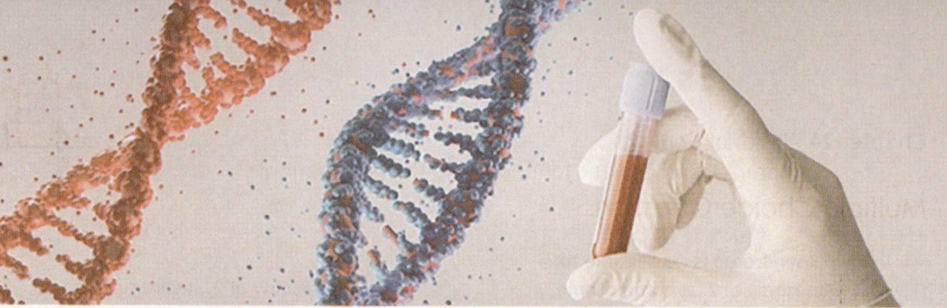

Chapter 25

Maternal and Genetic Influences on Development of Defects and Diseases

LEARNING OBJECTIVES

After the completion of the chapter, the readers will be able to:

- Understand the conditions affecting the mother, maternal drug therapy.
- Know about prenatal nutrition, food allergies and influence of maternal age.
- Discuss infertility and its treatment.
- Know about effect of radiation, drugs and chemicals on pregnancy.
- Discuss the spontaneous abortion.

CHAPTER OUTLINE

- Genetics and Infections
- Genetic Polymorphism
- Conditions Affecting the Mother
- Adverse Effect of Prenatal Infections in Newborn
- Consanguinity Atopy—Impact on Reproductive Health
- Prenatal Nutrition and Food Allergies
- Maternal Age
- Maternal Drug Therapy
- Effect of Radiation on Pregnancy
- Effects of Drugs and Chemicals on Pregnancy
- Infertility
- Spontaneous Abortion

KEY TERMS

Birth defects: Structural or functional abnormalities present at birth, which can result from genetic, environmental, or a combination of factors.

Congenital disorders: Conditions that are present at birth and may have genetic, environmental, or unknown causes.

Genetic disorders: Conditions caused by abnormalities in an individual's DNA, often inherited from parents.

Genetic factors: Inherited traits and genetic variations that can affect the susceptibility to certain diseases or conditions.

Maternal age: The age of the mother at the time of conception, which can influence the risk of certain genetic disorders.

Maternal health: The overall health and well-being of the mother during pregnancy.

Maternal nutrition: The impact of the mother's diet on fetal development.

Neonatal screening: Testing performed shortly after birth to identify genetic or metabolic disorders that may not be apparent at birth.

Prenatal development: The process of development that occurs from conception to birth.

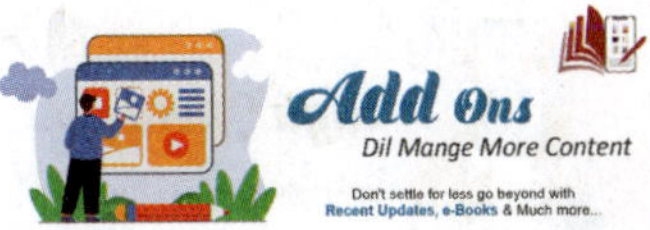

GENETICS AND INFECTIONS

Human infectious diseases have been widely misunderstood to be purely infectious. Genetics also play a role in infections. The mutated genes lower the immunity of a person. Genetic mutations may be harmful or beneficial.

Importance of genetics in prevention and prediction of risk:

- Using information about a person's genetic make-up to tailor strategies for detection, treatment, and prevention of diseases.
- Monitoring changes in CNPs (copy number polymorphisms) may help to recognize emerging drug resistance quickly and early.
- The cure for HIV probably lies in gene therapy.

GENETIC POLYMORPHISM

Genetic polymorphism determines the diversity of individuals. It leads to changes in the DNA sequence and an increased susceptibility to disease.

Genetic Polymorphism and Infections

Genetic polymorphism can manifest in the form of SNPs (single nucleotide polymorphisms), insertions, deletions, or other structural changes in the DNA sequence.

It involves allelic variation which is genetic polymorphism involving the presence of different alleles of a gene in a population:

When allele frequency is <1% = Rare variant

Genetic polymorphism is common in populations and there may be different versions of genes present in individuals within the group. Most common genetic polymorphism is single nucleotide polymorphism (SNPs). They involve a single nucleotide change in the DNA sequence. For example, an SNP may result in a change from adenine (A) to guanine (G), other genetic polymorphism types are RFLP (restriction fragment length polymorphism; variable number of tandem repeats (VNTRs); simple sequence repeats (SSRs).

Importance of Genetic Polymorphism

- Some genetic polymorphisms may have functional consequences. They can affect the structure or function of the encoded protein, influencing an individual's traits, susceptibility to infections or response to drugs. They contribute to the variability seen in traits within a population.
- The genetic polymorphism is inherited from one generation to the next. The genetic polymorphisms are associated with an increased risk of developing certain diseases. These associations are studied under genomics.
- Genetics polymorphism affects the resistance power of an individual toward a disease. For example, 1/3 of world's population is infected with *M. tuberculosis*; however, only a minority (10%) of those infected ever develop clinical disease.
- Epidemiological evidence accumulated, since the 1930s, that human genetic factors play a role in immunodeficiency and susceptibility to infectious diseases. The possibility of infectious diseases is higher in monozygotic twins than in dizygotic twins.

For example, tuberculosis

Several genes have now been associated with susceptibility to mycobacterium (TB and leprosy):

- Vitamin D receptor gene (VDR, which has over 490 single nucleotide polymorphisms)
- Natural resistance-associated macrophage protein-1 gene (NRAMP1)

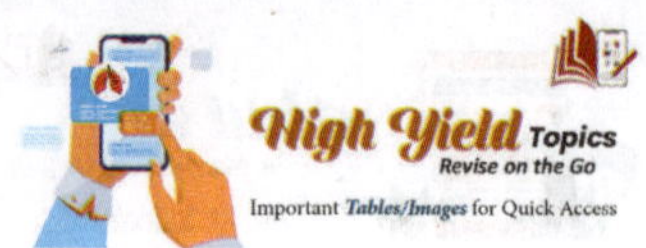

- Human Leukocyte Antigen gene (HLA-DR)
- Interferon gamma gene

For example, malaria

Genetic factors account for about 25% of the variability of the incidence of malaria in the general population. Malarial parasite shows resistance for artemisinin which is conferred by an increase in the number of gene copies for the multidrug resistance (pfmdr) gene. Mutations in pfcrt gene also multiply the pfmdr gene thus leading to chloroquine resistance.

Types of Genetic Polymorphisms

- **Single nucleotide polymorphisms (SNP):** Substitution of one or the other of 2 bases of DNA at a single location
- **Variable number of tandem repeat (VNTR):** The polymorphism is displayed by the relative migration of individual bands, alleles, according to the number of repeats
- **Restriction fragment length polymorphism (RFLP):** Refers to differences (or variations) among people in their DNA sequences at sites recognized by restriction enzymes
- **Simple sequence repeat (SSR):** The number of the tandem repeats of a specific microsatellite at a specific locus. SSRs are single locus markers and have a few to even more than ten alleles in each locus; thus, SSRs are highly polymorphic.

CONDITIONS AFFECTING THE MOTHER

Certain medical conditions may complicate a pregnancy. However, with proper medical care, most women can enjoy a healthy pregnancy in spite of medical challenges. Some of the important medical conditions affecting mothers are discussed ahead.

Diabetes and Pregnancy

Women having diabetes before or those who develop it during gestation require additional medical care. Diabetes can have serious consequences for mother and fetus.

Pre-gestational Diabetes

The symptoms and complications depend on the progression of diabetes.

Gestational Diabetes

The glucose level is elevated and other diabetic symptoms appear during pregnancy. The placenta produce estrogen, cortisol and human placental lactogen. Some of these hormones have a blocking effect on the mother's insulin. This condition is known as insulin resistance. In this case, there is high risk of developing diabetes later in life. It usually begins it about 20–24 weeks into pregnancy. Normally, the mother's pancreas is able to make additional insulin to overcome insulin resistance. However, if the mother's body is not producing enough insulin to overcome the effect of the placental hormones, gestational diabetes results.

Risk Factors of Gestational Diabetes

- Age (over 25-year-old).
- A family history of diabetes.

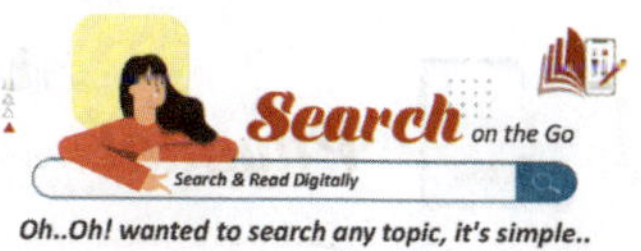

- Previous delivery of a very large infant, a stillborn or a child with certain birth defects.
- Obesity.

Treatment Plan

After diagnosing gestational diabetes (usually done between 24 and 28 weeks of pregnancy) specific treatment plan for gestational diabetes is made depending on:
- Personal preference.
- Condition and the severity of the disease.
- Age, overall health and medical history.
- Long-term expectations for the course of the disease.
- Tolerance for specific medicines, procedures or therapies.

Treatment

Treatment for gestational diabetes focuses on keeping blood glucose levels in the normal range and it includes:
- Exercise.
- A special diet.
- Daily blood glucose monitoring.
- Insulin injections or oral medications.

Fetal Complications from Gestational Diabetes

Infants of mothers with gestational diabetes are susceptible to electrolyte imbalances, such as low-serum calcium and low-serum magnesium levels. Additionally, it may cause the following complications:
- **Fetal macrosomia:** A baby that is considerably larger than normal. The nutrition provided through the placenta may contain high level of glucose. The extra glucose present in the blood of mother is converted into fat in the body of fetus and causes the baby to grow excessively large leading to a large size.
- **Birth injury:** If the baby is large in size, it may be difficult to deliver and can get injured in the process.
- **Hypoglycemia:** If mother's blood sugar level is consistently high right after delivery, it causes the fetus to have a high level of insulin in its circulation, although it no longer has the high level of sugar from mother. This drops the blood sugar level of the newborn. If the sugar level is very low, it may become necessary to administer glucose intravenously until the baby's blood sugar stabilizes.
- **Respiratory distress (difficulty breathing):** Too much insulin or too much glucose in a baby's system may delay lung maturation and cause respiratory problems (more likely if it is born before 37 weeks of pregnancy).

High Blood Pressure and Pregnancy

High blood pressure during pregnancy leads to placental complications and slows down fetal growth. If left untreated, severe hypertension may cause seizures, stroke and even death of the mother and fetus.
- **Chronic hypertension:** If mother has high blood pressure before pregnancy, then there is a need to continue taking antihypertensive medicine.
- **Gestational hypertension:** Gestational hypertension occurs most often during a young woman's first pregnancy. A woman is also more likely to develop gestational hypertension during a twin pregnancy or if she was having hypertension or hypotension during a previous pregnancy.
- **Pre-eclampsia (formerly called toxemia):** Pregnancy-induced high blood pressure. There will be protein in the urine and which may cause swelling due to fluid retention. Eclampsia, the most severe form of this

condition, is diagnosed when the mother has seizures in addition to the hypertension. Hospitalization, medications and often delivery is recommended to save mother and baby.

Maternal Infections During Pregnancy

Infections during pregnancy (prenatal) can pose a threat to the baby. An infection that goes untreated can lead to preterm labor and rupture of the membranes surrounding the fetus.

Toxoplasmosis

- Toxoplasmosis is an infection caused by a single-celled parasite called *Toxoplasma gondii (T. gondii).*
- **Complications:** Babies who become infected with toxoplasmosis before birth can be born with serious mental or physical problems, preterm delivery, and baby can born with liver, brain and eye-related disorders.
- Toxoplasmosis often causes flu-like symptoms, including swollen lymph glands or muscle aches and pains in mother which last for a few days to several weeks.
- Fetal testing may include ultrasound and/or testing of the amniotic fluid or cord blood.
- **Management:** Includes treatment with antibiotics and hand washing.

Food Poisoning

Ingesting food contaminated with bacteria or parasites may cause food poisoning.
- Food poisoning can dehydrate a mother and deprive the fetus of nourishment. It can lead to early labor, abortion or still birth.
- Food poisoning can cause meningitis and pneumonia in a fetus, resulting in possible death.
- **Management:** Pregnant mother should avoid eating undercooked or raw foods to avoid food poisoning.
- Keep following hand hygiene.

Sexually-Transmitted Disease

- **Chlamydia complications**: Associated with premature labor and rupture of the membranes.
- **HBV complications in fetus:** Infected pregnant women can pass the virus to their fetus during pregnancy and at delivery. If infection occurs later in pregnancy, the risk of infecting the baby is greater.
  - Babies of mothers with unknown HBV status should receive the hepatitis B vaccine in the first 12 hours of birth.
  - Infants of HBV-positive mothers should receive hepatitis B immunoglobulin and the hepatitis B vaccine during the first 12 hours of birth.
  - Babies of mothers with negative HBV status should be vaccinated before leaving the hospital.
  - All babies should complete the hepatitis B vaccine series to be fully protected from HBV infection.
  - Premature infants weighing <4.5 pounds, born to mothers with negative HBV status should have their first vaccine dose delayed until one month after birth or leaving the hospital.
- **HIV complications:** Adverse pregnancy outcomes in HIV positive women include increased rates of spontaneous early abortion, low birth weight babies, stillbirths, preterm labor, preterm rupture of membranes, other sexually transmitted diseases, bacterial pneumonia, urinary tract infections.
- **Genital Herpes complications:** If women become infected with genital herpes in the last three months of pregnancy, the virus is passed on to their babies in about 30–50 out of 100 births. Infection leads to brain damage, eye issues, or even infant death.

Summary of some common prenatal infection have been depicted in Table 25.1.

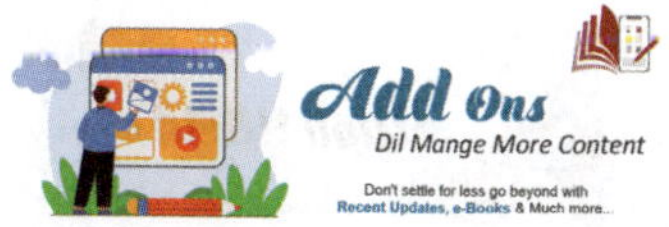

Table 25.1: Summary of some common prenatal infections, along with potential adverse effects on the fetus

Prenatal infection	Causative agent	Transmission	Adverse effects on fetus
Rubella (German Measles)	Rubella virus	Respiratory droplets	Congenital rubella syndrome: Heart defects, deafness, cataracts, intellectual disabilities, organ abnormalities. Increased risk if infection occurs in the first trimester.
Cytomegalovirus (CMV)	Cytomegalovirus	Saliva, urine, blood, and other body fluids	Hearing loss, intellectual disabilities, vision problems, microcephaly. Severity varies with the timing of infection during pregnancy.
Toxoplasmosis	Toxoplasma gondii (parasite)	Ingestion of contaminated food or water, contact with cat feces	Hydrocephalus, seizures, intellectual disabilities, vision problems. Severity depends on when the infection occurs during pregnancy.
Herpes Simplex Virus (HSV)	HSV-1 or HSV-2	Direct contact with infected lesions	Neonatal herpes: Skin, eye, or mouth infections; central nervous system damage; developmental delays. Cesarean delivery may be recommended if active lesions are present during labor.
Syphilis	Treponema pallidum (bacterium)	Sexual contact, congenital transmission	Congenital syphilis: Stillbirth, prematurity, developmental delays, bone deformities, hepatosplenomegaly. Early detection and treatment with penicillin can prevent complications.
Human Immunodeficiency Virus (HIV)	Human Immuno-deficiency Virus	Blood, sexual contact, perinatal transmission	Increased risk of premature birth, low birth weight, and neonatal HIV infection. Antiretroviral therapy during pregnancy can reduce the risk of transmission.
Zika Virus	Zika virus	Mosquito bites, sexual transmission	Microcephaly, brain abnormalities, eye defects. Most critical during the first trimester but can pose risks throughout pregnancy.
Parvovirus B19 (Fifth Disease)	Parvovirus B19	Respiratory secretions, blood	Anemia, fetal hydrops (severe swelling), miscarriage. Most significant risk during the first half of pregnancy.
Hepatitis B	Hepatitis B virus	Blood, sexual contact, perinatal transmission	Chronic hepatitis, liver disease. Vaccination of newborns born to infected mothers can prevent transmission.
Listeriosis	Listeria monocytogenes (bacterium)	Contaminated food (e.g., unpasteurized dairy, deli meats)	Miscarriage, stillbirth, premature birth, neonatal infections. Prevention through safe food handling practices.

ADVERSE EFFECT OF PRENATAL INFECTIONS IN NEWBORN

The prenatal infections, can increase the risk of a preterm birth, and serious health complications in the newborn which include specific organ damage, developmental delay, and even death. It further includes:

- **Phenylketonuria (PKU):** It is due to deficiency of phenylalanine hydroxylase (PAH). In this disorder, the body cannot properly process the amino acid phenylalanine due to a deficient enzyme called phenylalanine hydroxylase.

- **Noncancerous (benign) tumors:** Other inborn errors of metabolism such as tuberous sclerosis complex, is a rare genetic condition that causes mainly non-cancerous (benign) tumors to develop in different parts of the body. The tumors most often affect the brain, skin, kidneys, heart, eyes and lungs.
- **Other genetic disorders** include myotonic dystrophy (progressive muscle wasting and weakness); cystic fibrosis; Turner syndrome (Turner syndrome, a condition that affects only females, results when one of the X chromosomes (sex chromosomes) is missing or partially missing. It leads to developmental problems, including short height, failure of the ovaries to develop and heart defects) sickle cell disease, and connective tissue disorders.

The severity of adverse effects can vary based on factors such as the timing of infection during pregnancy, the health of the mother, and the presence of any pre-existing conditions. Pregnant mothers should take prompt medical help if they suspect that they have been exposed to or infected with any of the infectious agents.

CONSANGUINITY ATOPY—IMPACT ON REPRODUCTIVE HEALTH

Consanguinity

Consanguinity comes from two Latin words; 'con' means shared and 'sanguis' means blood. Therefore, consanguinity refers to relationship by blood (being from the same family) or by a common ancestor (Fig. 25.1). Socially, it means marrying blood relatives.

Consanguineous marriage: It is defined as marriage between close blood relatives who have at least one common ancestor. Consanguineous marriages remain culturally and socially favored and respected in many countries.

Consanguinity is a deeply-rooted cultural trend in certain communities because of the following reasons:

- It is more favorable for the women's status.
- The wife would have better relationship with her in-laws and could be protected by them in time of need.
- There is a general belief that marrying within the family reduces the possibilities of hidden health and financial uncertainties.
- Premarital negotiations regarding financial matters of marriage are more easily conducted, keeping the money and property within the family.
- Strengthens family ties, and enforces family solidarity.

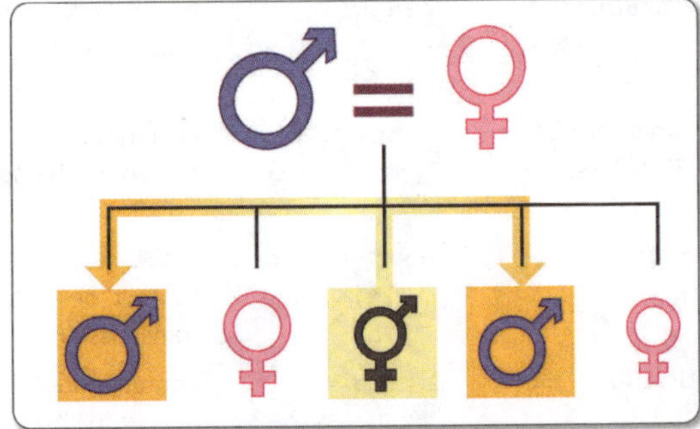

Figure 25.1: Consanguinity

Adverse Effects of Consanguinity

Genetic disorders: Among genetic disorders, only autosomal recessive disorders are strongly associated with consanguinity.

Stillbirth: Stillbirth rates are either similar or slightly higher among consanguineous couples than the non-related couples. There is a positive association between parental consanguinity and increased infant and childhood mortality.

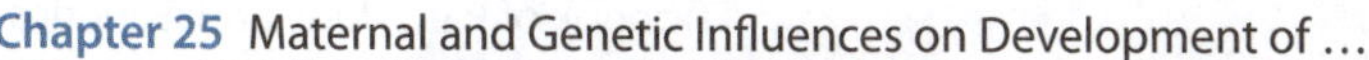

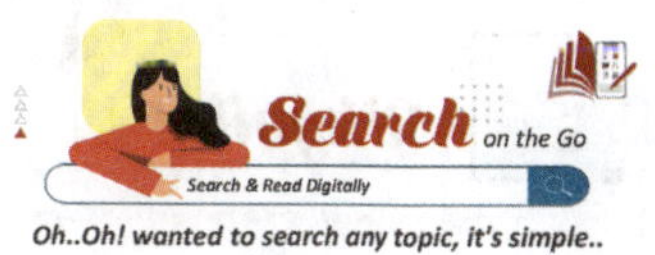

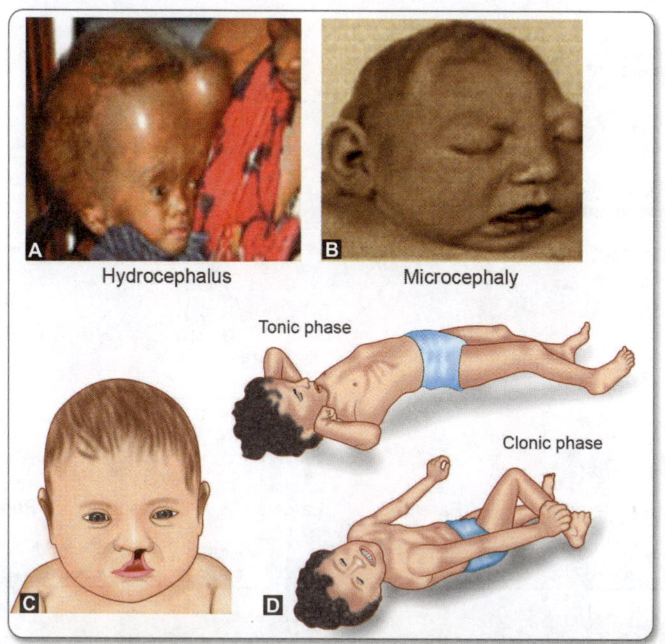

Figures 25.2A to C: **A.** Anencephaly; **B.** Microcephaly; **C.** Cleft lip; **D.** Seizures

- **Congenital malformations (Figs 25.2A to D):**
  - **For example:** Anencephaly, cleft lip, cleft palate, etc.
  - **Phenotypic characteristics:** Blindness, hearing loss, seizures.
- **Metabolic disorders:** Phenylketonuria is three times more common among consanguineous cases than in general population
  - **Other disorders:** Mental retardation, primary amenorrhea, etc.
  - Various disabilities.
  - Chronic adult non-communicable diseases.

Atopy

The term atopy was coined by Coca in 1923. Atopy is hereditary predisposition toward developing type I hypersensitivity reactions on exposure to specific antigens. Atopy includes allergic diseases such as hay fever, asthma, chronic urticaria. These allergic manifestations are due to abnormally high sensitivity to antigens known as allergens. Allergens may be inhaled, ingested or got by contact dermatitis. Atopy allergens induce IgE type of antibodies.

Causes

- **Genetic factors:** It may run in families. In atopic individuals, large quantities of IgE antibodies are produced.
- **Environmental factors:** Environment plays a role in the development of atopy. Bottle feeding tends to develop atopy in later life more often than the breast-fed babies
- **Maternal diet:** It may be a causal factor in atopic diseases in child, suggesting antioxidants, certain lipids, certain diet may cause atopic diseases.

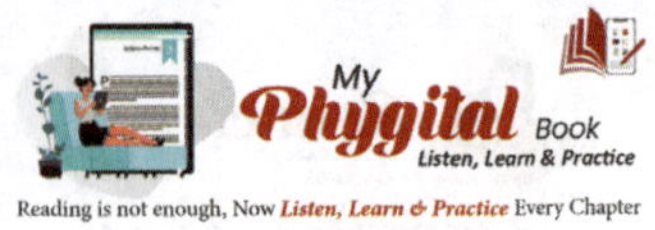

MUST KNOW

Genetic inheritance– degree of cousinhood

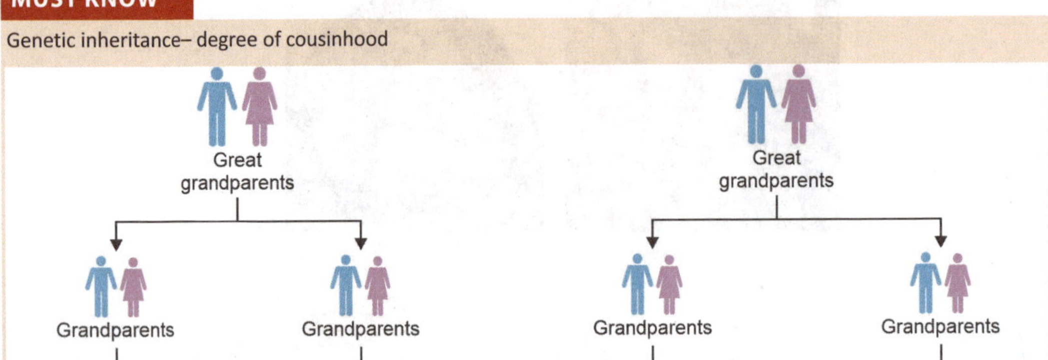

Note: On an average, first cousins share 1/8 of their genes inherited from their common ancestors.

Consanguinity Atopy

The relationship between atopy and consanguinity is complex and involves a combination of genetic and environmental factors. Consanguinity can contribute to the risk of atopy by increasing the likelihood of sharing specific genetic factors associated with allergic conditions. However, the association between genetics and environmental factors is complex, and not all individuals with consanguineous relationships will develop atopic conditions. It is essential to consider both genetic and environmental aspects when studying or discussing the risk of atopy in families with consanguinity.

Relationship Between Atopy and Consanguinity

- **Genetic factors:** Atopy has a strong genetic component, which means that individuals with a family history of atopic conditions (such as asthma, hay fever, or eczema) are more likely to develop these conditions themselves.
- **Environmental factors:** While genetics plays a significant role, environmental factors also contribute to the development of atopic conditions. These factors may include exposure to allergens, pollutants, and lifestyle factors.
- **Research findings:** Studies have investigated the relationship between consanguinity and the risk of atopy, and findings can vary. Some studies suggest that consanguinity may be associated with an increased risk of certain allergic conditions, while others may not find a clear association.

  The relationship is likely to be influenced by the specific genetic variations present in the family and the environmental context.

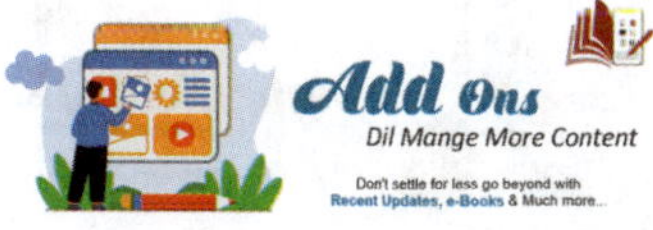

Role of a Nurse in Consanguinity Atopy

A nurse can play a significant role in addressing the challenges associated with consanguinity and atopy. Some specific aspects of the nurse's role are:

- **Assessment and family history:** Conduct thorough assessments to gather detailed family histories, especially focusing on atopic conditions such as asthma, allergies, and eczema. Identify if consanguinity is present within family.
- **Education and counseling:** Provide education to individuals and families about the potential genetic implications of consanguinity on atopic conditions. Explain the increased risk and help them understand the importance of early detection and management.
- **Genetic counseling referral:** Recognize the need for genetic counseling and refer individuals or families to genetic counselors for more in-depth information and guidance on the genetic aspects of atopic conditions associated with consanguinity.
- **Support for decision making:** Assist individuals and families in making informed decisions about family planning by providing support and resources. This may involve discussing the potential risks and benefits of various reproductive options.
- **Allergy management:** Be involved in the management of atopic conditions, including providing information on allergen avoidance, administering medications, and assisting with treatment plans. Work collaboratively with other healthcare professionals, such as allergists, to ensure comprehensive care.
- **Preventive measures:** Educate families on preventive measures to minimize the impact of atopic conditions. This may include recommendations for allergen-free environments, dietary considerations, and lifestyle modifications.
- **Promotion of healthy lifestyles:** Advocate for and promote healthy lifestyle choices that can positively impact atopic conditions. This may include encouraging breastfeeding, a balanced diet, and regular physical activity.
- **Advocacy and support:** Advocate for individuals and families within the healthcare system to ensure they receive appropriate care and support. Provide emotional support and resources to help cope with the challenges associated with atopic conditions.
- **Community education**: Engage in community education initiatives to raise awareness about the relationship between consanguinity and atopy. Disseminate information about preventive measures and early intervention strategies.
- **Cultural competence:** Be culturally competent and sensitive to the unique needs and beliefs of individuals and families. Understand the cultural context surrounding consanguinity and tailor care accordingly.
- **Documentation and collaboration:** Maintain thorough and accurate documentation of assessments, interventions, and education provided. Collaborate with other healthcare professionals to ensure continuity of care and a holistic approach to managing atopic conditions.
- **Clinical care:** Includes education, advocacy, and support, fostering a comprehensive and patient-centered approach.

PRENATAL NUTRITION AND FOOD ALLERGIES

Prenatal nutrition can play a role in the development of the fetal immune system and potentially impact the risk of food allergies later in life. While research in this area is ongoing and not all mechanisms are fully understood, however some points regarding prenatal nutrition and food allergies are as follows:

- **Maternal diet:** A mother's diet during pregnancy can influence the developing immune system of the fetus. Some studies suggest that certain nutrients, such as omega-3 fatty acids found in fish, may have a protective effect against the development of allergies.

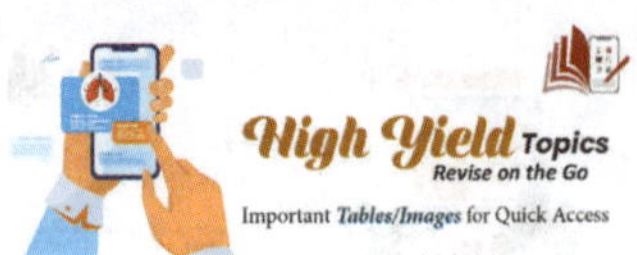

- **Diverse diet:** Encouraging pregnant women to consume a diverse and balanced diet that includes a variety of fruits, vegetables, whole grains, and lean proteins may contribute to a well-rounded nutritional profile. This diversity can expose the fetus to a range of nutrients that may support immune system development.
- **Probiotics and prebiotics:** Probiotics (beneficial bacteria) and prebiotics (substances promote the growth of beneficial bacteria) in maternal diets may influence the gut microbiota of both the mother and the developing fetus, potentially affecting immune system development.
- **Breastfeeding:** Breast milk contains antibodies and other immune factors that may support the infant's developing immune system. The introduction of allergenic foods during breastfeeding may also play a role in tolerance development.
- **Avoidance of allergic foods:** There is no clear evidence to support widespread avoidance, and some studies even suggest that early introduction of allergenic foods may be protective.

MUST KNOW

Food allergy—mechanism

Development of food allergies is a complex process, influenced by genetic, environmental, and immunological factors. While prenatal nutrition can play a role, it is not the sole determinant of food allergy risk.

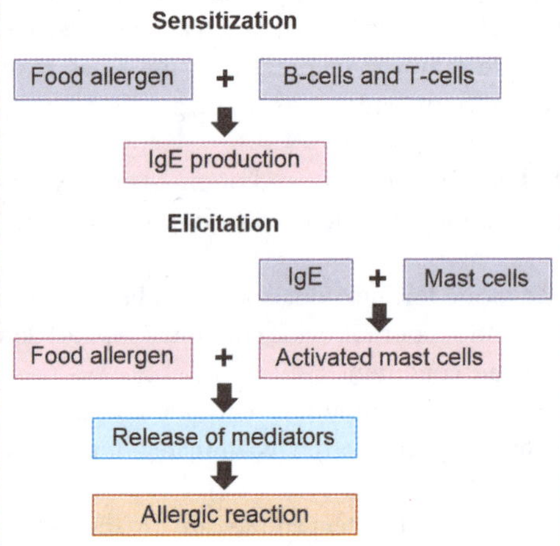

Most Common Food Allergens to Avoid in Prenatal Period

CASE SCENARIO 1

A pregnant woman came to OPD with complaints of vomiting and diarrhea. (This happened due to Lactose Intolerance.)

Food allergies (Table 25.2) can appear at any time during pregnancy. Symptoms may appear as soon as the allergen is tolerated or several hours later. Most common food allergens are – peanuts soyfish, shellfish, wheat, dairy products and fish.

- **Peanut:** Peanuts should be avoided by atopic pregnant women, breastfeeding moms, and their children. During pregnancy, allergic reactions and symptoms can fluctuate due to hormonal changes. Some women find their symptoms reduced by pregnancy; others find they increase.
- **Milk/dairy allergy:** The most common signs of lactose intolerance are abdominal pain, bloating, cramping and gas after ingesting dairy products.

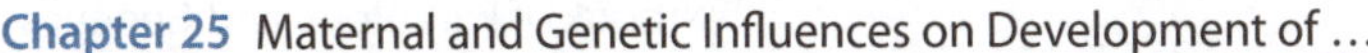

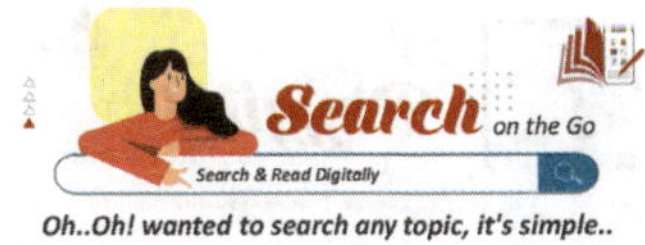

Table 25.2: Food allergy: Symptoms and testing methods

Allergy	Allergens	Antibodies	Symptoms	Testing
Egg allergy	Ovomucoid; Ovo transferrin; Conalbumin; Lysozymes; Ovalbumin; Alpha-livetin; Vitellus	IgE	Respiratory or cardiovascular symptoms, presenting with cough, wheezing, breathing difficulty, or pallor and floppiness are uncommon	Skin prick test, egg-specific IgE, and egg component testing
Fish allergy	Parvalbumins; Gelatin; Enolase; Aldolase; Vitellogenin; Tropomyosin	IgE	Anaphylaxis, nausea, gastrointestinal, and rhinitis	Skin prick test, Immuno-CAP, and immunoblotting
Peanut allergy	Ara h 1 and Ara h 3	IgE	Skin (e.g., urticaria, flushing, and angioedema), gastrointestinal tract (e.g., vomiting, nausea, abdominal pain, and diarrhea), respiratory system (e.g., rhinorrhea, sneezing, coughing), and the cardiovascular system (e.g., cardiovascular collapse)	Skin prick test and basophil activation test
Cashew nut allergy	Vicilin; Legumins	IgE	Respiratory and gastrointestinal indications	Skin prick test, double-blind placebo-controlled food challenge (DBPCFC)
Milk allergy	Casein protein and whey protein; alpha-lactalbumin and beta-lactalbumin	IgE	Hives; wheezing; Itching; or tingling feeling around the lips or mouth; swelling of the lips, tongue, or throat; coughing or shortness of breath; vomiting; and other digestive-related problems	Skin prick test; blood test; oral food challenge

- **Egg allergy:** Egg allergy symptoms usually occur a few minutes to a few hours after eating eggs or foods containing eggs. Signs and symptoms range from mild to severe and can include skin rashes, hives, nasal congestion, and vomiting or other digestive problems.
- **Fish/seafood allergy:** Seafood allergy in pregnant women sometimes has mild reactions, sometimes leading to many serious complications, the most severe is anaphylaxis. The mother's life can be at risk if an anaphylactic reaction is not detected in time.

Symptoms of Food Allergy

- Rashes, hives on the body.
- Blisters may appear and spread to other areas of the skin.
- Itchy skin which is often more at night.
- Other symptoms are cough, stuffy nose, itchy ears, itchy throat.

Effect of Food Allergies on a Pregnant Woman's Health

Food allergies can have serious effects on a pregnant woman's health:

- Mothers can have a miscarriage, premature birth or cause birth defects if they have allergies during 9 months of pregnancy.

- Pregnant women with allergies during pregnancy also increase the likelihood of children getting sick after birth.
- The symptoms of food allergy not only affect the mother's body but also have the risk of being transmitted to the fetus through the placenta.
- The allergic mechanism can also interfere with the growth, development or directly damage the lungs and bronchi of the fetus, which is extremely dangerous.

Role of Prenatal Nutrition in Prevention of Genetic Disorders

The prenatal nutrition plays a crucial role in the prevention of certain genetic disorders and the overall health of the developing fetus. Proper prenatal nutrition can influence the expression of genes and contribute to a healthy pregnancy.

- **Folate or folic acid and NTDs and Down syndrome:**
  - Folate is essential for DNA synthesis and repair, and a deficiency can lead to abnormalities in the developing neural tube. Trisomy 21 (T-21) (commonly known as Down syndrome can also be prevented by taking folic acid.
  - Deficiency of B vitamins and folic acid in maternal diet is another commonly associated cause of cleft lip and palate in the newborn.
  - Adequate intake of folate, a B-vitamin, is crucial in early pregnancy to prevent Down syndrome, cleft palate and neural tube defects (NTDs) such as spina bifida and anencephaly.
- **Iodine and thyroid:**
  - Iodine is essential for the production of thyroid hormones, which are critical for the development of the fetal brain and nervous system.
  - Inadequate iodine intake during pregnancy can lead to intellectual disabilities and developmental delays in the baby.
- **Omega-3 fatty acids and thyroid:**
  - Omega-3 fatty acids are important for cognitive function and can contribute to the prevention of neurodevelopmental disorders. Fish oil (omega-3 fatty acids) may also improve cognition functions.
  - Omega-3 fatty acids, particularly docosahexaenoic acid (DHA), play a crucial role in the development of the fetal brain and nervous system.
- **Iron and hemoglobin production:**
  - Iron deficiency during pregnancy can lead to anemia and negatively impact the baby's growth and development.
  - Iron is essential for the production of hemoglobin, which carries oxygen to the developing fetus.
- **Antioxidants and protection of DNA:**
  - Antioxidants, such as vitamins C and E, help protect developing cells from oxidative stress and damage to DNA.
  - Oxidative stress can contribute to genetic mutations, and adequate antioxidant intake may help mitigate these risks.
- **Protein and cellular development:**
  - Proteins are essential for the growth and development of cells, tissues, and organs.
  - A balanced intake of protein is crucial for normal fetal development and can help prevent certain genetic disorders related to cellular function.
- **Avoiding harmful eatables:**
  - Adequate prenatal nutrition involves avoiding substances that can harm fetal development, such as alcohol, tobacco, and certain medications.
  - Exposure to these substances can increase the risk of genetic and developmental disorders.

EXTRA EDGE

Myths about Food Allergies During Pregnancy

There are several myths and facts surrounding the topic of food allergies during pregnancy. Some common myths and corresponding facts are as follows:

Myth 1: Avoiding allergenic foods during pregnancy prevents allergies in the body.
Fact: No clear evidence to support widespread avoidance. The studies suggest that early introduction of allergenic foods may actually help prevent allergies in babies.
Myth 2: Eating peanuts during pregnancy will cause allergy in the baby.
Fact: Relationship between mother's diet during pregnancy and the development of allergies in the baby is complex. There is no clear evidence for this.
Myth 3: Breastfeeding increases the risk of allergies.
Fact: On the contrary, breastfeeding may provide immune factors that can support the infant's developing immune system.
Myth 4: Allergic reactions during pregnancy will harm the baby.
Fact: Allergic reactions in the mother are generally not harmful to the baby.
Myth 5: Allergies skip a generation.
Fact: It's not guaranteed that allergies will skip a generation. Environmental factors also play a significant role. It's possible for a child to have allergies even if the parents don't, and vice versa.
Myth 6: Allergies can only develop in childhood.
Fact: It is possible to develop allergies at any age, including during adulthood. Pregnancy does not confer immunity against the development of allergies.
Myth 7: A gluten-free diet is necessary for everyone during pregnancy.
Fact: Unless a woman has been diagnosed with celiac disease or a gluten sensitivity, a gluten-free diet is not necessary during pregnancy. Gluten-containing grains provide important nutrients, and unnecessary restriction may lead to nutritional deficiency.

MATERNAL AGE

Maternal age refers to the age of a woman when she gives birth to a child. It is a significant factor in various aspects of reproductive health, pregnancy outcomes, and the well-being of both the mother and the child. Some points are as follows:

- **Fertility:** Maternal age is closely linked to fertility. Generally, women are most fertile in their late teens to early 20s, and fertility tends to decline gradually with age. After the age of 35, fertility decline becomes more pronounced. Fertility generally starts declining slowly when a woman is in her early 30s, and after the age of 35, the decline speeds up. This is due to the effect of aging on the ovary and eggs.
- **Pregnancy risk:** Advanced maternal age, typically defined as being 35 years or older at the time of delivery, is associated with an increased risk of certain pregnancy complications. These may include gestational diabetes, preeclampsia, and chromosomal abnormalities, such as Down syndrome.
- **Late pregnancy issues:** Some obstetrical complications appear to be related to the aging process alone, while others are largely related to coexisting factors such as multiple gestation, higher parity, and chronic medical conditions, which are less likely to be observed in younger women.
- **Cesarean delivery:** Older women are more likely to deliver by cesarean section than younger women.
- **Risk of life:** Older women are at increased risk of maternal death.
- **Risk of aneuploidy in oocyte increases with age:**
  - **Monosomy:** Absence of one homologous chromosome. Autosomal monosomy is fatal.
  - **Trisomy:** Presence of three homologous chromosomes.
- **Multiple pregnancies:** The likelihood of having twins or higher-order multiples increases with maternal age, primarily due to factors, like changes in hormonal levels and increased use of assisted reproductive technologies (ART) like *in vitro* fertilization (IVF).

- **Ectopic pregnancy:** Maternal age ≥35 years is associated with increased risk of ectopic pregnancy compared with younger women. This high risk reflects an accumulation of risk factors over time, such as multiple sexual partners, pelvic infection, and tubal pathology.
- **Spontaneous abortion:** Older women experience an increased rate of spontaneous abortion. These losses are both trisomic and euploid and primarily due to decline in oocyte quality; changes in uterine and hormonal function. The vast majority of losses occur between in the first trimester of pregnancy.
- **Preterm birth and low birth weight:** Young maternal age (below 18 years) and advanced maternal age are both associated with an increased risk of preterm birth and low birth weight. Adequate prenatal care is essential to help manage these risks.
- **Social and economic factors:** Maternal age can be influenced by social and economic factors. Young maternal age may be associated with factors, like lower educational attainment and socioeconomic status, while advanced maternal age may be related to delayed childbearing for career or personal reasons.
- **Parenting challenges:** Both younger and older mothers may face unique challenges in parenting. Younger mothers may encounter difficulties related to balancing parenting responsibilities with educational and career pursuits, while older mothers may navigate concerns related to energy levels and potential health issues.
- **Personal choice and family planning:** Maternal age is often influenced by personal choice and family planning decisions. Factors such as relationship stability, career goals, and overall readiness for parenthood contribute to the timing of childbirth.

NOTE

It is important to note that while maternal age is a significant factor, individual health, lifestyle, and access to healthcare also play crucial roles in determining pregnancy outcomes. Women of all ages can have healthy pregnancies with proper prenatal care and attention to individual health needs. Regular consultations with healthcare providers are essential to address the unique considerations associated with maternal age.

Genetic Counseling at Advanced Age

Genetic counseling is often recommended for women of advanced maternal age. Genetic counselors can provide information about the specific risks associated with the mother's age, discuss available testing options, and help individuals make informed decisions about their pregnancy.

Genetic Abnormalities with Advanced Age

Advanced maternal age, typically defined as being 35 years or older at the time of delivery, is associated with an increased risk of chromosomal abnormalities in the fetus. This is primarily due to changes that occur in a woman's eggs (oocytes) as she ages.

The risk of chromosomal abnormalities is not uniform across all age groups but increases gradually. The risk becomes more pronounced after the age of 35 and further increases with each year of advancing maternal age.

Causes of Genetic Abnormalities

- **Errors in cell division:** The likelihood of errors in the division of cells (meiosis) during egg development increases with age leading to chromosomal abnormalities.
- **Single gene disorders** occur when a change in one gene causes a disease. Examples include cystic fibrosis, sickle cell anemia, Tay-Sachs disease, hemophilia, and Marfan syndrome.

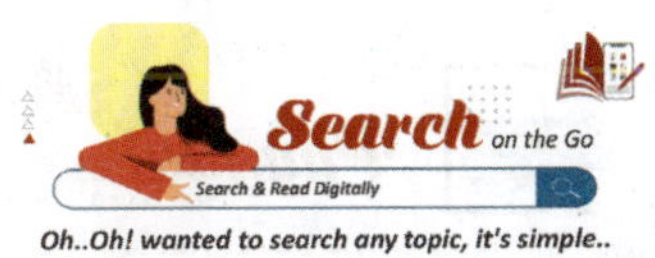

- **Chromosomal abnormalities:** Chromosomal abnormalities occur where there are missing or extra chromosomes, or pieces of chromosomes. Down syndrome, the most common chromosomal abnormality, is caused by an extra chromosome number 21. Chromosome abnormalities can be inherited from a parent or they can happen by chance.
- **Other trisomies:** Besides Down syndrome, advanced maternal age is also associated with an increased risk of other trisomies, where there is an extra copy of a specific chromosome. For example, trisomy 18 (Edwards syndrome) and trisomy 13 (Patau syndrome) are more likely to occur in pregnancies.
    - **Multifactorial or complex disorders** are caused by a combination of genetic predispositions and environmental factors, which makes it harder to predict who may be at risk. Examples include heart defects, cleft lip or cleft palate, and spina bifida.
    - **Teratogenic disorders** occur when the baby is exposed to substances during pregnancy that cause abnormalities, otherwise known as "teratogens". Babies are very sensitive in the first trimester, when all of the organs are developing. Teratogens include alcohol, drugs, lead, high levels of radiation exposure, and certain medications, infections and toxic substances.

Role of Nurse in Advanced Age Pregnancy

The roles of a nurse in supporting a woman of advanced maternal age during pregnancy involve:

- **Assessment and monitoring:** Conducting thorough assessments of the woman's health, including pre-existing medical conditions, to identify potential risks associated with advanced maternal age.
- **Education and counseling:**
    - Providing information about the potential risks and complications associated with pregnancy at an advanced age.
    - Discussing the importance of prenatal screening and testing to identify potential genetic abnormalities.
- **Support for emotional well-being:**
    - Recognizing and addressing any emotional or psychological concerns the woman may have regarding her age and the pregnancy.
    - Collaborating with other healthcare providers: Collaborating with obstetricians, perinatologists, and other healthcare professionals to a comprehensive care plan.
    - Ensuring that the woman receives specialized care and additional monitoring as required.
- **Monitoring fetal development:**
    - Monitoring fetal growth and development through regular ultrasounds and other diagnostic tests.
    - Assessing for any signs of fetal distress or complications.
- **Managing complications:** Being vigilant for potential complications, such as gestational diabetes, preeclampsia, and chromosomal abnormalities.
- **Postpartum support:**
    - Providing support and education during the postpartum period, addressing issues such as breastfeeding, postpartum recovery, and newborn care.
    - Monitoring for any postpartum complications that may be more prevalent in women of advanced maternal age.
- **Advocacy and empowerment:** Advocating for the woman's needs and preferences throughout the pregnancy and childbirth process.
    - Empowering the woman to actively participate in decision-making regarding health.
- **Continuing follow-up:**
    - Continuing to monitor the woman's health and the baby's development postpartum.
    - Facilitating appropriate follow-up care and addressing any ongoing health issues.

MATERNAL DRUG THERAPY

Maternal drug therapy during pregnancy requires careful consideration because both the mother and the developing fetus both can be affected:

- **Risk assessment:** conduct a thorough risk assessment to evaluate the potential risks of drug therapy. Attention should be focused on the specific trimester of pregnancy, as certain drugs may have different effects at different stages.
- **Teratogenicity:** The potential of a drug to cause congenital abnormalities in the developing fetus must be known to the healthcare providers so that the teratogenic drugs are avoided during pregnancy.
- **Individual treatment plans:** Individualized treatment plans based on the specific health condition of the pregnant woman should be followed. Some medical conditions may require ongoing medication management, and the risks of untreated conditions must be weighed against potential drug risks.
- **Informed consent:** Ensure that the pregnant woman understands the implications of taking a particular medication during pregnancy. Healthcare providers should discuss the potential risks and benefits of drug therapy, so as to take informed decisions about her treatment.
- **Monitoring and follow-up:** Regular monitoring of both the mother and the fetus is important throughout the course of drug therapy. This includes routine prenatal care, laboratory tests, and ultrasounds to assess fetal development and well-being.
- **Non-pharmacological alternatives:** Nonpharmacological alternatives or lifestyle modifications may be considered safer options during pregnancy, to avoid the harmful effect of drugs.
- **Update on latest research and guidelines:** It is important for healthcare providers to stay updated on the latest research and guidelines related to maternal drug therapy during pregnancy. A collaborative and patient-centered approach is essential to address the unique needs and circumstances of each pregnant woman.

Pharmacokinetics of Drugs Used During Pregnancy

- **Absorption:** Gastrointestinal changes, such as increased gastric emptying time and decreased acidity, influence the absorption of drug.
- **Distribution:** Changes in body composition, such as increased fat stores and total body water, can affect the volume of distribution of drugs. Plasma protein levels, particularly albumin, may decrease during pregnancy, potentially leading to increased levels of free (unbound) drug in the bloodstream.
- **Metabolism:** Hepatic metabolism, primarily mediated by enzymes in the cytochrome P450 system, can be altered during pregnancy such as—CYP3A4 and CYP2D6, may be induced or inhibited, affecting the rate at which drugs are metabolized. The activity of phase II metabolism for example, glucuronidation may also change.
- **Elimination:** Renal blood flow and glomerular filtration rate (GFR) increase during pregnancy, leading to increased renal elimination of drugs. Changes in tubular secretion and reabsorption may also impact drug elimination.
- **Placental drug transfer:** Drugs can cross the placenta and reach the fetal circulation, potentially affecting the developing fetus. The factors promoting placental drug transfer include molecular size, lipid solubility of drug and maternal and fetal blood flow, and placental barriers.
- **Changes in drug half-life:** Due to alterations in drug absorption, distribution, metabolism, and elimination, the half-life of certain drugs may be prolonged or shortened during pregnancy. This further affects the dosing frequency and overall drug exposure.

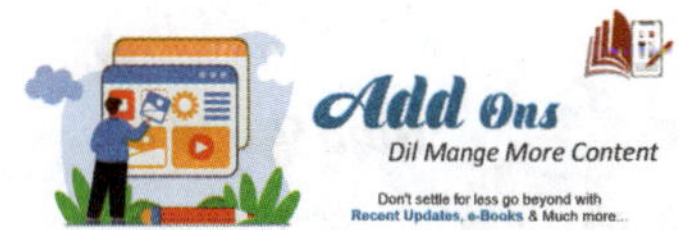

- **Fetal metabolism and excretion:** The fetus can metabolize and eliminate certain drugs, although the capacity for drug metabolism is generally lower compared to adults. Fetal drug exposure is influenced by the balance between maternal drug transfer across the placenta and fetal drug metabolism and elimination.
- **Timing and duration of pregnancy:** The pharmacokinetics of drugs can vary across different trimesters of pregnancy, so the timing of drug administration may be important. Some changes in drug metabolism and elimination may persist during the postpartum period.

Effects of various drugs on fetus at different stages of pregnancy have been discussed in Table 25.3.

Role of Nurse in Maternal Drug Therapy

Nurses play a crucial role in maternal drug therapy to ensure the health and safety of both the mother and the developing fetus. Their responsibilities in this case are as follows:

- **Assessment:**
  - Conduct a thorough assessment of the pregnant woman's health history, including pre-existing medical conditions, allergies, and medications.
  - Evaluate the potential risks and benefits of drug therapy based on the specific needs of the mother and the stage of pregnancy.
- **Education:**
  - Educate pregnant women about the importance of disclosing all medications, including over-the-counter drugs and herbal supplements, to ensure a comprehensive understanding of their health status.
  - Provide information about the potential risks associated with certain medications during pregnancy and discuss alternative options when necessary.
- **Collaboration with healthcare team:**
  - Collaborate with midwives, obstetricians, pharmacists, and other healthcare professionals to develop an individualized and safe drug therapy plan for pregnant women.

Table 25.3: Effects of various drugs on fetus at different stages of pregnancy

Class of drugs	Effects in first trimester	Effects in second trimester	Effects in third trimester
Antibiotics	Risk of fetal organ malformation	Limited impact on fetal development	Risk of neonatal complications
Antidepressants	Potential risk of congenital defects	Continued monitoring for fetal growth	Risk of neonatal withdrawal symptoms
Antihypertensive	Risk of fetal organ malformation	Continued monitoring for fetal growth	Potential risk of fetal renal function
Anticonvulsants	Increased risk of neural tube defects	Continued monitoring for fetal growth	Risk of neonatal withdrawal symptoms
Analgesics	Potential risk of heart defects	Continued monitoring for fetal growth	Risk of neonatal respiratory issues
Anticoagulants	Risk of bleeding disorders	Continued monitoring for fetal growth	Risk of bleeding complications
Antidiabetic	Risk of birth defects	Continued monitoring for fetal growth	Risk of neonatal hypoglycemia
Antiretrovirals	Potential risk of birth defects	Continued monitoring for fetal growth	Risk of vertical transmission

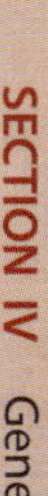

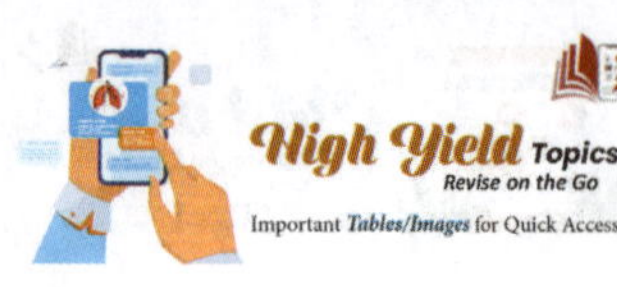

    - Participate in interdisciplinary discussions to address the unique needs and concerns of pregnant patients.
- **Administration of medication:**
    - Administer medications as prescribed by healthcare providers, ensuring accurate dosages and proper routes of administration.
    - Evaluate the effectiveness of the prescribed medications in managing the maternal condition.
- **Monitoring and evaluation:**
    - Monitor the mother for any adverse reactions or side effects and promptly report findings to the healthcare team.
    - Regularly monitor maternal vital signs, laboratory results, and other relevant indicators to assess the impact of drug therapy on both the mother and the fetus.
- **Support:**
    - Assist pregnant women in adhering to their medications by providing clear instructions, addressing concerns, and offering support.
    - Collaborate with the healthcare team to explore alternative medications or interventions that may be more suitable for pregnant women if noncompliance becomes an issue.
- **Advocacy:**
    - Advocate for the rights and well-being of pregnant women by ensuring that they receive appropriate and timely medical care, including necessary medications.
    - Advocate for the development of evidence-based guidelines and protocols related to maternal drug therapy.
- **Risk assessment and management:**
    - Assess the potential risks of medication exposure during different stages of pregnancy and contribute to risk management strategies.
    - Balance the benefits of treating maternal conditions with the potential risks to the fetus, while considering the overall health of both.
- **Education:**
    - Stay informed about current research and guidelines related to medications and their safety during pregnancy.
    - Engage in ongoing education to enhance knowledge and skills related to maternal drug therapy.
- **Communication with pregnant women:** Have open communication with pregnant women to address their concerns, provide information, and encourage active participation in decision-making regarding their drug therapy.

EFFECT OF RADIATION ON PREGNANCY

Exposure to radiation during pregnancy can have potential risks for the developing fetus. It is important to note that pregnant women should always consult with their healthcare providers to assess specific risks and receive personalized advice.

Exposure to Ionizing Radiation

Exposure to ionizing radiation during pregnancy can have potential risks to the developing fetus. Ionizing radiation has enough energy to remove tightly bound electrons from atoms, and this can damage living tissues. The effects of radiation on pregnancy depend on factors such as the dose, the gestational age at the time of exposure, and the type of radiations.

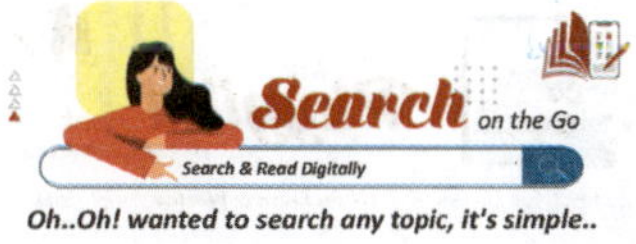

Teratogenic Effects

High Doses in Early Pregnancy

- **Risk of spontaneous abortion:** Exposure to high doses of ionizing radiation during the first two weeks after conception can increase the risk of spontaneous abortion or birth defects. This is because the developing organs and tissues are particularly susceptible during this period.
- **Organ development:** Exposure during the organ-forming stages (weeks 2–7 of pregnancy) can lead to structural abnormalities in organs, potentially causing birth defects.
- **Risk of childhood cancer:** Exposure to high doses of radiation in the later stages of pregnancy may not cause structural abnormalities, but it may increase the risk of childhood cancers, such as leukemia, later in the child's life.

High Doses in Late Pregnancy

Exposure to high doses of radiation in the later stages of pregnancy may not cause structural abnormalities, but it may increase the risk of childhood cancers, such as leukemia, later in the child's life.

Effects on Cognitive Development

High-dose Exposure

If the brain of the developing fetus is exposed to high doses of radiation, it may lead to intellectual and developmental disabilities.

Low-dose Exposure

Diagnostic imaging, such as X-rays and CT scans, involves much lower doses of radiation. In many cases, the benefits of the diagnostic information may outweigh the potential risks. Healthcare provider should carefully consider the necessity of the procedure and take steps to minimize radiation exposure.

Nonionizing radiation (such as that from ultrasound or MRI) does not carry the same risks as ionizing radiations.

MUST KNOW

- As general rule, the sensitivity of a tissue to ionizing radiation is directly proportional to its rate of proliferation.
- Healthcare providers follow the principle of ALARA (As Low As Reasonably Achievable) when using ionizing radiation in medical procedures involving pregnant women.
- Take steps to minimize radiation exposure and ensure that the benefits of the procedure outweigh the potential risks.
- Inform the pregnant women before performing any medical procedure involving radiations on them.

Effect of Ionizing Radiations on Fetus

Harmful effects on the fetus include:

- Miscarriage
- Teratogenicity
- Intrauterine Growth Retardation (IUGR)
- Induction of cancers (such as leukemia) that appear in childhood. The risk to the fetus is related to gestational age at exposure and the radiation dose.
- Mental teratogenicity
- Mental retardation

Risk of Ionizing Radiations According to Gestational Age

First trimester: It is the most radiation-sensitive stage because of very rapid fetal growth. Radiation injury produces an "all or nothing" effect and the harmful effect usually ends in a miscarriage. Many women are never aware that they are pregnant at the time of exposure or miscarriage. Therefore, it is difficult to estimate the incidence of fetal wastage due to radiation.

Second trimester: During this period, the fetus is in its most sensitive stage of development as major organ systems begin to differentiate, however the overall growth rate has slowed down. Doses above the threshold levels may cause gross congenital malformations and mental retardation.

Third trimester: Though the features are more resistant to radiation in the third trimester, a high dose of radiation >0.5 Gy or 50 rad may result in adverse effects including miscarriage; IQ reduction and severe mental disorders.

Precipitating Factors

- Gestational age at the time of exposure
- History of previous pregnancies including that of congenital malformations
- Other potentially harmful environmental factors (smoking, alcohol/drugs, malnutrition, etc.)
- Taking drugs (smoking, alcohol/drugs)
- Maternal/paternal age
- Assessing fetal exposure using dose reconstruction techniques
- Attitude of the mother toward the pregnancy.

Mechanism of Radiation Exposure to Cells

Thermal and nonthermal effects produced by radiations can cause the following destructive effects on the cells.

- **Genetic effects:** Ionizing radiation can directly interact with cellular molecules, particularly DNA and damage it. The most severe form of DNA damage is the induction of double-strand breaks, where both strands of the DNA helix are broken.
- **Cellular damage:** The majority of cellular damage from ionizing radiation occurs indirectly through the radiolysis of water molecules.
- **Cell cycle arrest:** The cells may undergo cell cycle arrest to allow time for repair mechanisms to operate.
- **Oxidative stress:** The production of free radicals during ionization events can lead to oxidative stress, causing damage to lipids, proteins, and other cellular components.
- **Mitochondrial dysfunction:** Ionizing radiation can affect mitochondrial function, leading to the release of reactive oxygen species and disruption of cellular energy production.

Exposure to Nonionizing Radiations

Exposure to nonionizing radiation, such as from cell phones, Wifi, and microwaves, is generally considered safe. However, it is advisable to use devices with caution and follow recommended safety guidelines.

EFFECTS OF DRUGS AND CHEMICALS ON PREGNANCY

Many drugs and chemicals may have carcinogenic effects on the developing fetus, e.g., diethyl-stilbestrol. Drugs may harm both the mother and the baby. All illegal drugs such as heroin and cocaine, and some legal

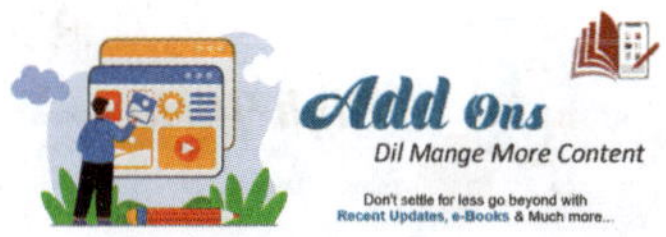

substances such as alcohol, tobacco and certain medical drugs are dangerous for the health of mother and her baby. Continuous use of drug increases the risk of miscarriage and premature delivery.

MUST KNOW

Stilbestrol is a hormone used for threatened abortion with vaginal bleeding, before 20 weeks of gestational age in some countries.

- **Alcohol:** It is number one fetal teratogen, especially in the early weeks. Intrauterine exposure to even a small amount of alcohol may result in fetal alcohol syndrome (FAS). The symptoms of FAS may include:
  - Slow growth before and after birth
  - Abnormal facial features (congenital abnormalities)
  - Defective heart and other organs
  - Malformed limbs
  - Genital abnormalities
  - Central nervous system damage
    - Behavioral problems, such as hyperactivity
    - Extreme nervousness
    - Reduced ability to concentrate
- **Cocaine and methamphetamine:** These are powerful stimulants of the central nervous system. They suppress mother's powerful stimulants of the central nervous system. They suppress mother's appetite, cause constriction of blood vessels, increase the heart beat and cause the blood pressure to soar. The adverse effects on the fetus are higher:
  - Retarded growth
  - Attention and orientation problems
  - Hyperirritability
  - A tendency to stop breathing
  - Malformed or missing organs
  - Strokes and seizures

  The risks of spontaneous abortion, premature birth and stillbirth also increase with fetal exposure to cocaine and methamphetamine. When these drugs are used late in pregnancy, the newborn may become drug dependent and suffer from withdrawal symptoms, such as tremors, sleeplessness, muscle spasm, and sucking difficulties. Learning difficulties sucking difficulties. Learning difficulties may develop later.
- **Cigarette smoking:** Smoking during pregnancy causes low infant birth weight. There is also a strong association between smoking and a higher fetal and infant mortality rate. Smoking women have a much higher risk of an ectopic pregnancy. Cigarette smoke may be teratogenic and may cause cardiac abnormalities as well as anencephaly.

  Maternal smoking is a significant factor in the development of cleft lip and palate and has been linked with Sudden Infant Death Syndrome (SIDS). Infants nursing by smoking mothers have also been found to have an increased incidence of gastrointestinal disturbances. Even a mother's exposure to second-hand cigarette smoke during pregnancy or while nursing predisposes her baby to increased incidence of respiratory problems including bronchitis and pneumonia, during the first year of life.
- **Heroin and other narcotics**: Use of heavy narcotics increases the danger of premature birth accompanied by low birth weight, breathing difficulties, low blood sugar (hypoglycaemia) and intracranial hemorrhage. The newborn becomes drug dependent and suffers from withdrawal symptoms, such as irritability, vomiting and diarrhea and joint stiffness.
- **Intravenous drug abuse**: Women who use contaminated needles to inject narcotics are prone to become HIV infected and obviously run a risk of passing the virus on to their babies.
- **Inhalants:** At least one inhalant, the organic solvent toluene that is widely used in paints and glues, appears to cause malformations, like those produced by alcohol. It is possible that all organic solvents may cause birth defects.

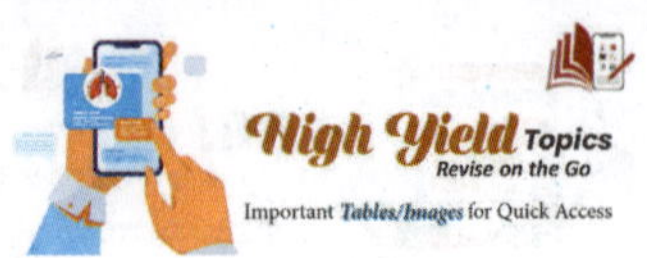

- **Over the counter drugs:** Some medications may pose risks during pregnancy, especially in the first trimester. Pregnant women should consult with their healthcare providers before taking any medication, including over-the-counter.
- **Other teratogens:** The category includes pesticides; industrial chemicals; some hormones; antibiotics; oral chemicals; some hormones; antibiotics; oral anticoagulants, anticonvulsants, antitumor agents, thýroid drugs, thalidomide, and numerous other prescription drugs cause birth defects.

INFERTILITY

Infertility is the failure to conceive even after 12 months period of unprotected intercourse. Infertility also refers to the inability of a sexually active noncontracepting couple to achieve pregnancy in one year. Infertility is a significant social and medical problem affecting couples worldwide. Infertility refers to an inability to conceive after having regular unprotected sex. Average incidence of infertility is about 15% globally which varies in different populations. Some causes can be detected and treated, whereas others cannot. Unexplained infertility constitutes about 10% of all cases.

Types of Infertility

Two types of infertility are primary infertility and secondary infertility:

1. **Primary infertility:** When a woman is unable to bear a child.
2. **Secondary infertility:** When a woman has been pregnant but failed to achieve live birth after having a live birth previously.

Causes of Infertility

Both men and women can experience infertility, and there are various factors that can contribute to this condition. It is important to note that infertility is a complex issue, often involving a combination of factors.

Causes of Female Infertility

- **Ovulatory disorders:** Problems with ovulation, where the ovaries fail to release eggs regularly, can be a major cause of female infertility. Conditions, like polycystic ovary syndrome (PCOS), can disrupt normal ovulation.
- **Fallopian tube blockage:** Blockages or damage to the fallopian tubes can prevent the egg from meeting the sperm, hindering fertilization. This can be caused by pelvic inflammatory disease, endometriosis, or previous pelvic surgeries.
- **Uterine issues:** Abnormalities in the structure or function of the uterus can affect fertility. Fibroids, polyps, or other uterine abnormalities may interfere with implantation.
- **Endometriosis:** This is a condition where tissue similar to the lining of the uterus grows outside the uterus. It can cause inflammation, scarring, and adhesions, impacting fertility.
- **Age:** Female fertility declines with age, especially after the age of 35. As a woman gets older, the quality and quantity of her eggs diminish, making it more difficult to conceive.
  - Premature ovarian failure (before age of 40).
- **Hormonal imbalance:** Disorders such as thyroid problems or problems with the pituitary or adrenal glands can disrupt the hormonal balance necessary for reproductive processes.
- **Previous sterilization treatment:** Illegal drugs have harmful effect on the fertility.

Causes of Male Infertility

- **Sperm disorders:** Problems with sperm production, motility (movement), or morphology (shape) can contribute to male infertility. Conditions such as varicocele, infections, or genetic disorders may affect sperm quality.
  - Low sperm count: <15 million sperm per mL of semen
  - Normal count is 20 million sperm per mL of semen or more
  - No sperm: Absence of sperms in semen
  - Low sperm motility
  - Abnormal sperms (Fig. 25.3) having unusual shape, cannot move and fertilize egg. Its causes can be testicular infections, testicular cancer or testicular surgery.

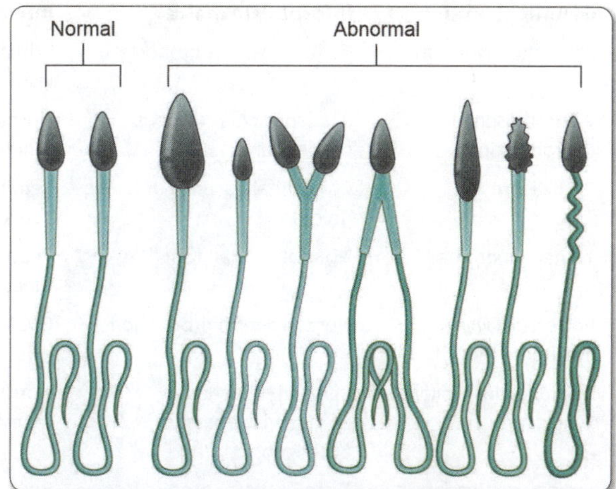

Figure 25.3: Abnormal shape of sperms

- **Testicular factors:** Issues affecting the testicles, such as undescended testicles or testicular injuries, can impact sperm production, such as:
  - Overheating of testicles
  - Undescended testicles
  - Hypogonadism
- **Ejaculation disorders:** Problems with ejaculation, including premature ejaculation or retrograde ejaculation (where semen enters the bladder instead of exiting the penis), can lead to infertility.
- **Genetic disorders:** Some genetic conditions can affect male fertility. Examples include Klinefelter syndrome or Y-chromosome microdeletions.
- **Hormonal imbalances:** Disorders affecting hormonal regulation, such as problems with the pituitary gland or the hypothalamus, can affect sperm production.
- **Environmental factors:** Exposure to certain environmental factors, like toxins, radiation, or excessive heat can also affect sperm production.
- **Infections:** Like mumps, hypospadias and chlamydia infection.

Common or Shared Causes of Infertility in Males and Females

Lifestyle factors: Both men and women may experience infertility due to lifestyle factors such as smoking, excessive alcohol consumption, drug use, poor nutrition, and obesity.

Chronic illness: Certain chronic conditions, such as diabetes, can affect fertility in both men and women.

Stress: While the relationship between stress and infertility is complex, high levels of stress can impact reproductive health in both men and women.

Genetic disorders: Genetic disorders play a significant role in infertility, affecting both men and women (Table 25.4).

- Turner syndrome or Klinefelter syndrome can affect the development of reproductive organs and may lead to infertility.

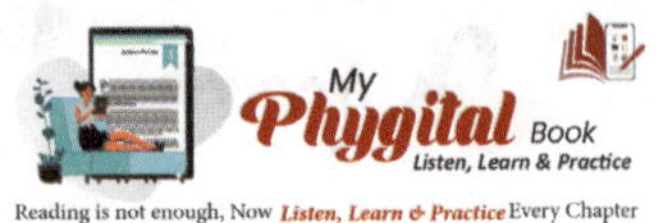

Table 25.4: Role of genetic disorders in the infertility in males and females

Genetic condition	Infertility in males	Infertility in females	Basic mode of mutation
Klinefelter Syndrome	Reduced sperm production	Primary ovarian insufficiency	Aneuploidy (extra X chromosome in males)
Y-Chromosomal Microdeletions	Azoospermia (no sperm production)	Normal ovarian function	Deletions on the Y chromosome
Cystic Fibrosis	Congenital absence of the vas deferens	Reduced fertility due to cervical mucus issues	CFTR gene mutations
Turner Syndrome	Normal ovarian function	Reduced ovarian function	Monosomy X (missing or partially missing X)
Polycystic Ovary Syndrome (PCOS)	Normal sperm production	Ovulatory dysfunction	Polygenic inheritance and environmental factors
Androgen Insensitivity Syndrome	Infertility due to unresponsiveness to androgens	Normal ovarian function	Mutations in the androgen receptor gene (AR)
Premature Ovarian Failure (POF)	Normal sperm production	Premature depletion of ovarian follicles	Various genetic factors, including mutations in specific genes
Congenital Adrenal Hyperplasia (CAH)	Normal sperm production	Irregular or absent menstrual cycles	Enzyme deficiencies due to mutations in certain genes

- Cystic fibrosis, a genetic disorder that affects the respiratory and digestive systems, can also cause infertility due to the absence or blockage of the vas deferens in men.
- Chromosomal abnormalities, such as alterations in the number or structure of chromosomes, can lead to infertility. These abnormalities may affect the development of eggs or sperm, increasing the risk of miscarriages or the birth of a child with developmental issues.
- Polycystic ovary syndrome (PCOS) is a common cause of female infertility.
- Y-chromosome microdeletions which involve the loss of genetic material on the Y chromosome and can lead to sperm production issues.
- Fragile X syndrome, a genetic condition that affects intellectual and developmental function, can also be associated with fertility problems. Female carriers of the fragile X gene may have a higher risk of ovarian dysfunction.
- Genetic mutations can affect the regulation of hormones involved in reproductive processes. Hormonal imbalances may disrupt menstrual cycles in women or impact sperm production in men.
- Familial patterns also affect fertility. Families with a history of reproductive issues may have a genetic predisposition that contributes to fertility challenge.

Genetic Basis of Infertility in Male and Female

Among various causes of infertility, genetic factors play a significant role in both male and female infertility as discussed ahead:

Genetic Basis of Male Infertility

- **Y chromosome microdeletions:** Deletions on the Y chromosome can lead to male infertility. The azoospermia factor (AZF) region on the Y chromosome is particularly important for spermatogenesis.

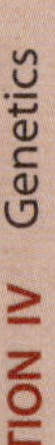

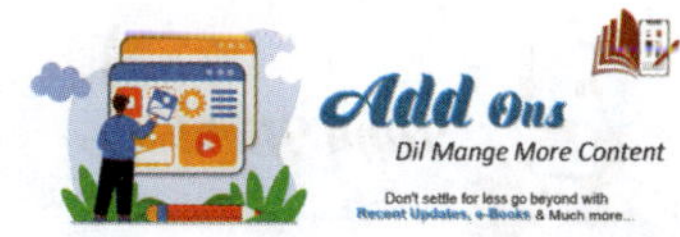

Microdeletions in these regions can result in the absence of sperm (azoospermia) or low sperm count (oligospermia).

- **Extra X chromosome:** Men with Klinefelter syndrome have an (XXY) instead of the typical XY chromosome configuration. This condition is associated with reduced fertility, testicular atrophy, and low testosterone levels.
- **Mutations in the CFTR (cystic fibrosis transmembrane regulator) gene:** Mutations in the CFTR gene, associated with cystic fibrosis, may also impact the function of the vas deferens, leading to obstructive azoospermia.
- **Androgen receptor gene mutation:** Mutations in the androgen receptor gene can lead to androgen insensitivity, impairing the normal development of male reproductive organs and causing infertility.
- **Mutations in genes involved in spermatogenesis:** Mutations in genes involved in spermatogenesis, such as SYCP3, TEX11, and others, can lead to impaired sperm production.

Genetic Basis of Female Infertility

- **Mutations in genes related to hormonal regulation:** Polycystic ovary syndrome (PCOS) is a common cause of female infertility and mutations related to hormonal regulation, insulin sensitivity, and ovarian function are linked to PCOS.
- **Premutation of the FMR1 gene:** Fragile X syndrome, has been linked to ovarian insufficiency and early menopause, caused by premutation of the FMR1 gene.
- **Partial or complete absence of one X chromosome:** Women with Turner syndrome have a partial or complete absence of one X chromosome (45X). This condition is associated with ovarian dysgenesis and infertility.
- **Mutations in oocyte specific genes:** Mutations in genes specific to oocyte development, such as FIGLA, NOBOX, and GDF9, can lead to ovarian dysfunction and infertility.
- **Gene polymorphisms:** Certain gene polymorphisms may increase the risk of developing endometriosis, which can be associated with infertility.
- **Chromosomal abnormalities:** Structural or numerical chromosomal abnormalities, such as translocations or aneuploidies, can lead to recurrent pregnancy loss and infertility.

Evaluation of Infertility

Medical History

- Detailed reproductive history for both partners.
- Any previous pregnancies, miscarriages, or fertility treatments.
- Information on menstrual cycles, sexual history, and contraceptive use.

Physical Examination

- Examination of the reproductive organs for both partners.
- Assessment of secondary sexual characteristics.
- Identification of any physical abnormalities or conditions.

Female Infertility Tests

- **Ovulation tracking:**
  - Basal body temperature charting
  - Monitoring cervical mucus changes
  - Ovulation predictor with the help of kits

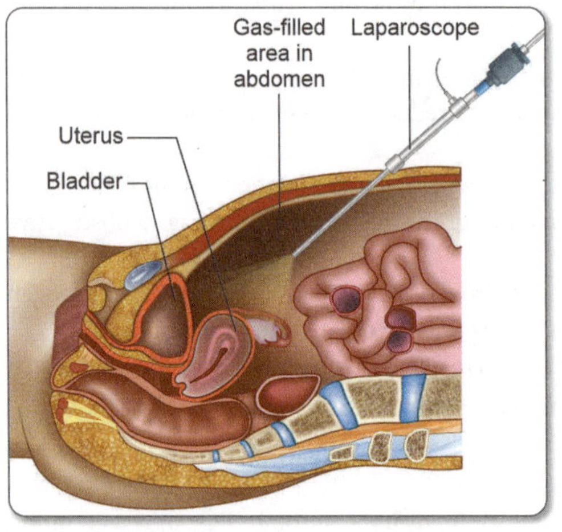

Figure 25.4: Transvaginal laparoscopy

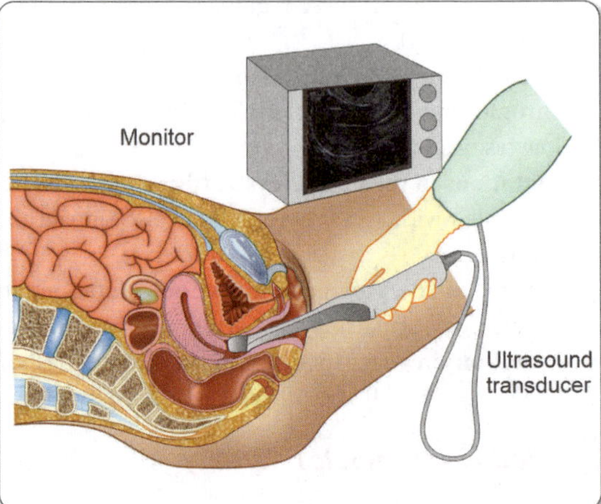

Figure 25.5: Ultrasound transducer

- **Hormone testing:**
  - Follicle-stimulating hormone (FSH) levels on specific days of the menstrual cycle
  - Luteinizing hormone (LH) levels
  - Estradiol levels
- **Hysterosalpingography (HSG):** X-ray to check for blockages or abnormalities in the fallopian tubes and the uterus.
- **Transvaginal laparoscopy:** Direct visual examination of the pelvic reproductive anatomy. Indicated for those with symptoms or risk factors or an abnormal HSG or ultrasonography who have no other clear indications for ART (e.g., severe male factor infertility) (Fig. 25.4).
- **Transvaginal ultrasonography:** It can be used to diagnose uterine pathology, including myomas. Transvaginal ultrasonography defines the size and shape of the uterine cavity and for detection of intrauterine pathology (endometrial polyps, submucous myomas, synechiae) (Fig. 25.5).
- **Ovarian reserve testing:**
  - Anti-Mullerian Hormone (AMH) levels
  - Antral follicle count via ultrasound

Male Infertility Tests

- **Semen analysis:**
  - Evaluation of sperm count, motility, and morphology
  - Assessment of liquefaction time and pH
  - Semen analysis (Table 25.5)—separately discussed as Examination of Semen in Chapter 21
- **Hormone testing:**
  - Testosterone levels
  - Follicle-stimulating hormone (FSH) and luteinizing hormone (LH) levels
- **Genetic testing:** Karyotype analysis to identify any genetic abnormalities

Shared Tests

- **Genetic tests:** Carrier screening for both partners.

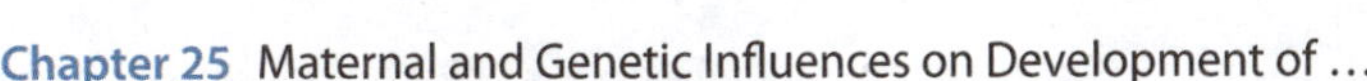

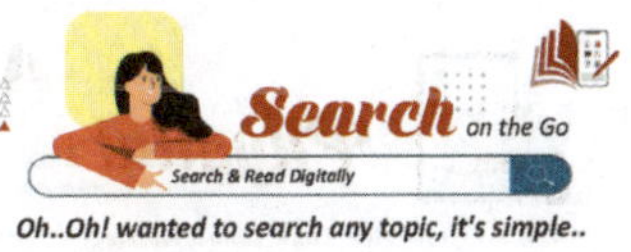

Table 25.5: Semen analysis—normal parameters

Volume	2.0 mL or more
Sperm concentration	20 million/mL or more
Motility	50% forward progression 25% rapid progression
Viscosity	Liquification in 30–60 min
Morphology	30% or more normal forms
pH	7.2–7.8
WBC	Fewer than 1 million/mL

- **Imaging studies:**
  - Transvaginal ultrasound for women
  - Scrotal ultrasound for men

Additional Tests

- **Thyroid function tests:** To assess thyroid hormone levels.
- **Prolactin levels:** Elevated levels may affect fertility.
- **Blood glucose levels:** To rule out diabetes, which may impact fertility.

Treatment of Infertility

The treatment of infertility depends on the underlying cause and may vary from lifestyle modifications to more advanced medical interventions.

Lifestyle modifications:

- **Weight management:** Achieving a healthy weight can improve fertility in both men and women.
- **Diet and exercise:** Adopting a balanced diet and engaging in regular physical activity can positively impact fertility.

Medications:

For women: For ovulation induction

- **Hormone therapy:**
  - Gonadotropins to stimulate the ovaries
  - Progesterone supplements to support the luteal phase
- **Surgery**
  - **Laparoscopic surgery:** To treat endometriosis, remove ovarian cysts, or address tubal blockages
  - **Hysteroscopic surgery:** To correct uterine abnormalities, like polyps or fibroids

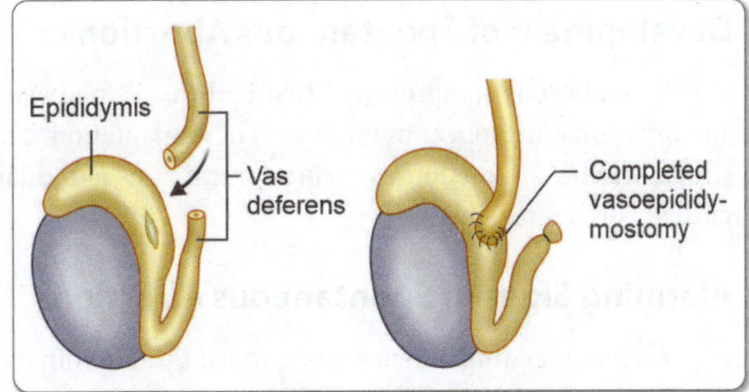

Figure 25.6: Vasoepididymostomy

For men:

- Medications to treat hormonal imbalances or improve sperm production
- **Surgery:** To correct varicoceles, blockages, or anatomical issues
- **Surgery for epididymal blockage:** A bypass of the blockage can be performed, called vasoepididymostomy (Fig. 25.6) (vas deferens is reconnected to epididymis).

Assisted reproductive technologies (ART):

- **Intrauterine insemination (IUI):** The sperm is directly placed into the uterus during the woman's fertile window
- **Invitro fertilization (IVF):** Eggs are retrieved from the ovaries, fertilized with sperm in a laboratory, and the resulting embryos are implanted into the uterus.
- **Intracytoplasmic sperm injections (ICSI):** A single sperm is directly injected into an egg during IVF.

Donor eggs or sperm: In case of severe male or female infertility, using donor eggs or sperm may be an option.

Surrogacy:

If carrying a pregnancy is not possible for the woman, a surrogate may carry the pregnancy on her behalf this this under as:

- **Preimplantation genetic testing (PGT):** Screening embryos for genetic abnormalities before implantation during IVF.
- **Counseling and support:** Emotional support and counseling can be beneficial throughout the infertility treatment process.
- **Continued monitoring and adjustments:** Regular monitoring of treatment progress and adjustments to the treatment plan as needed.

Alternative therapies:

People explore acupuncture, herbal treatments, or other alternative therapies although their effectiveness is not universally supported by scientific evidence. Research is ongoing to document their efficacy.

SPONTANEOUS ABORTION

Spontaneous abortion, commonly known as a miscarriage, refers to the natural loss of a pregnancy before the end of 28th week of pregnancy. It is a relatively common occurrence, and many miscarriages happen in the early weeks of pregnancy, often before a woman is aware that she is pregnant. The commonest chromosomal anomaly leading to spontaneous abortions is Trisomy 16.

Development of Spontaneous Abortion

Usually, embryo is compromised first and this is followed by hemorrhage into the decidua basalis. Necrosis and inflammation appear in the region of implantation. The detached conceptus is a foreign body and causes strong uterine contractions. Uterine contractions and dilatations of the cervix expel products of conception partially or completely.

Alarming Signs of Spontaneous Abortions

- **Vaginal bleeding:** Often accompanied by abdominal cramps
- **Pelvic pain:** Ranging from mild to severe
- **Tissue passing:** Passing of clots or tissue from the vagina

Causes of Spontaneous Abortion

The factors responsible for abortion are as follows:

Maternal factors:

- **Infections:** Microorganisms have a specific local effect on the conceptus which can cause systemic effects that may result in abortion, such as mycoplasma, listeria or toxoplasma.

- **Environmental exposure:** Exposure to mutagenic or teratogenic agents lead to abortion, e.g. as smoking and alcohol consumption which lead to an increased incidence of chromosomal disorders and abortions.
- **Psychological factors:** Spontaneous abortion is found to be associated with anxiety, panic disorders and depression.
- **Systemic disorders:** Systemic disorders, such as diabetes mellitus, hypothyroidism and systemic lupus erythematosus (SLE) are related to spontaneous abortion.
- **Maternal age:** Risk of abortion increases with maternal age. There is increased incidence of chromosomal abnormalities in older women.
- **Hormonal factors:** Inadequate production of progesterone will lead to inadequate development of the decidua and abortion.
- **Uterine abnormalities:** Abortion increases if the uterus is septate. Leiomyoma of the uterus may cause abortion. Lacerations of the cervix which extend deeper may result in abortion in second trimester or in premature labor.
- **Trauma:** Abortion may follow surgical operative procedures, like myomectomy or removal of an ovary containing the corpus luteum of pregnancy, or appendectomy

Fetal factors: Genetic abnormalities of the conceptus leads to spontaneous abortions.

Genetic Causes of Spontaneous Abortion

- Miscarriages frequently occur due to a complex interplay of genetic and environmental factors, spontaneous abortions, or miscarriages, result from:
  - Chromosomal abnormalities such as trisomies (extra chromosomes) or monosomies (missing chromosomes), affecting embryonic development. Trisomies are usually the result of chromosome nonseparation in maternal meiosis and commonly involve chromosomes 13, 16, 18, 21 and 22.
  - Aneuploidy is one of the most common causes of recurrent pregnancy loss (RPL). Balanced, reciprocal, and Robertsonian translocations in the fetus can predispose to spontaneous miscarriages.
  - Genetic mutations in critical developmental genes, parental chromosomal rearrangements, and blood clotting disorders, like Factor V Leiden contribute to pregnancy loss.
  - Genetic risk factors also include meiotic errors, mitotic errors, and abnormal parental chromosome structure.
- Other factors are:
  - Immune system disorders and environmental factors can also play a role.
  - Maternal age, especially advanced age, increases the risk of chromosomal abnormalities.

Diagnosis of Spontaneous Abortions

- **Ultrasound:** To confirm the loss of the fetus and determines if the miscarriage is complete.
- **Blood tests:** Measuring human chorionic gonadotropin (hCG) levels to monitor pregnancy hormones.
- **Vaginal or cervical swab:** for microbiological tests.

Types of Spontaneous Abortions and their Management

Spontaneous abortions can be categorized into different types based on the method used, the stage of pregnancy, and the reasons for the procedure. It implies the expulsion of all or any part of the placenta or membrane with or without fetus or with live born or still born infant weighing less than 1 kg. If abortion occurs before 12 weeks, it is referred to as early abortion and thereafter it is late abortion.

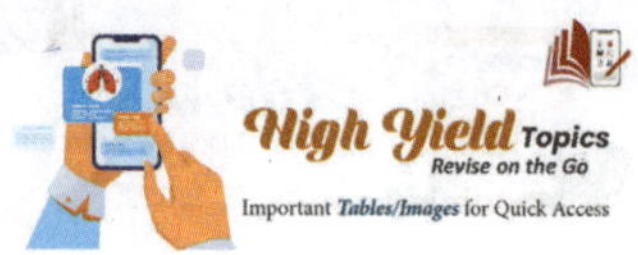

Threatened Abortion or Miscarriage

- Natural loss of a pregnancy before the 20th week of gestation.
- Closed soft cervix.
- Pain may not be a prominent feature although lower abdominal dull ache accompanied with bleeding is there (Fig. 25.7).
- Threatened abortion is often due to chromosomal abnormalities or other factors affecting fetal development.

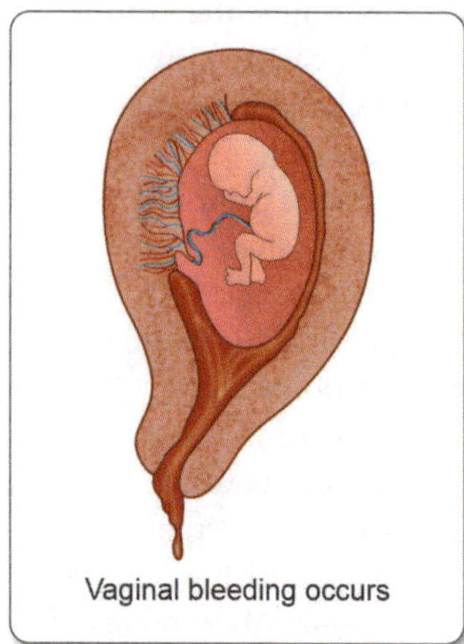

Figure 25.7: Threatened abortion

Management of Threatened Abortion

- Patient is kept at rest in bed until 2 days after blood loss has ceased.
- Intercourse is forbidden.
- As soon as the initial bleeding has stopped, an ultrasound is done to check the situation of pregnancy.

Inevitable Abortion

- A clinical pregnancy gets complicated by both vaginal bleeding and cramp, like lower abdominal pain.
- Rupture of membranes (Fig. 25.8).
- The cervix is frequently partially dilated, attesting to the inevitable abortion.

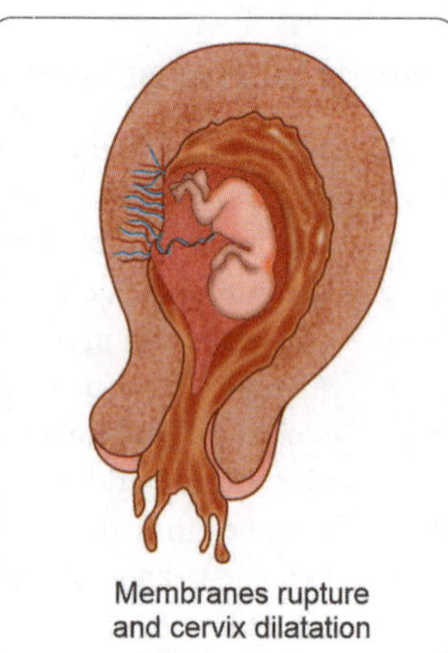

Figure 25.8: Inevitable abortion

Management of Inevitable Abortion

- The uterus is examined aseptically.
- If the abortion is not quickly completed, or if the hemorrhage becomes severe, the contents of the uterus are removed with a suction curettage

Incomplete Abortion

- In addition to vaginal bleeding, cramp-like pain and cervical dilatation is noted.
- It also involves passage of some of the products of conception (described as looking like pieces of skin or liver) (Fig. 25.9).

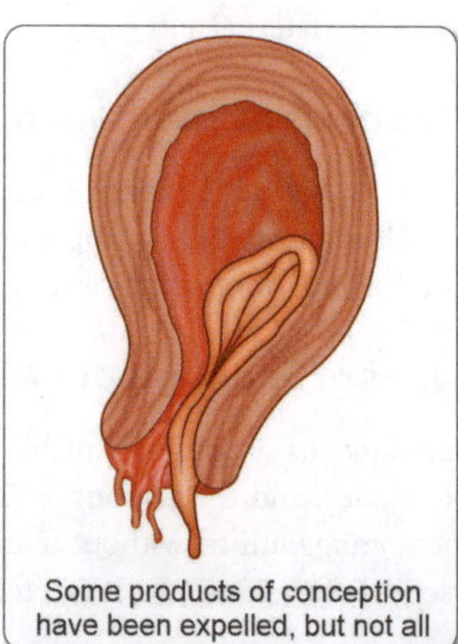

Figure 25.9: Incomplete abortion

Management of Incomplete Abortion

- Patient requires hospitalization.
- Treatment is focussed at preventing infection, controlling bleeding and obtaining an empty and involuting uterus.
- The main risk associated with retained products are hemorrhage and sepsis.

Complete Abortion

- After passage of all the products of conception, the uterine contractions and bleeding subsides, cervix closes (Fig. 25.10).
- The uterus becomes smaller than the stage of amenorrhea.
- The symptoms of pregnancy are no longer present. Pregnancy test becomes negative.

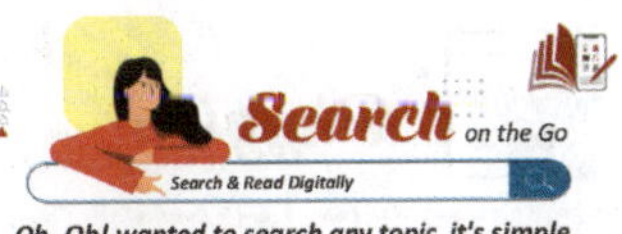

Missed Abortion

- In this case, fetus has died but retained in the uterus for few weeks. (It leads to problem because after 16 weeks' gestation, dilatation and curettage may become risky) (Fig. 25.11).
- Closed cervical os.
- No fetal cardiac activity or empty sac.
- Fibrinogen levels must be checked weekly until the fetus and placenta are expelled.

Management of Missed Abortion

- Once the diagnosis has been made the uterus should be emptied.
- Early in gestation, evacuation of the uterus is usually accompanied by suction curettage.

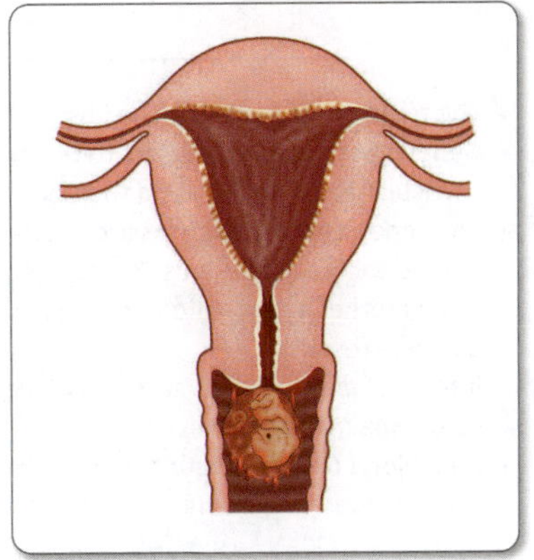

Figure 25.10: Complete abortion

Recurrent Abortion

- Recurrent abortion refers to any case in which there have been three consecutive spontaneous abortions.
- Possible causes are known to be genetic error, anatomic abnormalities of the genital tract, hormonal abnormalities, infection, immunologic factors, or systemic disease.

Management of Recurrent Abortion

- Paternal and maternal chromosomes must be evaluated
- Pelvic examination
- The mother must be ruled out for the systemic disorders such as DM, SLE and thyroid disorder
- Mother should be ruled out for the presence of Mycoplasma, Listeria, Toxoplasma diseases
- Emotional support

The algorithm for managing recurrent spontaneous abortions is as follows (Flowchart 25.1).

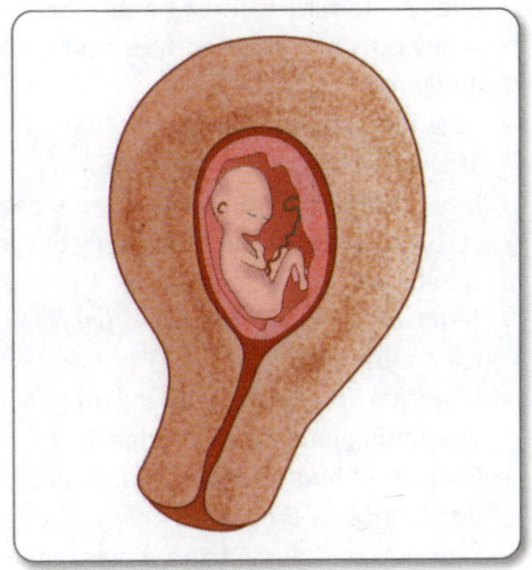

Figure 25.11: Missed abortion

Flowchart 25.1: Algorithm for managing recurrent spontaneous abortions

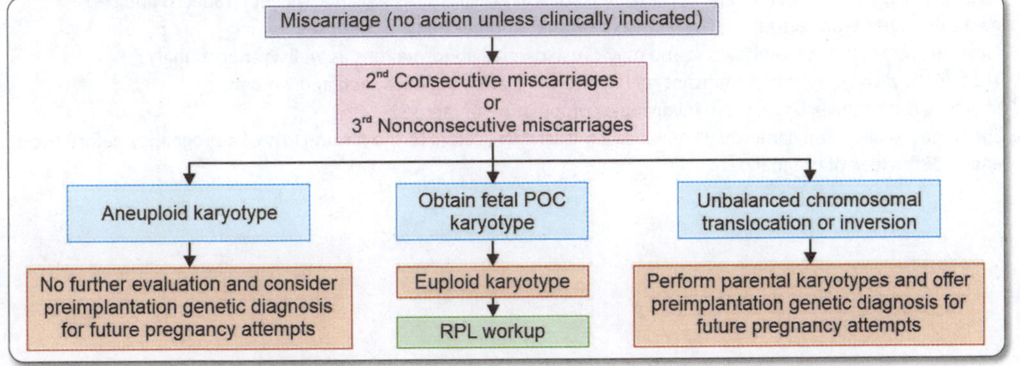

Abbreviation: POC, product of conception; RPL, recurrent pregnancy loss

SUMMARY

- The mutated genes lower the immunity of a person.
- Genetic polymorphism refers to the existence of multiple genetic variants (alleles) within a population, at a particular locus (location) in the DNA sequence of a gene.
- The genetic polymorphisms are associated with an increased risk of developing certain diseases.
- Diabetes can have serious consequences for mother and fetus.
- If the mother's production of insulin is not enough to overcome the effect of the placental hormones, gestational diabetes results.
- Infants of mothers with gestational diabetes are susceptible to imbalances, such as low-serum calcium and low-serum magnesium levels.
- High blood pressure during pregnancy leads to placental complications and slowed fetal growth.
- An infection that goes untreated can lead to preterm labor and a rupturing of the membranes surrounding the fetus.
- Infants of HBV-positive mothers should receive hepatitis B immunoglobulin and the hepatitis B vaccine during the first 12 hours of birth.
- Adverse pregnancy outcomes in HIV positive women include increased rates of spontaneous early abortion, low birth weight babies, stillbirths, preterm labor, preterm rupture of membranes.
- Phenylketonuria is three times more common among consanguineous cases than in general population.
- Atopy is hereditary predisposition toward developing type I hypersensitivity reactions on exposure to specific antigens.
- Consanguinity can contribute to the risk of atopy by increasing the likelihood of sharing specific genetic factors associated with allergic conditions.
- Most common food allergens are – peanuts, soy, fish, shellfish, wheat, dairy products and fish.
- Fertility generally starts to slowly decline when a woman is in her early 30s, and after the age of 35 the decline speeds up.
- Teratogens include alcohol, drugs, lead, high levels of radiation exposure, and certain medications, infections and toxic substances.
- Maternal drug therapy during pregnancy requires careful consideration because both the mother and the developing fetus have its impact.
- Changes in body composition, such as increased fat stores and total body water, can affect the volume of distribution of drugs.
- Exposure to radiation and certain chemicals during pregnancy can have potential risks for the developing fetus.
- Ionizing radiation has enough energy to remove tightly bound electrons from atoms, and this can damage living tissues.
- If the brain of the developing fetus is exposed to high doses of radiation, it may lead to intellectual and developmental disabilities.
- Non-ionizing radiation (such as that from ultrasound or MRI) does not carry the same risks as ionizing radiations.
- All illegal drugs such as heroin and cocaine, and some legal substances such as alcohol, tobacco and certain medical drugs are dangerous for the health of mother and her baby.
- Cigarette smoke may be teratogenic and may cause cardiac abnormalities as well as anencephaly.
- The genetic disorders play a significant role in infertility, affecting both men and women.
- Infertility is a complex issue, often involving a combination of factors.
- Spontaneous abortion, commonly known as a miscarriage, refers to the natural loss of a pregnancy before the end of 28th week of pregnancy.

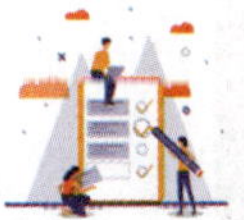

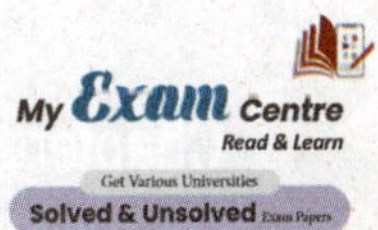

ASSESS YOURSELF

Long Answer Questions

1. Why is it that women exceeding 37 years of age have more chances of having a child with Down's syndrome? Discuss.
2. What is infertility? Explain the factors that contribute to infertility.
3. Discuss the effects of radiations during prenatal period.

Short Answer Questions

1. Write about the effects of drugs and chemicals on fetal growth.
2. What is consanguinity?
3. Write short notes on:
   i. Conditions affecting during prenatal period
   ii. Spontaneous abortions

Multiple Choice Questions

1. **An agent that can potentially cause a birth defect or negatively alter cognitive and behavioral outcomes refers to:**
   a. Carcinogens
   b. Teratogens
   c. Mutations
   d. All of these
2. **Which of the following period is most vulnerable to teratogens?**
   a. Germinal Period
   b. Embryonic Period
   c. Fetal Period
   d. None of these
3. **Infertility is when a couple fails to conceive after:**
   a. 4 years of unprotected sex
   b. 3 years of unprotected sex
   c. 2 years of unprotected sex
   d. 1 year of unprotected sex
4. **This condition impairs infertility**
   a. PCOD
   b. Fibroids
   c. Endometriosis
   d. All of these
5. **In women, this sexually-transmitted disease can result in infertility:**
   a. Human papillomavirus (HPV)
   b. Pelvic inflammatory disease
   c. Genital herpes
   d. None of these
6. **The effects of diabetic mother on infants is/are:**
   a. Brain enlargement as a part of macrosomia
   b. Hyperglycemia in infant
   c. First-trimester abortion
   d. All of these
7. **Abortion is the expulsion or extraction from the uterus, spontaneous or induced, or the fetus or embryo weighing:**
   a. <100 g
   b. <50 g
   c. <250 g
   d. <500 g
8. **Spontaneous abortions commonly occur during:**
   a. First week
   b. Second trimester
   c. Third trimester
   d. Before 16 weeks

Answer Key

1. b	**2.** b	**3.** d	**4.** d	**5.** b	**6.** c
7. d	**8.** d				

Chapter 26

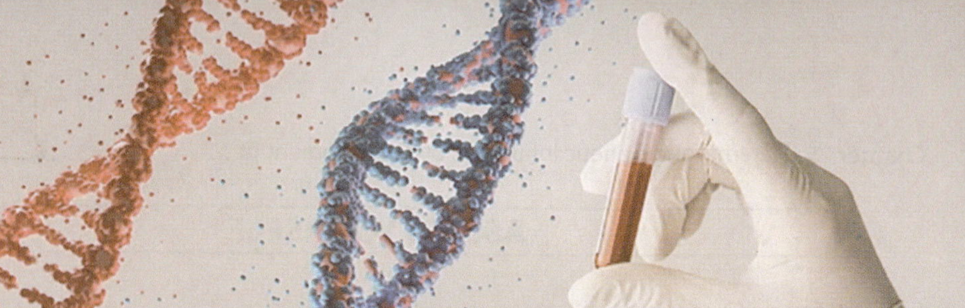

Prenatal Testing

LEARNING OBJECTIVES

After the completion of the chapter, the readers will be able to:

- Discuss prenatal tests.
- Explain and differentiate between invasive and non-invasive prenatal tests.

CHAPTER OUTLINE

- Introduction
- Indications for Prenatal Testing
- Benefits of Prenatal Testing
- Prenatal Tests

KEY TERMS

Autosomal recessive: Hereditary pattern in which the carrier of an altered gene does not show any characteristics of the disorder.

Chromosome abnormality: A change in the number of structural changes in the normal 23 pairs of chromosomes.

Cleft lip and palate: Developmental anomaly in babies when the upper lip or palate (roof of the mouth) is not joined properly.

Congenital anomaly: An anomaly which is present at birth, although not necessarily hereditary.

Critical period: The specific time during prenatal development when an organ or structure is most vulnerable to the effects of teratogens.

Fetoscopy: A special fiber optic instrument passed through the abdomen of a pregnant woman to examine the baby. If required, it is usually done in 18–20 weeks of pregnancy.

Genetic testing: Analyzing an individual's DNA to identify genetic variations associated with disease or the risk of developing certain conditions.

Single gene disorder (also called monogenic disorder): These are genetic conditions that are caused by a change in one gene. There are many different single gene disorders, two examples are cystic fibrosis and sickle cell disease. They can be inherited or passed down in families or can occur for the first time in a particular pregnancy.

Teratogens: Substances or factors that can cause malformations or functional abnormalities in the developing fetus, such as drugs, infections, and environmental factors.

Variant: It refers to an alteration in a DNA sequence. All humans have variants in their DNA which make each of us unique.

INTRODUCTION

Prenatal screening and diagnostic tests are offered to all pregnant women as part of routine antenatal care to determine if their fetus is at significant risk of having a particular disorder, e.g., Down's syndrome, sickle cell anemia. This helps in deciding about giving exceptional healthcare; and to continue or discontinue a pregnancy. Due to the increased risk, women at advanced maternal age are often offered additional prenatal screening and testing options. The tests used for prenatal testing may be noninvasive prenatal tests (NIPT) or invasive prenatal tests (IPT).

INDICATIONS FOR PRENATAL TESTING

- Advanced maternal age.
- Previous child with a chromosome abnormality.
- Women who are pregnant with multiple gestations (twins or more).
- Family history of single gene disorder of a neural tube defect or of other congenital structural abnormalities and abnormalities identified in pregnancy.
- Women who previously had miscarriages.
- Other high-risk factors, such as consanguinity, poor maternal health.

NOTE

In India, Prenatal Diagnostic Technique (Regulation and Prevention of Misuse) Act 1994, is followed. It was revised in April 2003. The incidence of major congenital abnormalities is 2–3% of pregnancies.

BENEFITS OF PRENATAL TESTING

The following are the benefits of prenatal testing:

- Prenatal testing can provide valuable information about the chromosomal health of the fetus. However, it is important to note that these tests are optional, and decisions about whether to undergo testing are based on individual preferences and values.
- Prenatal testing diagnoses genetic abnormalities and structural anomalies in early embryo and fetus in order to take timely prenatal counseling and appropriate interventions.
- It allows timely termination of pregnancy thereby preventing wastage and perinatal mortality.
- Timely medical treatment of a condition before or after birth.
- Parents can decide regarding whether to abort a fetus with a diagnosed condition.
- Parents can prepare psychologically, socially, financially, and medically for a baby with a health problem or disability.
- It can determine the outcome of pregnancy.

PRENATAL TESTS

Patient counseling: Before undergoing tests meant for prenatal diagnosis, healthcare providers must thoroughly counsel pregnant female about the potential risks and benefits of the procedure. Informed consent is obtained to ensure that the individual is aware of the potential risks and is making an informed decision.

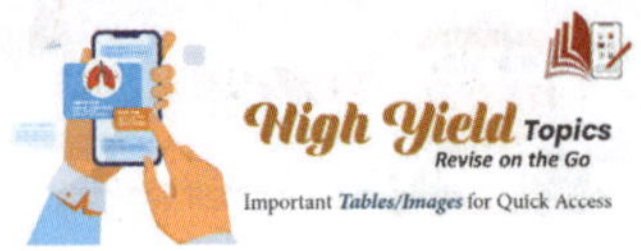

Invasive Prenatal Tests

Invasive prenatal diagnostic tests involve the extraction of fetal tissues or fluids for genetic testing to assess the health and development of the fetus.

Limitations of invasive prenatal tests: The invasive approach to obtaining fetal tissue and DNA is currently the gold standard for prenatal diagnosis. Many women are reluctant to undergo invasive testing, either due to the risk to the pregnancy, or because they would not terminate the pregnancy irrespective of the results.

Fetal Tissue Biopsy

It involves the removal and examination of a small sample of tissue from a developing fetus for diagnostic purpose. The choice of procedure depends on the specific information needed and the stage of pregnancy. The types of procedure to do fetal tissue biopsies include:

- Chorionic villus sampling.
- Amniocentesis.
- Cordocentesis or fetal blood sampling.

The detailed analysis of the above mentioned procedures is as follows:

Chorionic Villus Sampling (CVS)

This test is usually carried out between 11–14 weeks (in 2nd trimester) gestation. CVS may cause miscarriage in around 1–2% of cases.

Purposes:

- **Chromosomal analysis:** To detect numerical abnormalities such as Down syndrome (Trisomy 21), Edwards syndrome (Trisomy 18), or Patau syndrome (Trisomy 13).
- **Genetic testing:** To identify specific genetic disorders or mutations.

Procedure:

Chorionic Villus Sampling (CVS) (Fig. 26.1) involves the collection of a small sample of chorionic villi, in the placenta. A small sample of the placenta is taken for testing, either by inserting a needle through the abdominal wall or by passing a fine tube or forceps through the cervix. There are two main methods for performing CVS:

1. **Transabdominal CVS:** A thin needle is inserted through the abdominal wall to reach the chorionic villi under ultrasound guidance.
2. **Transcervical CVS:** A catheter is passed through the cervix to obtain a sample of chorionic villi.

Advantages:

- **Early detection:** CVS can be performed earlier in pregnancy compared to amniocentesis, providing results sooner.
- **Rapid results:** Chromosomal analysis and genetic testing results are available within a few days to a couple of weeks.

Risks:

- Miscarriage (estimated to be around 0.5%–1%).
- Infection or bleeding at the puncture site.

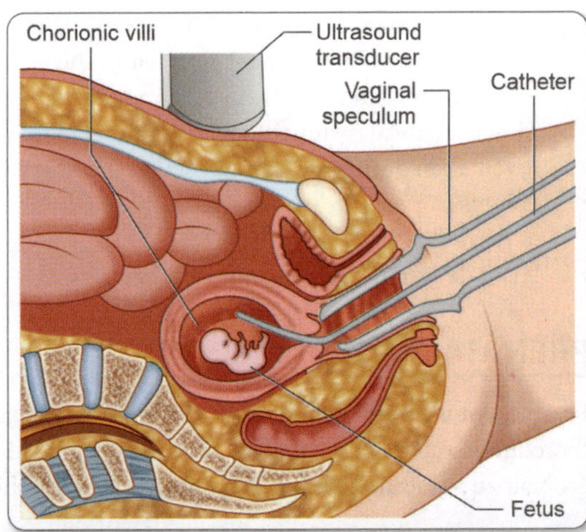

Figure 26.1: Chorionic villus sampling

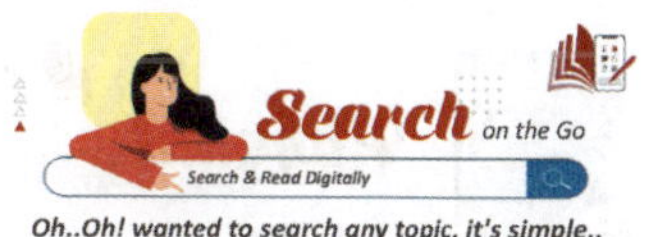

Amniocentesis

Obtain a sample of amniotic fluid from the amniotic sac surrounding the fetus. This sample contains cells shed by the fetus, and are analyzed by karyotyping (Fig. 26.2). This procedure is usually carried out after 15 weeks gestation (2nd trimester).

Procedure:

Involves insertion of a thin, hollow needle through the mother's abdominal wall and into the amniotic sac under ultrasound guidance. A small amount of amniotic fluid, which surrounds the fetus, is withdrawn and collected for further analysis.

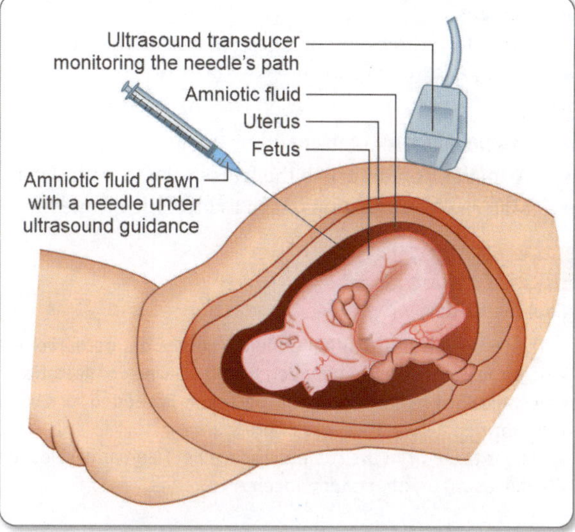

Figure 26.2: Amniocentesis

Advantages:

- **Chromosomal analysis:** Detailed information about the genetic makeup of the fetus.
- **Genetic testing:** Can be used for specific genetic testing based on family history or other factors.
- Detection of neural tube defects such as spina bifida.

Risks:

- Miscarriage.
- Bleeding or infection.
- **Rh sensitization:** Rh-negative individuals may be at risk of Rh sensitization, and Rh immunoglobulin may be administered.

Cordocentesis or Fetal Blood Sampling

It is also known as percutaneous umbilical blood sampling (PUBS). It is a prenatal diagnostic procedure (Fig. 26.3) that involves the direct sampling of fetal blood from the umbilical cord.

Purposes:

- To assess for chromosomal abnormalities.
- To diagnose or rule out blood disorders, such as hemoglobinopathies (e.g., thalassemia) or platelet disorders.
- To test fetal infections.

Indications:

When other diagnostic tests are inconclusive or when there is a high risk of certain blood disorders.

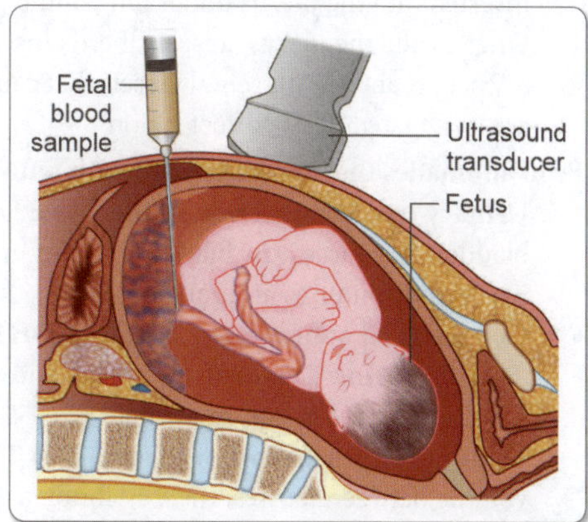

Figure 26.3: Cordocentesis

Procedure:

- Usually performed between the 18th and 24th weeks (after 18 weeks) of pregnancy.
- Involves the insertion of a thin needle through the mother's abdominal wall and into the umbilical cord, guided by ultrasound.
- Fetal blood is then drawn for analysis.

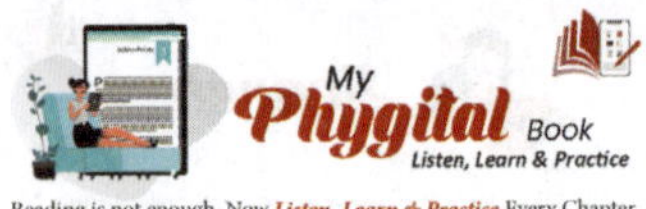

Advantages:
- Provides a direct and detailed analysis of the baby's blood.
- Rapid results.

Risks:
- Miscarriage risk.
- A small risk of injury to the fetus or the umbilical cord.
- Maternal complications, such as bleeding or infection.

RECENT UPDATE

Coelocentesis
- The test involves aspiration of fluid from the extraembryonic coelom.
- Test can be performed between 6- and 12-week of gestation.
- Technically it requires similar expertise as is needed for CVS or amniocentesis.
- Performed before 10 weeks of pregnancy.
- Fluid is taken from the coelomic space between amniotic membrane and uterine cavity.
- Fetal loss=0 or <that of amniocentesis.

Fetoscopy

Fetoscopy is an endoscopic method used during or after 18th week of pregnancy (Fig. 26.4). To allow surgical access to the fetus, the amniotic cavity, the umbilical cord and the fetal side of the placenta.

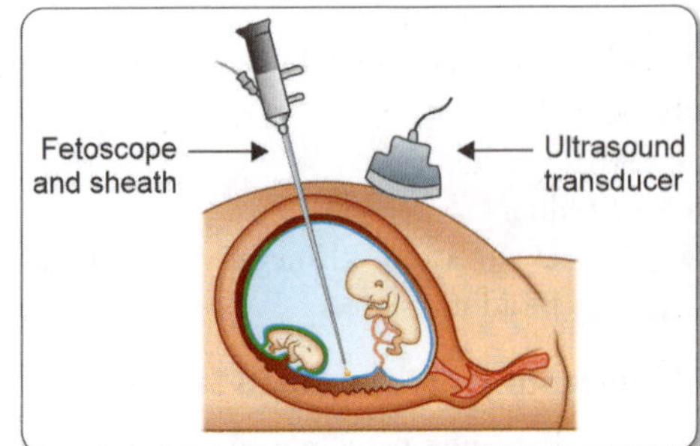

Figure 26.4: Fetoscopy

Procedure:
- Insertion site for fetoscope is selected with the help of ultrasound.
- After a small skin incision at that site, the fetoscope is inserted into the uterus under ultrasound guidance.
- Once inside the uterus, a laser fiber is inserted into the fetoscope, and the placental vessels that cause the TTTS are coagulated under direct vision.

Fetal anomalies that can be treated with fetoscopy are:
- **Urinary tract obstruction in the fetus:** Urine comes back up to the kidneys and damages the urinary bladder. It enlarges the bladder of fetus and also reduces the amount of amniotic fluid as fetal urine is main contributor to amniotic fluid.
- **Congenital diaphragmatic hernia (CDH):** In such cases diaphragm does not develop properly.
- **Acardiac twins:** One fetus has heart and other does not. So the heart has to supply blood to both the developing fetuses. Approximately 50–75% acardiac twins die.
- **Twin-twin transfusion syndrome (TTTS):** Twin fetuses share the placenta. Due to unequal blood volume between fetuses, there is abnormally low blood volume in the donor twin and high in the other one who is recipient twin. TTTS twins die without intervention.

Risk: Injuring and losing the fetus during the procedure.

Noninvasive Prenatal Techniques Tests

Noninvasive prenatal testing (NIPT) is an alternative way to screen for certain genetic conditions without the need for invasive procedures. NIPT involves analyzing cell-free fetal DNA circulating in the maternal blood.

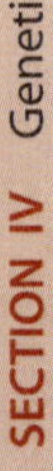

NIPT is highly accurate but is not a diagnostic test, and positive results should be confirmed with invasive diagnostic testing.

Advantage: These tests do not carry a risk of miscarriage or harm to the fetus.

Limitations of NIPT: The limitations of NIPT are as follows:

- NIPT is not a diagnostic test; it is a screening test for chromosomal abnormalities.
- It does not screen for structural defects.
- It is not designed to detect fetal genetic conditions other than the targeted aneuploidies.
- NIPT may give a high chance result when the fetus does not actually have the condition. For an instance if the results of NIPT are positive for Down syndrome, there is 20% chance that the result is wrong and the fetus does not have the condition.
- Expensive as compared to invasive tests.
- Only limited to testing three chromosomes and gender testing.
- Specific kits are required.

Cell-free Fetal DNA (cffDNA)

Cell-free fetal DNA (cffDNA) refers to small fragments of fetal DNA that circulate freely in the maternal bloodstream during pregnancy. This DNA is released from the placenta and represents genetic material from the developing fetus. cffDNA can first be observed as early as seven weeks (as early as the first-trimester) of gestation, and the amount of cffDNA increases as the pregnancy progresses.

Sample for cffDNA is collected by venipuncture on the mother.

The test is recommended for the following groups:

- Women aged 35 years or older at delivery.
- Those with sonographic findings indicating increased risk for fetal aneuploidy.
- Those with a prior pregnancy complicated by trisomy 21, 18, or 13.
- Patient or partner carries a balanced Robertsonian translocation indicating increased risk for fetal trisomy 21 or 13.
- Those with an abnormal first-, second-, or combined first and second-trimester screening test result for aneuploidy.

Clinical Applications of cffDNA Test:

- Fetal sex determination (in the case of sex-linked disorders and certain endocrine disorders).
- Certain autosomal single gene disorders (particularly where the paternal disease-causing allele differs from the maternal one).
- Routine antenatal screening at a population level, e.g., testing for Down's syndrome and other aneuploidies (Trisomy 21), Edwards syndrome (Trisomy 18), and Patau syndrome (Trisomy 13).
- Management of pregnancies at risk of specific complications, e.g., fetal RhD testing in RhD negative women (currently receive anti-D prophylaxis without testing).
- To decide when to deliver exceptional healthcare, which is to be personally delivered.

Ultrasound Imaging

The frequency range of 1–12 megahertz is used for ultrasound imaging. Developing embryo can be visualized at about 6 weeks of gestation (Fig. 26.5). The sonographic findings of genetic conditions are tabulated in Table 26.1.

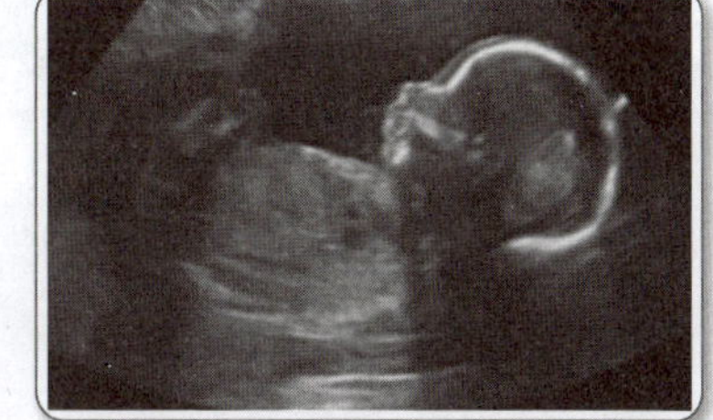

Figure 26.5: Ultrasonography

Basic Ultrasound

It is commonly used to monitor fetal development, identify the fetas position, and screen for structural abnormalities

3D and 4D Ultrasound

This advanced ultrasound technique provides more detailed, three-dimensional images of the fetus, allowing for better visualization of its features.

Table 26.1: Sonographic findings: 99% of fetuses with open spina bifida have one or more of tabulated findings

Condition	Characteristics	Sonographic findings
Frontal notching (Lemon sign)	Small biparietal diameter	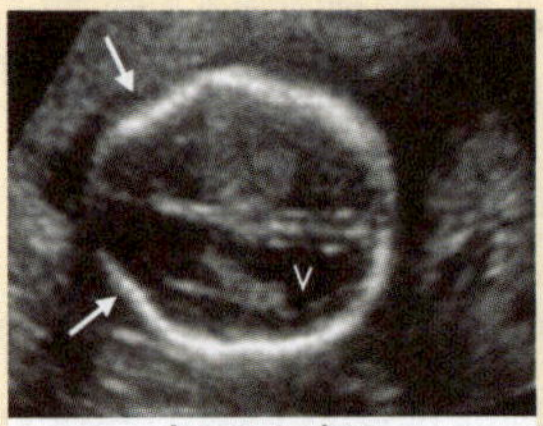 Lemon sign; 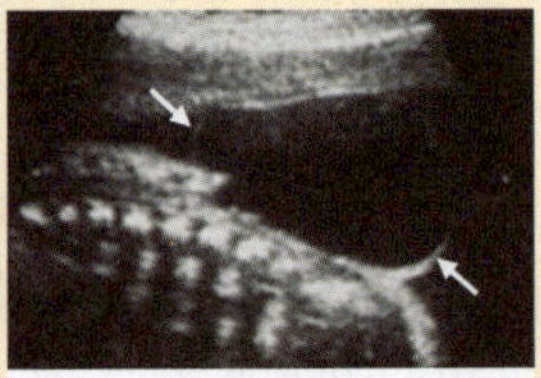 Spina bifida
Banana sign due to cerebellar herniation	Obliteration of cisterna magna, ventriculomegaly	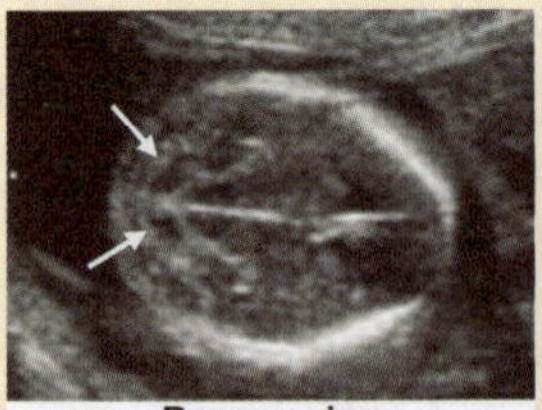 Banana sign; 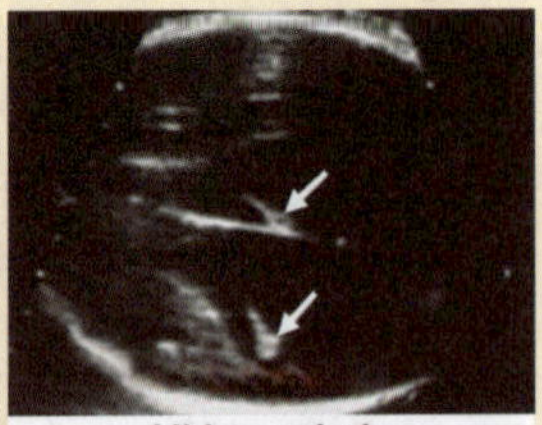 Hidrocephaly
Anencephaly Too much fluid in the amniotic sac (polyhydramnios)	Missing parts of the skull and brain. Exposed areas of brain tissue (no skin or skull covering it). Smaller head size than expected.	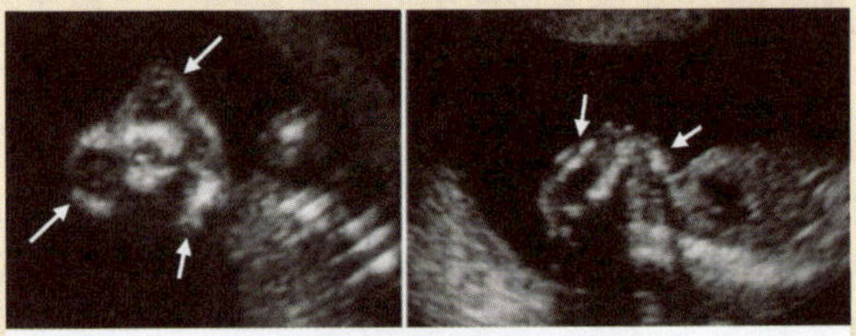 Anencephaly
Encephalocoele a purely cystic mass or may contain echoes from herniated brain tissue.	A defect in the calvarium containing a cystic or solid mass with a gyral pattern that is contiguous with the brain.	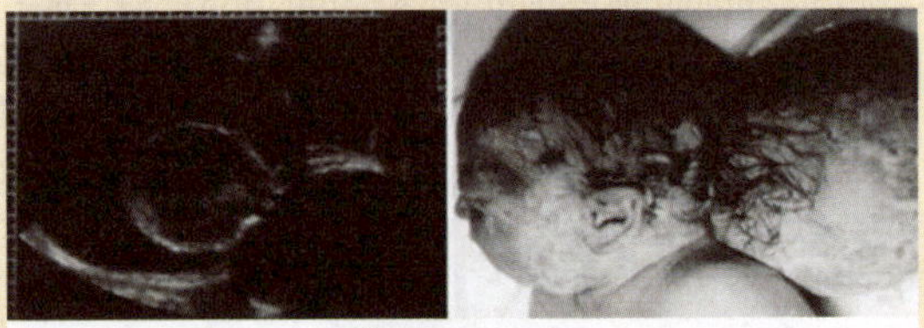 Encephalocele

Magnetic Resonance Imaging

- MRI is combined with ultrasound usually at or after 18 weeks of gestation.
- MRI is a risk-free method.
- MRI (Fig. 26.6) can provide detailed images of fetal anatomy and is often used when additional information is needed after an abnormal ultrasound finding.
- It is particularly useful for assessing the central nervous system and other structures.

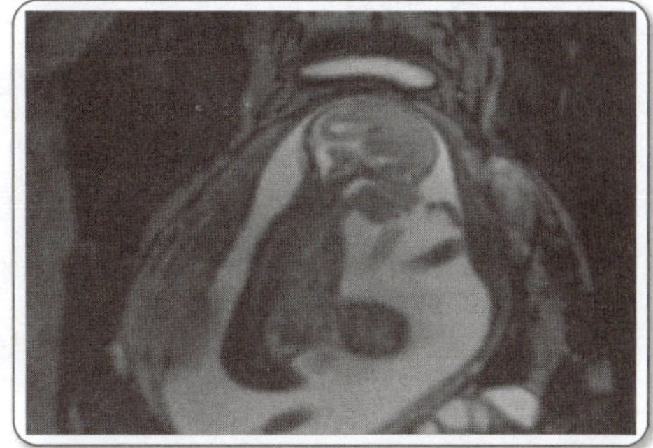

Figure 26.6: Magnetic Resonance Imaging

Triple Test

Triple test measures:

- Alpha-fetoprotein (AFP)
- Human chorionic gonadotropin (hCG)
- Unconjugated estriol (UE3)

Positive test is indicated when:

- AFP ↓
- hCG ↑
- Unconjugated estriol ↓

The triple test screens (table) for fetal disorders such as open NTD, Down syndrome, trisomy 18 are given in Table 26.2.

Quadruple Screen Test

AFP, hCG, estriol and inhibin are measured.

Umbilical Artery Doppler Blood Flow Studies

Umbilical artery doppler blood flow assessment provides information about increased vascular resistance, allowing for the identification of high-risk pregnancies. It is a noninvasive method of studying hemodynamic patterns to determine fetal well-being. This is especially important in any fetus with known or suspected intrauterine growth restriction (IUGR) or cord compression from a nuchal cord or knots.

PCR

There is bidirectional traffic between mother and fetus through placenta. Fetal derived cell-free DNA from mother DNA is distinguished by:

- QF-PCR
- Digital PCR

Table 26.2: Screening of fetal disorders by triple test

Disorders	MSAFP	uE3	Beta hCG	Inhibin A
Open NTD	Increased	No change	No change	No change
Downs syndrome	Decreased	Decreased	Increased	Increased
Trisomy 18	Decreased	Decreased	No change	No change

Abbreviations: hCG, human chorionic gonadotropin; MSAFP, maternal serum alpha-fetoprotein; uE3, unconjugated estriol

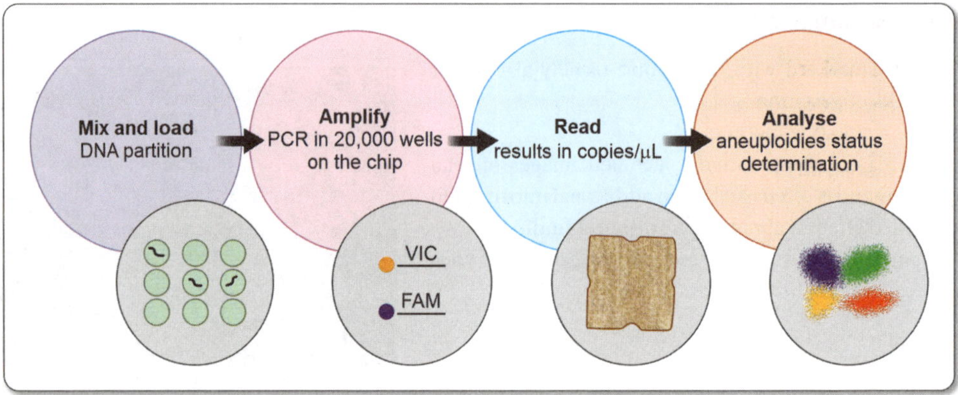

Figure 26.7: Digital PCR for prenatal testing

Note: FAM and VIC—dyes

QF-PCR (Quantitative Fluorescent - PCR)

Fully automated technique that provides rapid diagnoses of selected chromosomal anomalies (Commonly trisomy 13, 18, 21) by eliminating the need to culture fetal cells. QF-PCR provides rapid (within 24–48 hours) diagnosis of whether there is aneuploidy of the analyzed chromosomes. The advantage of this over FISH is that it can make the diagnosis with fewer cells.

Digital PCR

Enriched single template DNA or RNA molecules are isolated by dilution and then amplified the sample is partitioned into multiple duplicates and analyzed. Digital PCR (Fig. 26.7) allows detection of fetal chromosomal aneuploidy utilizing uncultured amniocytes and chorionic villus tissue in <6 hours.

RECENT UPDATE

SAFE and RAPID

The special non-invasive Advances in fetal and neonatal evaluation (SAFE) is a Reliable Accurate Prenatal Non-Invasive Diagnosis (RAPID) of UK National Program, funded by the National Institute for Health Research. The test includes targeted new generation sequencing (MALDI-TOF mass spectrometry) and digital PCR. More rapid tests include:
- Rapid-FISH (rapid fluorescence *in situ* hybridization),
- Multiple ligation PCR amplification (MLPA),
- Quantitative fluorescent polymerase chain reaction (QF-PCR)

Fetal Heart Echocardiography

A fetal echocardiogram might be done for many reasons, including a family history of certain heart problems. The fetal echocardiogram helps to know about any major problem that may be affecting the developing baby's heart walls and valves, the blood vessels leading to and from the heart, and the heart's pumping strength.

Laboratory Markers

During pregnancy, various biochemical markers are often measured in maternal serum to assess the health of both the mother and the developing fetus (Table 26.3).

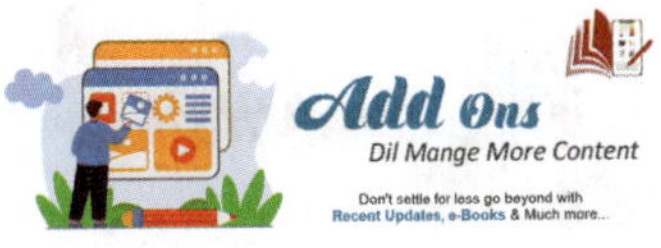

Table 26.3: Markers in maternal serum/blood/plasma to assess fetomaternal health

Biochemical marker	Normal reference range
Human Chorionic Gonadotropin (hCG)	**Varies by gestational age:** Elevated levels are expected during pregnancy.
Alpha-fetoprotein (AFP)	**Varies by gestational age:** Elevated levels may indicate neural tube defects or other fetal abnormalities.
Estriol (E3)	**Varies by gestational age:** A decrease may indicate a problem with the fetus or the placenta.
Inhibin A	Elevated levels may be associated with chromosomal abnormalities, such as Down syndrome.
Progesterone	**Varies by gestational age:** Essential for maintaining pregnancy.
Pregnancy-associated plasma protein A (PAPP-A)	Lower levels may be associated with chromosomal abnormalities.
Thyroid-stimulating hormone (TSH)	Reference range may be narrower in pregnancy. Abnormal levels may indicate thyroid dysfunction.
Free thyroxine (FT4)	Important for monitoring thyroid function during pregnancy.
Glucose	Fasting and postprandial levels. Abnormal levels may indicate gestational diabetes.
Complete Blood Count (CBC)	Hemoglobin, hematocrit, platelet count, white blood cell count. Abnormalities may indicate anemia or infection.
Blood Type and Rh Factor	Rh-negative mothers may require Rh immune globulin to prevent Rh incompatibility issues.

Human chorionic gonadotropin: hCG is a critical hormone in the early stages of pregnancy, and its levels can be detected in the blood and urine. This hormone can be detected in the blood as early as 11 days after conception and in the urine a few days later. This is crucial for the maintenance of the uterine lining to support the growing embryo. In a healthy pregnancy, hCG levels generally double every 48–72 hours during the early weeks.

Maternal serum alpha-fetoprotein (MSAFP): Alpha-fetoprotein (AFP) or MSAFP is a glycoprotein synthesized by the fetal yolk sac and later by the fetal gastrointestinal tract and liver. in defects if fetal integument, such as in case of neural-tube and ventral wall defects, AFP leaks into the amnionic fluid, resulting in dramatically increased maternal serum AFP levels. Screening (Fig. 26.8) is generally performed from 15th to 20th weeks.

- **Causes:** Three common causes of AFP level elevation are underestimation of gestational age, multifetal gestation, and fetal demise.
- Virtually all cases of anencephaly and many cases of spina bifida may be detected or suspected during a standard second-trimester evaluation of MSAFP levels.
- **Cut-off value:** 2.0 or 2.5 MoM.

Estriol: Estriol is one of the three main naturally occurring estrogens in the human body, along with estradiol and estrone. Estriol levels can be measured to monitor the health of the fetus, especially in situations where there is concern about fetal distress or complications.

PAPP-A: (First trimester screening) Combining blood tests with ultrasound measurements, this screening assesses the risk of chromosomal abnormalities, including Down syndrome. It typically involves measuring

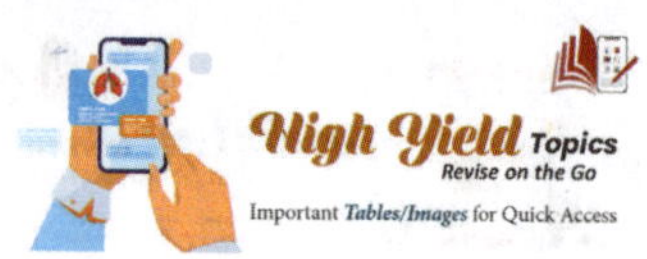

serum markers such as free beta-human chorionic gonadotropin (β-hCG) and pregnancy-associated plasma protein-A (PAPP-A).

EXTRA EDGE

Down syndrome screening: In combination with other markers, such as PAPP-A, hCG is used for screening purposes to assess the risk of Down syndrome and other chromosomal abnormalities.

Inhibin-A, alpha-fetoprotein (AFP), human chorionic gonadotropin (hCG), estriol (Quadruple screen): Conducted in the second trimester, this blood test measures levels of alpha-fetoprotein (AFP), human chorionic gonadotropin (hCG), estriol, and inhibin-A. It is used to assess the risk of neural tube defects and chromosomal abnormalities.

NOTE

While non-invasive prenatal testing is valuable for screening, a definitive diagnosis of certain conditions may require invasive procedures. The choice of prenatal diagnostic methods depends on factors such as maternal age, medical history, and the presence of risk factors.

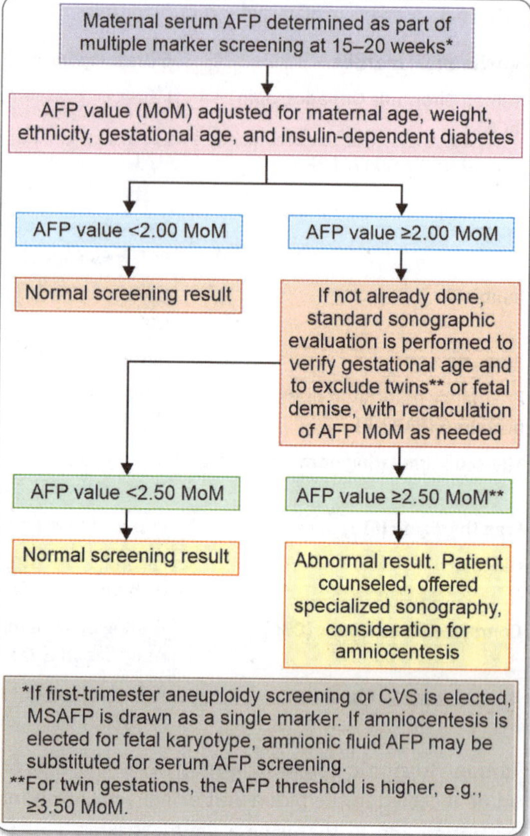

Figure 26.8: Algorithm for AFP testing

SUMMARY

- Prenatal screening and diagnostic tests help in deciding about giving exceptional healthcare; and to continue or discontinue a pregnancy.
- Invasive prenatal diagnostic tests involve the extraction of fetal tissues or fluids for genetic testing to assess the health and development of the fetus.
- NIPT involves analyzing cell-free fetal DNA circulating in the maternal blood.
- 3D and 4D ultrasound advanced techniques provide more detailed, three-dimensional images of the fetus, allowing for better visualization of its features.
- Chorionic villus sampling involves the collection of a small sample of chorionic villi, in the placenta.
- Amniocentesis is a prenatal diagnostic procedure used to obtain a sample of amniotic fluid from the amniotic sac surrounding the fetus.
- Cordocentesis is a prenatal diagnostic procedure that involves the direct sampling of fetal blood from the umbilical cord.
- MRI can provide detailed images of fetal anatomy and is often used when additional information is needed after an abnormal ultrasound finding.
- Umbilical artery doppler assessment provides information about increased vascular resistance, allowing for the identification of high-risk pregnancies.

Contd...

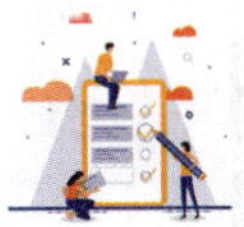

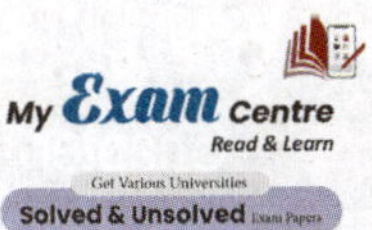

- QF-PCR provides rapid (within 24–48 hours) diagnosis of whether there is aneuploidy of the analysed chromosomes.
- In a healthy pregnancy, hCG levels generally double every 48–72 hours during the early weeks.
- Defects in fetal integument, such as neural-tube and ventral wall defects, permit AFP to leak into the amnionic fluid, resulting in dramatically increased maternal serum AFP levels.
- Measuring estriol levels can be used to monitor the health of the fetus, especially in situations where there is concern about fetal distress or complications.

ASSESS YOURSELF

Long Answer Question

1. Discuss prenatal testing techniques.

Short Answer Questions

1. Define amniocentesis.
2. Differentiate between CVS and amniocentesis.
3. Write short notes on:
   i. NIPT
   II. Triple test

Multiple Choice Questions

1. Amniocentesis, chorionic villi and alpha-fetoprotein sampling are performed to determine ________________.
   a. The most likely date of birth of the fetus
   b. Whether the baby will be normal or abnormal
   c. Whether the mother has a genetic abnormality
   d. Both a and b

2. Which of the following can be examined by amniocentesis procedure?
   a. Chromosome analysis
   b. Detecting genetic defects
   c. Maturity of fetal lungs
   d. All of these

3. The fluid sample required for performing the amniocentesis test is ________________.
   a. The amnion
   b. The placenta
   c. The liquid surrounding the fetus
   d. All of these

4. Which of these procedures has the least risk for an unborn child?
   a. Amniocentesis
   b. Alpha-fetoprotein sampling
   c. Chorionic villi sampling
   d. All have the same risk level

5. Which of the following sentence is true for the chorion?
   a. The organ in the uterus connected to the fetus by the umbilical cord
   b. The sac- or pouch-like organ within uterus containing the amniotic fluid surrounding the fetus
   c. A membrane developing around an embryo, contributing to the formation of the placenta
   d. None of the above

6. Which of the following medical conditions are responsible for producing incorrect Alpha-fetoprotein (AFP) screening results and indicating a fetus has genetic defects?
   a. The mother is anemic
   b. The mother has Rh-negative blood
   c. The date of conception has been miscalculated
   d. All of these

Answer Key

1. b **2.** d **3.** c **4.** b **5.** c **6.** b

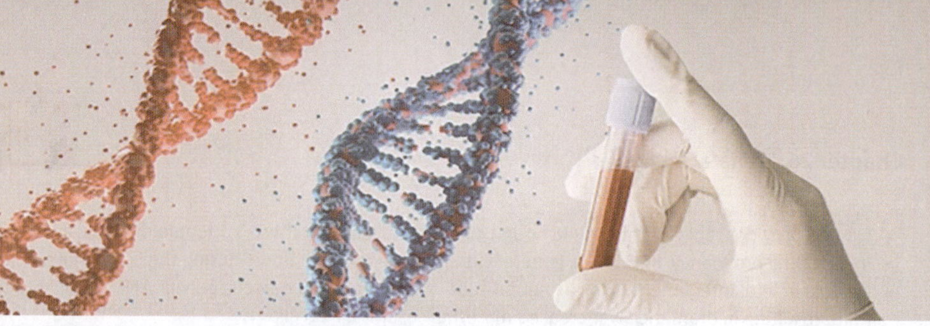

Chapter 27

Genetic Testing in the Neonates and Children

LEARNING OBJECTIVES

After the completion of the chapter, the readers will be able to:

- Explain genetic testing, its types, and needs.
- Discuss developmental delay and approaches for screening it.
- Understand dysmorphism.

CHAPTER OUTLINE

- Introduction
- Types of Genetic Tests
- Genetic Screening and Testing
- Clinical Tests in Genetics
- Screening for Congenital Abnormalities
- Developmental Delay
- Dysmorphism

KEY TERMS

Arachnodactyly: A condition in which the fingers are long, slender, and curved.

Arthrogryposis: A term describing a number of conditions that affect the joints.

Brachydactyly: Short digits.

Clitoromegaly: Enlarged clitoris.

Lactic acidosis: A type of metabolic acidosis that occurs when lactic acids are built in the blood.

Macroglossia: A rare condition that and has enlarged tongue.

Otoacoustic emission test: Measures hair cell function in the inner ear.

Skeletal dysplasia: A category of rare genetic disorders that cause abnormal development of a baby's bones, joints, and cartilage.

INTRODUCTION

Genetic testing in neonates and children involves examining their DNA to identify potential genetic disorders or conditions. This type of testing can provide valuable information about a child's health, guide treatment decisions, and offer insights into its future health risks.

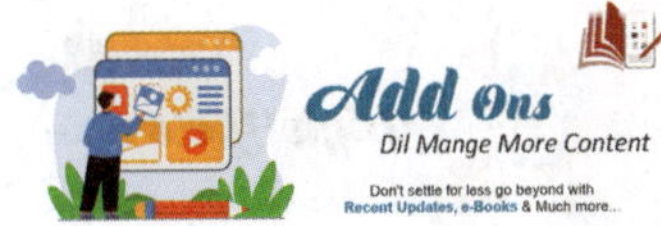

TYPES OF GENETIC TESTS

Main types of genetic testing methods are as follows:

- **Chromosome study** (Blood sample, prenatal sample, skin biopsy, or other tissue sample): Chromosome studies may be done when a child is born with multiple birth defects. The chromosomes need to be stained in order to see them with a microscope.
- **DNA study:** Errors in DNA amino acid sequences is assessed. There are two ways to analyze the DNA:
  1. **Direct DNA study** (Blood samples): It looks directly at the gene in question for an error. This technology is called FISH or PCR. Errors in the DNA may include:
     - Deletion—when a piece of the gene's DNA is lost.
     - Duplication—when the gene's DNA is replicated.
     - Point mutation—change in a single unit (base pair) of the gene's DNA.
     - Trinucleotide repeat—a repeated replication of a small sequence of the DNA.
  2. **Indirect DNA study** (From blood samples): It involves using markers (DNA sequences located close to or even within the gene of interest) to find out whether a person has inherited the important region of the genetic code that is passing through the family with the disease.
- **Biochemical genetic study:** From blood sample urine sample, spinal fluid, or other tissue sample, depending on the disorder. Biochemical genetic testing involves the study of enzymes in the body that may be abnormal. The enzymes may be deficient or absent, unstable, or have altered activity that can lead to signs of diseases.
- **Protein truncation study** (From blood sample): A mutation in a gene causes it to make a protein that is shortened (truncated). With the protein truncation test, it is possible to "measure" the length of the protein in a gene.

GENETIC SCREENING AND TESTING

Congenital anomalies are a leading cause of infant mortality. There are over 4500 Mendelian disorders that have a known genetic etiology at present. The genetic screening and diagnostic tests are required for the following reasons:

- It is difficult to decide a plan of care without a certain diagnosis.
- Obtaining a genetic diagnosis often assists in patient management.
- Families dealing with serious medical issues in their children often endure years of diagnostic uncertainty therefore, early diagnosis helps them in coping with the problem.
- Prevention of genetic disease in future children.

MUST KNOW

Screening versus Diagnostic Testing

- **Screening:** This is a standard procedure conducted shortly after birth to screen for a range of genetic disorders that may not be apparent at birth but can cause serious health issues if not detected early. It typically involves a blood test and, in some cases, additional tests based on the initial results.
- **Diagnostic testing:** Diagnostic testing involves more in-depth analysis of the child's DNA.

Genetic Screening

Newborn screening involves testing newborns for certain genetic, metabolic, hormonal, and functional disorders. Children are screened when a genetic disorder is suspected. Newborn screening typically occurs

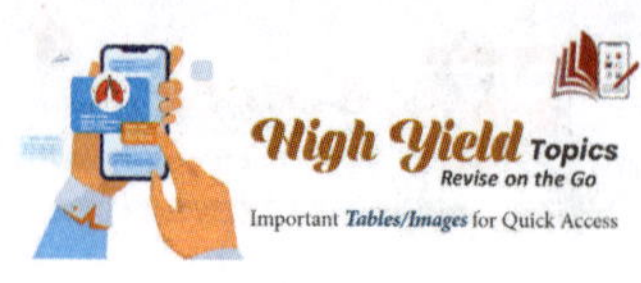

within the first few days of a baby's life. Early detection and intervention through newborn screening have proven to be highly effective in preventing or minimizing the impact of certain conditions. The heel stick blood sample is drawn from a neonate within 48 hours of birth and aids screening of up to 50 diseases including sickle cell disease, hypothyroidism, and phenylketonuria.

Genetic Testing

Genetic testing is a type of medical test that identifies changes in genes, chromosomes, or proteins. The results of a genetic test can confirm or rule out a suspected genetic condition or help determine a person's chance of developing or passing on a genetic disorder. The following points are kept in mind while going for genetic screening and testing:

- **Ethical considerations:** Particularly regarding privacy, consent, and the potential psychological impact of knowing one's genetic information.
- **Advances in genetic technologies:** Next-generation sequencing has enhanced the speed and accuracy of genetic analyses, making it more accessible for diagnosing rare genetic disorders.
- **Ongoing monitoring:** Regular monitoring and follow-up testing is necessary to assess a child's development and health over time.
- **Research and precision medicine:** Genetic data from neonates and children contribute to research in understanding genetic diseases, facilitating the development of targeted therapies and personalized medicine approaches.

Characteristics of Genetic Testing

- Genetic counseling is important before advising for any test with genetic implications.
- Genetic testing is voluntary and it has both benefits and limitations.
- Genetic testing is different from the other tests done in clinical practice.
- Genetic test of the patient may also provide results for family members. It may open up ethical or psychological problems.

Purpose of Genetic Testing

To confirm a clinical diagnosis: When a genetic disorder is suspected from physical characteristics or symptoms, genetic tests are required for either confirmation of genetic disease or to rule out a suspected genetic disorder.

Carrier testing/screening: Carrier of particular genetic disorder carries one copy of a mutated gene of a disease. Carrier testing is done in unaffected genes for individuals who have a family history of a genetic disorder.

Predictive and presymptomatic testing: Presymptomatic testing is most commonly done for individuals, who have a family member with a genetic disorder, but are not having features of the disorder themselves at the time of testing.

Barriers of Genetic Testing

- Atypical presentation of a typical genetic disorder in the newborn period.
- Sequential testing may be time consuming in a critically ill child.
- Infants on life support—comprehensive clinical assessment can be difficult in such cases.
- Complex phenotype issues such as:
  - Small for gestational age.

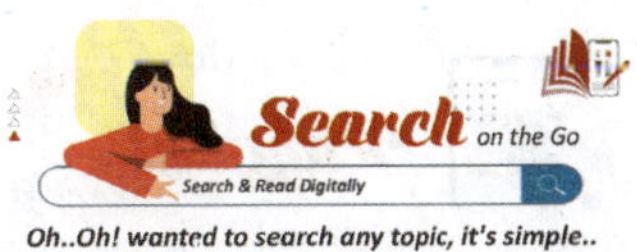

- Bilateral microphthalmos, microcornea, small palpebral fissures, iris colobomas, pulmonary hypoplasia.
- Atrial septal defect.
- Left-sided multicystic dysplastic kidney (pelvic), small right kidney.
- Anal atresia.
- Ambiguous genitalia.

CLINICAL TESTS IN GENETICS

The tests which can be done to find out genetic basis of anomalies in pregnant woman include amniotic fluid or the placenta testing.

The algorithm followed to test a newborn and children can be seen in the Figure 27.1.

- **Whole genome sequencing (WGS):** Examines the entire DNA sequence, including noncoding regions, providing a comprehensive analysis of a person's genetic makeup
- **Other tests to find out genetic basis of anomalies are:**
  - Karyotyping
  - FISH
  - Metabolic testing—Plasma amino acids, urine organic acids, acylcarnitine profile, lactate, and ammonia
  - Global metabolomic associated pathway screen for diagnosing inborn errors of metabolism (MAPS)
  - Nuclear Mito NGS test—for diagnosing mitochondrial disease
  - Methylation study
  - Single gene testing (CFTR, SMA, CHD7)

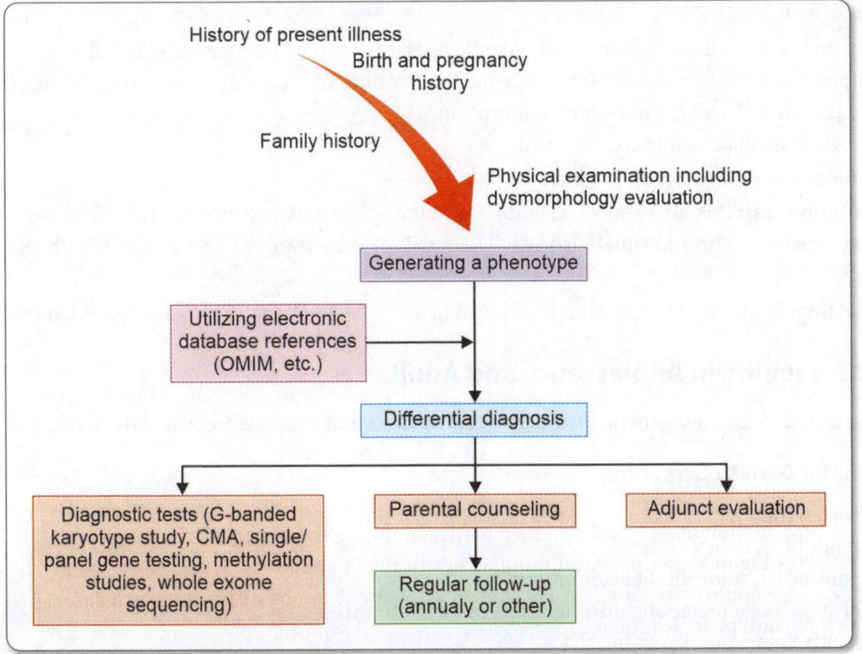

Figure 27.1: Algorithm of genetic testing of a newborn

Abbreviations: CMA, chromosomal microarray analysis; OMIM, online Mendelian inheritance in man

SECTION IV Genetics

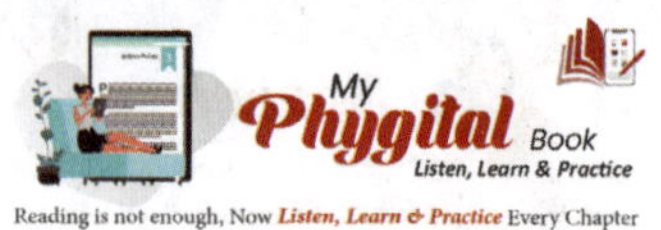

RECENT UPDATE

Rapid Genetic Testing

Chromosomal Microarray Analysis (CMA) and Whole Exome Sequencing are powerful diagnostic tools in the evaluation of critically ill infants suspected to have genetic disorders. Neonates often present with atypical presentation of recognizable disorders making clinical diagnosis more difficult. Rapid genetic testing (critical exome sequencing) provides earlier diagnosis in infants in ICUs, affecting clinical decision-making.

- **Chromosomal microarray analysis (CMA):** Checks for smaller deletions/duplications in the genome—an entire gene may be missing along with other genes.
- **Whole exome sequencing:** The exome ("sum total" of exons) makes up about 1.5% of the whole genome, but is predicted to harbor 85% of disease-causing variants. Exome sequencing is ordered when there is:
  - No clinical diagnosis.
  - Extensive differential diagnosis.
  - All other previous testings have been nondiagnostic.
  - Rapid testing is needed for determining patient's diagnosis and prognosis.

CMA checks for:	Exome checks for:
• Missing genes • Duplicated genes • Large chunks of missing genes	• Misplaced amino acid sequence • Missing sequences • Extra amino acid sequence

SCREENING FOR CONGENITAL ABNORMALITIES

Genetic testing before a pregnancy is ideal, because this provides the wide range of choices if an increased risk of a deleterious genetic condition is detected. However, most of the genetic tests are done after the woman becomes pregnant.

Depending on the time of performing these genetic tests, they can be divided into the following four types:

- Preimplantation: Before conception (i.e., when one or both of the parents are carriers of a certain trait).
- Prenatal testing: These are done after conception.
- Newborn or neonatal, childhood screening.
- Screening tests in adolescence and adulthood.

Preimplantation test: It is also known as embryo screening. This can reduce the risk of having a child with a particular genetic or chromosomal disorder. The test is also used in IVF techniques to rule out unhealthy embryos.

Prenatal testing: Summary of prenatal tests is given in Table 27.1. (Prenatal tests are discussed in Chapter 26)

Genetic Screening in Adolescence and Adults

The tests are used to identify genetic disorders after birth, so that it can be treated early in life.

Indications for Genetic Screening

- **Newborn with:**
  - Major birth defects
  - Unusual (dysmorphic) facial features
  - Suspicion of a metabolic disorder (e.g., phenylketonuria)
  - Positive newborn screening test
  - Congenital hypothyroidism

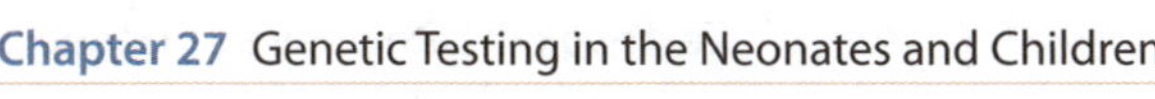

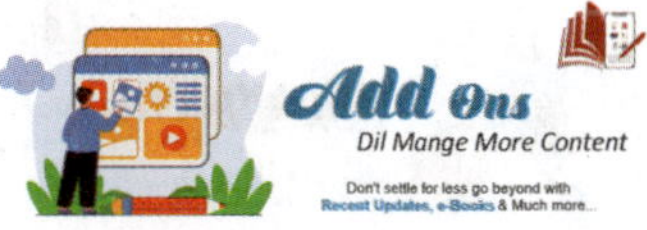

Table 27.1: Summary of prenatal tests

Method	Use	Risk
Preimplantation genetic diagnosis	Identify genetic abnormalities before implantation	Requires IVF Protocol
Ultrasonography	• Determine fetal age • Assess growth of fetus • Detection of birth defects/structural abnormalities • Sex determination (It is prohibited by law to reveal the sex to couples)	None
Amniocentesis • Procedure risk 0.5–1.0% • Performed in second trimester (15–20 weeks)	• **Amniotic fluid:** Biochemical analysis to analyze proteins and measure enzymes • Cells of fetal origin for chromosomal analysis	<0.5% risk of miscarriage
Chorionic villus sampling (CVS) performed during 9–11 weeks	**Fetal cells:** DNA analysis, chromosomal analysis	<2% risk of miscarriage
Umbilical vein blood sampling (cordocentesis) • Procedure risk 1–2% • Performed in the first-trimester • Specialized technique	Fetal blood cells for chromosomal analysis and DNA analysis **Fetal blood serum:** Measure serum enzymes and proteins	<2% risk of miscarriage
Fetoscopy	To visualize the fetus *in utero*	Risk of miscarriage

- Suspected aneuploidy, e.g.,
  - Features of Down syndrome
  - Unbalanced autosome (e.g., Prader-Willi syndrome)
  - Sex chromosomal abnormality (e.g., Turner syndrome)
  - Fragile-X syndrome

- **Child with:**
  - Developmental delay and/or unexplained mental retardation
  - Unusually tall or short stature, or growth delays
  - Known chromosomal abnormality

Types of Genetic Tests

Mainly two types of genetic tests are used:

1. **Exome sequencing:** Looks for all the genes in the DNA or just focuses on the genes related to medical condition (critical exome).
2. **Whole genome sequencing:** The most comprehensive genetic test and it looks for all genes of a person even beyond the DNA.

Applications of Genetic Screening Tests

Screening of blood for:

- **Phenylketonuria (PKU):** PKU is an inherited disorder that affects the breakdown of the amino acid phenylalanine. It can lead to intellectual disabilities. The blood sample is collected from the baby's heel.
- **Hypothyroidism:** This test screens for congenital hypothyroidism. Early detection and treatment are crucial for normal development.

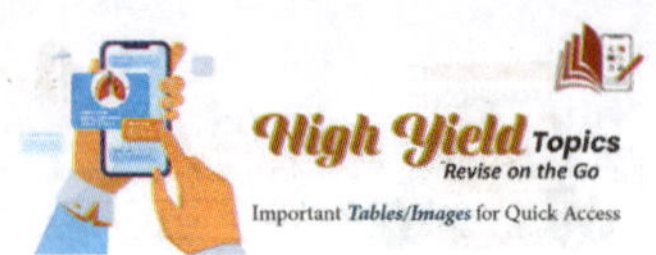

- **Galactosemia:** A metabolic disorder that impairs the body's ability to process galactose, a sugar present in milk. It can lead to serious complications.

Screening of ears for:

- **Otoacoustic emissions (OASE) and Auditory brainstem response (ABR):** OAE measures the sounds produced by the inner ear, while ABR measures the electrical activity in the auditory nerve and brainstem.

Screening of heart for:

- **Critical congenital heart disease (CCHD) screening:** This test uses pulse oximetry to measure the oxygen levels in the baby's blood. Low oxygen levels may indicate a potential heart defect.

Genetic screening for diseases:

- **Cystic fibrosis:** Some regions include screening for cystic fibrosis, a genetic disorder that affects the respiratory, digestive, and reproductive systems. Testing may involve blood samples or, in some cases, genetic testing.
- **Metabolic disorders:** In addition to PKU and galactosemia, some newborn screening programs include tests for other metabolic disorders, such as maple syrup urine disease, homocystinuria, and others.
- **Sickle cell disease and other hemoglobin disorder:** Testing for hemoglobinopathies, including sickle cell disease and thalassemia, especially in regions with a higher prevalence of these conditions.
- **Cystic fibrosis:** This is a genetic disorder that affects the respiratory, digestive, and reproductive systems. Testing may involve blood samples or, in some cases, genetic testing.

Other diseases which are screened:

- Multiple congenital anomalies
- Neonatal hypotonia, feeding difficulties
- Neonatal seizures
- Congenital heart disease
- Cardiomyopathy
- Brain malformations
- Skeletal dysplasia
- Arthrogryposis
- Liver failure
- Immunodeficiency
- Lactic acidosis

NOTE

- Before undergoing genetic testing, families receive genetic counseling.
- Genetic counselors help explain the benefits, limitations, and potential implications of testing.
- They also assist in interpreting results and making informed decisions about further medical management.

DEVELOPMENTAL DELAY

Developmental delay is when a child is slow in reaching the milestones of child's developmental areas. The developmental areas include physical, cognitive, social, behavioral skills. Some common examples of developmental delay observed are in the area of speaking ability, ability to smile, ability to respond back and ability to walk, etc. Developmental delay occurs when children have not reached these milestones by the expected time period. Developmental delays can be further understood as follows.

Types of Developmental Delay

Cognitive Delays

These include the ability to learn and affect intellectual abilities of children. These are often noticed when a child starts going to school and is difficult to diagnose. Down syndrome is a known cause of cognitive delay caused due to genetic defects.

Motor Delays

Normal child has motor milestones over developmental time, as given in Table 27.2. Children with motor delays have affected abilities to coordinate group of muscles. The group of muscles include both small (hands and fingers) and large (arms and legs). Infants with gross motor delays are unable to crawl or roll, similarly the older kids have difficulties in walking or using the stairs. Few people (with a fine motor delay) have difficulty in holding small objects. Some of the examples of motor delays caused by the genetic disorder are achondroplasia, muscular dystrophy, and cerebral palsy.

Social, Emotional and Behavioral Delays

Almost all social, emotional, and behavioral delays are related to neurobehavioral disorders. These disorders are due to abnormal development of the brain which takes place because of various reasons including genetic variations. These delays impact the ability of children to interact, communicate and learn. The normal social developmental milestones are as given in Table 27.3. Some of the well-known examples of social developmental delays are spectrum of disorders related to autism and attention deficit hyperactivity disorders.

Speech Delays

Disorders associated with language receptiveness or expression are referred to as speech delays. The normal speech developments over the time are given in Table 27.4. In this, a child faces difficulties understanding words, colors, shapes, body parts and concepts. In case of delays in language expression a child is unable to babble, talk and create sentences. Usually, receptive language disorder and language expression disorders appear together in most cases.

Table 27.2: Normal motor milestones over developmental time

Age in months	Gross motor milestones	Fine motor milestones
3	Neck holding	Rattling
4		Bidextrous grasp (holding objects with both hands)
5	Sitting with support	
7		Palmar grasp (holding objects using palm)
8	Sitting independently	
9	Trying to stand up with support	Pincer grasp (holding objects using thumb and index finger)
10	Trying to walk	
12	Standing independently	
13	Walking independently	
18	Running	

Table 27.3: Social developmental milestones with age in months

Age in months	Social milestones
2	Social smiles
3	Recognizes mother
6	Smiles at mirror image
9	Hand waves as bye-bye
12	Plays simple ball games
36	Knows gender

Table 27.4: Normal speech developments over the time

Age in months	Speech developments
1	Responds to sound and babbles
3	Cooing or first voice by baby other than crying
6	Coos and babbles
9	Babbles along with repetitive sounds, like babababa
12	Learns new words starting with p, b, m, h, w
24	Has words everything, imagines, words start with k, g, f, t, d and n.
36	Answers questions with who, what and where questions

Risk Factors

The risk factors fall in two categories:

1. **Genetic factors:** Children are placed at genetic risk by being born with a genetic or chromosomal abnormality. For example, Down syndrome.
2. **Environmental factor:** Environmental risk results from exposure to harmful agents either before or after birth, and things, like poor maternal nutrition, or exposure to toxins, e.g., lead, or drugs, or infections that can be passed from mother to baby during pregnancy, e.g., measles or HIV.

Approaches for Screening Developmental Delay

Three approaches to screening include the following:

1. **Informal screening:** Informal screening is based on observing the child during a routine pediatric check-up and asking parents about their concerns about child's development.
2. **Routine formal screening:** Routine formal screening is systematic developmental screening of all children with the help of standardized screening instruments.
3. **Focussed screening:** It involves developmental screening of the following groups of children:
   - Children whose parents express developmental concerns or in whom teachers and physicians suspect problems.
   - Newborns with conditions that have known to have high risk for developmental delay.
   - High risk infants: Those who need periodic assessments are:
     - Very low birth weight (<1500 g)
     - Neurologic conditions
     - Intraventricular hemorrhage
     - Periventricular leukomalacia
     - Hypoxic ischemic encephalopathy
     - APGAR score 0–3 at 10, 15 and 20 min
     - Meningitis
     - Persistent seizures
     - Apnea beyond term
     - Abnormal neurological condition during first week of life
     - Hyperbilirubinemia
     - Symptomatic hypoglycemia with seizures
     - Septicemia

Note: At-risk newborn has a low "optimality score" and are likely to develop neurodevelopmental disabilities later in life in most of the cases.

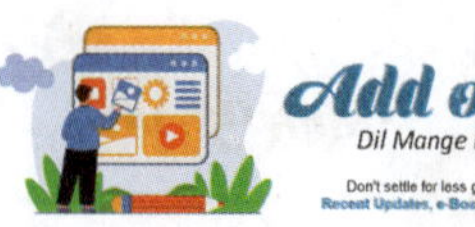

Screening of Developmental Delay

The popular screening tests are as follows:

Baroda Development Screening Test (BDST) for Infants

India introduced the first development screening tool in 1991, the Baroda Development Screening Test (BDST). Baroda Development Screening Test for Infants is based on Baroda Norms on BSID-Research Form 1961 (were studied at the Child Development Unit of the Department of Pediatrics in the K.E.M. Hospital, Pune). It is used for the assessment of the motor-mental development of infants.

Developmental Assessment Scale for Indian Infants (DASII)

It is an Indian adaptation of Bayley Scales, is considered a standard assessment tool for developmental delay. The tool contains motor development items which cover the child's development from supine to erect posture, neck control, locomotion and basic locomotive skills. It includes the record for manipulative behavior such as reaching, picking up things, and manipulating, etc.

Bayley Scales

Bayley scale is designed for screening high risk infants aged 3–24 months. Five domains included in the Bayley Scales of Infant Development are:

1. **Language scale:** Including receptive and expressive subdomains.
2. **Social emotional:** Self-regulation, manipulation, communicating needs, using emotional signals.
3. **Cognitive scale:** Visual preference, attention, memory, sensorimotor, manipulation, exploration, and content formation.
4. **Motor scale:** Fine motor and gross motor skills.
5. **Adaptive behavior:** Listening, self-care, understanding, relating to others and playing.

Trivandrum Development Screening Chart (TDSC)

The Trivandrum Development Screening Chart (TDSC) is an assessment method to check cognitive and motor milestones for children 0–6-year-old (Fig. 27.2). A vertical line is drawn, or a pencil is kept vertically, at the level of the age of the child (in months) being tested. If the child fails to achieve any item that falls short on the left side of the vertical line, the child is considered to have a developmental delay. The tool is designed as a simple method for community health workers to assess a child's development and recommend interventions as necessary. It is not for assessing the developmental age of the child or for the diagnosis of a developmental disability.

Denver Developmental Screening Test (DDST)

Denver developmental screening test (DDST) is a tool that combines direct observation and parental report. The tool consists of 125 items, organized in four developmental domains, namely gross motor, fine motor, adaptive language, personal and social.

Battelle Developmental Inventory Screening Test (BDIST)

Battelle developmental inventory screening test (BDIST) can be used to screen children aged 12–96 months, using a combination of direct assessment, observation and parental interview.

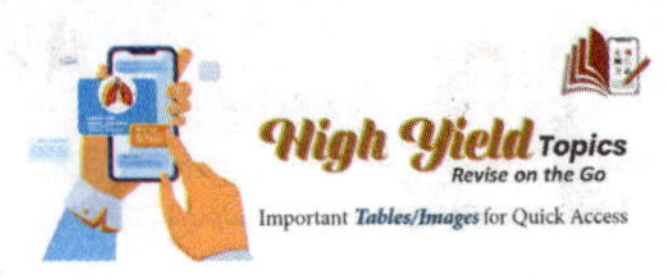

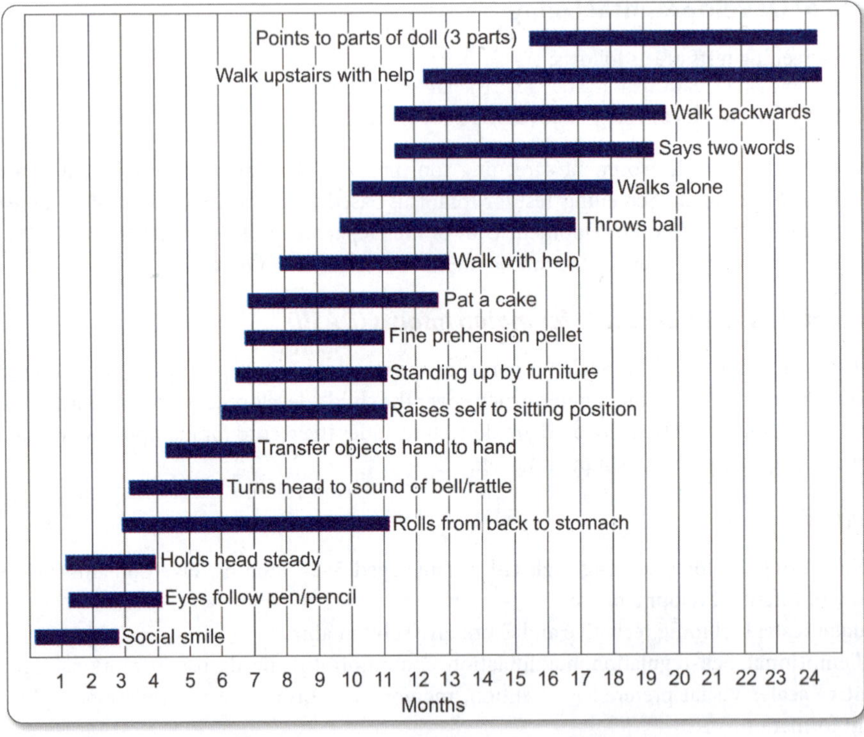

Figure 27.2: Trivandrum development screening chart

Child Development Inventories (CDI)

Child development inventories (CDI) known as the Minnesota Child Development Inventory, was created to provide a systematic, standardized method for parents to report on their children's strengths, problems and present development. CDI measures a child's development in eight areas, namely social, self-help, gross motor, fine motor, expressive language, language comprehension, letters and numbers. It consists of 300-item booklet and answer sheet for the parent to complete and profile sheet for recording the results.

Interventions for Managing Developmental Delay

- Counseling and training for a family
- Educational programs
- Medical services
- Nursing services
- Nutritional services
- Occupational therapy
- Physical therapy
- Psychological services

DYSMORPHISM

The term "dysmorphism" is associated with morphological disorders or abnormalities observed during the development. This may be because of genetic variations or environmental effects. In simple words a noticeable structural feature not formed correctly is known as dysmorphism. Some of the common examples are dysmorphism in nose shape, upper lip, large head, hypertelorism and hypotelorism (wide or narrow space between the eyes respectively). Chromosome aneuploidy and single gene abnormalities are common genetic causes of dysmorphism.

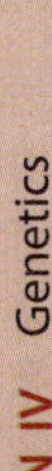

Screening for Dysmorphism

Diagnosis of body dysmorphic disorder is typically based on:
- A psychological evaluation that assesses risk factors and thoughts, feelings, and behaviors related to negative self-image.
- Personal, social, family and medical history.

History

History of the patient and his family is noted along with medical history at various levels (Table 27.5).

Table 27.5: Levels of history personal, family and medical

Level of history	Features	Figures
Pedigree	Consanguinity increases the risk for an autosomal recessive (AR) disorder.	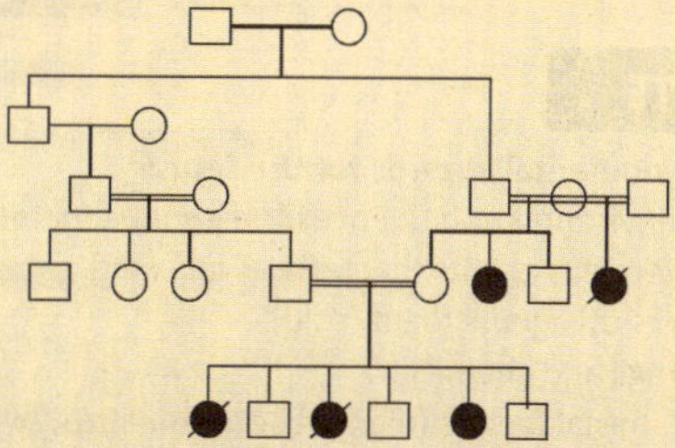 Family pedigree suggestive of autosomal recessive disorder
	Male patient with similarly affected male siblings or maternal male relatives suggests X-linked disorder.	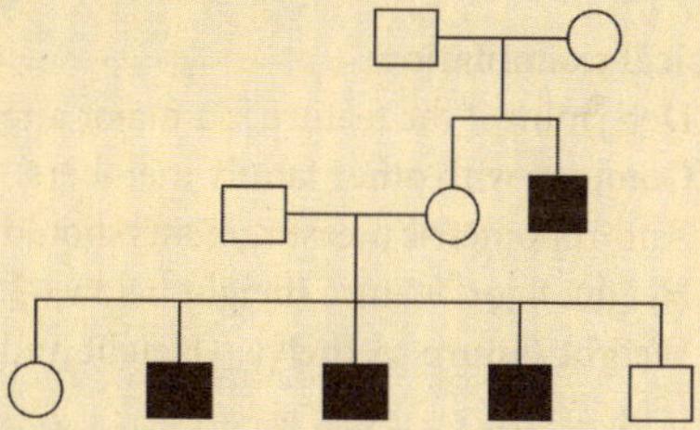 Family pedigree suggestive of an X-linked disorder
	Vertical transmission suggests an autosomal dominant (AD) disorder, especially male to male transmission.	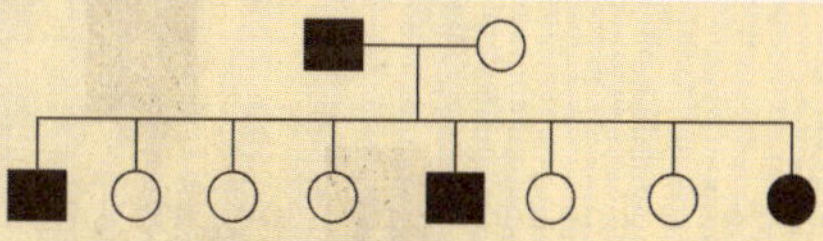 Family pedigree suggestive of an AD disorder
History of miscarriages	Stillbirths or early neonatal deaths suggests the possibility of a parental balanced chromosome rearrangement.	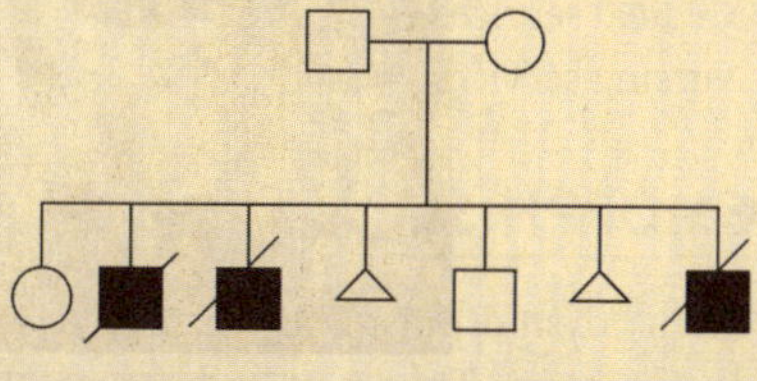 Family pedigree with multiple stillbirths and abortions

Contd...

Level of history	Features	Figures
Pregnancy and family history	• History of uterine malformations or oligohydramnios may be suggestive of causing malformation. • Abnormal fetal position or weak fetal movements suggest abnormal fetal tone. • Placental morphology may give clue to the diagnosis (e.g., large placenta in Beckwith-Wiedemann. • Birth measurements, as symmetrical intrauterine growth retardation (IUGR) suggests early onset whereas, asymmetrical IUGR suggests late onset.	

NOTE

Environmental hazards for the fetus:

The environment influences the genetic material by the effect of:

- Infectious agents (bacteria, virus, etc.).
- Physical agents (heat, cold).
- Drugs and chemicals.
- Maternal factors (e.g., diabetes mellitus, hypertension).

History of Growth and Development

Physical examination:

- Determine if the feature is a major anomaly, minor anomaly or a normal variant.
- Compare with other family members.
- Anthropometric measurements should be used whenever possible to quantitatively identify abnormalities.
- Height: Short stature (height below –3SD) (Figs 27.3 and 27.4) or tall stature (height above +3SD)
- **Weight failure to thrive:** (Height and weight below –3SD) (Fig. 27.5) or obesity (weight above +3SD) (Fig. 27.6).

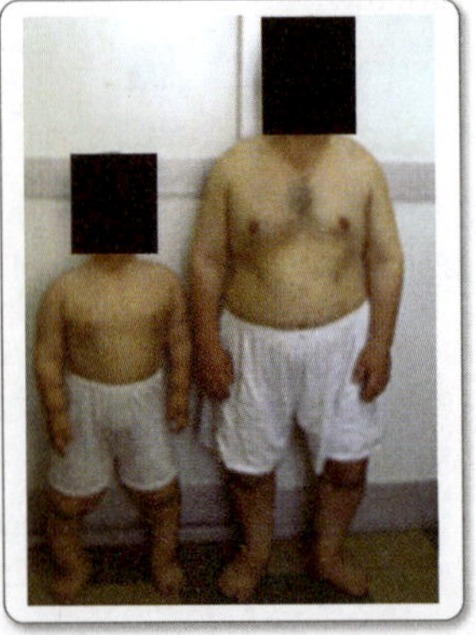

Figure 27.3: A short father and son with spondylo-epi-metaphyseal dysplasia

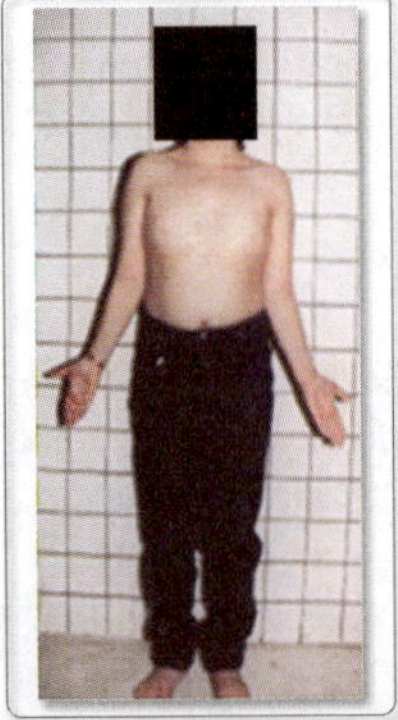

Figure 27.4: Short female with Turner syndrome

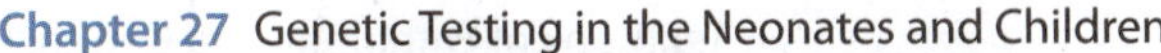

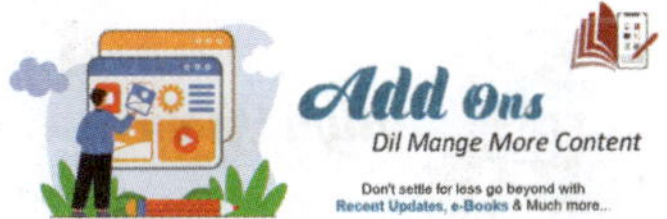

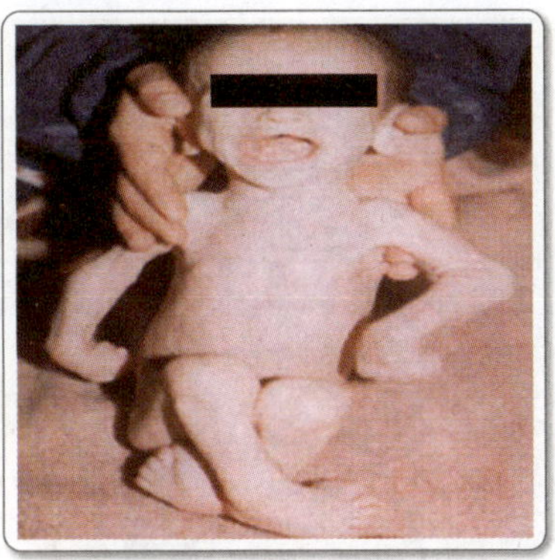

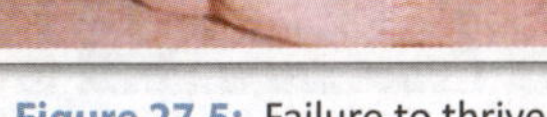

Figure 27.5: Failure to thrive

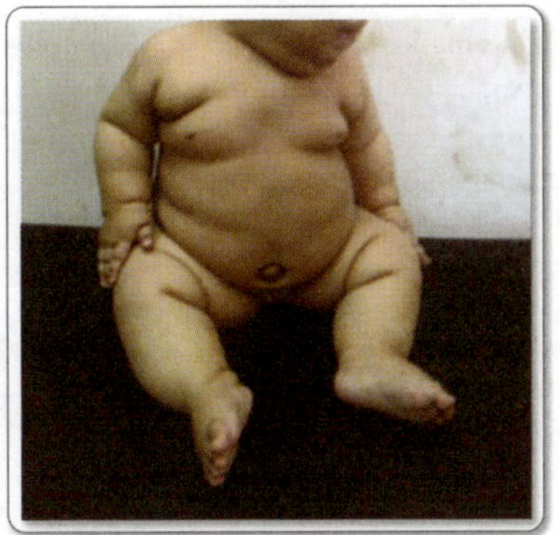

Figure 27.6: Obesity

Conditions Showing Dysmorphism

Some of the genetic anomalies showing dysmorphism are shown in Table 27.6.

Table 27.6: Dysmorphism showing anomalies

Specific organ anomalies	Examples
Unusual head shape Small head 'microcephaly' (head circumference below –3SD) or large head 'macrocephaly') (head circumference above +3SD)	**A.** Microcephaly; **B.** Macrocephaly
Body proportions: E.g., short spine, short limbs or long limbs	Disproportionate shortening—autosomal recessive spondyloepimetaphyseal dysplasia

Contd...

Specific organ anomalies	Examples
Mouth and lips: Abnormal lips (thin/full, tented, down turned, cleft) Cleft lip; microstomia, macrostomia	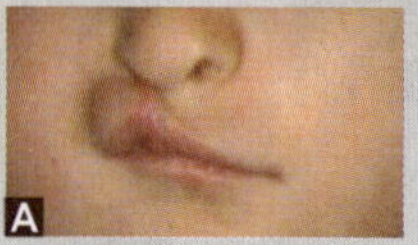 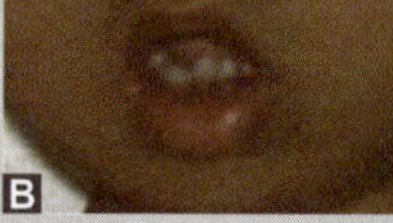 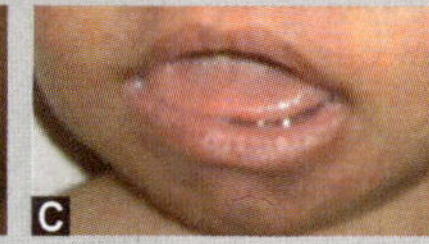 **A.** Cleft lip; **B.** Microstomia; **C.** Macrostomia
Hands & feet anomalies: Brachydactyly, Arachnodactyly, Syndactyly	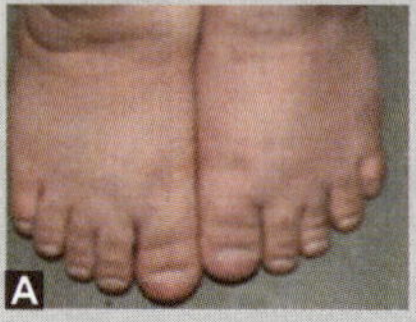 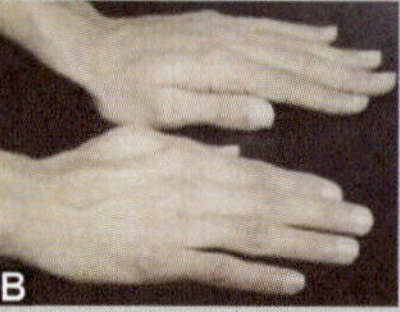 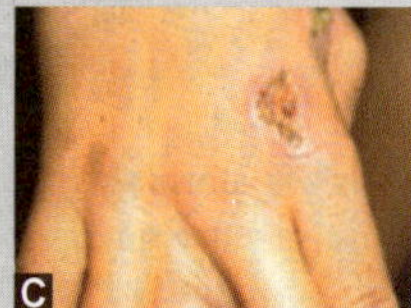 **A.** Brachydactyly; **B.** Arachnodactyly; **C.** Syndactyly
Nose: Short or long nose (the nose is usually ⅔–¾ the length of the distance between the nasal bridge and the upper lip).	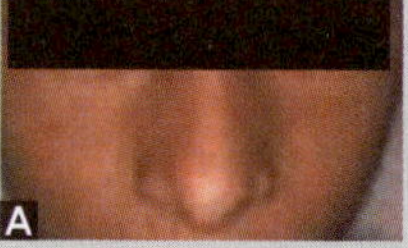 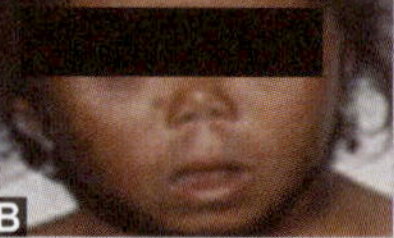 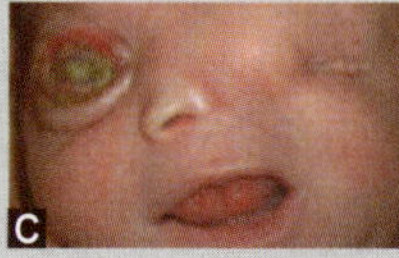 **A.** Long nose; **B.** Short nose; **C.** Heminasal aplasia
Eyes: Corneal opacities, heterochromia or other eye abnormalities.	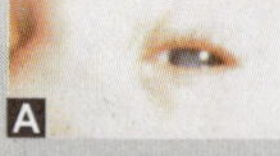 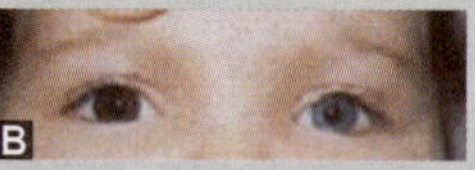 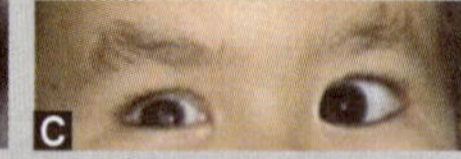 **A.** Corneal opacity; **B.** Heterochromia; **C.** Squint
Ears: Abnormal ear position (low-set, posteriorly rotated).	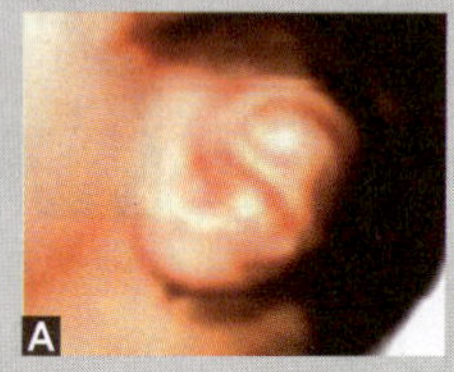 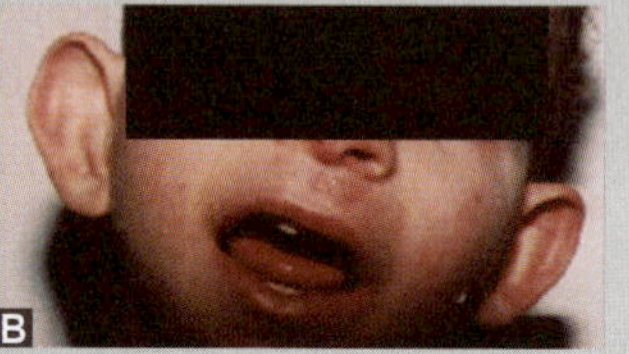 **A.** Low-set, posteriorly rotated ear; **B.** Low-set ears
Eyebrows: E.g., synophrys (fused eyebrows) hypertelorism (increased distance)	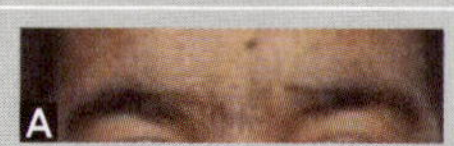 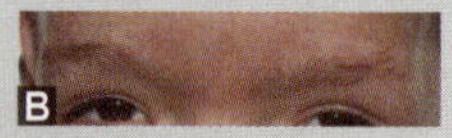 **A.** Synophrys; **B.** Hypertelorism
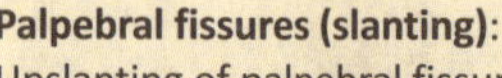**Palpebral fissures (slanting)**: Upslanting of palpebral fissures (e.g., Down syndrome) or downslanting of palpebral fissures (e.g., Noonan syndrome and Rubinstein-Taybi syndrome)	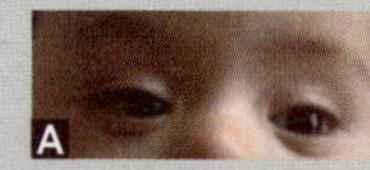 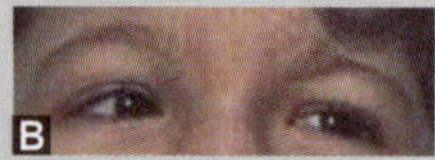 **A.** Upslanting of palpebral fissures; **B.** Downslanting of palpebral fissures
Oral cavity, tongue, palate and mandible anomalies: Macroglossia, Bifid uvula	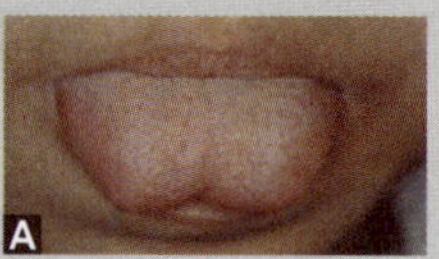 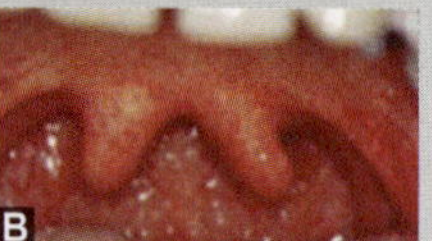 **A.** Macroglossia; **B.** Bifid uvula

Contd...

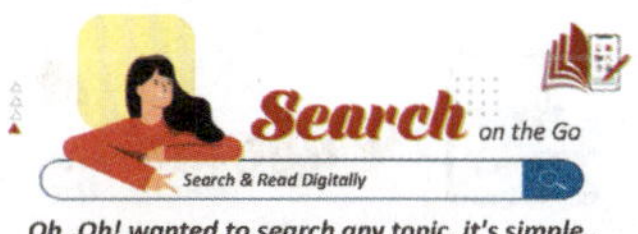

Specific organ anomalies	Examples
Reduction defects: Hemimelia, Ectrodactyly, Axial hand reduction	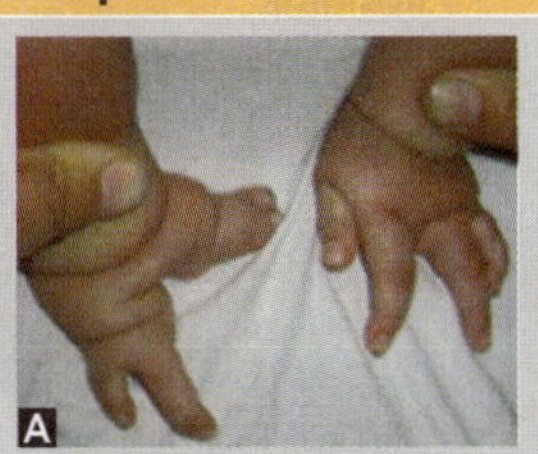 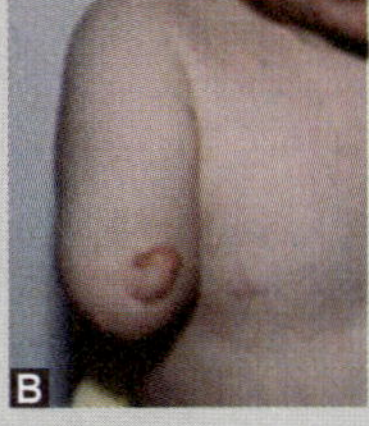 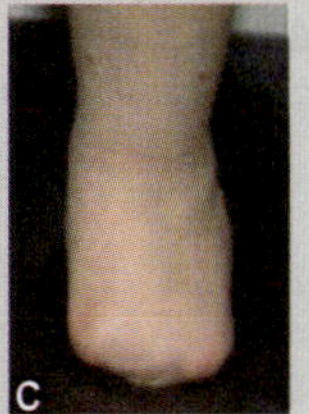 **A.** Hemimelia; **B.** Ectrodactyly; **C.** Axial hand reduction
Nails and dermatoglyphics anomalies: Abnormal flexion creases, Dysplastic nails with polydactyly, Clasped hand	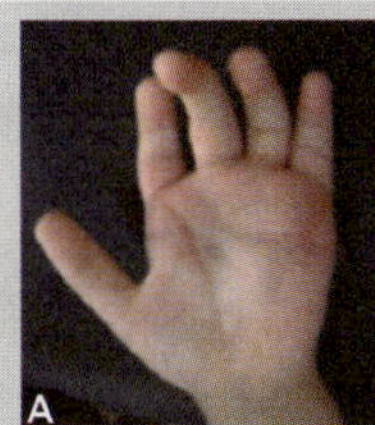 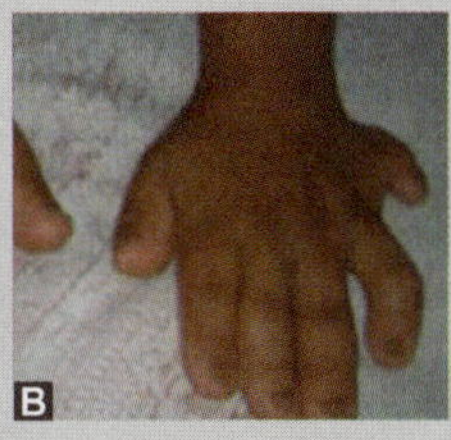 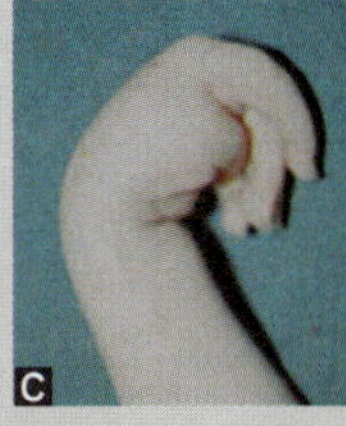 **A.** Abnormal flexion creases; **B.** Dysplastic nails with polydactyly; **C.** Clasped hand
Skin anomalies: E.g., pigmentation, scales, pterygium, appendages, skin nevus	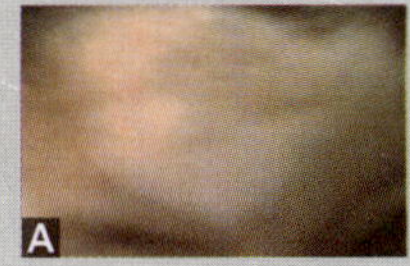 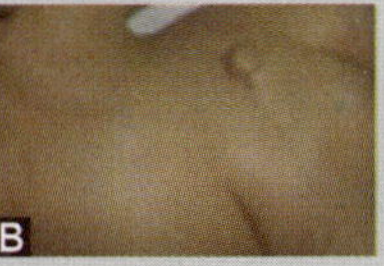 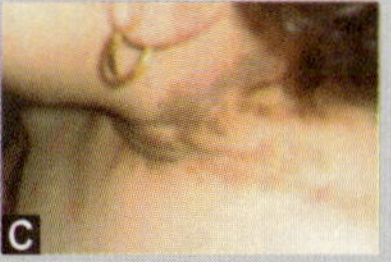 **A.** Hypopigmented skin; **B.** Skin appendage; **C.** Skin nevus
Hair anomalies: Hirsutism, alopecia, hypertrichosis	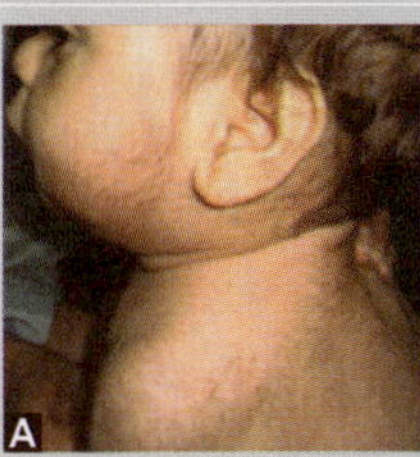 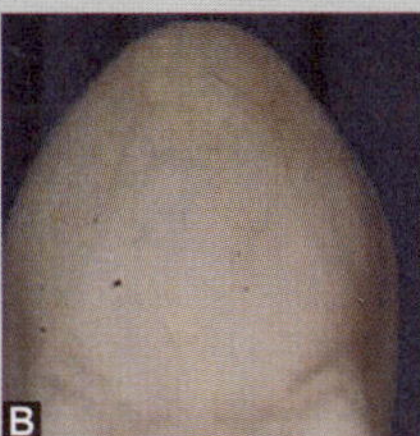 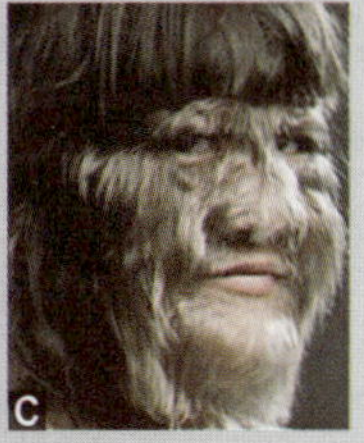 **A.** Generalized hirsutism; **B.** Alopecia; **C.** Hypertrichosis
Other anomalies: Short neck, abnormal chest, myelomeningeocele	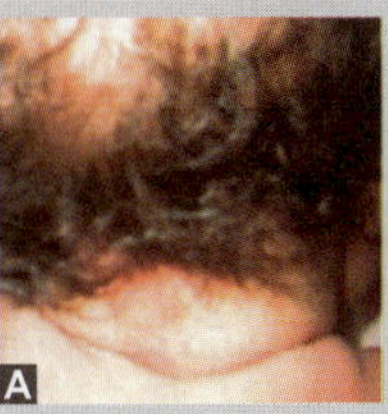 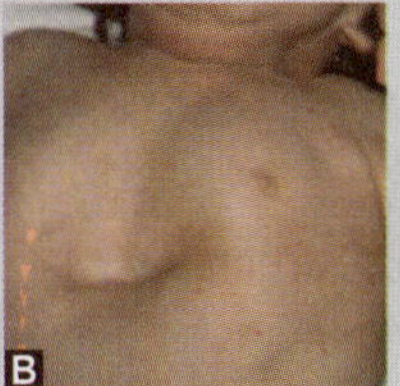 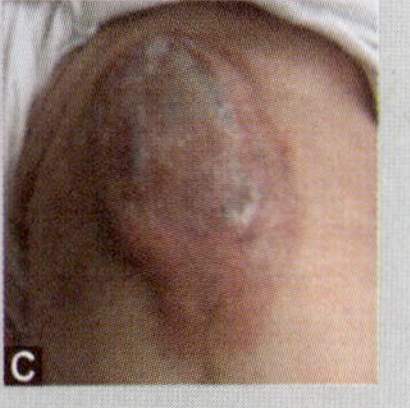 **A.** Short neck; **B.** Abnormal chest; **C.** Myelomeningeocele

Contd...

Specific organ anomalies	Examples
Genital anomalies: E.g., ambiguous genitalia—micropenis, clitromegaly	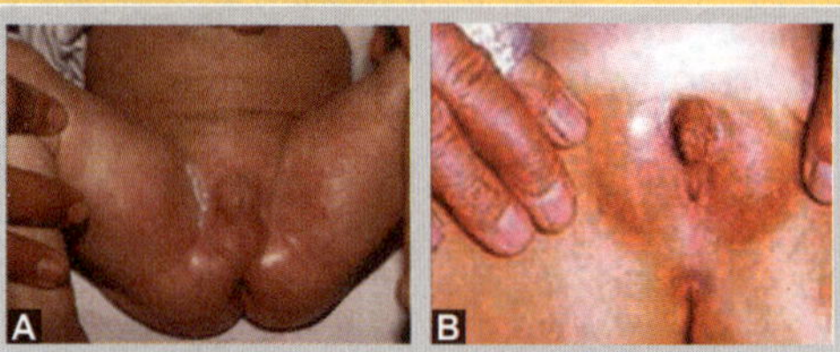 **A.** Micropenis; **B.** Clitromegaly
Abnormal joint shape or mobility: Hypermobility of wrist, dislocated knee joints	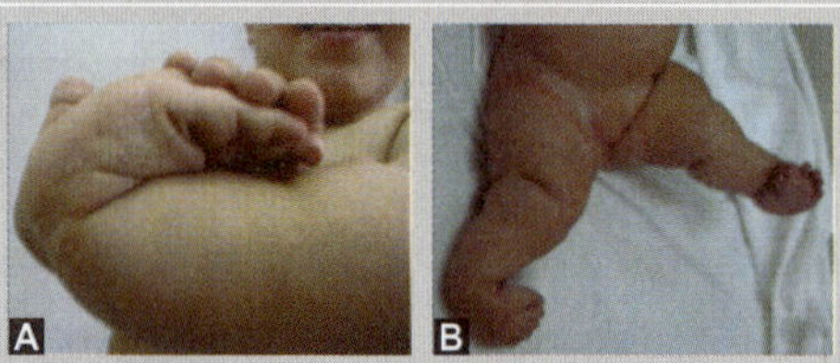 **A.** Hypermobility of wrist; **B.** Dislocated knee joints
Abdomen anomalies: Umbilical hernia, gastroschisis	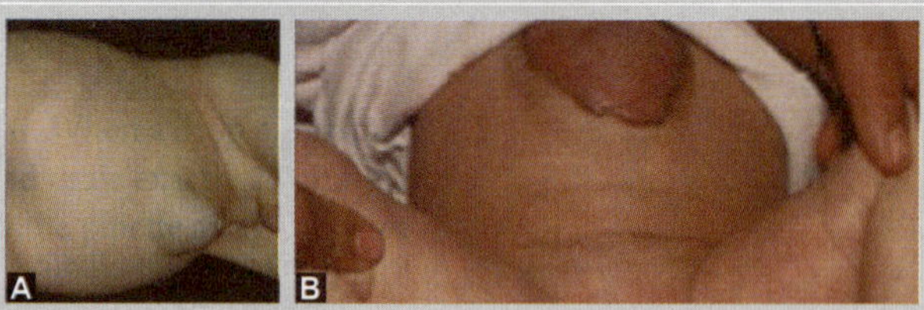 **A.** Umbilical hernia; **B.** Gastroschisis

Indications of Dysmorphism Screening

- **Indications for chromosome analysis:**
  - Multiple congenital anomalies
  - Ambiguous genitalia
  - Developmental delay with major and/or minor anomalies
  - History of >2 miscarriages
- **Indications for metabolic screening:**
  - Metabolic disorders known to cause dysmorphism are lysosomal disorders, and peroxisomal disorders, disorders of cholesterol synthesis

Diagnosis of Dysmorphism

- **Karyotyping:** Chromosomes in sample are examined. The sample can be taken from blood, bone marrow, pleural tissue, ammotic fluid, etc.
- **Radiological examination for bony changes and neuroimaging of brain structures.**
  - Clinical course
  - Screening history of similarly affected family members

Interventions for Management of Dysmorphism

- **Treatment of:**
  - Symptoms
  - Underlying cause

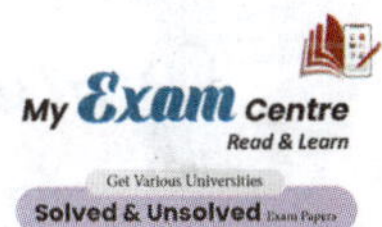

- **Counseling about:**
  - Diagnosis, natural history, prognosis, management
  - Recurrence risk
  - Reproductive complications
- **Follow-up:**
  - Identification and counseling of at-risk family members
  - Surveillance for complications
  - Correction

SUMMARY

- Chromosome studies may be done when a child is born with multiple birth defects.
- The heel stick blood sample is drawn from neonate within 48 hours of birth and screened for up to 50 diseases including sickle cell disease, hypothyroidism, and phenylketonuria.
- The results of a genetic test can confirm or rule out a suspected genetic condition or help determine a person's chance of developing or passing on a genetic disorder.
- Genetic data from neonates and children contribute to research in understanding genetic diseases
- Carrier testing is done in unaffected genes for individuals who have a family history of a genetic disorder.
- CMA and whole exome sequencing are powerful diagnostic tools in the evaluation of critically ill infants suspected to have genetic disorders.
- Genetic testing before a pregnancy is ideal, because this provides the wide range of choices if an increased risk of a deleterious genetic condition is detected.
- Preimplantation test is also known as embryo screening.
- Newborn and childhood genetic screening tests are used to identify genetic disorders just after birth, so that it can be treated early in life.
- Critical congenital heart disease (CCHD) screening test uses pulse oximetry to measure the oxygen levels in the baby's blood.
- Genetic counselors help explain the benefits, limitations, and potential implications of testing.

ASSESS YOURSELF

Long Answer Questions

1. Discuss genetic testing done for newborns and children.
2. What are the indications and which genetic issues can be analyzed by genetic testing?

Short Answer Questions

1. What are the types of genetic tests?
2. Write about barriers in genetic screening of newborns.
3. What is newborn genetic screening tests?

Multiple Choice Questions

1. **Which of the following are NOT elements of counseling prior to routine prenatal genetic testing?**
   a. Review of family history
   b. Review of medical history
   c. Review of the patient's use of medication or controlled substances
   d. Discussion of patient's values and preferences

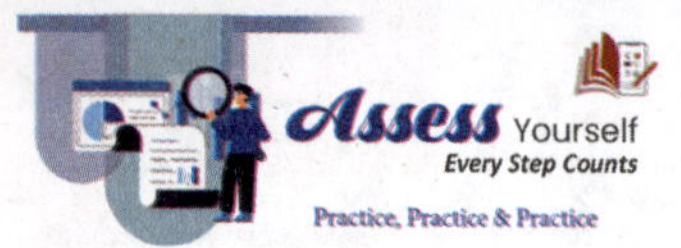

2. **Which of the following statements are true regarding genetic screening?**
   a. Screening tests help the patient define her risks of passing along a genetic disorder.
   b. Screening tests usually involve an invasive procedure such as amniocentesis or chorionic villi sampling.
   c. Screening tests are more comprehensive and accurate than diagnostic tests.
   d. All of the above statements are true.
3. **When considering the patient's preferences with regard to prenatal genetic testing:**
   a. The practitioner should draw blood for genetic testing as part of the routine prenatal visit and discuss the results with the patient afterwards.
   b. The practitioner should take steps to ensure that the patient understands the difference between genetic screening and diagnostic testing
   c. Some patients may decide that they wish to forego screening tests based on their values, needs, and desires.
   d. Both (b) and (c) only
4. **Newborn infants commonly have:**
   a. Capillary hemangioma on the forehead
   b. Posterior cranial fontenalle.
   c. Metopic sutures
   d. All of these
5. **The following cause the onset of persistent vomiting in a 3-week-old child:**
   a. Disaccharidase intolerance
   b. Duodenal atresia
   c. Pyloric stenosis
   d. Hiatus hernia
   e. Lactose intolerance
6. **Neonatal convulsion can be caused by:**
   a. Maternal hyperparathyroidism
   b. Subdural hematoma
   c. Birth asphyxia
   d. Hyponatremia
   e. All of the above
7. **The following maternal condition can cause disease in the fetus/newborn:**
   a. Hyperparathyroidism
   b. ITP
   c. Myasthenia gravis
   d. Diabetus mellitus
   e. All of the above
8. **One should be concerned about term infant who has not passed meconium stool:**
   a. During the process of birth
   b. By 24 hours of life
   c. By 1–2 hour of life
   d. By 6–12 hours of life
   e. All of the above

Answer Key

1. c	**2.** a	**3.** d	**4.** d	**5.** c	**6.** e
7. e	**8.** b				

Chapter 28

Genetic Conditions of Adolescent and Adults

LEARNING OBJECTIVES

After the completion of the chapter, the readers will be able to:

- Discuss congenital abnormalities.
- Explain inborn errors of metabolism.
- Discuss hematological disorders.
- Understand familial cancer.

CHAPTER OUTLINE

- Introduction
- Congenital Abnormalities
- Neural Tube Defects
- Down Syndrome (Trisomy 21)
- Turner Syndrome
- Klinefelter Syndrome
- Huntington Disease
- Mental Illness
- Alzheimer's Disease
- Attention Deficit Hyperactivity Disorder
- Autism Spectrum Disorder
- Generalized Anxiety Disorder
- Inborn Errors of Metabolism
- Cancer Genetics—Familial Cancer
- Conditions of Inherited/Familial Cancers
- Blood Groups Alleles
- Hematological Disorders

KEY TERMS

Atresia: A body part that is tubular in nature, and without a normal opening, or lacking the ability to allow material to pass through it.

Congenital: Existing at birth or before birth.

Congenital hyperthyroidism: Excess thyroid hormone in the bloodstream that leads to the body's metabolism being too active.

Craniorachisis: Combination of anencephaly with a contiguous bony defect of the cervical spine.

Encephalocele: A congenital type of neural tube defect, where a sac containing brain/meninges/cerebrospinal fluid forms outside the skull due to a bone defect.

Gastroschisis: A birth defect where a hole in the abdominal (belly) wall beside the belly button allows the baby's intestines to extend outside of the baby's body.

Hypospadias: A birth defect in boys in which the opening of the urethra is not located at the tip of the penis.

Microcephaly: A birth defect where a baby's head is smaller than expected when compared to babies of the same sex and age.

Orofacial clefts: Birth defects that occur when a baby's lip or mouth does not form properly during pregnancy.

INTRODUCTION

A genetic condition occurs when an altered (changed) gene is inherited from parents that increases the risk of developing a particular condition. However, not all genetic conditions are passed down from parents, some genetic changes occur randomly before birth. Most genetic disorders are rare. There are over 6,000 known genetic disorders. Genetic disorders can be caused by a mutation in one gene (monogenic disorder), by mutations in multiple genes (multifactorial inheritance disorder), by a combination of gene mutations and environmental factors, or by damage to chromosomes (changes in the number or structure of entire chromosomes).

CONGENITAL ABNORMALITIES

According to World Health Organization (WHO), in a year 240,000 newborns affected by congenital disorder will die within 28 days of birth. Various types of abnormalities ranging from deformities in body structure or loss of functions that are present at the time of birth and are of prenatal origin.

Types of Congenital Abnormalities

Examples of congenital abnormalities are divided into two types based on either affecting internal or external organs (Table 28.1).

Identification of congenital disorders can be done by preconception screening, peri-conception screening, and neonatal screening. Most of the congenital abnormalities can be identified during pregnancy and can be prevented with appropriate treatment. Prevention of congenital defects is possible with intake of adequate folic acid or iodine, staple food with supplementation and vaccination. Some congenital abnormalities can be treated with surgical interventions, for example, congenital heart defects, cleft lips, or cleft palate. On the contrary, some of the congenital abnormalities can be treated with medical interventions one example is congenital hyperthyroidism.

NEURAL TUBE DEFECTS

Normally, during first month of pregnancy, the two sides of the fetus's spine (backbone) join together to cover and protect the spinal cord, spinal nerves and meninges. As development progresses, the top of the neural tube becomes the brain, and the rest of the tube becomes the spinal cord. An NTD happens when this tube

Table 28.1: Examples of internal or external congenital abnormalities

Internal	External
• Atresia or stenosis ▪ Esophageal atresia ▪ Large intestine stenosis/atresia ▪ Anorectal atresia/stenosis • Congenital Heart Disease ▪ Tricuspid valve atresia ▪ Pulmonary valve atresia ▪ Interrupted aortic arch. ▪ Common truncus • Renal hypoplasia	• Microcephaly • Orofacial clefts ▪ Cleft lip ▪ Cleft palate ▪ Cleft lip and palate • Neural tube defects ▪ Anencephaly ▪ Craniorachischisis ▪ Iniencephaly • Limb reduction defects • Gastroschisis • Hypospadias

doesn't close completely somewhere along its length. Neural tube defects develop early in the pregnancy, even before a woman knows about her pregnancy.

Development of neural tube defects is due to genetic and nongenetic factors. Nongenetic factors indirectly affect the neural tube formation. The following are the few examples of nongenetic factors and their functions in developing neural tubes.

Types of Neural Tube Defect

The most prevalent types of NTDs are anencephaly, craniorachischisis, open spina bifida and encephalocele.

- **Anencephaly:** Anencephaly happens when the fetus's neural tube doesn't close at the top during fetal development. The skull, scalp and brain do not develop properly, and portions of the brain and skull are missing (Fig. 28.1A). In anencephaly, the absence of the brain and calvaria can be total or partial.
    - **Craniorachischisis** (Fig. 28.1B) is characterized by anencephaly accompanied by a contiguous bony defect of the spine and exposure of neural tissue. Infants with anencephaly are either stillborn or die soon after birth.
- **Spina bifida:** It happens when the neural tube doesn't close completely somewhere along the spine during fetal development.
    - **Open spina bifida or myelomeningocele:** A bony defect of the posterior vertebral arches (the lower thoracic vertebrae) is accompanied by herniation of neural tissue and meninges and is not covered by skin (Fig. 28.1C).
    - **Meningocele**: Characterized by a sac of fluid that protrudes through an opening in the baby's back, but the spinal cord is not involved or damaged.
    - **Closed spina bifida or spina bifida occulta:** Characterized by a small gap in the baby's spine, but there is no opening or sac on the back (the bony defect is of lumbar vertebrae), the herniated meninges and neural tissue are covered by skin.
- **Encephalocele:** The neural tube does not close near the brain and there remains an opening in the skull. The brain and the membranes that cover it can protrude through the skull, forming a sac-like bulge (Fig. 28.1D).
- **Iniencephaly:** This happens when the spine is severely malformed. It often causes lack of a neck, and baby's head is bent severely backward. Babies with iniencephaly are usually stillborn.

Causes of NTD

Exact cause of neural tube defects (NTDs) is not known but it is believed that it is a complex combination of genetic, nutritional and environmental factors. Although the factors believed to affect before and during the

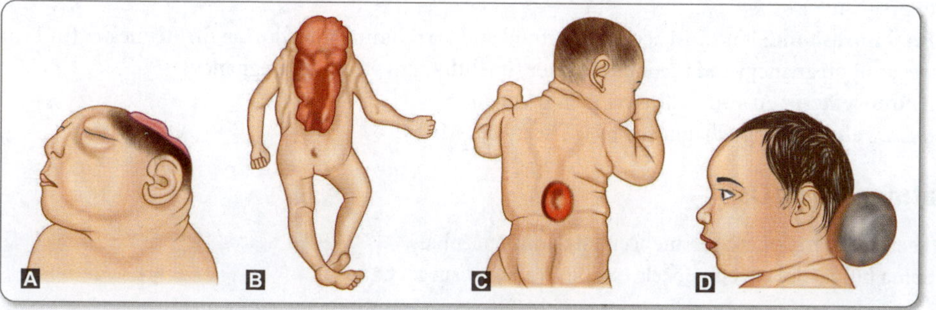

Figures 28.1A to D: **A.** Anencephaly; **B.** Craniorachischisis; **C.** Open spina bifida; **D.** Encephalocele

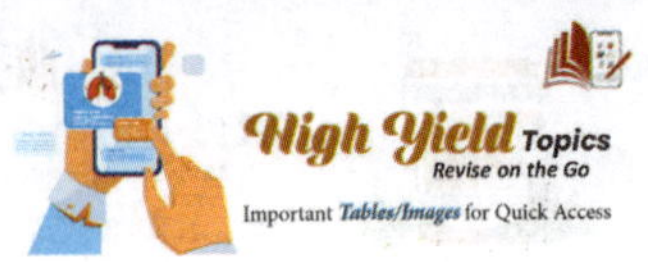

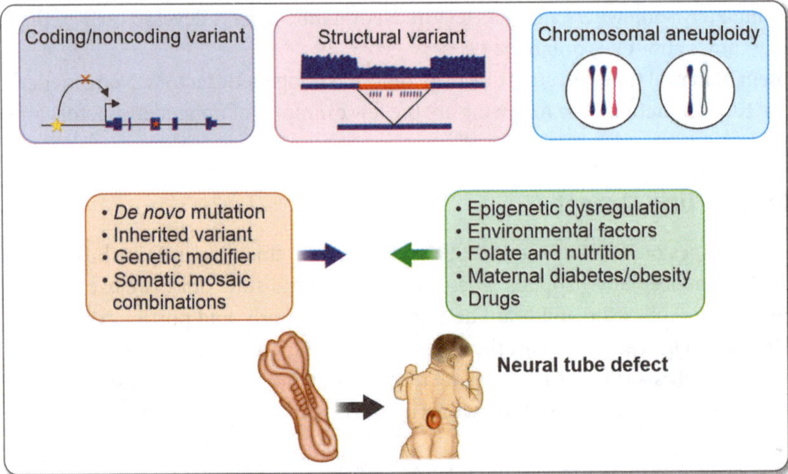

Figure 28.2: Genetic basis of neural tube defect

first trimester of pregnancy are the use of certain medicines such as epilepsy medications; maternal diabetes and genetic factors.

Obesity diabetes, using opioids, having high temperature in first trimester are some of the other factors that may cause NTD.

Hyperthermia: Other than nutrition, hyperthermia (increased body temperature of a pregnant woman >40°C), pesticides, arsenic, polyaromatic hydrocarbons and antibiotics are known to cause neural defects. Development of neural tube defects are multifactorial and involve multiple factors that include physical and genetic.

Environmental factors: Other than nutrition, hyperthermia (increased body temperature of pregnant woman >40°C), pesticides, arsenic, polyaromatic hydrocarbons and antibiotics are known to cause neural tube defects.

Genetic basis of NTDs: There is de novo mutation in the presence of genetic modifiers and it forms structural variants to cause neural tube defects. Maternal nutrition, obesity and diabetes or consumption of some drugs contribute in the occurrence of NTD (Fig. 28.2).

Diagnosis of NTD

- **Blood test:** α-fetoprotein (AFP) in maternal blood increases if the test is positive (in 16th to 18th weeks of pregnancy).
- **Fetal ultrasound:** It is most accurate method and is recommended during first trimester (in 11th to 14th weeks of pregnancy) and second trimester (in 18th–22th weeks of pregnancy).
- **Amniocentesis:** At 15th–20th weeks of pregnancy
(NTDs after birth are diagnosed by CT scan and MRI.)

Treatment of NTDs

- There is no treatment for anencephaly or iniencephaly.
- Spina bifida and encephalocele can be treated by surgery.

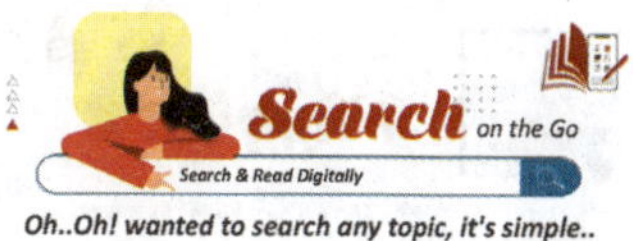

Prevention of NTDs

Maternal Nutrition

Taking folic acid can prevent NTD in the baby. NTDs happen in the first month of pregnancy, before a woman knows about her pregnancy. This is the reason that it is important to take supplements folic acid before a woman conceives.

Role of Folic Acid in Lowering the Risk of NTD

- At the cellular level, supplementation with folic acid has an effect on the differentiation, proliferation, and junction formation during fetal development.
- Deficiency of folate is supplemented with folic acid which is a stable alternative. Folate or folic acid is an important nutrient required for multiple functions such as nucleotide synthesis, serine glycine interconversion, methyl group biogenesis. Several studies have shown that polymorphism of folate metabolism genes MTRR and MTHFR is associated with increased risk of development of neural tube defects.
- It is recommended for women of reproductive age to consume 400 mcg of folic acid each day to help prevent the birth defects in the children. Further if a woman is planning to become pregnant and had previous history of childbirth with neural defects, then such woman should consume 4000 mcg of folic acid per day recommended by CDC.

DOWN SYNDROME (TRISOMY 21)

Down syndrome (DS) is genetic condition in which an individual is born with an extra chromosome. More precisely there will be an extra copy of chromosome 21, that gives the name Trisomy 21 to this disorder. This genetic disorder is named after Down, who first time described its clinical symptoms in 1866 although the relationship between extra chromosome and symptoms of Down syndrome were reported in 1959. Downs syndrome affects multiple organ systems of the body such as musculoskeletal, neurological and cardiovascular systems. Individuals with Down syndrome are likely to develop certain disorders such as autoimmune disorders, epilepsy, hearing and vision problems, hypothyroidism, recurrent infections, anxiety and Alzheimer's.

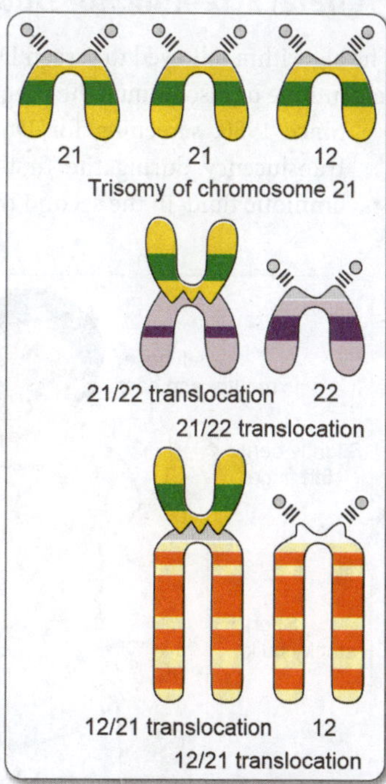

Figure 28.3: Genetic base of Down syndrome or Trisomy 21

Risk Factors

Advanced maternal age is associated with segregation errors in meiosis I and meiosis II. Further errors during various stages of cell cycle correspond to development of trisomy, these are meiosis I (~66%) meiosis II (~21%) paternal meiosis I (~3%) or meiosis II (5%); mitosis (5%).

Down's Syndrome is caused by a spontaneous genetic mutation that occurs very early in zygote development. It happens in one of the following ways (Fig. 28.3):

- **Trisomy:** Where there is an extra chromosome 21

- **Translocation:** Sometimes one chromosome is acquired when it is misplaced from another, (called translocation)
- **Mosaicism:** When only a percentage of cells has the mutation. Coexist with normal cells. Mosaicism occurs later in development, relative to the other forms.

Causes

- Women over 35 are more likely to carry a child with Down syndrome but it is not due to health factors in the mother or father. It is not caused by drinking or drug use. It is a spontaneous genetic mutation.
- If a Down's female had a child, the condition can be passed on and is not considered a mutation; males are thought to be sterile.
- In the case of hereditary translocation Down syndrome (a rare one), an extra chromosome 21 is inherited from one of the parents.

Characteristic Features

Physical features (Figs 28.4A and B): People with DS have an IQ which is mildly-to-moderately low range and have delayed speech and language development. The common physical features are given in Table 28.2.

Clinical problems: Children with DS experience various degrees of intellectual disability and are more vulnerable to health complications, including respiratory disease, hearing problems, and vision impairment, among many other congenital abnormalities (Table 28.3).

Prenatal Screening for Down Syndrome

The algorithm followed to screen DS is as shown in Figure 28.5. It helps the parents to take a further decision to continue or discontinue the pregnancy, in case the test is positive.

- Since 1980, screening for Down syndrome involved screening of maternal serum and fetal nuchal translucency during the first trimester, and levels of alpha-fetoprotein in the maternal serum and amniotic fluid, in the second trimester.

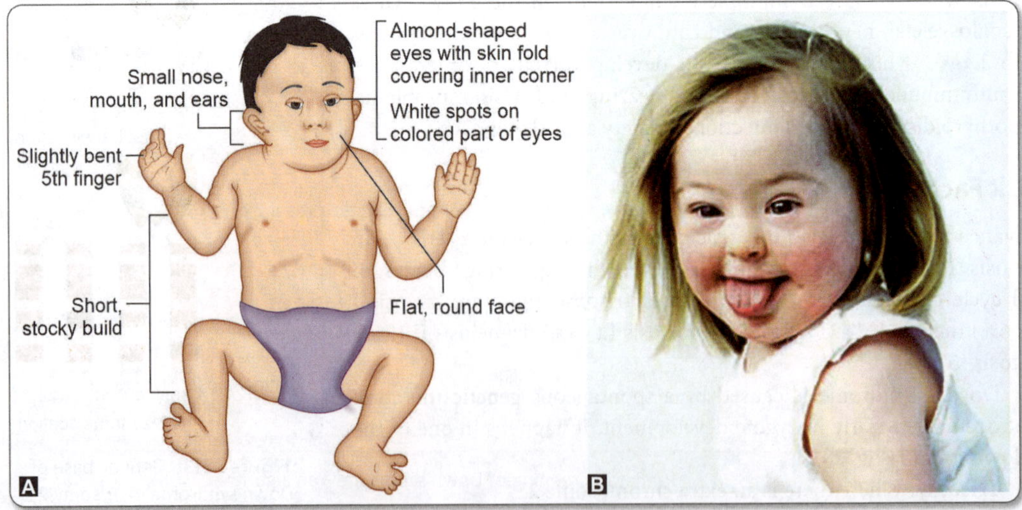

Figures 28.4A and B: Physical features in Down syndrome

Table 28.2: Clinical features of Down syndrome

Most reliable and discriminative signs	Small ears Wide space in between the 1st and 2nd toe ("Sandal gap") Small internipple distance Brushfield spots Nuchal skin fold
Reliable and discriminative signs	Brachycephaly Hypotonia Flat face Upward slant of the eye Transverse line in the palm of the hand ("Simian fold")
Age-dependent signs	Epicanthic fold
Difficult to differentiate	Low, flat nose bridge Small mouth

Table 28.3: Clinical problems in children with Down syndrome

Congenital heart defects	Obesity
Vision disorders	Transient myeloproliferative disorder
Hearing disorders	Thyroid disorders
Obstructive sleep apnoea syndrome	Atlanto-axial instability
Wheezing airway disorders	Urinary tract anomalies
Congenital defects of gastrointestinal tract	Skin problems
Coeliac disease	Behavior problems

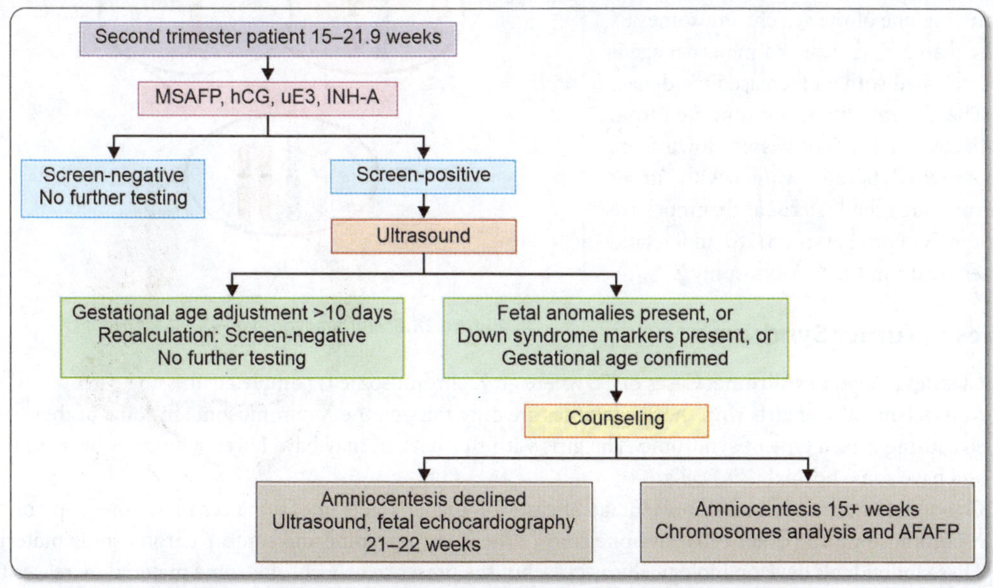

Figure 28.5: Prenatal screening of Down syndrome—an algorithm

Abbreviations: AFAFP, amniotic fluid alpha-fetoprotein; DNH-A, inhibin A; hCG, human chronic gonadotropin; MSAFP, maternal serum alphafactoprotein; µE3, unconjugated estriol produced

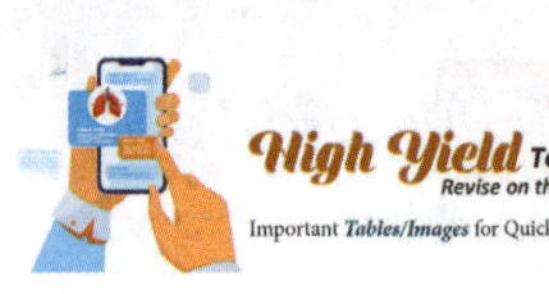

- Recently, new tests have been added to the panel, which are beta-human chorionic gonadotrophin, pregnancy associated plasma protein A and inhibin A.
- Further ultrasonography is helpful to evaluate the correct date of pregnancy to correlate with these tests, making ultrasonography a routine mandatory test.

Prenatal Management

A pregnant woman carrying fetus with confirmed Down syndrome needs special attention in terms of support and care. These women are at higher risk of miscarriage about 30% at 12 weeks of gestation. These higher risk of miscarriages increases with maternal age.

TURNER SYNDROME

Turner syndrome (TS) was named after Dr Henry Turner, who discovered the condition in 1938. TS is a genetic condition that affects only females. The condition is caused by an abnormal chromosome and affects about one in every 2,500 baby girls, but is much more common among pregnancies, such as miscarriages and stillbirths.

Cause

Turners syndrome is typically caused by nondisjunction of a pair of sex chromosomes (fail to separate) during the formation of an egg (or sperm), so, when an abnormal egg unites with a normal sperm to form an embryo, that embryo may end up missing one of the sex chromosomes (X rather than XX). Advanced maternal age is not associated with an increased incidence.

The abnormality is not inherited from an affected parent (not passed down from parent to child) because women with Turner syndrome are usually sterile and cannot have children. Refer to Figure 28.6 to understand Turner syndrome 45X–Monosomy X.

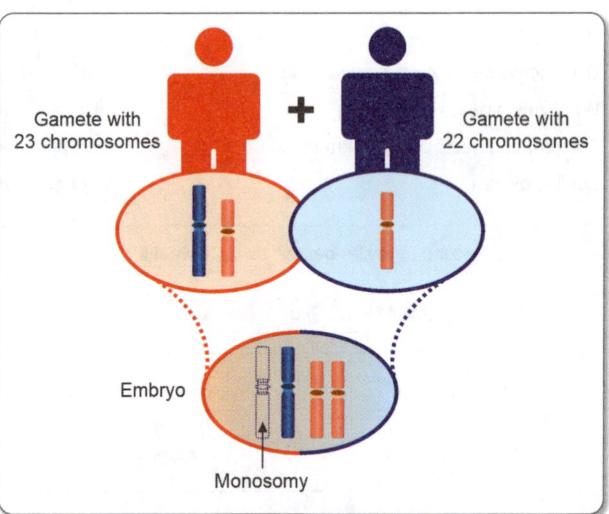

Figure 28.6: Turner syndrome 45X–Monosomy X

Types of Turner Syndrome

- **Classical Turner syndrome:** Cases of TS where an X chromosome is completely missing.
- **Mosaicism:** 30% of girls with the TS disorder are only missing the X chromosome in some of their cells so causing mixed type of syndrome. The girls with this pattern may have fewer symptoms because they still have some normal (XX) cells.
- **Gonadoblastoma:** In a small percentage of cases of Turner syndrome, some cells have one copy of the X chromosome and other cells have one copy of the X chromosome and some Y chromosome material. These individuals develop biologically as girls, but the presence of Y chromosome material increases the risk of developing a type of cancer called gonadoblastoma.

Table 28.4: Inclination of Turner syndrome

45,X	50%
46,X,i(Xq)	15%
45,X/46,XX mosaics	15%
45,X/46,X,i(Xq) mosaics	About 5%
45,X, other X abnormality	About 5%
Other 45,X/? mosaics	About 5%

The inclination of Turner syndrome is about 50% cases with 45X; whereas 15% each can be 46X and 45X or 46XX mosaics (Table 28.4).

Characteristic Physical Features

Girls and women who have TS, have two main characteristic features:

1. Being shorter than average in height.
2. A lack of development of the ovaries, leading to infertility.

Overall characteristic features of TS are shown in Figure 28.7.

Features in older females include:

A combination of the following symptoms are seen:

- A broad chest and widely spaced nipples.
- Absent or incomplete development at puberty.
- Drooping eyelids, dry eyes.
- Infertility.
- No periods (absent menstruation).
- Short height.
- Vaginal dryness.
- Arms that turn out slightly at the elbow.

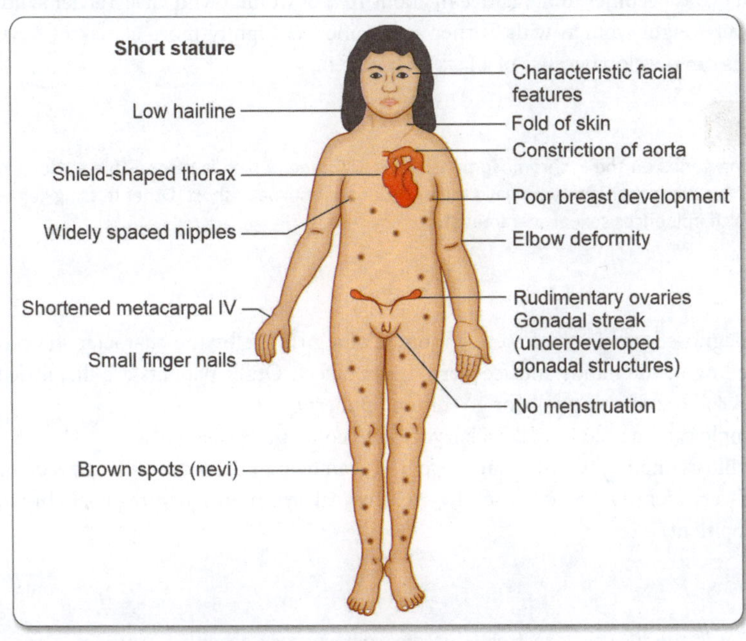

Figure 28.7: Features of Turner syndrome

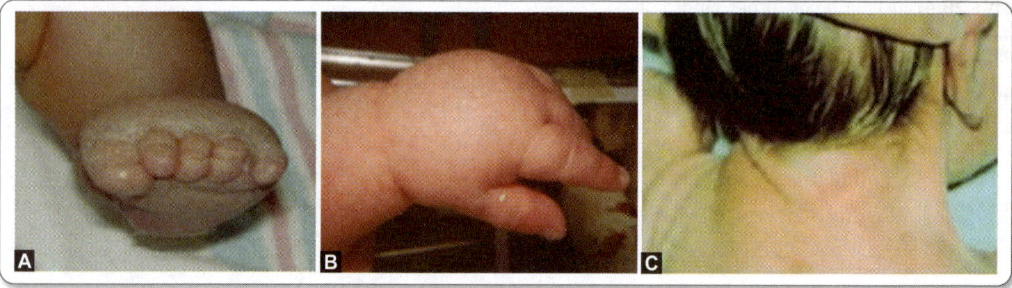

Figures 28.8A to C: Symptoms in young infants **A and B.** Swollen foot and hand; **C.** Indistinct hairline

- Short stature (143–145 cm tall)
- Loss of ovarian function
- Hormone imbalances (thyroid, diabetes)
- Stress and emotional deprivation
- Diseases affecting the kidneys, heart, lungs or intestines
- Bone diseases
- Learning problems (especially in maths)

Features in young infants (Figs 28.8A to C) include:

- Swollen hands and feet.
- Wide and webbed neck and a low or indistinct hairline.

Clinical Features

- Heart murmur, sometimes associated with narrowing of the aorta.
- A tendency to develop high blood pressure.
- Scoliosis occurs in 10 percent of adolescent girls.
- The thyroid gland becomes under active in about 10% of women who have Turner syndrome.
- Older or over-weight women with Turner syndrome are slightly more at risk of developing diabetes. Osteoporosis can develop because of a lack of estrogen.

EXTRA EDGE

One of the missing genes on the X chromosome is the SHOX gene, which is responsible for long bone growth. The missing SHOX gene is the reason girls who have the disorder are unusually short. Other missing genes regulate ovarian development, which influences sexual characteristics.

Diagnosis

- Cases are diagnosed within the first few months of a girl's life by the characteristic physical symptoms such as swelling of the hands and feet, or a heart defect. Other patients are diagnosed in adolescence because they fail to grow normally or go through puberty.
- A blood sample can be used to make a karyotype to confirm the diagnosis.
- Chorionic villus sampling (CVS) or amniocentesis can help in diagnosis during pregnancy
- Ultrasound can identify the disorder by its physical symptoms before the baby is born (signs of underdevelopment).

Treatment

Hormone therapy is the best way to treat this disorder such as growth hormones, androgen or estrogen depending on the symptoms.

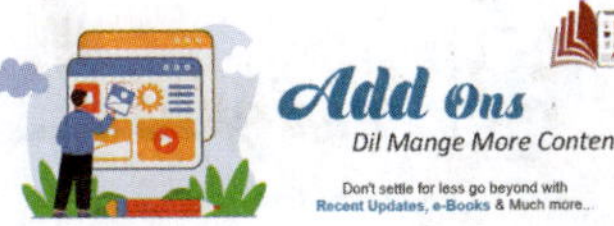

KLINEFELTER SYNDROME

Klinefelter syndrome (KS) is a genetic disorder in which there is at least one extra X chromosome to a standard human male karyotype. 47XXY is the most common sex chromosome aneuploidy in males and the second most common condition caused by the presence of extra chromosomes. Other mammals also have the XXY syndrome, including mice. The syndrome was named after Harry F. Klinefelter in 1942.

Frequency: Roughly between 1:500 and 1:1000 live male births

Cause

- Meiotic nondisjunction of chromosome pairs during the first or second division of gametogenesis.
- Mitotic nondisjunction on the developing zygote.

Types

- Mosaic: Males having 47XXY/46XY.
- 48XXYY and 48XXXY occur in 1 in 18,000–50,000 male births.
- 49XXXXY occurs 1 in 85,000–100,000 male births

MUST KNOW

Additional chromosomal material can contribute to cardiac, neurological, orthopedic and other anomalies.

Diagnosis

By prenatal diagnosis:

- In adults, often the diagnosis is made accidentally as a result of examinations and medical visits for reasons not linked to the condition.
- The analysis of the chromosomes' karyotype on lymphocytes is a standard test.
- Clinical sample is dermal fibroblasts or testicular tissue.

Characteristics Features

Features in baby, child, and teen:

- May sit up, crawl, and walk later than other infants.
- Weaker muscles and reduced strength.
- They tend to be taller than average as they grow up.
- They may have less muscle control and coordination.
- Entering puberty, these males don't make as much testosterone.
- **Mental ability:**
  - Speech/language deficits, learning disabilities/academic issues and/or behavioral issues.
  - Tend to be quiet and undemanding.
- **Delays in language acquisition and development:**
  - Have greatest difficulty with expressive language, that is the ability to put thoughts, ideas, and emotions into words.
  - Face problems during adolescence such as emotional and behavioral, and difficulties at school.

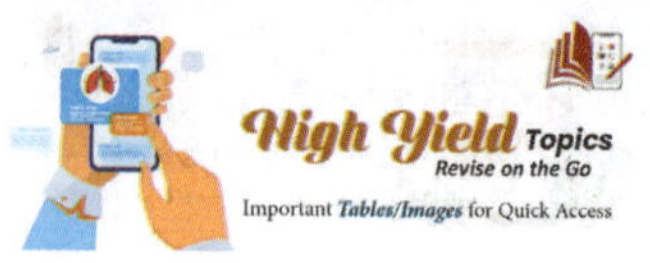

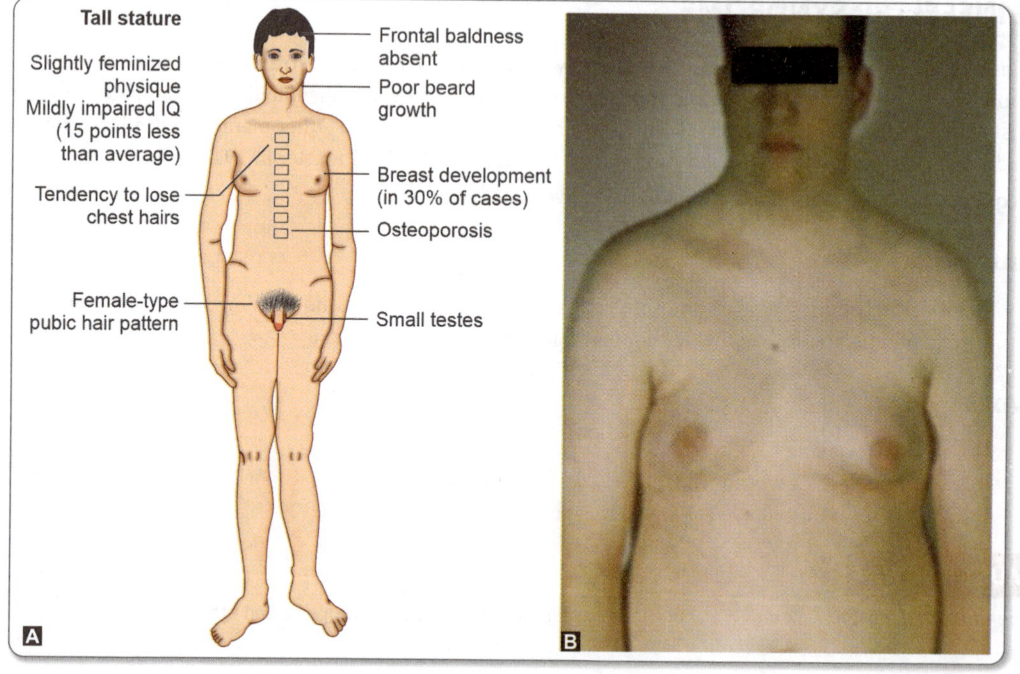

Figures 28.9A and B: Characteristic features in Klinefelter syndrome

Features in adults (Figs 28.9A and B):

- Tall body stature, increased length of extremities and narrow shoulders.
- Decreased facial and body hair (due to less testosterone).
- Increased FSH, LH and normal/decreased testosterone levels.
- Gynecomastia (increase in breast tissue).
- Increase of fatty tissue, especially in abdomen and pelvis.
- Atrophic testicular volume: 2–3 mL.
- Decreased IQ levels.
- Osteoporosis.
- Increased risk of breast cancer, autoimmune disorders, and hypothyroidism.

Treatment

The genetic variation is irreversible, only signs and symptoms can be treated:

- Cosmetic surgery for gynecomastia (increase in breast tissue).
- Males with Klinefelter's syndrome are given testosterone therapy, around the age of puberty.
- Planned and timed psychosocial support.
- IVF technologies to help father children.

HUNTINGTON DISEASE

Huntington disease (HD) is a neurodegenerative disorder that causes the progressive breakdown of nerve cells in the brain, especially damage in the basal ganglia (Figs 28.10A and B). Huntington disease has a broad

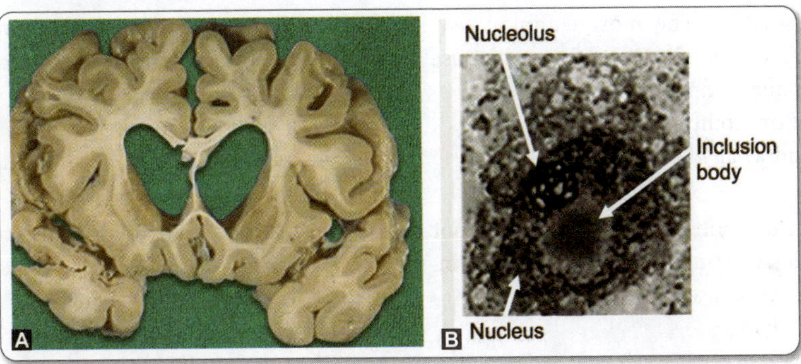

Figures 28.10A and B: Huntington disease—inclusion body in cell of brain

impact on a person's functional abilities and usually results in movement, thinking (cognitive) and psychiatric disorders.

Most people with Huntington disease develop signs and symptoms in their 30s or 40s, but the onset of disease may be earlier or later in life. When disease onset begins before the age of 20, the condition is called juvenile Huntington's disease.

Causes

Huntington disease involves defect in neurotransmitters and is believed to be caused by loss of cell bodies of GABA-secreting neurons in the caudate nucleus and putamen and acetylcholine-secreting neurons in many parts of the brain. It is caused by an inherited defect in a single gene. Huntington disease is an autosomal dominant disorder, which means that a person needs only one copy of the defective gene to develop the disorder. A parent with a defective Huntington gene could pass along the defective copy of the gene or the healthy copy. Each child in a family, therefore, has a 50 percent chance of inheriting the gene that causes the genetic disorder.

Characteristic Features

Huntington disease usually causes movement, cognitive and psychiatric disorders with a wide spectrum of signs and symptoms. Which symptoms appear first, varies greatly among affected people. During the course of the disease, some disorders appear to be more dominant or have a greater effect on functional ability.

Movement disorders: The movement disorders, associated with Huntington disease, include both involuntary movements and impairments in voluntary movements:

- Involuntary jerking or writhing movements (chorea).
- Muscle problems, such as rigidity or muscle contracture (dystonia).
- Slow or abnormal eye movements.
- Impaired gait, posture and balance.
- Difficulty with the physical production of speech or swallowing.

Cognitive disorders: Cognitive impairments often associated with Huntington's disease include:

- Difficulty in focusing on tasks.
- Lack of flexibility or the tendency to get stuck on a thought, behavior or action (perseveration).
- Lack of awareness of one's own behaviors and abilities.
- Slowness in processing thoughts or "finding" words.
- Difficulty in learning new information.

Psychiatric disorders: The most common psychiatric disorder associated with Huntington disease is depression. Depression appears to occur because of injury to the brain and subsequent changes in brain function. Signs and symptoms may include:

- Feelings of irritability, sadness.
- Social withdrawal.
- Insomnia.
- Fatigue and loss of energy.
- Frequent thoughts of death, dying or suicide.

Dementia: The dementia start probably does not result from the loss of GABA neurons but from the loss of acetylcholine-secreting neurons, especially in the thinking areas of the cerebral cortex. Dementia in Huntington disease causes:

- Emotional changes.
- Depression.
- Lack of manners.
- Extreme eccentricity.
- Obsessive compulsive symptoms.
- **Complications:**
  - Depression associated with Huntington's disease may increase the risk of suicide.
  - Lack of physical activity, dietary problems, and eating and swallowing problems can cause constipation, incontinence, and weight loss.
  - Psychiatric and cognitive problems can lead to social isolation and deep depression.
  - The patient is usually bedridden in the final stages.
  - Common causes of death include pneumonia or other infections, injuries related to falls and complications related to the inability to swallow.

Diagnosis

The diagnosis of Huntington disease is based on:

- General physical examination and review of family medical history.
- **Neurological examination:** Motor nerve coordination helps to assess by observing reflexes, muscle strength, muscle tone, coordination, balance, sensory symptoms, sense of touch, vision and eye movement, hearing.
- **Psychiatric symptoms:** Such as mental status, mood.
- **Neuropsychological testing:** Standardized tests are used to assess memory, reasoning, mental ability, language and spatial reasoning.
- **Psychiatric evaluation:** To check emotional state, patterns of behaviors, quality of judgment, coping skills, signs of disordered thinking, evidence of substance abuse.
- **Brain imaging and function:** The imaging technologies may include MRI, or CT (Fig. 28.11) which shows atrophy of the caudate nuclei.

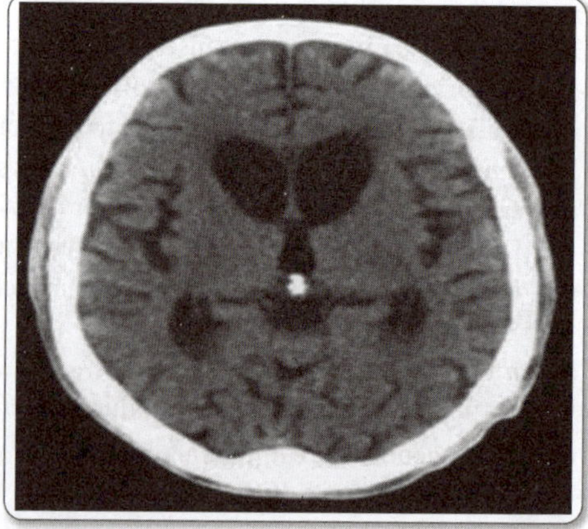

Figure 28.11: Atrophy of the caudate nuclei (bilaterally)

Treatment

- No treatments can alter the course of Huntington's disease.
- Symptomatic relief providing supportive measures
- Preventing complications.

MENTAL ILLNESS

Mental health is defined as a state of complete physical, mental and social well being and not merely the absence of disease or infirmity. Mental illness can occur when the brain or part of the brain is not working well or is working improperly which is abnormal brain functioning. It leads to disruption of the brain function. Mental illness is rarely caused by stress alone.

Causes of Mental Illness

- It is not the consequence of poor parenting or bad behavior.
- It is not the result of personal weakness or deficits in personality.
- It is not the manifestation of malevolent spiritual intent (Devil or evil effects). In exceptional cases it is caused by nutritional factors.
- It is not caused by poverty.

Complications of Mental Illness

- Thinking difficulties or problems.
- Extreme emotional problems.
- Focusing attention highs and lows.

Disorders of Mental Illness

EXTRA EDGE

Mental disorders are the result of both genetic and environmental factors. There is no single genetic switch that when flipped, causes a mental disorder. It is difficult for doctors to determine a person's risk of inheriting a mental disorder or passing on the disorder to his or her children.

Schizophrenia

Schizophrenia is a serious mental illness that affects the person's thoughts, feelings and behaviors. People suffering from schizophrenia may seem like they have lost touch with reality, which can be distressing for them and for their family and friends. It is heritable:

- **Clinical symptoms:** Hallucinations, disorganized thoughts and behavior, disorganized thinking, lack of motivation, slow movement, change in sleep patterns, poor grooming or hygiene, changes in body language and emotions.
- **Genetic basis:** Possible gene defects linked to schizophrenia are on the chromosomes—1, 6, 8, 10, 13, 18, 22, and the X chromosome; or it may be polygenic (caused by a combination of gene defects).

Mental Health Bill

The government has published a new draft of mental health bill for overstretching the mental health services. The National Mental Health Program helps:

- To prevent and treat mental disorders.
- To apply mental health technology to improve general health services.

Bipolar Disorder

Bipolar disorder is highly prevalent disorder, which is genetically inherited. Familial transmission is seen. It is a mental health condition that causes extreme mood swings that include emotional highs (mania or hypomania) and lows (depression). Significant marker in BD is only one gene (CACNA1C).

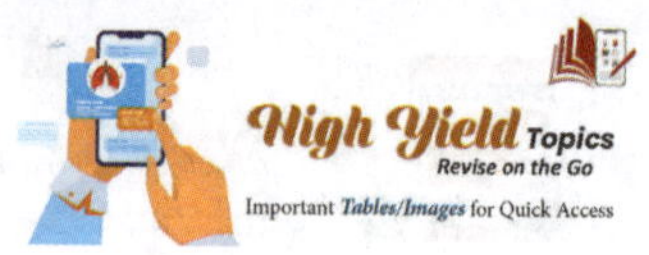

Causes

Genes responsible for the disorder are:

- GRK-3 gene, on chromosome 22
- FAT-1 gene on chromosome 4
- AY070435 gene (Slynar) on chromosome 12
- Genes on 18, 21, 1, 6, 7, 10, 22, 11
- X-chromosome
- Polymorphisms

Characteristic Features

Depressive episodes may include symptoms, such as low energy, low motivation and loss of interest in daily activities. Mood episodes last days to months at a time and may also be associated with suicidal thoughts.

Treatment

Treatment is usually lifelong and often involves a combination of medications and psychotherapy.

Depression

- The serotonin transporter gene is linked to depression. It controls two parts of the brain: amygdala and cingulate.
- It is of two types—the long and short version. Those with two copies of the long version show better connectivity between the amygdala and cingulate.
  Example: The identical twins have identical genetic material. If twins are raised together and one twin develops clinical depression, the other twin also develops clinical depression (76%). If twins are raised apart and one twin develops clinical depression, the other twin also develops clinical depression 67% of the time.
- The disorder goes through families.

ALZHEIMER'S DISEASE

There is progressive deterioration of cognitive abilities, agitation and hallucinations in AD. It is a neurodegenerative disease and expected cause is neuritic amyloid plaques. The shape of tau protein becomes tangled. APP (amyloid precursor protein), presenilin1, presenilin 2 are a known cause of early-onset of Alzheimer disease (EOAD) (onset below age 65). 95% Alzheimer disease (AD) is sporadic and polygenic. Late-onset is associated with apolipoprotein E 4 allele risk factor.

MUST KNOW

Alzheimer's disease (AD) differs from age related memory problems as in age-related memory issues, only a part of memory is lost but in AD, entire experience of the life is forgotten. Some main differences between AD and age-related memory loss are as follows:

Differences between Alzheimer's and age related memory loss

Alzheimer's disease	Age-related memory loss
• Forgets entire experiences	• Forgets part of an experience
• Is gradually unable to care for self	• Is usually able to care for self
• Rarely remembers later	• Often remembers later
• Is gradually unable to follow written/spoken directions	• Is usually able to follow written/spoken directions

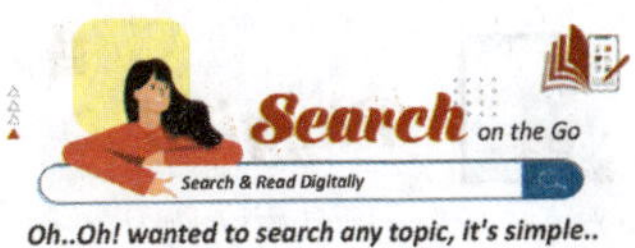

Characteristic Features

Progressive deterioration of cognitive abilities:
- Agitation
- Hallucinations

Risk Factors

Increasing age may increase the likelihood of developing AD.

RECENT UPDATE

Researchers have identified one Alzheimer risk gene called apoliprotein APOE4 which in another rare gene when inherited and it, will develop the disorder. The APOE4 gene is considered a "risk factor" gene for AD and appears to influence the age of onset of the disease. Rare genes that directly cause Alzheimer have been found in only a few hundred extended families worldwide.

Diagnosis

Genetic tests are available or both APOE4 and the rare genes that directly cause AD, yet health professionals do not currently recommend routine genetic testing for AD.

ATTENTION DEFICIT HYPERACTIVITY DISORDER

Attention deficit hyperactivity disorder (ADHD) tends to run in families and, in most cases, it is proposed that the genes for ADHD are inherited from the parents. Most cases are diagnosed when children are under 12 years old, but sometimes it is diagnosed later in childhood.

Causes

- Research shows that parents and siblings of someone with ADHD are more likely to have ADHD themselves. Although, the way ADHD is inherited is likely to be very complex and is not thought to be related to a single genetic fault.
- It has been observed by scans that people with ADHD have certain areas of the brain smaller, whereas other areas may be larger. Other studies have suggested that people with ADHD may have an imbalance in the level of neurotransmitters in the brain, or these may not work properly.

Characteristic Features

- Inattentiveness (difficulty concentrating and focusing).
- Hyperactivity and impulsiveness.
- People with ADHD may also have additional problems, such as sleep and anxiety disorders.

AUTISM SPECTRUM DISORDER

Some children show autism spectrum disorder (ASD) symptoms within the first 12 months of life. In others, symptoms may not show up until 24 months of age or later.

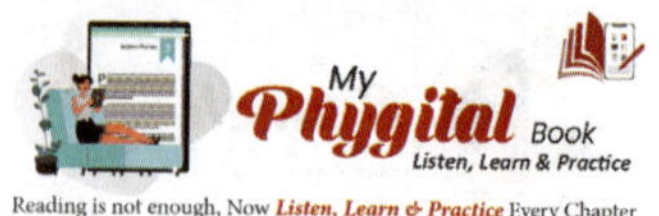

EXTRA EDGE

Genetic Disorders Associated with Autism as a Feature

Single gene disorders which include both autosomal and X-linked defects associated with autism as a feature include:

- Tuberous sclerosis (*TSC1* and *TSC2* genes).
- X-linked Rett (*MECP2* gene).
- Neurofibromatosis (*NF1* and *NF2* genes).
- Fragile X (*FMR1* gene) syndromes.
- Other syndromic conditions associated with autism include Sotos, Moebius, Noonan, Cohen, Joubert, De Lange, oculo-auriculo-vertebral spectrum, myotonic dystrophy and, *PTEN* gene disturbances with extreme macrocephaly.

Causes

Autism is highly heritable. It is estimated that at least 50% of genetic risk is predicted by common genetic variation, due to spontaneous mutations or predictable inheritance patterns. The remaining genetic risk is yet to be determined. Both genetic and non-genetic factors modulate the penetrance of risk genes, resulting in a highly heterogeneous disease phenotype for similar pathogenic variants.

Characteristic Features

People with ASD often have problems with social communication and interaction, and restricted or repetitive behaviors or interests. People with ASD may also have different ways of learning, moving, or paying attention.

Diagnostic Criteria

To meet diagnostic criteria of autism, according to DSM-5, a child must have persistent deficits in each of the three areas of social communication and interaction (A.1. through A.3.) plus at least two of four types of restricted, repetitive behaviors:

A.1. Deficits in social-emotional reciprocity, ranging, for example, from abnormal social approach and failure of normal back-and-forth conversation; to reduced sharing of interests, emotions, or affect; to failure to initiate or respond to social interactions.

A.2. Deficits in nonverbal communicative behaviors used for social interaction, ranging, for example, from poorly integrated verbal and nonverbal communication; to abnormalities in eye contact and body language or deficits in understanding and use of gestures; to a total lack of facial expressions and nonverbal communication.

A.3. Deficits in developing, maintaining, and understanding relationships, ranging, for example, from difficulties in adjusting behavior to suit various social contexts; to difficulties in sharing imaginative play or in making friends; to absence of interest in peers.

GENERALIZED ANXIETY DISORDER

Severe, ongoing anxiety that interferes with daily activities is known as generalized anxiety disorder (GAF). The disorder can occur at any age.

Clinical Features

Features may include:

- Constant worry
- Restlessness
- Trouble with concentration

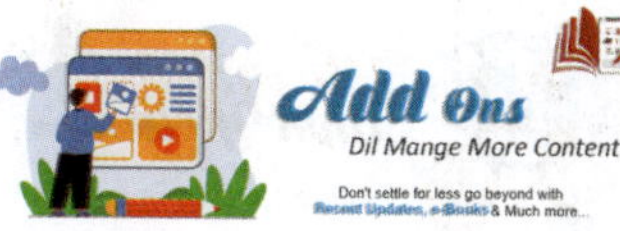

Treatment

Treatment may include:
- Counseling
- Antidepressants

INBORN ERRORS OF METABOLISM

Metabolism errors are rare genetic (inherited) disorders in which the body cannot properly turn food into energy. The disorders are usually caused by defects in specific proteins (enzymes) that help break down (metabolize) parts of food. In most of the disorders, problems arise due to accumulation of substances which are toxic or interfere with normal function, or due to the effects of reduced ability to synthesize essential compounds. Inborn errors of metabolism are now often referred to as congenital metabolic diseases or inherited metabolic diseases.

Indications of Inborn Errors of Metabolism

- Illness presentation within first 48 hours of age
- Family history of:
  - Neonatal death of unclear etiology.
  - History of child with neurologic deterioration.
  - History of multiple miscarriages.
  - Consanguinity.

Characteristic Features of Neonates with Inborn Errors of Metabolism

General:
- Poor oral intake and/or vomiting.
- Lethargy coma, seizures, changes in tone or reflexes.
- Hepatosplenomegaly, dysmorphic features.
- Cataracts.

Characteristic symptoms:

The characteristic symptoms depend on the system involved which are as follows (Table 28.5):

Table 28.5: Characteristic symptoms of inborn errors of metabolism

System	Signs and symptoms
Neurological	Ataxia, seizures, arthrogryposis, movement disorders, myopathy, hypotonia, encephalopathy, myelopathy, leukodystrophy, intellectual impairment, autism, regression (loss of acquired skills), white matter changes, hydrocephalus, acroparaesthesia
Gastrointestinal	Hepatomegaly, liver failure and fibrosis, jaundice, hyperammonemia, splenomegaly, abdominal pain, gastrointestinal insufficiency, nausea/vomiting
Cardiac	Arrhythmias, valve disease, cardiomyopathy
Endocrine	Adrenal failure, hypoglycaemia, hypocalcaemia, ambiguous genitalia, hypo/hyperketosis
Skeletal	Joint restriction, dysostosis multiplex, short/tall stature, osteochondrosis
General	Failure to thrive, dysmorphism, hypo/hyperhidrosis
Eye	Cataracts, retinopathy, gaze palsy, lens dislocation

The inborn errors of metabolism are mainly inherited biochemical disorders with specific enzyme defect that interferes with the normal metabolism of protein, fat or carbohydrate.

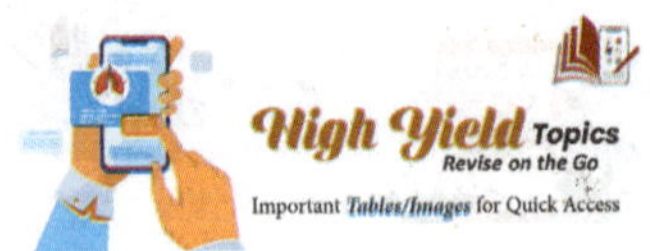

Diagnosis of Inborn Errors of Metabolism

The inherited metabolic disorders are not evident at the time of birth. These errors are diagnosed when some symptoms appear. Lab patterns are noted as shown in the Table 28.6.

Table 28.6: Some examples showing lab patterns in inborn errors of metabolism

	Protein metabolism defects			Carbohydrate defects	Lipid defects	
	Urea cycle disorders	**Organic acidemias**	**Amino acdiopathies**	**Disorders of carbohydrate metabolism**	**Fatty acid oxidation disorders**	**Mitochondrial/ congenital lactic acidoses**
Examples	OTC deficiency, citrullinemia (arginine synthetase deficiency)	Methylmalonic acidemia, propionic acidemia, glutaric acidemia	PKU (Phe), tyrosinemia, homocyst-inuria, maple syrup urine disease (leu-cine)	Galactosemia, hereditary fructose intol-erance, glyco-gen storage disorders	Medium-chain acyl- CoA dehydrogenase (MCAD) deficiency, carnitine deficiency	Mitochondrial encephalopa-thy, lactic acido-sis, and stroke-like episodes (MELAS)
AG Metabolic Acidosis	- (Respiratory alkalosis)	++	±	±	±	±
Hyperam-monemia	+++	++	±	--	±	--
Hypogly-cemia	--	±	±	++	++	±
Ketones	--	Inappropriately high	Appropriate to inappropri-ately high	Appropriate to inappropriately high	Inappropriately low	Appropriate to inappropriately high
Lactic acidosis	--	±	±	+	±	+++
Diagnos-tic tests	PAA, UOA, orotic acid for OTC def	UOA, ACP	PAA, UOA, ACP	Enzyme testing Liver biopsy	ACP	mtDNA NGS, muscle biopsy, enzyme tests

Note: *Red circle – primary finding*

CANCER GENETICS—FAMILIAL CANCER

Change or mutation in a specific gene may have been inherited and it may predispose a person to a particular type of cancer. Cancer due to an inherited trait results from a change in at least one gene that occurred before conception, and at least one additional change in a gene occurring after conception. Cancer linked to an inherited trait can be passed on to a person's family members. Gene mutation increases the chance to develop one or more cancers.

Most hereditary cancer syndromes exhibit autosomal dominant inheritance. The most common hereditary cancer syndromes related to women's cancer include hereditary breast and ovarian cancer syndrome, Lynch syndrome, Li–Fraumeni syndrome, Cowden syndrome, Peutz–Jeghers syndrome, and hereditary diffuse gastric cancer.

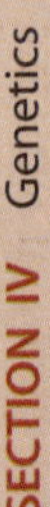

Risk Factors

- Familial cancers have increased risk to first-degree relatives.
- The interplay of hereditary and environmental factors, e.g., in lung cancer and breast cancer. Women at risk are, who have:
  - **Mutation of BRCA1 and 2:** If a parent passes a mutated BRCA1 or BRCA2 gene to their child, the child will have a much higher risk of developing breast and several other cancers.
  - **Ovarian cancer:** Closely related with breast cancers. Both occur in many dominant families and often in same individual.
  - Colorectal carcinomas.

Indications

- When an individual has a reasonable likelihood of carrying a cancer predisposing gene change.
- Clustering of cancer in one family.
- Onset of adult type of carcinoma at early ages.
- Multiple independent carcinomas arising in individual.
- Bilateral cancer in paired organs.
- Presence of a rare cancer.
- Presence of the same or associated cancers that comprise a syndrome.

Screening for Common Inherited/Familial Cancers

Genetic testing

- **For breast cancer:** Mammography—self-examination and regular clinical examination.
- For ovarian cancers, colorectal carcinomas, and familial melanomas: Monthly skin exams, and twice-yearly dermatologic evaluation and early excision of suspicious lesions.

Steps followed to analyze familial cancer in a patient are as follows:

1. Selection of a patient.
2. Pretest counseling.
3. Review of family history.
4. Informed consent.
5. Testing of patient.

CONDITIONS OF INHERITED/ FAMILIAL CANCERS

Lynch Syndrome

Lynch syndrome is a type of inherited cancer syndrome associated with a genetic predisposition to different cancer types. People with Lynch syndrome have a higher risk of certain types of cancer. Lynch syndrome is also known as hereditary nonpolyposis colorectal cancer (HNPCC).

Cancer begins when normal cells begin to change and grow out of control, forming a mass called tumor. A tumor can be benign (non-cancerous) or malignant (cancerous), which means it can spread to other parts of the body. A benign tumor means the tumor can grow but will not spread.

Lynch syndrome is among the most common hereditary cancer syndrome. Lynch syndrome significantly increases the risk of developing colorectal cancer. There is also an increased risk of developing cancers of endometrium, gastric, ovarian, small intestine, pancreas, prostate, urinary tract and bile duct. It also enhances the possibility of occurrence of sarcomas, sebaceous skin tumors of skin and brain cancers. Research indicates that 1 in every 300 people may be carriers of a gene associated with Lynch syndrome.

Genetic Basis of Lynch Syndrome

The cancers associated with Lynch syndrome have a specific pattern of mutations known as microsatellite instability (MSI), or mismatch repair deficiency (MMR-D). The genes included are *MLH1*, *MSH2*, *MSH6*, *PMS2*, and *EPCAM*.

Screening

Genetic testing to diagnose for colorectal, endometrial, ovarian, and/or other cancers in multiple relatives on the same side of a family.

The cancers associated with Lynch syndrome are more likely to be diagnosed at a young age.

Hereditary Breast and Ovarian Cancer (HBOC)

Hereditary breast and ovarian cancer (HBOC) is hereditary, meaning that it is caused by a mutation (genetic change) that can be passed down in families.

Causes

Hereditary breast and ovarian cancer (HBOC) is most often caused by mutations (genetic changes) in the breast cancer 1 (BRCA1) and breast cancer 2 (BRCA2) genes. Mutations in other, less common genes have also been associated with HBOC. However, most breast and ovarian cancers are not related to HBOC.

If there are BRCA mutation, the patient is likely to get cancers, such as:

- Breast cancer by age of 70 years (about 6 out of 10 women).
- Ovarian cancer by age of 70 years (about 4 out of 10).
- Increased risks for other cancers including prostate, pancreatic, and male breast cancers.

Management

In case a person is found to have HBOC, steps may be taken to reduce the cancer risks, including:

- Screenings for cancer by having earlier, more frequent, testing.
- Taking preventive medications that can decrease the risk of cancer.
- Undergoing preventive surgery to remove breasts, ovaries, and fallopian tubes.

Dominant Inherited Cancer Syndromes

Single mutant gene is inherited. Usually, it is a point mutation of tumor suppressor gene.

- **Retinoblastoma:**
  - Mutation of Rb tumor suppressor gene.
  - Bilateral.
  - Increased risk of developing second cancer.
- **Familial adenomatous polyposis:** (FAP) is a family cancer syndrome caused by certain inherited changes in the APC gene. People with FAP have a very high chance of developing colorectal cancer at an early age and are also at risk of developing other kinds of cancer.
  - Mutation of APC Tumor suppressor gene.
  - Polypoid adenomas.

- **Li-Fraumeni syndrome:** It is a rare hereditary disorder that increases the risk of familial cancer. Researchers estimated that the syndrome affects 5 in 20,000 families, worldwide. Li-Fraumeni syndrome cannot be prevented. But early and consistent cancer screenings and treatment can limit the syndrome's impact on life.
- **Cause:** Germ line mutation of p53 gene which is a tumor suppressor. The mutated gene keeps the cells from dividing and growing too quickly or in an uncontrolled way, to form tumors.

It increases the chances of breast, sarcomas, brain tumors and childhood adrenocortical carcinomas and acute leukemias. Female born with Li-Fraumeni syndrome have a 100% chance of developing breast cancer.

MUST KNOW

MEN1 and MEN2

- **MEN1:** Increased risk for developing parathyroid tumors, pancreatic tumors and/or pituitary tumors.
- **MEN2:** Mutation of RET proto-oncogene.
  - Increased risk to develop medullary thyroid cancers
  - Also have increased risk to develop pheochromocytoma, parathyroid tumors, and/or mucosal neuromas on the lips and tongue. The diagnosis and classification of MEN depends on family and medical history, clinical examination and genetic testing.

Hereditary Nonpolyposis Colorectal Cancer

Increased risk of cancers of colon, ovary, stomach, endometrium, small intestine and bile duct

Von Hippel Lindau Disease

Characterized by abnormal growth of blood vessels in certain parts of the body:

- Increased risk to develop growths in blood capillaries called angiomas or hemangioblastomas.
- These growths may develop in the retinas, certain areas of brain, spinal cord, adrenal glands and other parts of body retinal detachment and blindness.
- Angiomas in brain or spinal cord—the symptoms are headaches, problems with balance in walking, or weakness of arms and legs. Development of cysts and tumors in kidney, pancreas, liver or adrenal glands or in some cases RCC.

Neurofibromatosis Type 1

- Principally affects the Schwann cells.
- Neurofibromas in nerve sheaths, tumors of CNS, autonomous nervous system, meninges and eyes, skeletal developmental defects; also tumors, like lipomas, rhabdomyosarcomas, sebaceous adenomas and chromaffinomas.
- Increased incidence of meningiomas and gliomas.

Peutz-Jeghers Syndrome

- Multiple polyps throughout GIT.
- Cutaneous pigmentation around lips, oral mucosa, face, genitalia.

Cowden Syndrome

Increased risk of breast and thyroid cancers.

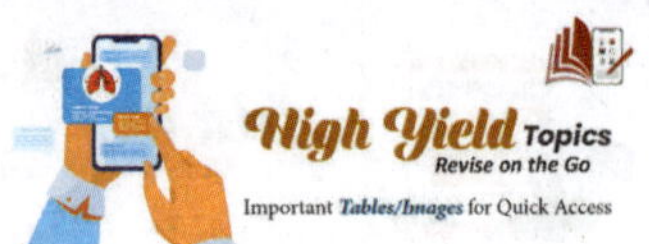

Familial Melanomas

The genes involved are CMM1, CMM2, (CDKN2), CDK4:

- Approximately 5–7% patients are from genetically high-risk families.
- Characterized by invasive melanoma in at least two first degree relatives.
- Some have 10–100 moles on upper trunk and limbs.

Cancers Due to Defective DNA Repair

Defective DNA repair results in DNA instability.

Autosomal Recessive

- **Xeroderma pigmentosa**:
  - Defect in mucleotide excision stage of repair.
  - Damage induced by UV radiations
- **Bloom's syndrome**:
  - Defect in the repair enzymes DNA ligase
  - Increased risk of all forms of cancers
- **Ataxia telangiectasia:**
  - Defect in repair of gamma radiation damage to nucleotide bases.
  - Reduced CMI.
  - Cerebellar ataxia, telangiectasia in conjunctiva, sclera.
  - Predisposition to cancers, like malignant lymphomas, ovarian dysgerminomas and tumors of brain.

BLOOD GROUPS ALLELES

More than 20 genetically determined blood group systems are known today. The ABO and Rhesus (Rh) systems are the most important ones used for blood transfusions.

Inheritance of Blood Group

ABO and Rh genes are not linked. ABO and Rh(D) type are inherited independently For example: An A Rh(D) positive mother and a B Rh(D) positive father could have an O Rh(D) negative child ABO and Rh(D) (Table 28.7).

Table 28.7: Inheritance of ABO and Rh (D)

Mother Group A *AO* Rh(D) pos *Dd*		Father Group B *BO* Rh(D) pos *Dd*
Group A AO Rh(D) pos *Dd*	Group B *BO* Rh(D) pos *Dd*	Group O OO Rh(D) neg *dd*

Two major blood group systems relevant to hematological disorders are the ABO system and the Rh system.

Role of ABO Group System

- **Blood transfusion compatibility:** ABO system plays role in blood transfusion compatibility. Incompatible transfusions can lead to a severe immune reaction, known as a hemolytic reaction.
- **Hemolytic disease of newborn (HDN):** In cases where an expectant mother has a different blood type from her fetus (especially if the mother is O and the baby is A, B, or AB), there is a risk of HDN. This condition occurs when maternal antibodies attack fetal red blood cells, leading to anemia and other complications in the newborn.

Role of Rh System

- **Rh incompatibility:** Rh-negative mothers carrying Rh-positive fetuses may develop antibodies against Rh-positive blood cells, leading to hemolytic disease of the newborn (similar to ABO incompatibility). Rh immunoglobulin (RhIg) is administered to Rh-negative pregnant women to prevent the development of antibodies.
- **Blood transfusions and organ transplants:** The Rh factor is also considered during blood and organ transplants. A mismatch in the Rh factor can trigger immune responses.

Significance of Blood Group Alleles

Blood group alleles play a significant role in hematological disorders, influencing susceptibility, severity, and treatment.

HEMATOLOGICAL DISORDERS

Sickle Cell Anemia

Sickle cell anemia is an inherited form of anemia.

Cause

It is due to a point mutation in the Hb gene, encoding hemoglobin. This mutation causes the substitution of glutamic acid with valine, leading to the production of abnormal hemoglobin (HbS). In homozygous individuals inheriting HbS from both parents, red blood cells assume a sickle shape, causing vascular blockages, anemia, and organ damage. Heterozygotes may exhibit milder symptoms, possessing one normal and one mutated gene. The genetic basis involves autosomal recessive inheritance, highlighting the importance of both parents carrying the sickle cell trait for a child to develop the disorder.

Effect of Sickle Cells

There are not enough healthy red blood cells to carry adequate oxygen throughout the body. In sickle cell anemia, the red blood cells become rigid and sticky, and are shaped like sickles or crescent moons. These irregularly-shaped cells can get stuck in small blood vessels, which can slow or block blood flow and oxygen to parts of the body.

Complications include heart attack, stroke, jaundice, increased infections, gallstones, deterioration of retina which may lead to blindness, delay in growth.

Thalassemia

Thalassemia, also known as Mediterranean anemia, is a condition which is inherited.

Cause

Thalassemia is a hereditary blood disorder arising from mutations in the HBB gene, affecting hemoglobin production. Autosomal recessive inheritance of mutated genes from both parents results in reduced or absent synthesis of globin chains, leading to abnormal hemoglobin formation. The severity varies depending on the number and nature of mutated alleles. Thalassemia major manifests in homozygotes, causing severe anemia, while heterozygotes may display a milder condition (thalassemia minor).

Types of Thalassemia

It is of two types:

1. **α-thalassemia:** α-thalassemia occurs when one or more of the four alpha chain genes fails to function. The "failed" genes are almost invariably lost from the cell due to a genetic misfunction.

   Impact of α-thalassemia:
   - Loss of one gene diminishes the production of the alpha protein only slightly—silent carrier.
   - Loss of two alpha genes produces a condition with small red blood cells—mild anemia. People with this condition look and feel normal.
   - Loss of three alpha genes produces a serious hematological problem—severe anemia, and often require blood transfusions to survive. There is severe imbalance between the alpha chain production and beta chain production (which is normal). It causes an accumulation of beta chains inside the red blood cells. Beta chains begin to associate in groups of four, producing an abnormal hemoglobin, called "hemoglobin H" - condition is called "hemoglobin H disease".
   - Loss of all four alpha genes produces a condition that is incompatible with life. The gamma chains produced during fetal life associate in groups of four to form an abnormal hemoglobin called "Hemoglobin Barts". Most people with four-gene deletion alpha thalassemia die in utero or shortly after birth.

2. **β-thalassemia:** β-thalassemia occurs when the beta globin chains are either produced inadequately or not at all. A person suffers from beta thalassemia when he inherits one defected beta globin chain from each parent.

   There are two types of β-thalassemia:
   - β-thalassemia minor occurs when only one of the beta chains is defected. This results in low levels of hemoglobin production in the blood. It produces mild anemia caused by an iron deficiency although the levels of iron in the blood appear normal.
   - β-thalassemia major, also called Cooley's anemia, occurs when both beta chains are defected. There is no production of hemoglobin. It is a serious life-threatening condition. Patients with major thalassemia and hemoglobin H disease suffer from many complications if not treated properly and on time.

Hemolytic Disease of the Newborn (HDN)

Hemolytic disease of newborns is primarily caused by Rh incompatibility between the mother and the fetus. If an Rh-negative mother is carrying an Rh-positive fetus, and there is an exposure to Rh-positive blood during pregnancy or delivery, the mother's immune system may produce antibodies against the Rh-positive red blood cells of the fetus. In subsequent pregnancies with Rh-positive fetuses, these antibodies can cross the placenta, leading to hemolysis (destruction of red blood cells) in the newborn.

Genetic Basis of HDN

Rh incompatibility is due to genetic variation in the Rh factor, inherited from the parents.

- **Hereditary spherocytosis:** Genetic mutation leads to the formation of spherocytic red blood cells, which are more prone to destruction. The symptoms are anemia, jaundice, and an enlarged spleen due to increased red blood cell breakdown.
- **Genetic basis of hereditary spherocytosis:** caused by mutations in genes encoding proteins involved in red blood cell membrane structure, such as ANK1, SPTB, SPTA1, or others.

G6PD Deficiency

The deficiency results in a deficiency of the enzyme glucose-6-phosphate dehydrogenase, making red blood cells vulnerable to oxidative stress. The symptoms are hemolytic episodes triggered by certain drugs, infections, or fava bean consumption.

- **Genetic basis of G6PD deficiency:** X-linked recessive disorder caused by mutations in the G6PD gene
- **Autoimmune hemolytic anemia:** Immune system attacks its own red blood cells, leading to hemolysis. The symptoms are fatigue, pallor, jaundice, and enlarged spleen.
- **Genetic basis of autoimmune hemolytic anemia:** Associated with certain genetic factors predisposing individuals to autoimmune diseases.

Genetic Hemochromatosis

Hemochromatosis is a genetic disorder characterized by excessive absorption of dietary iron, leading to iron overload in various organs of the body. The most common type of hemochromatosis is hereditary hemochromatosis (HH), and it has several subtypes, with the most prevalent being known as HFE-associated hemochromatosis.

Symptoms

Common symptoms and complications associated with hemochromatosis include:

- **Fatigue and joint pain:** Due to excess iron accumulation in various organs.
- **Abdominal pain:** Due to overload of iron in liver.
- **Skin changes:** A bronze or grayish skin coloration, often referred to as “bronze diabetes” due to iron deposition.
- Heart problems and diabetes.

Cause

The majority of hereditary hemochromatosis cases are linked to mutations in the HFE gene. The HFE gene is located on the short arm of chromosome 6 and plays a crucial role in regulating iron absorption in the small intestine. The two most common mutations associated with hereditary hemochromatosis are C282Y and H63D.

1. **C282Y mutation:** This mutation is the most strongly associated with hereditary hemochromatosis. Individuals who inherit two copies (homozygous) of the C282Y mutation (one from each parent) are at an increased risk of developing iron overload.
2. **H63D mutation:** This mutation is less common and is usually associated with milder forms of hemochromatosis. Having two copies of the H63D mutation can contribute to iron overload, although the risk is generally lower.

MUST KNOW

Not everyone with these genetic mutations will develop hemochromatosis. The condition typically manifests when a person inherits two copies of the C282Y mutation or a combination of C282Y and H63D mutations.

Management

Early detection and therapeutic interventions such as phlebotomy.

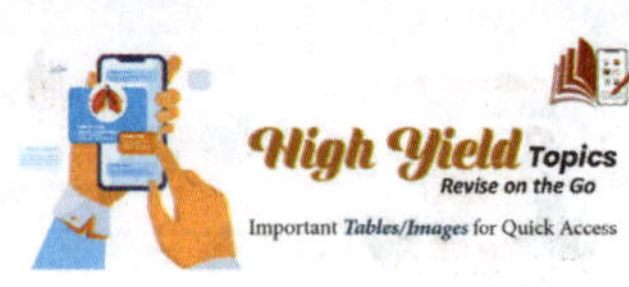

SUMMARY

- A genetic condition occurs when an altered (changed) gene is inherited from parents that increases the risk of developing a particular condition.
- Prevention of congenital defects is possible with intake of adequate folic acid or iodine, stapple food with supplementation and vaccination.
- Neural tube defects develop early in the pregnancy, even before the woman knows about her pregnancy.
- Development of neural tube defects are due to genetic and nongenetic factors.
- The most prevalent types of NTDs are anencephaly, encephalocele and spina bifida.
- Exact cause of neural tube defects (NTDs) is not known but it is believed that it is a complex combination of genetic, nutritional and environmental factors.
- Development of neural tube defects are multi factorial.
- Down syndrome is genetic condition in which an individual is born with an extra chromosome.
- Down syndrome is caused by a spontaneous genetic mutation that occurs very early in zygote development.
- In the case of hereditary translocation Down syndrome (a rare one), an extra chromosome 21 is inherited from one of the parents.
- Children with DS experience various degrees of intellectual disability and are more vulnerable to health complications.
- Turner syndrome is typically caused by nondisjunction of a pair of sex chromosomes (fail to separate) during the formation of an egg (or sperm).
- The abnormality is not inherited from an affected parent (not passed down from parent to child) because women with Turner syndrome are usually sterile and cannot have children.
- Klinefelter syndrome is a genetic disorder in which there is at least one extra X chromosome to a standard human male karyotype.
- Huntington disease is a neurodegenerative disorder that causes the progressive breakdown of nerve cells in the brain especially damage in the basal ganglia.
- Huntington disease usually causes movement, cognitive and psychiatric disorders with a wide spectrum of signs and symptoms.
- Mental illness can occur when the brain or part of the brain is not working well or is working improperly—abnormal brain functioning.
- Schizophrenia is a serious mental illness that affects how a person thinks, feels, and behaves.
- Bipolar disorder is a highly prevalent disorder which is genetically inherited.
- The serotonin transporter gene is linked to depression. It controls two parts of the brain: amygdala and cingulate.
- ADHD tends to run in families and, in most cases, it is proposed that the genes for ADHD are inherited from the parents.
- Autism is highly heritable.
- People with ASD may also have different ways of learning, moving, or paying attention.
- Inborn errors of metabolism are now often referred to as congenital metabolic diseases or inherited metabolic diseases.
- The inborn errors of metabolism are mainly inherited biochemical disorders with specific enzyme defect that interferes with the normal metabolism of protein, fat or carbohydrate.
- Most hereditary cancer syndromes exhibit autosomal dominant inheritance.
- Lynch syndrome is a type of inherited cancer syndrome associated with a genetic predisposition to different cancer types.
- HBOC is most often caused by mutations (genetic changes) in the breast cancer 1 (BRCA1) and breast cancer 2 (BRCA2) genes.
- Female born with Li-Fraumeni syndrome have a 100% chance of developing breast cancer.
- Von Hippel Lindau disease is characterized by abnormal growth of blood vessels in certain parts of the body.
- ABO and Rh(D) type are inherited independently.

Contd...

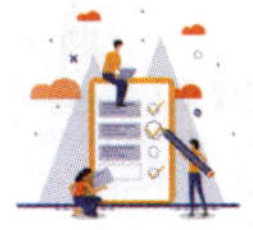

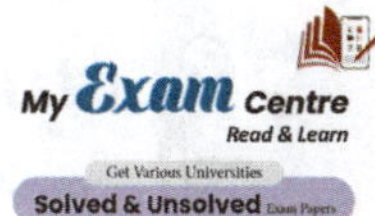

- In cases where an expectant mother has a different blood type from her fetus (especially if the mother is O and the baby is A, B, or AB), there's a risk of HDN.
- Rh immunoglobulin (RhIg) is administered to Rh-negative pregnant women to prevent the development of antibodies.
- Blood group alleles play a significant role in hematological disorders, influencing susceptibility, severity, and treatment.
- Blood group alleles play a significant role in hematological disorders, influencing susceptibility, severity, and treatment.
- In sickle cell anemia, the red blood cells become rigid and sticky and are shaped like sickles or crescent moons.
- Thalassemia is a hereditary blood disorder arising from mutations in the HBB gene, affecting hemoglobin production.
- Thalassemia major manifests in homozygotes, causing severe anemia, while heterozygotes may display a milder condition.
- Alpha thalassemia occurs when one or more of the four alpha chain genes fails to function.
- Beta thalassemia occurs when the beta globin chains are either produced inadequately or not at all.
- Hemolytic disease of newborn is primarily caused by Rh incompatibility between the mother and the fetus.
- Genetic mutation leads to the formation of spherocytic red blood cells, which are more prone to destruction.
- X-linked recessive disorder caused by mutations in the G6PD gene.
- Hemochromatosis is a genetic disorder characterized by excessive absorption of dietary iron, leading to iron overload in various organs of the body.
- The two most common mutations associated with hereditary hemochromatosis are C282Y and H63D.

ASSESS YOURSELF

Long Answer Questions

1. Discuss inborn errors of metabolism.
2. Describe the blood alleles and any three hematological disorders.

Short Answer Questions

1. What are familial cancers?
2. Write about hemolytic disease of newborns.
3. Write short notes on:
   i. Thalassemia
   ii. Hemochromatosis
   iii. Turner syndrome
   iv. Down syndrome
   v. Neural tube defects

Multiple Choice Questions

1. **Inborn errors of metabolism are the following; except:**
   a. Phenylketonuria
   b. Tay-Sachs disease
   c. Cystic fibrosis
   d. Turner's syndrome
2. **Down's syndrome is congenital chromosome abnormality and is also known as:**
   a. Trisomy 20
   b. Trisomy 31
   c. Trisomy 21
   d. None of these
3. **Children with Down's syndrome have what is known as brachycephaly. This means that the shape of the back of the head is:**
   a. Rounded
   b. Flattened
   c. Pointed
   d. None of these

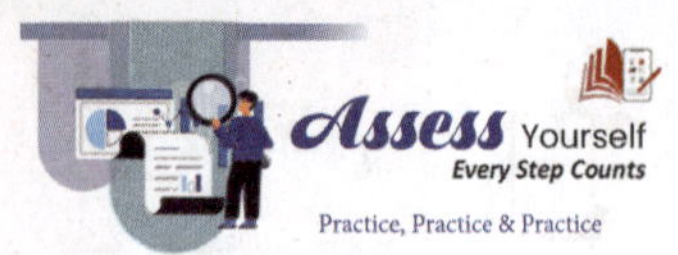

4. **A physical feature Down's syndrome is that the fifth finger may be slightly curved toward the other fingers. What is this known as?**
   a. Clinodactyly
   b. Clubbing
   c. Dupuytren's contracture
   d. Phalanges
5. **Which of the following statement is true about thalassemia?**
   a. There is a type of thalassemia depending on the number of mutations in genes
   b. It is caused by mutations in the DNA of cells which make up the haemoglobin
   c. Mild thalassemia may not need treatment
   d. All of the above
6. **Which type of thalassemia disease is Cooley anemia?**
   a. Alloimmunization
   b. β-thalassemia
   c. Alpha-thalassemia
   d. None of these
7. **The complications that can occur in severe thalassemia is:**
   a. Enlarged spleen
   b. Bone deformities
   c. Problems with the heart
   d. All of these
8. **A human female with Turner's syndrome:**
   a. Has one additional X chromosome
   b. Has 45 chromosomes with XO
   c. Is able to produce children with a normal husband
   d. Exhibit male characters

Fill in the blanks:

9. **Inborn errors of metabolism are a group of metabolic __________ which can be formed as a result of the lack of a single ________ in a single metabolic pathway.**
10. **Maple syrup urine disease is recognized by central nervous system manifestations of __________ and attacks of flaccidity and ____________.**

Answer Key

1. d	**2.** c	**3.** b	**4.** a	**5.** d	**6.** b
7. d	**8.** b	**9.** Disease; Enzyme		**10.** Convulsions; Apnea	

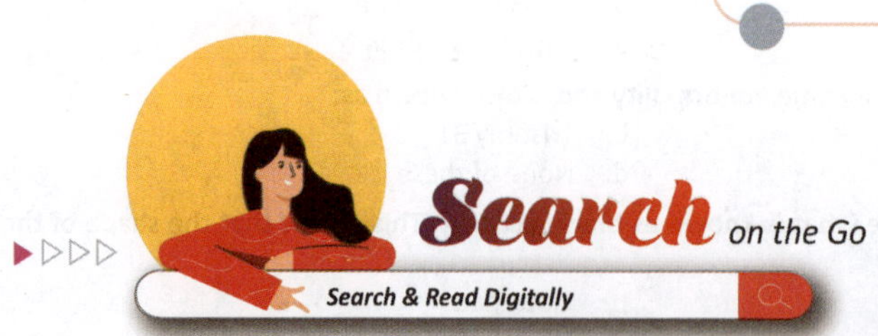

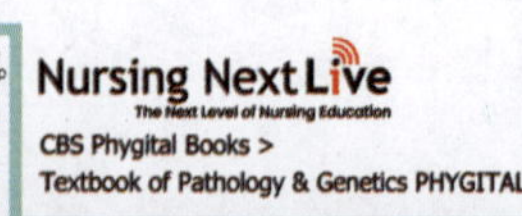

Chapter 29

Services Related to Genetics

LEARNING OBJECTIVES

After the completion of the chapter, the readers will be able to:
- Explain human genome project.
- Discuss the gene therapy and eugenic movement.
- Understand genetic counseling and role of nurse in genetical conditions.
- Know about legal and ethical issues as a genetics nurse.

CHAPTER OUTLINE

- Human Genome Project
- Gene Therapy
- Methods of Gene Transfer
- Applications of Gene Therapy for Inherited Disorders
- Genetic Testing
- The Eugenics Movement
- Genetic Counseling
- Role of Nurse in Genetic Counseling

KEY TERMS

Electroporation: The use of short high-voltage pulses to overcome the barrier of the cell membrane.

Euphenics: A symptomatic treatment of genetic diseases of human beings.

Euthenics: The study of the control of the environment, especially with a view to improving the health and living standards of the human race.

Functional genomics: The study of how genes and intergenic segments of the genome contribute to different metabolic pathways.

Gene augmentation: Adding a new protein coding gene to a cell.

Germ line: Refers to the sex cells (eggs and sperm) that sexually reproducing organisms use to pass on their genomes from one generation to the next (parents to offspring).

Pharmacogenomics: The study of how genes affect a person's response to drugs.

Sonoporation: The formation of small pores in cell membranes by using ultrasound for the transfer of nucleic acid materials.

HUMAN GENOME PROJECT

Human Genome Project (HGP) was an international scientific research project that aimed to determine the complete sequence of nucleotide base pairs that make up human DNA and all the genes it contains. It remains the world's largest collaborative biological project.

Participating Countries and Funding Agencies

- **Objective:** Determining the DNA sequence of the entire euchromatic human genome
- **Started:** In 1990
- **Time:** 15-year-long
- **Budget:** $3-billion project
- **Participants:**
  - Two major funding agencies, the US Department of Energy (DOE) and National Institute of Health (NIH)
  - The government-sponsored sequencing was performed in 20 universities and research centers in the United States, the United Kingdom, Japan, France, Germany, Canada, and China.
  - A parallel project was conducted outside the government sponsorship by the Celera Corporation or the Celera Genomics in 1998.

Aims of HGP

- To identify and map all the 20,000–25,000 genes (approximately) in the human DNA from a physical and functional standpoint.
- To determine the sequences of the 3 billion chemical base pairs that make up the human DNA.
- To store the information in databases.
- To discover more efficient technologies for data analysis.
- To allow access to the information and technologies to the private sectors. This information arise, HGP and also to sequence the genomes of other organisms that are important in medical research such as mouse, Drosophila, etc.

Factors Determining HGP

- **Kind (genetic makeup) of people:** Genetic makeup of people can help identify risks due to shared genes.
- **Type of marriage practices:** Interbreeding increases homozygosity, which can increase the chances of expression of harmful or beneficial recessive alleles. This may increase or decrease the fitness o the person.
- **Percentage of existing children born out of excellent genetic composition:** It can improve the races with incorporation of quality genes such as intelligency.

Process of HGP

The process involves genome mapping, or characterizing the chromosomes—a genetic map. The next step is DNA sequencing, or determining the order of DNA bases on a chromosome-physical maps.

- **First genetic mapping:** Genetic markers are invaluable for genome mapping. A genetic map shows the relative locations of these specific markers on the chromosomes. The genetic markers are any inherited physical or molecular characteristics that are different among individuals of a population (polymorphic). For example, restriction fragment length polymorphisms (RFLP).
- **Second DNA is amplified, or increased in quantity:** Two types of DNA amplifications are—cloning and Polymerase Chain Reactions (PCR).

- **Third is sequencing and the techniques used in HGP are:**
  - **Shotgun sequencing method:** The method involves randomly breaking up the genome into small DNA fragments that are sequenced individually.
  - **Sanger sequencing method:** This is chain termination method. This technique for DNA sequencing is based on the selective incorporation of chain-terminating dideoxynucleotides (ddNTPs) by DNA polymerase during in vitro DNA replication.

Sequencing determines the order of DNA bases on a chromosome.

Outcomes of HGP

- **Genome sequencing:** Provided a comprehensive map of the human genetic code.
- **Identification of genes:** The project led to the identification and mapping of approximately 20,000–25,000 protein-coding genes in the human genome.
- **Functional genomics:** HGP contributed to the emerging field of functional genomics, which focuses on understanding the functions of genes and how they interact within the biological systems. It provided insights into gene expression patterns, regulatory elements, and the complex networks that govern cellular processes.
- **Development of diagnostic tests:** It has facilitated the development of diagnostic tests, targeted therapies, and personalized medicine based on an individual's genetic makeup. Genetic information is now used in the diagnosis and treatment of various genetic disorders and cancers.
- **Comparative genomics:** The project allowed for comparative genomics, enabling researchers to study similarities and differences in the genomes of different species provided insights into evolutionary relationships.
- **Technological advances:** HGP played a crucial role in the development of faster and more cost-effective sequencing technologies has made large-scale genomic studies more accessible.
- **Ethical, legal and social implications (ELSI):** HGP led to the establishment of the ELSI program, which aimed to anticipate and address the ethical, legal, and social implications of genomic research.

Applications of HGP

- **Disease diagnosis and prediction:** HGP has enabled the identification of genetic markers associated with various diseases. This knowledge has facilitated the development of genetic tests for diagnosing and predicting the risk of certain genetic disorders, such as cystic fibrosis, Huntington's disease, and certain types of cancer.
- **Personalized medicine:** The sequencing of the human genome holds benefits for many fields, from molecular medicine to human evolution. Physicians can tailor treatment plans based on a patient's genetic makeup, optimizing therapeutic outcomes while minimizing adverse effects.
- **Pharmacogenomics:** Studying an individual's genetic makeup influences their response toward drugs. This knowledge is utilized to develop drugs that are more effective and have fewer side effects by considering genetic variations in drug metabolism and efficacy.
- **Genetic counseling:** Genetic counselors use information from the HGP to help individuals and families understand their genetic risks. This is especially important in cases where there is a family history of genetic disorders or when individuals are planning to have children. Genetic counseling assists in making informed decisions about family planning and healthcare.
- **Functional genomics and gene therapy:** Human genome project (HGP) has enhanced our understanding of gene function and regulation. Gene therapy holds promise for treating conditions with a genetic basis, such as certain types of muscular dystrophy and inherited blindness.

- **Biotechnology and agriculture:** Human genome project (HGP) allows for advances in agriculture through genetic modification to yield healthier, more disease-resistant crops. Manipulation of plant and animal genomes to improve agricultural crops, enhance livestock traits, and develop disease-resistant organisms. This contributes to advancements in food production and environmental sustainability.
- **Forensic applications:** It benefitted the advancement of forensic science. DNA fingerprinting, based on the variability in individual genomes, is widely used for criminal investigations, paternity testing, and establishing identity in mass disasters.
- **Evolutionary studies:** Understanding the similarities and differences in genomes helps researchers trace the evolutionary history of organisms.

EXTRA EDGE

Time line of HGP

1970: Fredrick Sanger developed a technique for DNA sequencing, known as the Sanger's method of DNA sequencing.
1985: Robert Sinsheimer at UCSC proposed the idea of sequencing the human genome.
1986: The US Department of Energy and the National Institute of Health came forward to fund the HGP.
1989: UK's Medical Research Council (MRC) joined the HGP.
1990: HGP was officially launched with James Watson as its Project Director. The 1st gene to be mapped was BRCA1, which is the gene for breast cancer.
1993: First 5-year-plan for HGP was published. Sanger Institute (UK) joins HGP.
1994: HGP's Human genetic mapping goal was achieved.
1995: Genetic Privacy Act was passed. 1st bacterial genome was sequenced (Hemophilus influenzae)
1996: 1st Human Gene map was published.
Yeast genome was sequenced.
HGP's mouse genetic mapping goal was achieved.
1997: NIH becomes NHGRI.
E. coli genome sequenced.
Genoscope, French National Genome Sequencing Centre was established.
1998: Second 5-year-plan for HGP was published.
Japan's RIKEN Genomic Services Center was established.
Genome of the roundworm Caenorhabditis elegans was sequenced.
SNP sequencing was initiated.
The Chinese National Human Genome Centers were established in Beijing and Shanghai.
1999: Sequencing of human chromosome 22 was completed and was published in "The Nature".
2000: Working draft of human genome completed. US president Clinton & UK's PM Blair support free access to genome information. Genomes of D. melanogaster and A. thaliana were sequenced and published in "The Nature".
2001: Working draft of human genome sequence was published in "The Nature" and "Science".
2002: Working draft of mouse genome sequence was completed and published.
2003: Finished version of human genome sequence was completed. HGP ended with all the goals achieved.

GENE THERAPY

Gene therapy is the insertion of genes into an individual's cells and tissues to treat a disease, such as a hereditary disease in which a deleterious mutant allele is replaced with a functional one (Fig. 29.1).

Types of Gene Therapy

- **Germline therapy:** It is not permitted in any country and is considered unethical.
- **Germline gene therapy:** In this case, germ cells, i.e., sperm or eggs are modified by the introduction of functional genes, which are integrated into their genomes. The change due to therapy would be heritable and would be passed on to future generation.

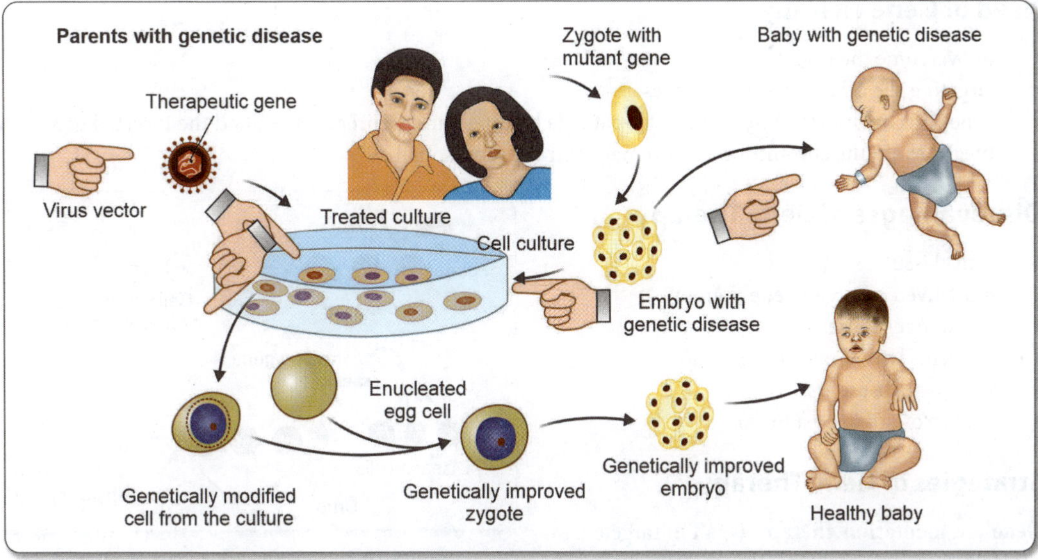

Figure 29.1: Germline gene therapy

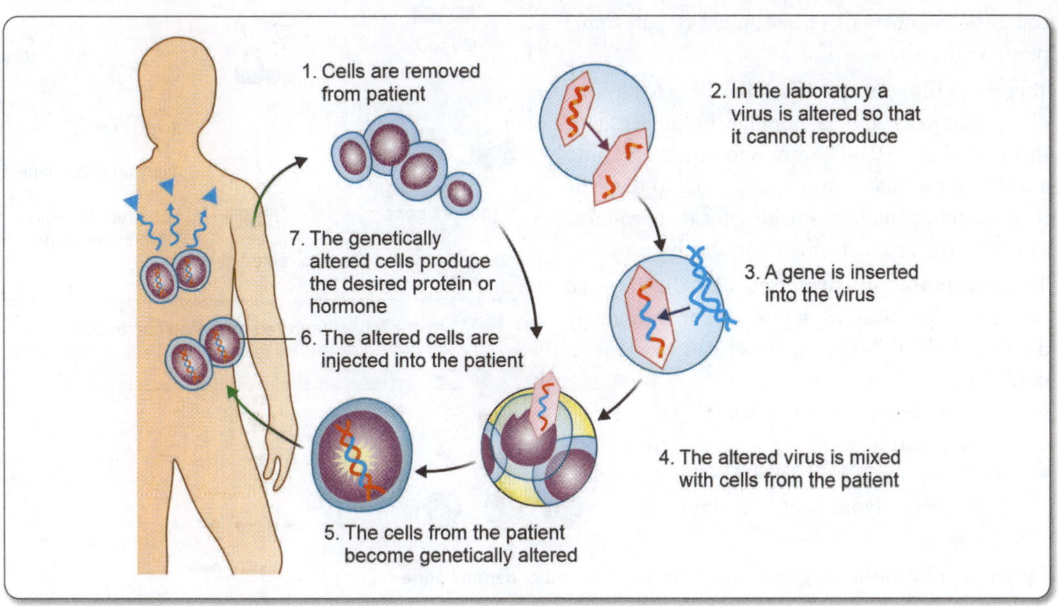

Figure 29.2: Somatic gene therapy

- **Somatic gene therapy:** In this, therapeutic genes are transferred into the somatic cells of a patient. Any modification and effects will be restricted to the individual patient only, and will not be inherited. Mainly, it aims to cure a disease only in the patient, not in patient's descendants (Fig. 29.2).

Need of Gene Therapy

- To overcome the disease.
- Targeting the cells of diseased tissues.
- Genes can be inserted into the cells of patients by direct and indirect routes, and the inserted genes can integrate into the chromosomes or remain extra chromosomal.

Disadvantages of Gene Therapy

- Ethical issues.
- Short-lived nature of gene therapy.
- Immune response.
- Problems with viral vectors.
- Multigene disorders.
- Chance of inducing a tumor.

Strategies of Gene Therapy

Gene augmentation therapy (GAT): Targeted to clinical disorders where the pathogenesis is reversible. GAT is applicable to the diseases caused by loss of function of a gene by introducing extra copies of the normal gene. Applied to autosomal recessive disorders.

Targeted killing of specific cells: Targeted killing of specific cells and is popular in cancer gene therapies (Fig. 29.3). The aim is to insert DNA into a diseased cell that causes specific cell to die. The inserted gene contains a suicide gene that produces a highly toxic product which kills the diseased cell.

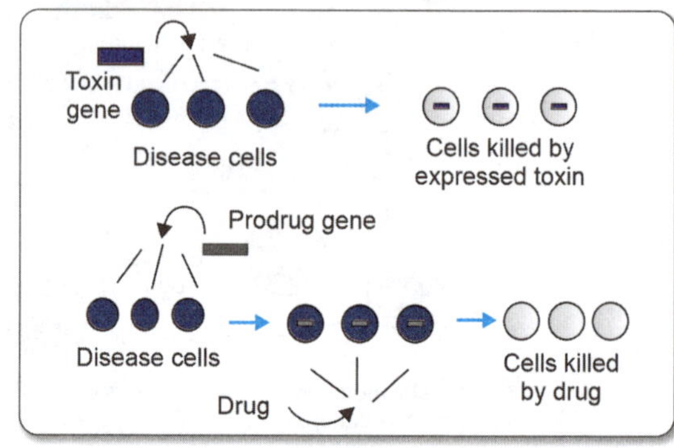

Figure 29.3: Targeted killing of specific cells

Targeted mutation correction (TMC): Targeted correction provides a template for homology directed TMC. TMC (Fig. 29.4) can be done at different levels:

- At gene level, based on homologous recombination.
- At RNA transcript level, by using particular types of therapeutic ribozymes.

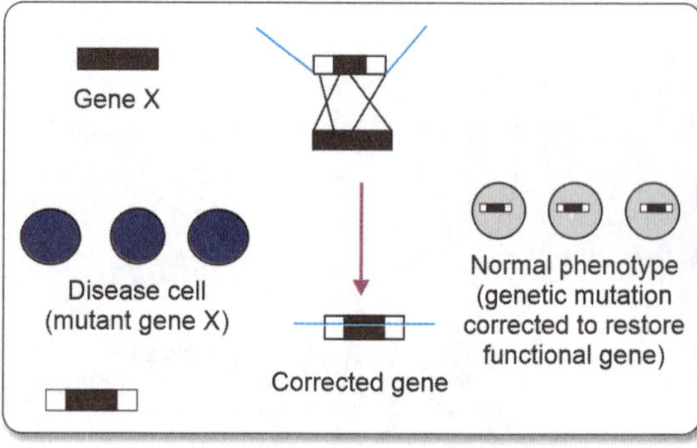

Figure 29.4: Targeted mutation correction

Targeted inhibition of gene expression: If disease cells display an inappropriate expression of a gene (in case of many cancers), a variety of different system can be used specifically to block the expression of a single gene at the DNA, RNA or protein levels (Fig. 29.5).

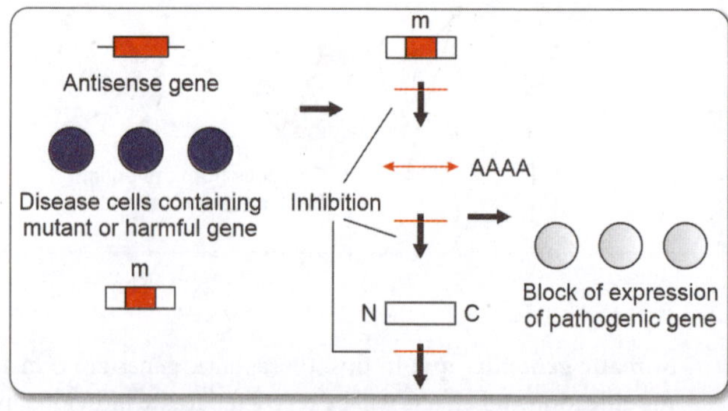

Figure 29.5: Targeted inhibition of gene expression

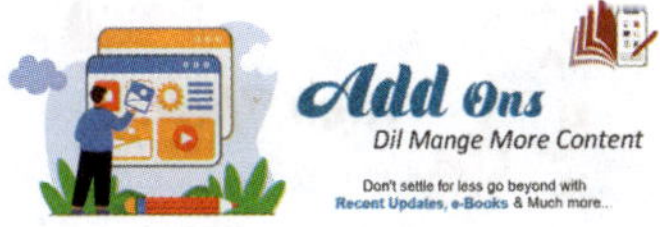

METHODS OF GENE TRANSFER

Viral Methods

Viral vectors are modified viruses engineered to carry and deliver specific genetic material into target cells. Commonly used viral vectors include retroviruses, lentiviruses, adenoviruses, adeno-associated viruses (AAVs), and herpes simplex viruses.

- **Retroviruses and lentiviruses:** Retroviruses and lentiviruses are capable of integrating their genetic material into the host cell's genome. This feature is advantageous for stable, long-term expression of the introduced gene.
- **Adenoviruses:** Adenoviruses are efficient at infecting a wide range of dividing and non-dividing cells but do not integrate into the host genome. They are often used for short-term expression of the introduced gene and are suitable for applications where transient gene expression is sufficient.
- **AAV:** Adeno-associated viruses (AAV) are small, non-pathogenic viruses that can establish long-term expression without integrating extensively into the host genome. AAVs are often used for gene therapy due to their low immunogenicity and ability to infect both dividing and nondividing cells.
- **Herpes simplex viruses:** Herpes simplex viruses are neurotropic and can be used for gene transfer to neurons. They are explored for applications in neuroscience and gene therapy for neurological disorders.

Disadvantage of Viral Methods

Viral methods face challenges such as immunogenicity, the risk of insertional mutagenesis (especially with integrating vectors), and limited cargo capacity for the genetic material.

Nonviral Methods

- **Lipid based:** Liposomes, which are lipid-based vesicles, can encapsulate and deliver genetic material. Cationic lipids or liposomes can form complexes with negatively charged DNA or RNA, facilitating their transport into target cells. Lipid nanoparticles provide a non-viral alternative for gene delivery.
- **Polymeric nanoparticles:** Polymeric nanoparticles, such as polyethyleneimine (PEI) and poly (lactic-co-glycolic acid) (PLGA), can be used to encapsulate and deliver genetic material. These particles protect the genetic payload and aid in its release within target cells.
- **Naked DNA or RNA:** Direct administration of naked DNA or RNA into cells is a simple non-viral approach. This can be achieved through techniques such as electroporation, where an electric field is applied to temporarily disrupt cell membranes, allowing genetic material to enter.
- **Peptides:** Peptides, short chains of amino acids, can be designed to form complexes with nucleic acids and facilitate their entry into cells. These peptides possess cell-penetrating properties, helping in the transport of genetic material across cell membranes.
- **CRISPR-Cas9:** Researchers have explored delivering CRISPR-Cas9 components as ribonucleoprotein complexes (RNPs) rather than using viral vectors. This involves directly introducing the Cas9 protein and guide RNA into cells to edit specific genomic sequences.
- **Electroporation:** Electroporation involves applying electrical pulses to cells, creating temporary pores in the cell membrane. This allows the uptake of genetic material. Electroporation is a versatile technique used for both in vitro and in vivo gene delivery.
- **Hydrodynamic:** This method involves the rapid injection of a large volume of naked DNA into the bloodstream. The sheer force of the injection leads to the uptake of genetic material by cells in the organ. The method is primarily used in preclinical research.

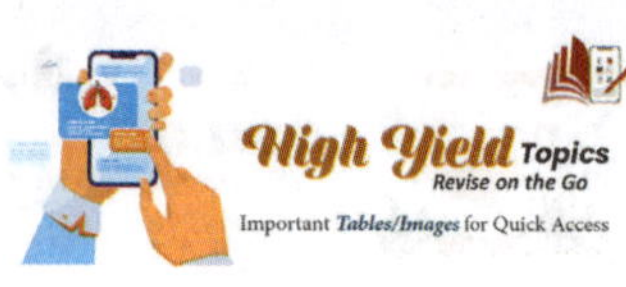

Table 29.1: Successful gene therapy for inherited disorders

Disorder	Cells altered	Gene therapy strategy
ADA deficiency	T-Cells and hematopoietic stem cells	Ex Vivo GAT Using Recombinant Retroviruses Containing an ADA Gene
Cystic fibrosis	Respiratory epithelium	In Vivo GAT Using Recombinant Adenoviruses or Liposome-to deliver the CFTR Gene
Familial	Liver cells	Ex Vivo GAT Using Retrovirus
Hypercholestemia		To Deliver the LdL Receptor Gene
Gaucher's disease	Hematopoietic stem cells	Ex Vivo GAT Using Retroviruses to Deliver the Gluco-Cerebrosidase gene

- **Sonoporation:** Sonoporation uses ultrasound to create transient pores in cell membranes, enabling the uptake of genetic material. This technique is being explored for its potential in localized and controlled gene delivery.

APPLICATIONS OF GENE THERAPY FOR INHERITED DISORDERS

Recessively inherited disorders are conceptually the easiest inherited disorders to treat by gene therapy. The first apparently successful gene therapy (Table 29.1) was initiated in 1990 for adenosine deaminase deficiency, cystic fibrosis, familial hypercholesterolemia (FH), Gaucher's diseases, for neoplastic disorders and infectious disease.

GENETIC TESTING

The topic has already been discussed in detail in Chapters 27 and 28. Kindly refer to these chapters.

THE EUGENICS MOVEMENT

Eugenics is an immoral and pseudoscientific theory that claims it is possible to perfect people and groups through genetics and the scientific laws of inheritance. Eugenicists worldwide believed that they could perfect human beings and eliminate so-called social ills through genetics and heredity.

The theory got popularity during the early 20th century. Eugenics can be positive and negative (Fig. 29.6).

Definition: Eugenics is the science that works on a set of beliefs and practices that aim to improve the genetic quality of a human population.

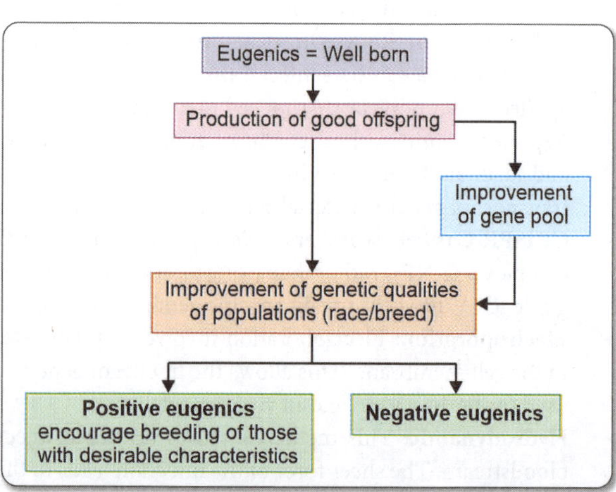

Figure 29.6: Concepts of eugenics

EXTRA EDGE

Euthenics is manipulating the environment in order to improve the genotype. The environmental factors involved are such as smoking, diet , obesity and lack of exercise in producing disease such as cancer, hypertension, diabetes mellitus and heart.

Principle of Eugenics

The term "eugenic" was coined in 1883 by Francis Galton. It has been derived from two Greek words meaning "good in birth," the term eugenics refers to a controversial area of genetic science based on the belief that the human species can be improved by encouraging only people or groups with "desirable" traits to reproduce, while discouraging or even preventing reproduction among people with "undesirable" qualities.

Aims of Eugenics

According to Galton, eugenics is required:

- To save the resources.
- To create healthy people/healthy community.
- To have intelligent people or to have the community free from mentally retarded people.
- To decrease the human suffering.

Factors Determining Eugenics

- The genetic makeup of people which contributes to the ancestors of future generation.
- Type of marriage practices.
- The percentage of existing children born out of excellent genetic composition.

Types of Eugenics

The eugenics may be positive and negative.

Positive Eugenics

Positive eugenics refers to the promotion and implementation of measures aimed at encouraging the reproduction of individuals with desirable or advantageous genetic traits in order to improve the overall genetic quality of a population.

Purpose

Main purpose of positive eugenics was to achieve healthy population. Positive eugenics encourages reproduction among genetically advantageous population. For example, *in-vitro* fertilization, egg transplant and cloning.

Methods

To encourage reproduction among genetically advantages population. Various ways of positive eugenics are:

- *In vitro* fertilization.
- Egg transplant.
- Cloning.

Measures to have Positive Eugenics

The percentage of desirable traits can be increased by adopting the following measures:

- **Early marriage of those having desirable traits:** Subsidizing the fit because highly endowed persons lead a well-planned life and prefer to have small number of children. Therefore, selected young men and women should be encouraged to increase their birth rate.
- **Germinal choice:** The eugenically sound persons should not only increase their family size but through artificial insemination an outstanding man can also serve as father to many more children than would be otherwise possible. In a modern technique, a woman's ovum is taken out and artificially fertilized in a test-tube.
- **Education:**
  - For the eugenically oriented reforms in the society, the people should be educated about the basic principles of human biology, human genetics, eugenics and sex.
  - The children should be instructed about basic laws of health and they should be encouraged to develop a physically and mentally healthy body.
- **By avoiding germinal waste:** The wastage of best type of germplasm can be avoided by adopting the following measures:
  - The selection of marriage partners should be made with intelligence.
  - The wars must be avoided because in wars the best germplasm of the society is wasted.
- **Improvement of environmental conditions:** Both heredity and environment have interrelated role in the development of eugenically better persons.
- **Promotion of genetic research:** To have advanced knowledge in the field of genetics.
- **Genetic engineering:** It has become possible to produce various blood clotting factors, complement proteins (part of immune system) and other substances for the correction of genetic deficiency diseases (euphenics).

Negative Eugenics

Negative eugenics is concerned with decreasing or lowering the fertility among genetic Negative eugenics involves measures aimed at reducing the prevalence of undesirable or perceived "undesirable" genetic traits in a population, often through policies or practices that limit the reproduction of individuals considered to have such traits. The various ways of negative eugenics are abortion, sterilization, adoption of family planning methods. Negative eugenics is considered immoral because it enforces sterilization among genetically defective individuals.

Purpose

Negative eugenics is concerned with decreasing or lowering the fertility among genetic disadvantages.

Methods

The various ways of negative eugenics are:

- Abortion.
- Sterilization.
- Adoption of family planning methods.

Measures to Attempt Negative Eugenics

- **Sexual separation of the defective:** The defective persons may have various sex-linked diseases such as night blindness, hemophilia, color blindness, etc., which may be regulated by dominant or recessive genes. To avoid these issues, sexual separation of the defective persons is done.

- **Sterilization:** The sterilization is the best means to deprive an individual from his power of reproduction without interfering with any of his normal functions.
- **Control of immigration:** Through immigration there are enough chances that undesirable or defective genes of different races and nationalities may intermingle with the normal germplasm of the population.
- **Regulation of marriage:** Presently most human societies are money-minded and for a marriage or relationship like the wealthy or highly placed persons, who however, may have several defective genetical traits, are preferred over those who are economically weak but having eugenically sound hereditary traits.
- **Birth control:** People possessing more of undesired, dysgenic traits should be encouraged to have small families if at all allowed to reproduce. Their fetuses possessing dysgenic traits may be destroyed by abortion.
- **Statutory ban on marriage among close relatives:** Marriages among close relatives are called consanguineous marriages. The hidden recessive deleterious (e.g., lethal) traits can appear in the progeny in full view if both the parents carry them.
- **Genetic counseling:** A voluntary restriction of child bearing by couples with inherited genetic disorders (e.g., albinism, sickle cell anaemia, etc.) can be brought about through proper counseling by well qualified persons in the field.

GENETIC COUNSELING

Genetic counseling plays a crucial role in integrating genetic information into medical care and empowering individuals to make informed decisions about their health and the health of their families. Genetic counseling is a specialized process that provides individuals and families with information about the genetic aspects of medical conditions, helping them make informed decisions about healthcare, family planning, and genetic testing.

Definition: A process in aiding people to comprehend and adapt to the medical, psychological and familial implications of genetic contribution to diseases.

Aims of Genetic Counseling

It helps the individual or family:

- To comprehend the medical facts, including the diagnosis, the probable course of the disorder, and the available management.
- To appreciate the way heredity contributes to disorder, and the risk of recurrence in specified relatives
- To understand the options for dealing with the risk of recurrence.
- To choose the course of action which seems appropriate to them in view of their risk and the family goals and in accordance with the decision.
- To make the best possible adjustment to the disorder in the affected family member and/or the risk of recurrence of that disorder.

Criteria to Refer Patient to Genetic Counseling

- **A person with a known genetic condition within their family:** In order to know about the risks that threatens their family and/or those of offspring.
- Parents who have children with genetic defects, referred to a possible diagnosis.
- **A person with family history of cancer:** It is necessary to know increased risks and relevant options.
- **A person with a known genetic condition:** To see an expert counselor to understand more about their condition.

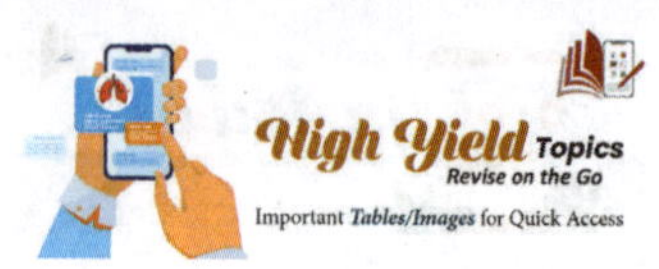

- **A person with potential genetic defects in the family:** To know if a diagnosis is available, along with relevant risks and options.
- **A pregnant couple with abnormal test results:** To help them understand their position biologically but then make personal decisions that they can live with their abnormal baby for a long term.

Types of Genetic Counseling

- **Prenatal genetic counseling:** Involves counseling for individuals or couples during pregnancy to assess the risk of genetic conditions in the developing fetus.
- **Pediatric genetic counseling:** Focuses on assessing and managing genetic conditions in children, including diagnosis, treatment, and long-term care.
- **Reproductive genetic counseling:** Focuses on assisting individuals or couples with family planning decisions and reproductive options.
- **Adult genetic counseling:** Addresses genetic conditions that may affect adults, including those with a family history of certain disorders.
- **Cancer genetic counseling:** Addresses the risk of hereditary cancers, providing information about genetic testing and risk reduction strategies.

Team Involved in Genetic Counseling

- **Medical geneticists:** Physicians with expertise in medical genetics who may be involved in complex cases.
- **Genetic counselors:** Those who hold specialized degrees in genetic counseling and work directly with individuals and families.
- **Other healthcare professionals:** Depending on the situation, a team may include obstetricians, pediatricians, oncologists, and other specialists.

Steps of the Genetic Counseling

1. **Referral and intake:** Individuals may be referred to genetic counseling by healthcare providers or self-refer based on family history or concerns. An initial intake involves collecting information about the individual's medical history, family history, and concerns.
2. **Risk assessment:** The genetic counselor assesses the likelihood of a genetic condition based on family and medical histories, ethnicity, and other relevant factors.
3. **Education:** Genetic counselors provide information about the nature of genetic conditions, inheritance patterns, and available testing options. They help individuals understand the medical, psychological, and social implications of genetic information.
4. **Counseling and support:** Emotional support is a crucial aspect. Genetic counselors help individuals cope with the psychological impact of genetic information and its potential implications for themselves and their families.
5. **Testing decision:** Genetic counselors assist individuals in making decisions about genetic testing, explaining the benefits, risks, and limitations associated with different testing options.
6. **Test coordination and interpretation:** If genetic testing is chosen, the genetic counselor coordinates the testing process and interprets the results. They explain the meaning of positive, negative, or inconclusive results.
7. **Family planning and decision making:** Genetic counselors help individuals explore family planning options, including prenatal testing, preimplantation genetic diagnosis (PGD), and adoption.
8. **Follow-up:** Ongoing support and follow-up are provided to address any additional questions, concerns, or changes in the individual's situation.

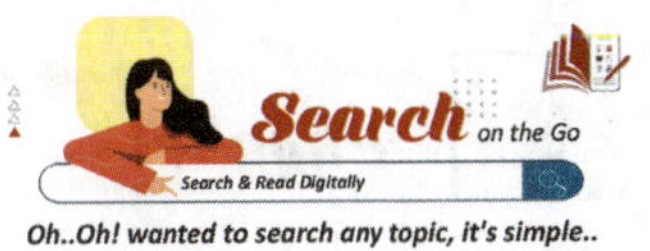

Applications of Genetic Counseling

- **Identifying and managing genetic risks:** Helping individuals understand and manage risks associated with genetic conditions.
- **Prenatal and reproductive decision-making:** Assisting with family planning decisions, prenatal testing, and reproductive options.
- **Cancer risk assessment:** Assessing the risk of hereditary cancers and providing guidance on surveillance and risk reduction strategies.
- **Assessing pediatric genetic disorders:** Assisting families in understanding and managing genetic disorders affecting children.

Legal and Ethical Issues in Genetic Counseling

Team involved in genetic counseling must be aware of some of the common ethical issues in genetics counseling.

Ethical Issues in Genetic Counseling

Major ethical issues are presented here with guidelines by The National Society of Genetic Counselors (NSG) Code of Ethics.

- **Informed consent:**
  - Providing thorough and comprehensible information about the purpose, benefits, risks, and alternatives of genetic testing or counseling.
  - Ensuring that individuals understand the potential implications of the information they may obtain.
- **Autonomy:**
  - Respecting the autonomy of individuals in making decisions about genetic testing and counseling.
  - Avoiding coercion and undue influence in the decision-making process.
- **Disclosing genetic information:**
  - Going through the ethical challenges of disclosing genetic information that may have implications for the health of relatives.
  - Balancing the duty to warn family members with the duty to respect patient confidentiality.
- **Cultural diversity:**
  - Addressing cultural beliefs and values that may influence the acceptance or refusal of genetic testing.
  - Recognizing and respecting cultural diversity in clients and adapting counseling approaches accordingly.
- **Financial constraints:** Considering the ethical implications of resource allocation, especially when dealing with limited healthcare resources and the cost of genetic testing.
- **Ongoing professional education:**
  - Staying informed about advancements in genetics and genomics to provide accurate and up-to-date information to clients.
  - Ensuring ongoing professional development to maintain competence and ethical practice.

ETHICAL CODE
Section I: Genetic Counselors Themselves
Genetic councelors must value professionalism, competence, integrity, objectivity, veracity, dignity, accountability and self-respect in themselves as well as in each other.

Contd...

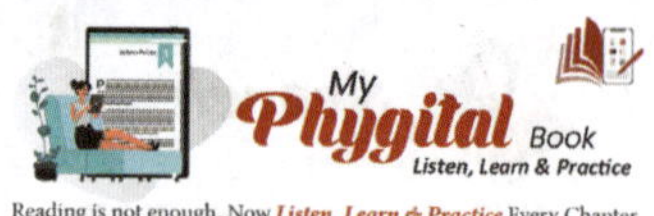

NSGC Code of Ethics

The National Society of Genetic Counselors (NSGC) has created a code of ethics to guide genetic counselors in caring of people. The NSGC Code of Ethics is based upon the distinct relationships genetic counselors have with themselves, their clients, their colleagues, and society.

- Seek out and acquire balanced, accurate and relevant information required for a given situation.
- Continue their education and training to keep abreast of relevant guidelines, regulations, position statements, and standards of genetic counseling practice.
- Work within their scope of professional practice and recognize the limits of their own knowledge, expertise, and competence.
- Accurately represent their experience, competence, and credentials, including academic degrees, certification, licensure, and relevant training.
- Identify and adhere to institutional and professional conflict of interest guidelines and develop mechanisms for avoiding or managing real or perceived conflict of interest when it arises.
- Acknowledge and disclose to relevant parties the circumstances that may interfere with or influence professional judgment or objectivity, or may otherwise result in a real or perceived conflict of interest.
- Assure that institutional or professional privilege is not used for personal gain.
- Be responsible for their own physical and emotional health as it impacts their professional judgment and performance, including seeking professional support, as needed.

Section II: Genetic Counselors and their Clients

- Provide genetic counseling services to their clients within their scope of practice regardless of personal interests or biases, and refer clients, as needed, to appropriately qualified professionals.
- Clarify and define their professional role(s) and relationships with clients, disclose any real or perceived conflict of interest, and provide an accurate description of their services.
- Provide genetic counseling services to their clients regardless of their clients' abilities, age, culture, religion, ethnicity, language, sexual orientation and gender identity.
- Enable their clients to make informed decisions, free of coercion, by providing or illuminating the necessary facts, and clarifying the alternatives and anticipated consequences.
- Respect their clients' beliefs, inclinations, circumstances, feelings, family relationships, sexual orientation, religion, gender identity, and cultural traditions.
- Refer clients to an alternate genetic counselor or other qualified professional when situations arise in which a genetic counselor's personal values, attitudes and beliefs may impede his or her ability to counsel a client.
- Maintain the privacy and security of their client's confidential information and individually identifiable health information, unless released by the client or disclosure is required by law.
- Avoid the exploitation of their clients for personal, professional, or institutional advantage, profit or interest.

Section III: Genetic Counselors and their Colleagues

- Share their knowledge and provide mentorship and guidance for the professional development of other genetic counselors, employees, trainees and colleagues.
- Respect and value the knowledge, perspectives, contributions, and areas of competence of colleagues, trainees and other professionals.
- Encourage ethical behavior of colleagues.
- Assure that individuals under their supervision undertake responsibilities that are commensurate with their knowledge, experience and training.
- Maintain appropriate boundaries to avoid exploitation in their relationships with trainees, employees, employers and colleagues.
- Take responsibility and credit only for work they have actually performed and to which they have contributed
- Appropriately acknowledge the work and contributions of others.
- Make employers aware of genetic counselors' ethical obligations as set forth in the NSGC Code of Ethics.

Contd...

Section IV: Genetic Counselors and Society

- Promote policies that aim to prevent genetic discrimination and oppose the use of genetic information as a basis for discrimination.
- Serve as a source of reliable information and expert opinion on genetic counseling to employers, policymakers, payers, and public officials. When speaking publicly on such matters, a genetic counselor should be careful to separate their personal statements and opinions made as private individuals from statements made on behalf of their employers or professional societies.
- Participate in educating the public about the development and application of technological and scientific advances in genetics and the potential societal impact of these advances.
- Promote policies that assure ethically responsible research in the context of genetics.
- Adhere to applicable laws and regulations. However, when such laws are in conflict with the principles of the profession, genetic counselors work toward change that will benefit the public interest.

Legal Issues in Genetic Counseling

Genetic counseling involves certain legal issues, however no specific laws are currently in place for guidance. In most of the cases, mixed laws are followed such as for data protection, Digital Personal Data Protection (DPDP) Act, 2023 is applied. There is a need of specialized laws for genetic counseling to avoid its misuse and to protect the information from going in public. The legal issues in genetics are as follows:

- **False results:** The likelihood of false negative and false positive results is one of the ethical issues in genetic counseling. For example, when testing pregnant women for Down syndrome markers, the results are only 60–80% accurate. This may result in a woman terminating her pregnancy without knowing that the results of the test were false.
- **Lack of treatment:** Another issue that some counselors may deal with, occurs when they test for conditions that have no known treatments. For example, Alzheimer's disease. Genetic testing can reveal whether a patient has a high risk of suffering from Alzheimer's later. As there is no known cure for the disease, counselors will find themselves in the position of telling patients about the disease and then making them more depressed.
- **Data security and storage:** Laws governing data protection and cyber security may apply to the storage and transmission of genetic information. Professionals must take appropriate measures to secure and protect patient data.
- **Nondiscrimination:** Addressing concerns related to potential discrimination based on genetic information, including insurance coverage, employment, and social stigma.
- **Genetic testing of minors:**
  - Balancing the rights of parents to make decisions for their children with the rights of the child to autonomy and privacy.
  - Ensuring that testing is in the best interest of the child and that the child's assent is considered when appropriate.
- **Genetic counseling for gender choices:**
  - Discussing the ethical considerations surrounding prenatal testing, preimplantation genetic diagnosis (PGD), and other reproductive technologies.
  - Balancing the desire for information with the potential emotional and psychological impact on individuals and couples.
- **Inappropriate testing:** With genetic testing, couples can now visit doctors, go through testing and then terminate pregnancies that do not result in perfect children or even pregnancies that result in a child of the gender they do not want.

- **Confidentiality:**
  - Safeguarding the privacy and confidentiality of genetic information and test results
  - Balancing the need for confidentiality with the obligation to disclose information that may have impact on the health of family members.
- **Regulation of genetic testing and counseling services:** Compliance with any licensing or accreditation requirements is crucial for professionals in this field. Regulatory bodies may oversee the provision of genetic testing and counseling services.
- **Consumer protection:** Laws related to consumer protection may apply to genetic testing services offered directly to consumers. Ensuring the accuracy and reliability of genetic tests is essential.
- **Research ethics:** If genetic counseling involves research activities, professionals must adhere to ethical guidelines and obtain necessary approvals from ethical review boards.
- **Professional standards and licensing:** Genetic counselors and therapists may be subjected to licensing requirements and professional standards. Adherence to these standards is essential to ensure the quality and ethics of the services provided.
- **Liability issues:** Professionals may be held liable for any harm caused by negligence or errors.

ROLE OF NURSE IN GENETIC COUNSELING

Nurses play a crucial role in genetic counseling, contributing to the multidisciplinary approach to patient care. While genetic counselors are typically specialized professionals in the field, nurses provide valuable support and assistance in various aspects of genetic counseling. Here are some roles that nurses may play in the context of genetic counseling:

- **Patient education:** Nurses educate patients and families about genetic conditions, inheritance patterns, and the implications of genetic testing. This includes providing information on the benefits, risks, and limitations of genetic testing.
- **Pretest counseling:** Before genetic testing, nurses assist in the counseling process by explaining the testing procedure, addressing patient concerns, and ensuring that individuals have realistic expectations about the potential outcomes.
- **Coordination of genetic testing:** Nurses are involved in coordinating genetic testing, including scheduling appointments, ensuring proper sample collection, and liaising with laboratory services.
- Planning and implementation of care during diagnosis and management of genetic disorders.
- Receiving the client and family and make them comfortable in assessment room for genetic counseling
- Obtain detail prenatal phase and family from the patient and family.
- **Collection of family health history:** Nurses can gather detailed family health histories, which are essential for identifying patterns of inheritance and assessing the risk of genetic conditions within families.
- Prepare and analyze pedigree to establish information about hereditary pattern.
- **Supportive care:** Information, counseling and support services to persons affected by or at risk for genetic disorders. Providing emotional support to individuals and families undergoing genetic counseling, especially when dealing with sensitive or difficult information.
- **Provide psychosocial support to individual and family throughout the counseling:** Sensitivity to cultural differences and adapting communication and care approaches accordingly to meet the diverse needs of patients and their families.
- **Post-test counseling:** Assisting with the communication of genetic test results to patients and their families, ensuring they understand the implications and helping them make informed decisions based on the results.

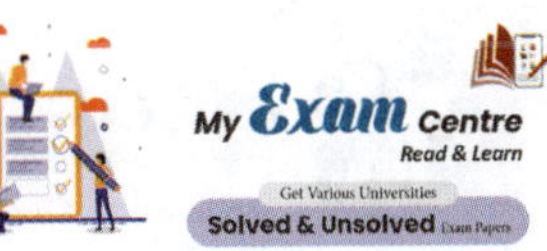

- **Referral to genetic counselors:** Recognizing when individuals need more specialized genetic counseling and facilitating referrals to genetic counselors or other relevant specialists.
- **Advocacy:** Advocating for patients and families within the healthcare system, ensuring their needs are met, and facilitating communication between different healthcare providers involved in the patient's care.
- **Documentation and record keeping:** Maintaining accurate and detailed records of genetic counseling sessions, including family histories, test results, and any recommendations made during the counseling process.
- **Long-term follow-up:** Collaborating with other healthcare providers to ensure appropriate follow-up care and interventions based on genetic counseling recommendations.

SUMMARY

- Determine the complete sequence of nucleotide base pairs that make up human DNA and all the genes it contains.
- The process involves genome mapping, or characterizing the chromosomes—a genetic map.
- HGP has enabled the identification of genetic markers associated with various diseases.
- Physicians can tailor treatment plans based on a patient's genetic makeup, optimizing therapeutic outcomes while minimizing adverse effects.
- Genetic counselors use information from the HGP to help individuals and families understand their genetic risks.
- Gene therapy is the insertion of genes into an individual's cells and tissues to treat a disease, such as a hereditary disease in which a deleterious mutant allele is replaced with a functional one.
- Viral vectors are modified viruses engineered to carry and deliver specific genetic material into target cells.
- Recessively inherited disorders are conceptually the easiest inherited disorders to treat by gene therapy.
- Eugenics is an immoral and pseudoscientific theory that claims it is possible to perfect people and groups through genetics and the scientific laws of inheritance.
- Main purpose of positive eugenics was to achieve healthy population.
- Negative eugenics involves measures aimed at reducing the prevalence of undesirable or perceived "undesirable" genetic traits in a population, often through policies or practices.
- Genetic counseling is a specialized process that provides individuals and families with information about the genetic aspects of medical conditions, helping them make informed decisions about healthcare, family planning, and genetic testing.
- Regulatory bodies may oversee the provision of genetic testing and counseling services.
- While genetic counselors are typically specialized professionals in the field, nurses provide valuable support and assistance in various aspects of genetic counseling.
- While genetic counselors are typically specialized professionals in the field, nurses provide valuable support and assistance in various aspects of genetic counseling.

ASSESS YOURSELF

Long Answer Questions

1. Discuss genetic counseling in detail.
2. What do you know about human genome project? Discuss.
3. What are the measures of positive and negative eugenics? Explain.
4. Describe the role of nurse in genetics.
5. What do you know about gene therapy? Write in detail.

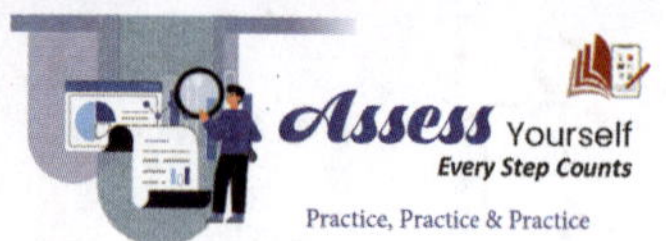

Short Answer Questions

1. Define eugenics and explain.
2. What is human genome project?
3. Write about genetic counseling.
4. Write short notes on:
   i. Eugenics movement
   ii. NSGC code of ethics

Multiple Choice Questions

1. **Which of the following methodology is used to identify all the genes that are expressed as RNA in HGP?**
   a. Sequence Annotation
   b. Expressed sequence tags
   c. Karyotyping
   d. Ammonification
2. **Which of the following is a suitable host for the process of cloning in HGP?**
   a. Virus
   b. All types of fungi
   c. Bacteria
   d. Protozoan
3. **Margaret Sanger, founder of Planned Parenthood, was criticized for:**
   a. Not advocating for a superior race
   b. Not advocating for the euthanasia of Harlem residents
   c. Advocating for eugenic practices
   d. Advocating for a superior race
4. **Eugenics means:**
   a. Genetic preventive measures
   b. Improvement of genetic endowment
   c. Improvement of environment
   d. Genetic counseling
5. **A person with the hereditary disease can be cured with the help of ________________.**
   a. Gene therapy
   b. Cloning
   c. Dialysis
   d. Chemotherapy
6. **A collection of methods that allows correction of a gene that has been diagnosed in child/embryo is called ________________.**
   a. Cloning
   b. Gene therapy
   c. Chemotherapy
   d. Dialysis
7. **In gene therapy, the gene defects are cured in a child or ________________ stage.**
   a. Adult
   b. Teenage
   c. Old
   d. Embryo
8. **Genetic conditions:**
   a. Are most commonly present in newborn infants.
   b. Always become worse as a person ages.
   c. Are directly attributable to a mutation in the genes.
   d. Are always diagnosed after others have determined that a genetic condition is present in the family.
9. **When considering genetic diseases, a key ethical consideration is the concept of:**
   a. Confidentiality
   b. Grief
   c. Caring
   d. Care giving

Answer Key

1. b	**2.** c	**3.** c	**4.** c	**5.** b	**6.** a
7. b	**8.** d	**9.** d			

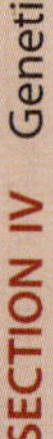

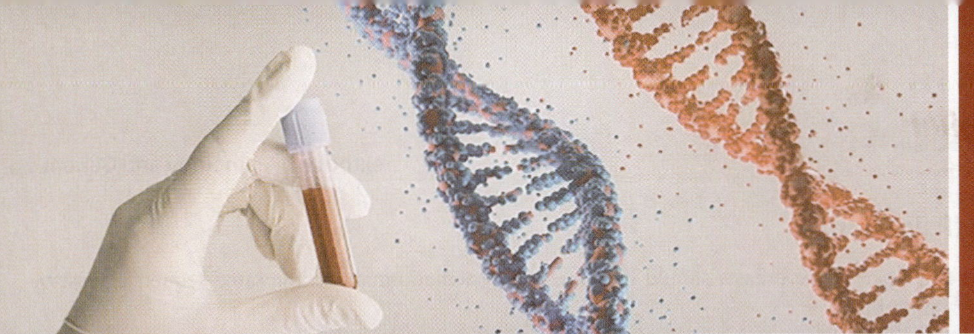

Annexures

ANNEXURE I Breast Self-Examination (BSE)

In an era where breast cancer incidence in the country is on the rise, a number of health education and awareness initiatives are being devised to facilitate the early detection of this lesion.

An important part of such programs includes the performance of breast self-examination that is assessment of breast abnormalities or lumps by the patients themselves. Nursing professionals can play a key role in enabling both awareness and correct performance of this technique as they serve as a compassionate bridge between the physician and the patient.

It must be highlighted that the current status of breast self-examination as stated in medical literature is that the *self-examination performed alone as a screening tool has no obvious benefit in reducing the risk of breast cancer-related morbidity*. However, **in combination with mammography and clinical breast evaluation, it is definitely of great benefit**. In this context, it is beneficial for all medical personnel to know about this technique.

WHEN SHOULD A BREAST SELF-ASSESSMENT BE DONE?

Breast self-examination (BSE) is usually is done a week after a woman's period as the premenstrual phase may physiologically cause the breasts to be swollen.

It should ideally be done every month so that the woman can detect changes she sees in her breasts, if any. The self examination is done in two parts—Visual Inspection and Touch (Palpation).

1. Visual Inspection

The subject should remove all garments prior to examination and preferably should stand in front of a mirror to enable better delineation of the breasts and armpits (axillae).

The visual inspection is to be done keeping one's hands on the hips to observe the breasts properly as well as after keeping the arms outstretched above the head to inspect the axillary region.

Points to note are:

1. The presence or absence of any obvious breast lump.
2. The nipples—whether inverted/retracted or whether any patch of erosion or discoloration or oozing discharge is present.
3. Overlying skin—inspect the presence or absence of any puckering or peau d' orange-like appearance or any redness/other signs of inflammation/any ulceration.
4. Any changes seen from the previous month's examination.

2. Touch (Palpation)

The exercise of palpating the breasts should be done in a systematic manner, the same sequence must be followed every month.

Palpation should be done using the flat surface of the middle three fingers of the hand. The subject should be instructed not to palpate using her fingertips as that would likely miss potential lesions.

Palpation should be done using varying degrees of pressure-low/medium/firm.

Both breasts are examined at a time, the three fingers of one hand being used to palpate all quadrants of the breast one at a time and then switched over for the other breast.

In subjects who have large breasts, it may be more beneficial to palpate the breast while lying down, following the same sequence as in standing position.

After palpating all the four quadrants, the subject should not forget to palpate beneath the areola region, squeezing the nipple on each side to examine if any discharge is elicited on doing so.

The woman should then using the flat of her fingers palpate the axilla to feel change in consistency, if any.

Advantages

The benefits of a self-examination are that as a screening tool it is:

- Non-invasive
- Not costly
- Can easily be done at home by the woman herself at her ease and convenience.
- It is confirmed or trusted only when supplemented by a clinical evaluation and mammographic assessment.

Disadvantages

- The detection of any changes, some of which may be insignificant may cause anxiety and distress to the subject.
- Breast self examination is not a substitute for clinical evaluation and should not delay taking clinical opinion when required.

ANNEXURE II ADA Update 2018-Diagnostic Criteria for Diabetes

- FPG ≥126 mg/dL (7.0 mmol/L)
- In a patient with classic symptoms of hyperglycemia or hyperglycemic crisis, a random plasma glucose ≥200 mg/dL (11.1 mmol/L)
- 2-hour Plasma glucose ≥200 mg/dL (11.1 mmol/L) during oral glucose tolerance test (OGTT)
- Glycated hemoglobin HbA1C ≥6.5%

Who to screen for diabetes mellitus?

In overweight or obese (BMI ≥25 kg/m^2), adults having one/more of the following risk factors:

- First-degree relative with diabetes
- High-risk race/ethnicity (African American, Latino, Native American, Asian American)
- History of CVD
- Hypertension (≥140/90 mm Hg or on therapy for hypertension)
- HDL cholesterol level <35 mg/dL and/triglyceride level >250 mg/dL
- Women with polycystic ovary syndrome
- Physical inactivity
- Other conditions associated with insulin resistance (e.g., severe obesity, acanthosis nigricans)
  - Patients with prediabetes (A1C ≥5.7% IGT, or IFG) should be tested yearly.
  - Women who were diagnosed with GDM should have lifelong testing at least every 3 years
  - For all others, testing should begin at the age of 45.

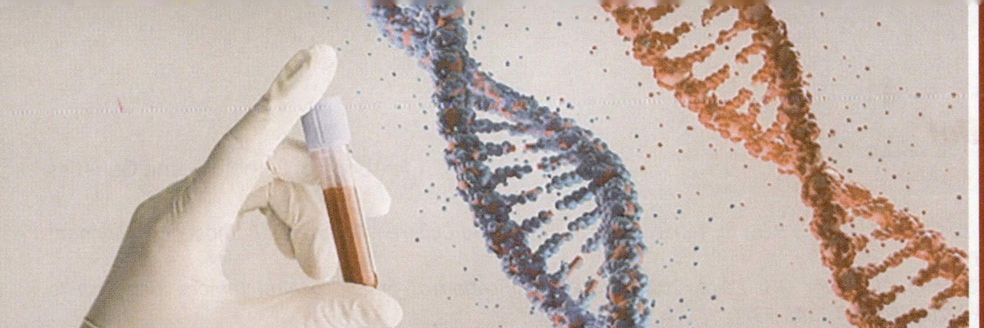

Further Readings

- *Almadani YH, Vorstenbosch J, Davison PG, et al. Wound healing: a comprehensive review. Semin Plast Surg. 2021;35(3):141-4.*
- *Balk RA. Systemic inflammatory response syndrome (SIRS): where did it come from and is it still relevant today? Virulence. 2014;5(1):20-6.*
- *Barletta JF, Muir J, Brown J, et al. A systematic approach to understanding acid-base disorders in the critically ill. Ann Pharmacother. 2024;58(1):65-75.*
- *Bennett JM, Reeves G, Billman GE, et al. Inflammation–nature's way to efficiently respond to all types of challenges: implications for understanding and managing "the epidemic" of chronic diseases. Front Med (Lausanne). 2018;5:316.*
- *Bhandari J, Thada PK, DeVos E. Typhoid Fever. In: StatPearls [Internet]. Treasure Island (FL): StatPearls Publishing; 2024.*
- *Birt MC, Anderson DW, Bruce Toby E, et al. Osteomyelitis: recent advances in pathophysiology and therapeutic strategies. J Orthop. 2016;14(1):45-52.*
- *Chakraborty RK, Burns B. Systemic Inflammatory Response Syndrome. In: StatPearls [Internet]. Treasure Island (FL): StatPearls Publishing; 2024.*
- *Chen L, Deng H, Cui H, et al. Inflammatory responses and inflammation-associated diseases in organs. Oncotarget. 2018;9(6):7204-18.*
- *Cheung AK, Chang TI, Cushman WC, et al. KDIGO 2021 Clinical Practice Guideline for the management of blood pressure in chronic kidney disease. Kidney Int. 2021;99(3S):S1-87.*
- *D'Arcy MS. Cell death: a review of the major forms of apoptosis, necrosis and autophagy. Cell Biol Int. 2019;43:582-92.*
- *Devine JF. Chronic obstructive pulmonary disease: an overview. Am Health Drug Benefits. 2008;1(7):34-42.*
- *Fink SL, Cookson BT. Apoptosis, pyroptosis, and necrosis: mechanistic description of dead and dying eukaryotic cells. Infect Immun. 2005;73(4):1907-16.*
- *Foucher J, Chanteloup E, Vergniol J, et al. Diagnosis of cirrhosis by transient elastography (FibroScan): a prospective study. Gut. 2006;55(3):403-8.*
- *Fowler VG, Durack DT, Selton-Suty C, et al. The 2023 Duke-International Society for Cardiovascular Infectious Diseases Criteria for Infective Endocarditis: updating the modified Duke Criteria. Clin Infect Dis. 2023;77(4): 518-26.*
- *Furman D, Campisi J, Verdin E, et al. Chronic inflammation in the etiology of disease across the life span. Nat Med. 2019;25:1822-32.*
- *Gill CM, Dolan L, Piggott LM, et al. New developments in tuberculosis diagnosis and treatment. Breathe (Sheff). 2022;18(1):210149.*
- *Gonzalez AC, Costa TF, Andrade ZA, et al. Wound healing: a literature review. An Bras Dermatol. 2016;91(5): 614-20.*
- *Hamilton PK, Morgan NA, Connolly GM, et al. Understanding acid-base disorders. Ulster Med J. 2017;86(3): 161-6.*

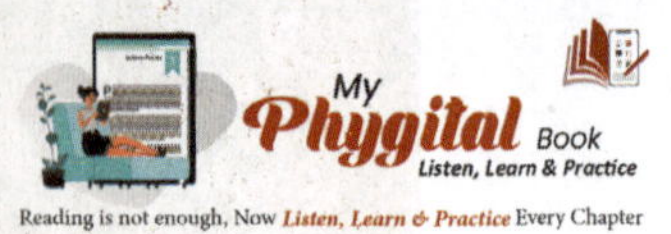

- *Heemskerk D, Caws M, Marais B, et al. Tuberculosis in Adults and Children. Chapter 2: Pathogenesis. London: Springer; 2015.*
- *Höhn AK, Brambs CE, Hiller GG, et al. 2020 WHO classification of female genital tumors. Geburtshilfe Frauenheilkd. 2021;81(10):1145-53.*
- *Huang Y, Ai L, Wang X, et al. Review and updates on the diagnosis of tuberculosis. J Clin Med. 2022;11(19):5826.*
- *Jameson J, Fauci AS, Kasper DL, Hauser SL, Longo DL, Loscalzo J. Harrison's Principles of Internal Medicine, 20th edition. New York: McGraw-Hill Education; 2018.*
- *Kay J, Upchurch KS. ACR/EULAR 2010 rheumatoid arthritis classification criteria. Rheumatology. 2012;51:vi5-9.*
- *Kellum JA, Romagnani P, Ashuntantang G, et al. Acute kidney injury. Nat Rev Dis Primers. 2021;7:52.*
- *Khalid N, Azimpouran M. Necrosis. In: StatPearls [Internet]. Treasure Island (FL): StatPearls Publishing; 2024.*
- *Koulaouzidis A, Bhat S, Karagiannidis A, et al. Spontaneous bacterial peritonitis. Postgrad Med J. 2007;83(980): 379-83.*
- *Kuhajda I, Zarogoulidis K, Tsirgogianni K, et al. Lung abscess—etiology, diagnostic and treatment options. Ann Transl Med. 2015;3(13):183.*
- *Kumar V, Abbas A, Aster J. Robbins and Cotran Pathologic Basis of Disease, 10th edition. Amsterdam: Elsevier; 2020.*
- *Long R, Divangahi M, Schwartzman K. Chapter 2: Transmission and pathogenesis of tuberculosis, Can J Respir Crit Care Sleep Med. 2022;6:sup1:22-32.*
- *Lusis AJ. Atherosclerosis. Nature. 2000;407(6801):233-41.*
- *Malfertheiner P, Camargo MC, El-Omar E, et al. Helicobacter pylori infection. Nat Rev Dis Primers. 2023;9:19.*
- *Momodu II, Savaliya V. Osteomyelitis. In: StatPearls [Internet]. Treasure Island (FL): StatPearls Publishing; 2024.*
- *Nagtegaal ID, Odze RD, Klimstra D, et al. The 2019 WHO classification of tumours of the digestive system. Histopathology. 2020;76(2):182-8.*
- *National Cancer Institute. (2021). Alcohol and Cancer Risk. [online] Available from https://www.cancer.gov/about-cancer/causes-prevention/risk/alcohol/alcohol-fact-sheet [Last accessed February, 2024].*
- *Patel R, Mueller M. Alcoholic Liver Disease. In: StatPearls [Internet]. Treasure Island (FL): StatPearls Publishing; 2024.*
- *Pfeifer JD, Humphrey PA, Ritter JH, Dehner LP. The Washington Manual of Surgical Pathology, 3rd edition. Gurugram: Wolters Kluwer India; 2019.*
- *Rajani R, Klein JL. Infective endocarditis: a contemporary update. Clin Med (Lond). 2020;20(1):31-35.*
- *Scallan J, Huxley VH, Korthuis RJ. Capillary Fluid Exchange: Regulation, Functions, and Pathology. Chapter 4: Pathophysiology of edema formation. San Rafael (CA): Morgan and Claypool Life Sciences; 2010.*
- *Severino P, D'Amato A, Pucci M, et al. Ischemic heart disease pathophysiology paradigms overview: from plaque activation to microvascular dysfunction. Int J Mol Sci. 2020;21(21):8118.*
- *Shrimanker I, Bhattarai S. Electrolytes. In: StatPearls [Internet]. Treasure Island (FL): StatPearls Publishing; 2024.*
- *Stern E, Sugumar K, Journey JD. Peptic Ulcer Perforated. In: StatPearls [Internet]. Treasure Island (FL): StatPearls Publishing; 2024.*
- *Thompson LD, Fitzpatrick SG, Müller S, et al. Proliferative verrucous leukoplakia: an expert consensus guideline for standardized assessment and reporting. Head Neck Pathol. 2021;15(2):572-87.*
- *Tsoris A, Marlar CA. Use of the Child Pugh Score in Liver Disease. In: StatPearls [Internet]. Treasure Island (FL): StatPearls Publishing; 2024.*
- *Vig T, Das P, Sakhuja P, Gaur K, Majumdar K, Pulimood A. Pathology of Inflammatory Bowel Diseases and Its Mimickers, Immunodeficiency and Vascular Gastrointestinal Lesions, and Drug-Induced Bowel Pathologies. In: Das P, Majumdar K, Datta Gupta S (Eds). Surgical pathology of the gastrointestinal system. Singapore: Springer; 2022. pp. 405-80.*
- *Walter JB, Talbot IC. Walter and Israel General Pathology, 7th edition. Edinburgh: Churchill Livingstone; 1996.*

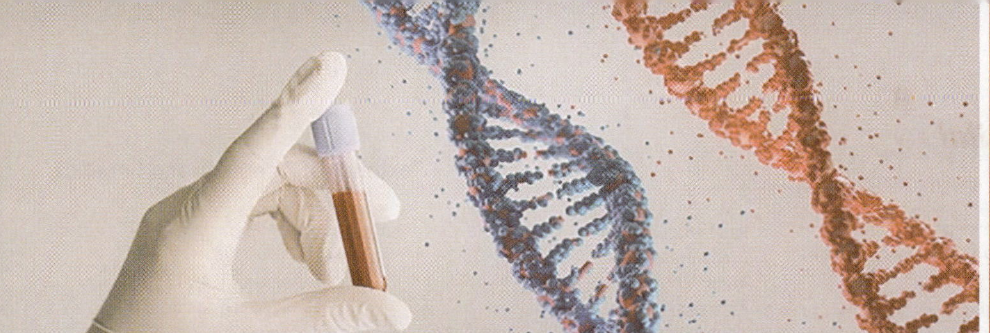

Index

Refer 'f' for figure and 't' for table, respectively.

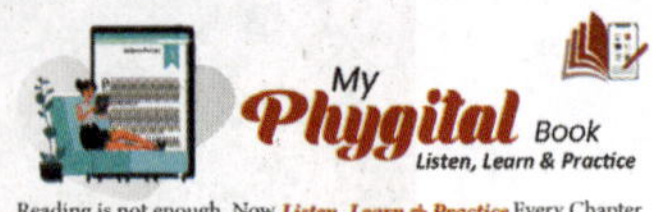
My
Phygital Book
Listen, Learn & Practice
Reading is not enough, Now Listen, Learn & Practice Every Chapter

B

C

INDEX

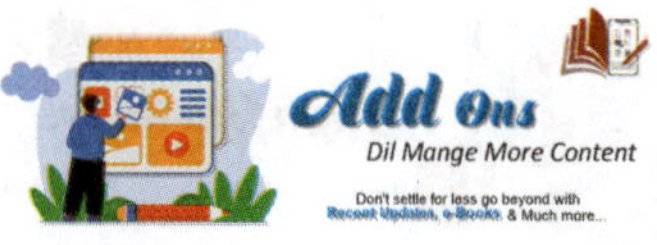
Add Ons
Dil Mange More Content
Don't settle for less go beyond with Recent Updates, e-Books & Much more...

D

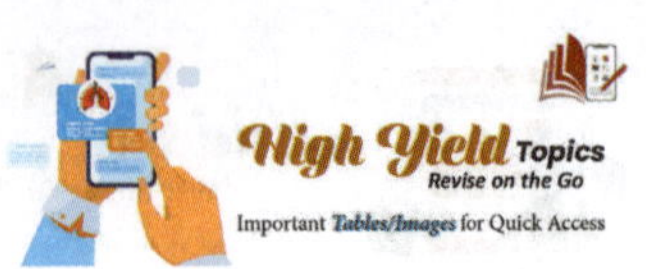

E

F

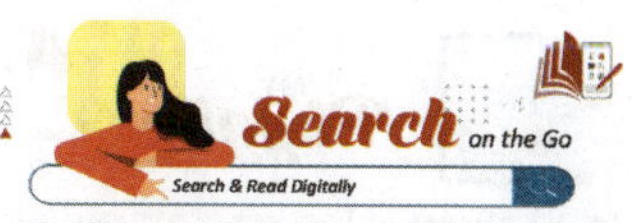
Search on the Go
Search & Read Digitally
Oh..Oh! wanted to search any topic, it's simple..

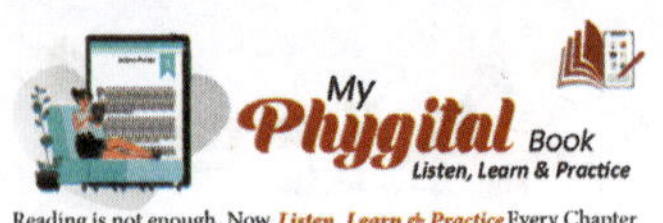
My
Phygital Book
Listen, Learn & Practice
Reading is not enough, Now Listen, Learn & Practice Every Chapter

I

J

K

L

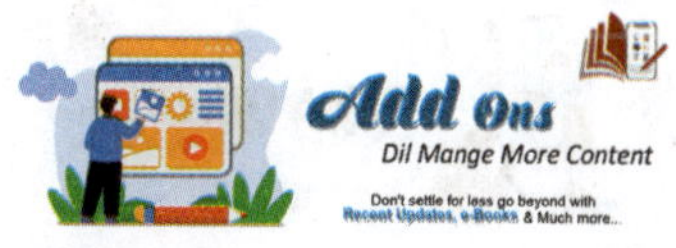
Add Ons
Dil Mange More Content

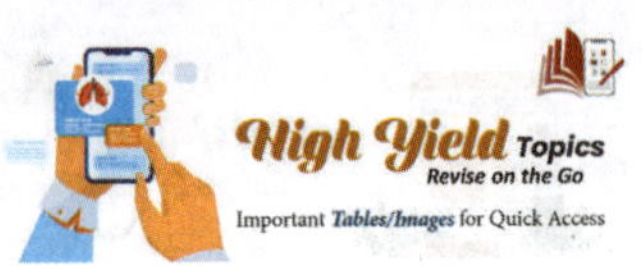

O

P

R

S

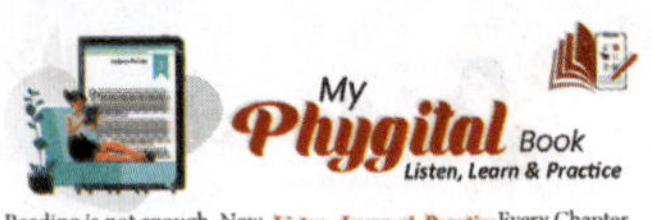
My
Phygital Book
Listen, Learn & Practice
Reading is not enough, Now Listen, Learn & Practice Every Chapter

T

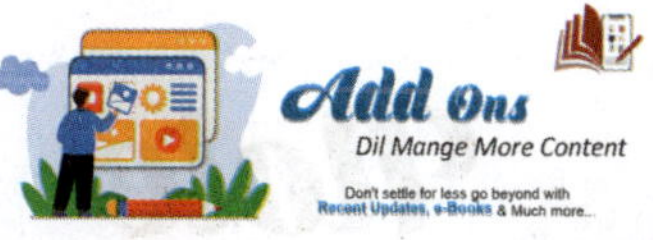
Add Ons
Dil Mange More Content
Don't settle for less go beyond with
Recent Updates, e-Books & Much more...

U

V

W

X

Y

Z

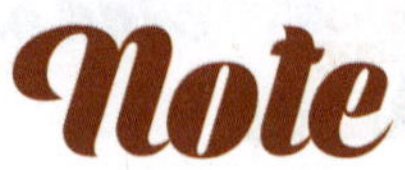
Note

Note

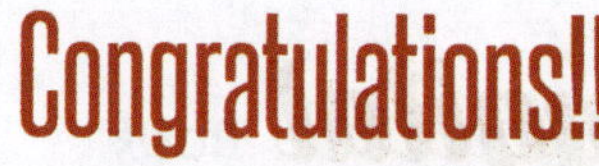

*You have completed the CHAPTER thoroughly, now it's time to assess your knowledge and learn more through **My Phygital Book***

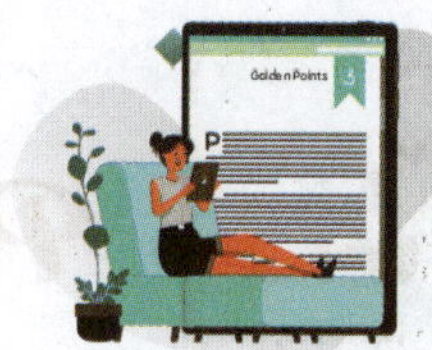

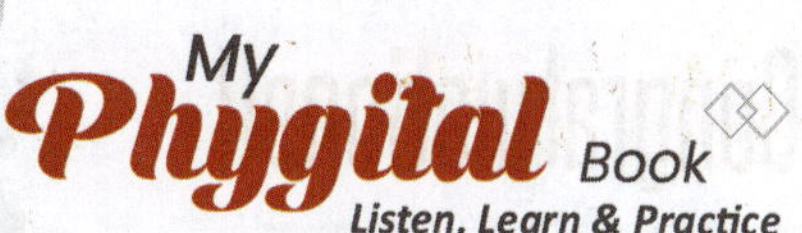

Reading is not enough, Now ***Listen, Learn & Practice*** Every Chapter

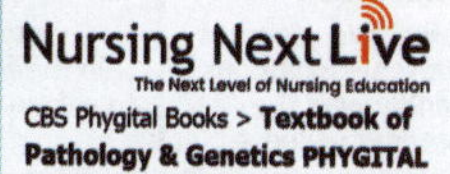

Golden Points	Solved Exercises	MCQs
Get One Liners of Chapter summary in the PODCAST form	Subjective and objective exercises given in book with their solutions to evaluate and assess the complete chapter knowledge	Chapter-wise extra MCQs in the form of Practice test to give in-depth concept clarity

Note